T0362404

Advances in Occupational and Environmental Lung Diseases

Editors

KRISTIN J. CUMMINGS
PEGGY S. LAI
CARRIE A. REDLICH

CLINICS IN CHEST MEDICINE

www.chestmed.theclinics.com

December 2020 • Volume 41 • Number 4

ELSEVIER

1600 John F. Kennedy Boulevard • Suite 1800 • Philadelphia, Pennsylvania, 19103-2899

http://www.theclinics.com

CLINICS IN CHEST MEDICINE Volume 41, Number 4
December 2020 ISSN 0272-5231, ISBN-13: 978-0-323-71289-7

Editor: Colleen Dietzler
Developmental Editor: Casey Potter

Clinics in Chest Medicine (ISSN 0272-5231) is published quarterly by Elsevier Inc., 360 Park Avenue South, New York, NY 10010-1710. Months of issue are March, June, September, and December. Periodicals postage paid at New York, NY and additional mailing offices. Subscription prices are $388.00 per year (domestic individuals), $766.00 per year (domestic institutions), $100.00 per year (domestic students/residents), $423.00 per year (Canadian individuals), $952.00 per year (Canadian institutions), $484.00 per year (international individuals), $952.00 per year (international institutions), $100.00 per year (Canadian Students), and $230.00 per year (International Students). International air speed delivery is included in all Clinics subscription prices. All prices are subject to change without notice. **POSTMASTER:** Send address changes to Clinics in Chest Medicine, Elsevier Health Sciences Division, Subscription Customer Service, 3251 Riverport Lane, Maryland Heights, MO 63043. **Customer Service: Telephone: 1-800-654-2452** (U.S. and Canada); **1-314-447-8871** (outside U.S. and Canada). **Fax: 1-314-447-8029. E-mail: journalscustomerservice-usa@elsevier.com (for print support); journalsonlinesupport-usa@elsevier.com (for online support).**

Reprints. For copies of 100 or more of articles in this publication, please contact the Commercial Reprints Department, Elsevier Inc., 360 Park Avenue South, New York, NY 10010-1710. Tel.: 212-633-3874; Fax: 212-633-3820; E-mail: reprints@elsevier.com.

Clinics in Chest Medicine is covered in *MEDLINE/PubMed (Index Medicus), Current Contents/Clinical Medicine, EMBASE/Excerpta Medica, Science Citation Index,* and *ISI/BIOMED.*

Contributors

EDITORS

KRISTIN J. CUMMINGS, MD, MPH
Chief, Hazard Evaluation System and Information Service, Occupational Health Branch, California Department of Public Health, Richmond, California, USA

PEGGY S. LAI, MD, MPH
Assistant Professor of Medicine, Division of Pulmonary and Critical Care Medicine, Massachusetts General Hospital, Harvard Medical School, Department of Environmental Health, Harvard T.H. Chan School of Public Health, Boston, Massachusetts, USA

CARRIE A. REDLICH, MD, MPH
Professor of Medicine, Pulmonary Section and Occupational and Environmental Medicine, Director, Yale Occupational and Environmental Medicine Program, Yale School of Medicine, New Haven, Connecticut, USA

AUTHORS

GARY ADAMKIEWICZ, PhD
Department of Environmental Health, Harvard T.H. Chan School of Public Health, Boston, Massachusetts, USA

KASSANDRA ALLBRIGHT, MD
Osler Medical Resident, Department of Medicine, Johns Hopkins University, Baltimore, Maryland, USA

STEPHEN R. BALDASSARRI, MD, MHS
Department of Internal Medicine, Section of Pulmonary, Critical Care, and Sleep Medicine, Yale School of Medicine, New Haven, Connecticut, USA

JOHN R. BALMES, MD
Professor, Department of Medicine, University of California, San Francisco, San Francisco, California, USA; Professor, School of Public Health, University of California, Berkeley, Berkeley, California, USA

EMILY BRIGHAM, MD, MHS
Assistant Professor of Medicine, Division of Pulmonary and Critical Care, Johns Hopkins University, Baltimore, Maryland, USA

ROBERT A. COHEN, MD
Clinical Professor, Division of Environmental and Occupational Health Sciences, University of Illinois at Chicago School of Public Health, Department of Medicine, Northwestern University Feinberg School of Medicine, Chicago, Illinois, USA

PAUL CULLINAN, MD
National Heart and Lung Institute, Imperial College London, London, United Kingdom

KRISTIN J. CUMMINGS, MD, MPH
Chief, Hazard Evaluation System and Information Service, Occupational Health Branch, California Department of Public Health, Richmond, California, USA

SARA DE MATTEIS, MD, MPH, PhD
Associate Professor, Department of Medical Sciences and Public Health, University of Cagliari, Cagliari, Italy; Honorary Senior Lecturer, NHLI, Imperial College London, London, United Kingdom

MARIE A. DE PERIO, MD
Medical Officer, Division of Field Studies and Engineering, National Institute for Occupational Safety and Health, Centers for Disease Control and Prevention, Cincinnati, Ohio, USA

BRITTANY DICKENS, BA
Research Coodinator, Barry Commoner Center for Health and the Environment, Queens College, City University of New York, Flushing, New York, USA

JOHANNA FEARY, MD
National Heart and Lung Institute, Imperial College London, London, United Kingdom

JONATHAN M. GAFFIN, MD, MMSc
Division of Pulmonary Medicine, Boston Children's Hospital, Harvard Medical School, Boston, Massachusetts, USA

LEONARD H.T. GO, MD
Research Assistant Professor, Division of Environmental and Occupational Health Sciences, University of Illinois at Chicago School of Public Health, Department of Medicine, Northwestern University Feinberg School of Medicine, Chicago, Illinois, USA

PHILIP HARBER, MD, MPH
Professor of Public Health, Mel and Enid Zuckerman College of Public Health, University of Arizona, Tucson, Arizona, USA

DREW HARRIS, MD
Assistant Professor of Medicine, Division of Pulmonary and Critical Care and Public Health Sciences, University of Virginia, Charlottesville, Virginia, USA

R. REID HARVEY, DVM, MPH
Respiratory Health Division, National Institute for Occupational Safety and Health, Centers for Disease Control and Prevention, Morgantown, West Virginia, USA

STEPHEN HOBBS, MD, FSCCT
Associate Professor of Radiology and Medicine, Vice-Chair, Radiology Informatics and Integrated Clinical Operations, Chief, Division of Cardiovascular and Thoracic Radiology, Medical Director, UK Healthcare Imaging Informatics, University of Kentucky, Lexington, Kentucky, USA

EFIA JAMES, MD, MPH
Instructor, Department of Medicine, Yale Occupational and Environmental Medicine Program, Yale School of Medicine, New Haven, Connecticut, USA

MIWAKO KOBAYASHI, MD
Medical Officer, Division of Bacterial Diseases, National Center for Immunization and Respiratory Diseases, Centers for Disease Control and Prevention, Atlanta, Georgia, USA

SILPA KREFFT, MD, MPH
Assistant Professor of Medicine, Division of Environmental and Occupational Health Sciences, National Jewish Health, Denver, Colorado, USA; Division of Pulmonary and Critical Care Medicine, VA Eastern Colorado Health Care System, Division of Pulmonary and Critical Care Medicine, University of Colorado Anschutz Medical Campus, Department of Environmental and Occupational Health, Colorado School of Public Health, Aurora, Colorado, USA

PEGGY S. LAI, MD, MPH
Assistant Professor of Medicine, Division of Pulmonary and Critical Care Medicine, Massachusetts General Hospital, Harvard Medical School, Department of Environmental Health, Harvard T.H. Chan School of Public Health, Boston, Massachusetts, USA

AMBROSE LAU, MD
Department of Medicine, Toronto Western Hospital, St Michael's Hospital, Toronto, Ontario, Canada

GONDY LEROY, PhD
Professor of Management Information Systems, Eller College of Management, University of Arizona, Tucson, Arizona, USA

JAHRED LIDDIE, BA
Department of Environmental Health, Harvard T.H. Chan School of Public Health, Boston, Massachusetts, USA

BRIAN LINDE, MD, MPH
Instructor, Department of Medicine, Yale Occupational and Environmental Medicine Program, Yale School of Medicine, New Haven, Connecticut, USA

STEVEN B. MARKOWITZ, MD, DrPH
Professor, Barry Commoner Center for Health and the Environment, Queens College, City University of New York, Flushing, New York, USA

MEREDITH C. McCORMACK, MD, MHS
Associate Professor of Medicine, Department of Medicine, Division of Pulmonary and Critical Care Medicine, Johns Hopkins University, Johns Hopkins School of Medicine, Baltimore, Maryland, USA

KATHLEEN NAVARRO, PhD, MPH
National Institute for Occupational Safety and Health, Centers for Disease Control and Prevention, Cincinnati, Ohio, USA

BENOIT NEMERY, MD, PhD
Emeritus Professor, Department of Pulmonary Medicine, Clinic for Occupational and Environmental Medicine, University Hospitals Leuven, Leuven, Belgium; Emeritus Professor, Toxicology and Occupational Medicine, Department of Public Health and Primary Care, Centre for Environment and Health, KU Leuven, Leuven, Belgium

RANDALL J. NETT, MD, MPH
Respiratory Health Division, National Institute for Occupational Safety and Health, Centers for Disease Control and Prevention, Morgantown, West Virginia, USA

SARATH RAJU, MD, MPH
Assistant Professor, Department of Medicine, Division of Pulmonary and Critical Care Medicine, Johns Hopkins University, Johns Hopkins School of Medicine, Baltimore, Maryland, USA

CARRIE A. REDLICH, MD, MPH
Professor of Medicine, Pulmonary Section and Occupational and Environmental Medicine, Director, Yale Occupational and Environmental Medicine Program, Yale School of Medicine, New Haven, Connecticut, USA

CARL REYNOLDS, MD
National Heart and Lung Institute, Imperial College London, London, United Kingdom

MARY B. RICE, MD, MPH
Department of Medicine, Beth Israel Deaconess Medical Center, Harvard Medical School, Boston, Massachusetts, USA

STEVEN RONSMANS, MD
Consultant Physician, Department of Pulmonary Medicine, Clinic for Occupational and Environmental Medicine, University Hospitals Leuven, PhD Candidate, Department of Public Health and Primary Care, Centre for Environment and Health, KU Leuven, Leuven, Belgium

CECILE ROSE, MD, MPH
Professor of Medicine, Division of Environmental and Occupational Health Sciences, National Jewish Health, Denver, Colorado, USA; Division of Pulmonary and Critical Care Medicine, University of Colorado Anschutz Medical Campus, Department of Environmental and Occupational Health, Colorado School of Public Health, Aurora, Colorado, USA

HARI M. SHANKAR, MD
Division of Pulmonary, Allergy and Critical Care, University of Pennsylvania, Philadelphia, Pennsylvania, USA

TRISHUL SIDDHARTHAN, MD
Assistant Professor, Department of Medicine, Division of Pulmonary and Critical Care Medicine, Johns Hopkins University, Johns Hopkins School of Medicine, Baltimore, Maryland, USA

SUSAN M. TARLO, MB BS
Professor, Department of Medicine, Dalla Lana School of Public Health, University of Toronto, Toronto Western Hospital, St Michael's Hospital, Toronto, Ontario, Canada

LARA WALKOFF, MD
Assistant Professor of Radiology, Divisions of Thoracic and Cardiovascular Radiology, Mayo Clinic College of Medicine, Rochester, Minnesota, USA

MOLLY WOLF, MD
Division of Pulmonary and Critical Care Medicine, Massachusetts General Hospital, Harvard Medical School, Boston, Massachusetts, USA

JENNA WOLFF, BA
Clinical Research Coordinator II, Division of Environmental and Occupational Health Sciences, National Jewish Health, Denver, Colorado, USA

JONATHAN M. WORTHAM, MD
Medical Officer, Division of Tuberculosis Elimination, National Center for HIV/AIDS, Viral Hepatitis, STD, and TB Prevention, Centers for Disease Control and Prevention, Atlanta, Georgia, USA

Contents

Preface: Occupational and Environmental Contributions to Lung Disease **xiii**

Kristin J. Cummings, Peggy S. Lai, and Carrie A. Redlich

Master Clinician and Public Health Practitioner: Selected Occupational and Environmental Pulmonary Cases **567**

Efia James, Brian Linde, and Carrie A. Redlich

Occupational and environmental exposures contribute to the development and progression of most lung diseases, yet their impact is greatly under-recognized in clinical practice. Clinicians caring for patients with respiratory diseases should maintain a high index of suspicion for occupational and environmental contributing factors. Mastering occupational and environmental medicine clinical decision making requires specialized clinical skills. These skills include obtaining an appropriate work and exposure history; making an assessment of the magnitude and relevance of exposures and their contribution to a patient's respiratory disease; utilizing appropriate resources for evaluation and management of exposure-related disease; and considering socioeconomic and public health factors.

Chest Imaging in the Diagnosis of Occupational Lung Diseases **581**

Lara Walkoff and Stephen Hobbs

Imaging plays a crucial role in the diagnosis and monitoring of occupational lung diseases (OLDs); however, the sensitivity and specificity of detection and diagnosis vary greatly depending on the imaging modality used. There is substantial overlap in appearance with non–occupation-related entities. OLDs should be considered in the differential even in the absence of a provided exposure history. Because many findings are not specific, a multidisciplinary approach is important in arriving at the diagnosis and will continue to be important as workplace-related pulmonary diseases evolve with changing industrial practices and workplace regulations.

Informatics Approaches for Recognition, Management, and Prevention of Occupational Respiratory Disease **605**

Philip Harber and Gondy Leroy

Computer and information systems can improve occupational respiratory disease prevention and surveillance by providing efficient resources for patients, workers, clinicians, and public health practitioners. Advances include interlinking electronic health records, autocoding surveillance data, clinical decision support systems, and social media applications for acquiring and disseminating information. Obstacles to advances include inflexible hierarchical coding schemes, inadequate occupational health electronic health record systems, and inadequate public focus on occupational respiratory disease. Potentially transformative approaches include machine learning, natural language processing, and improved ontologies.

Health Disparities in Environmental and Occupational Lung Disease 623

Emily Brigham, Kassandra Allbright, and Drew Harris

Pulmonary health disparities disproportionately impact disadvantaged and vulnerable populations. This article focuses on disparities in disease prevalence, morbidity, and mortality for asthma, chronic obstructive pulmonary disease, pneumoconiosis, and lung cancer. Disparities are categorized by race, age, sex, socioeconomic status, and geographic region. Each category highlights differences in risk factors for the development and severity of lung disease. Risk factors include social, behavioral, economic, and biologic determinants of health (occupational/environmental exposures, psychosocial stressors, smoking, health literacy, health care provider bias, and health care access). Many of these risk factors are complex and inter-related; strategies proposed to decrease disparities require multilevel approaches.

Respiratory Health Effects of Exposure to Cleaning Products 641

Sara De Matteis, Steven Ronsmans, and Benoit Nemery

There is consistent and growing evidence of an epidemic of "asthma-like" symptoms among professional cleaners. Questions include how big is this problem worldwide, which cleaning agents are dangerous, how do they affect the lungs, and is it really asthma? This issue is important to public health because of the increasing number of professional cleaners, many from vulnerable categories. There are implications for anybody exposed to cleaning products during housekeeping, including children. This article uses available evidence to give a broad but concise overview on what we know so far and how we can prevent the cleaning-associated respiratory public health burden.

Work-Related Upper-Airway Disorders 651

Ambrose Lau and Susan M. Tarlo

Work-related rhinitis and laryngeal disorders are common and can significantly contribute to work absences and presenteeism. Each can cause respiratory symptoms that may be misdiagnosed as asthma symptoms, and each may occur as an isolated disorder or may also accompany asthma. Suspicion of these disorders and correct management require a careful medical and occupational history. Investigations for work-related rhinitis include examination of the nose, allergy skin tests, and in some cases, monitoring of peak inspiratory nasal flows at work and off work, or specific challenge tests. Work-related laryngeal disorders require assistance from an otolaryngologist and speech language pathologist.

Occupational Bronchiolitis: An Update 661

Randall J. Nett, R. Reid Harvey, and Kristin J. Cummings

Occupational bronchiolitis is characterized by inflammation of the small airways following a range of inhalation exposures. Workers in industries producing or using flavorings ontaining diacetyl or 2,3-pentanedione are at risk. Cases of constrictive bronchiolitis also have been associated with military deployments, but the causative exposure(s) have not been identified. Multiple reports in recent years have drawn attention to previously unrecognized risk factors for occupational bronchiolitis in several settings, such as fiberglass-reinforced plastic boatbuilding. Both current and past occupational exposures should be considered in patients undergoing

evaluation for unexplained dyspnea. Diagnostic testing should include a thorough assessment of the small airways.

Coal Workers' Pneumoconiosis and Other Mining-Related Lung Disease: New Manifestations of Illness in an Age-Old Occupation 687

Leonard H.T. Go and Robert A. Cohen

Coal workers' pneumoconiosis (CWP) and other mining-related lung diseases are entirely preventable, yet continue to occur. While greater attention has been given to CWP and silicosis, mining exposures cause a broad spectrum of respiratory disease, including chronic bronchitis, emphysema, and pulmonary fibrosis. Physicians must obtain a detailed ccupational and exposure history from miners in order to make an accurate diagnosis and determine the risk of disease progression. Mining-related lung diseases are incurable and difficult to treat. Therefore, primary prevention by limiting dust exposure and secondary prevention through chest imaging and physiologic screening should be the primary focus of disease control.

Occupational Contributions to Interstitial Lung Disease 697

Carl Reynolds, Johanna Feary, and Paul Cullinan

Historically well-recognized occupational threats such as coal workers pneumoconiosis, silicosis, and asbestosis remain important and are very likely underestimated in measures of global disease burden. Studies of occupational exposure related to idiopathic pulmonary fibrosis, the most common interstitial lung disease, are limited but there is moderate evidence for metal, wood, and stone dust being significant contributors. Vigilance is required to identify causes, such as hypersensitivity pneumonitis due to microbial contamination of metalworking fluid (now responsible for greater than 50% of occupational hypersensitivity pneumonitis cases in the United Kingdom) in an everchanging workplace environment.

Silicosis: An Update and Guide for Clinicians 709

Silpa Krefft, Jenna Wolff, and Cecile Rose

This overview provides an update on silicosis epidemiology with review of exposures and emerging trends in acute and accelerated silicosis in the twenty-first century. The silicosis epidemics in mining, denim sandblasting, and engineering stone industries are highlighted. Clinical presentations of silicosis and silica-related conditions such as autoimmune, kidney, and mycobacterial disease, as well as lung cancer, are discussed. Important aspects of the new OSHA 2017 Silica Standard are presented. This review also includes practical guidance for clinicians to address questions that may arise when evaluating silica-exposed patients and to the public health responses needed following a diagnosis of silica-related disease.

Screening for Occupational Lung Cancer: An Unprecedented Opportunity 723

Steven B. Markowitz and Brittany Dickens

Selected occupational populations are at the highest risk of lung cancer, because they smoke at increased rates and are concurrently exposed to workplace lung carcinogens. Low-dose computed tomography (CT)–based lung cancer screening has an enormous potential to reduce lung cancer mortality in these populations, as shown both in the lung cancer screening studies in the general population and in studies of workers at high risk of lung cancer. Pulmonologists can play a key role

CLINICS IN CHEST MEDICINE

FORTHCOMING ISSUES

March 2021
Pulmonary Hypertension
Aaron B. Waxman and Inderjit Singh, *Editors*

June 2021
Next-generation Interstitial Lung Disease
Harold Collard, Luca Richeldi and Kerri A. Johannson, *Editors*

RECENT ISSUES

September 2020
Chronic Obstructive Pulmonary Disease (COPD)
Gerard J. Criner and Bartolome R. Celli, *Editors*

June 2020
Lung Cancer: Part II
M. Patricia Rivera and Richard A. Matthay, *Editors*

Preface
Occupational and Environmental Contributions to Lung Disease

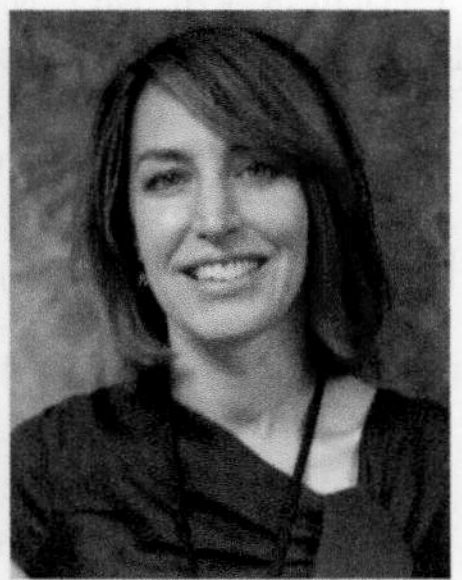

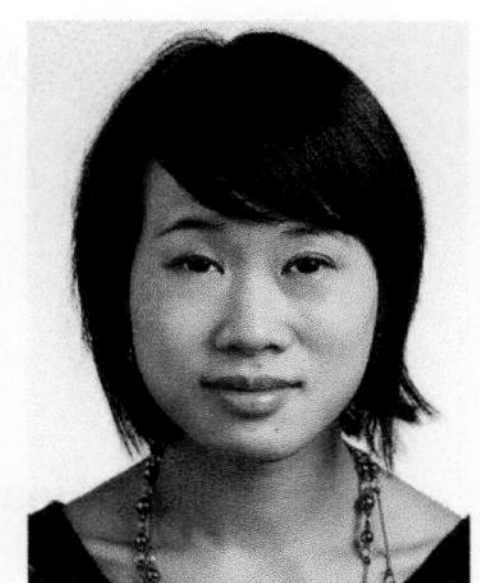

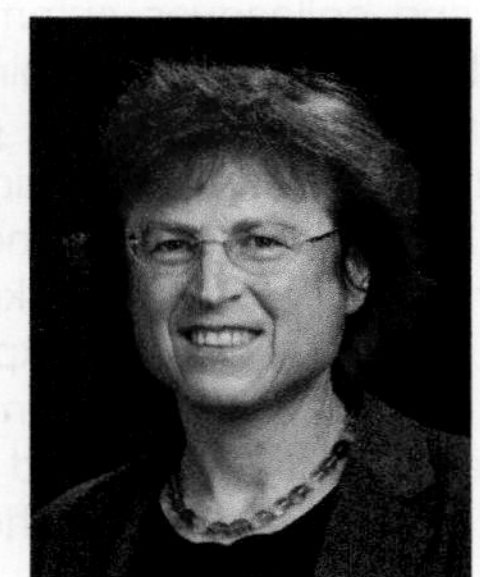

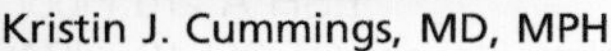

Kristin J. Cummings, MD, MPH   Peggy S. Lai, MD, MPH   Carrie A. Redlich, MD, MPH
Editors

It has been nearly a decade since the last issue of *Clinics in Chest Medicine* focused on Occupational and Environmental Lung Disease was published.[1] In the ensuing years, we have witnessed appalling outbreaks of preventable pneumoconioses and come to recognize that the implications of climate change for respiratory health are myriad, complex, and already well underway.[2–4] In light of such developments and the advances in our understanding of the impact of work and environmental exposures on respiratory health, it is important to revisit the topic.

It is perhaps fitting that we write during the COVID-19 pandemic, an event whose origin and overwhelming consequences are both linked to changing environmental and workplace factors. The coronavirus that causes COVID-19, severe acute respiratory coronavirus 2 (SARS-CoV-2), is the latest and most devastating in a long line of zoonotic viruses: SARS, Middle East respiratory syndrome, and Ebola among them, whose reach is increasing as climate change, population growth, work practices, and travel across borders bring people in closer contact with wildlife and one another.[5] Furthermore, the global spread of COVID-19 has led to infections and deaths among those whose work must continue despite the risk of transmission: health care workers, correctional officers, meat processors, and others deemed "essential."[6–8] Arguably, no other event in recent memory has so vividly highlighted the relevance of environment, occupation, and racial and income disparities to respiratory disease. The COVID-19 pandemic also reinforces the importance of prevention, early recognition, and surveillance, cornerstones of occupational health practice.

We attempt to integrate practical clinical approaches throughout the issue. Dr Redlich and colleagues present a collection of cases that highlights the importance of considering occupational and environmental factors for both diagnosis and effective management. Drs Hobbs and Walkoff provide a practical guide to radiologic findings of occupational lung disease, complete with an outstanding collection of images. Dr Markowitz explores occupational contributions to lung cancer and opportunities for screening. Dr De Perio and colleagues address the role of work in respiratory infections. Drs Harber and Leroy discuss the advances in informatics that are impacting practice today and those that hold promise for the future.

Occupational exposures collectively impact the entire respiratory system. Drs Lau and Tarlo examine the upper airway with a focus on work-related rhinitis and laryngeal disorders, increasingly recognized for their adverse impact on productivity and quality of life. Dr Nett and colleagues discuss recent advances in our understanding of occupational bronchiolitis, including new risk factors. Drs Reynolds and colleagues focus on the lung parenchyma, building on a recently published review[9] to describe the state

Clin Chest Med 41 (2020) xiii–xv
https://doi.org/10.1016/j.ccm.2020.09.001
0272-5231/20/© 2020 Published by Elsevier Inc.

of knowledge regarding occupational contributions to interstitial lung disease.

Drs Guo and Cohen provide an update on mining-related lung diseases, emphasizing the resurgence of coal workers' pneumoconiosis. Dr Krefft and colleagues provide a focused review of silicosis for the practicing clinician, including discussion of underrecognized clinical presentations. Dr De Matteis and colleagues summarize the growing body of literature on the respiratory health effects of cleaning and disinfecting products for professional cleaners. Their article is particularly timely in light of COVID-19 and the expanded use of such products in the workplace and by the general public.[10] Dr Navarro explores the respiratory effects of smoke exposure on wildland firefighters, who are increasingly called upon year round as climate change extends the fire season.

Another group of articles focuses on the important impact of environmental exposures on lung disease in the broader population. Dr Balmes, in a companion piece to Dr Navarro's, details the effects of wildfire smoke on the public and provides practical recommendations for vulnerable subpopulations on how to minimize exposure. Drs Shankar and Rice review the effects of climate change on environmental exposures and respiratory health. Drs Wolf and Lai discuss the ways that next-generation sequencing has shifted our understanding of how bacterial and fungal exposures impact health. Dr Adamkiewicz and colleagues detail the effects of outdoor air pollution on health, and Dr Raju and colleagues highlight the adverse impact of indoor air pollution, stratified by studies in high- versus low- and middle-income settings. Dr Baldassarri reviews the impact of electronic cigarettes on smoking cessation and nicotine addiction, as well as the risks of vaping-associated lung disease, with detailed answers to patient-centered questions about this new and widely prevalent exposure. Finally, there is growing awareness of disparities in harmful environmental exposures that impact lung disease, which is reviewed by Dr Brigham and colleagues.

It is clear that a wide range of work and environmental exposures plays a vital role in the development and progression of most lung diseases. Yet, the clinical impact of these exposures is greatly underappreciated, hindering treatment and broader preventive efforts. We must do better. We hope this issue on Occupational and Environmental Lung Disease will help clinicians and public health practitioners recognize, manage and prevent work and environmental-related lung diseases.

Kristin J. Cummings, MD, MPH
California Department of Public Health
850 Marina Bay Parkway P-3
Richmond, CA 94804, USA

Peggy S. Lai, MD, MPH
Massachusetts General Hospital
Pulmonary/Critical Care
Bulfinch 148
55 Fruit Street
Boston, MA 02114, USA

Carrie A. Redlich, MD, MPH
Yale School of Medicine
Occupational Health and Environmental Medicine
367 Cedar Street
ESH A 2rd Floor
New Haven, CT 06510, USA

E-mail addresses:
Kristin.Cummings@cdph.ca.gov (K.J. Cummings)
PSLAI@hsph.harvard.edu (P.S. Lai)
carrie.redlich@yale.edu (C.A. Redlich)

REFERENCES

1. Redlich CA, Blanc PD, Gulati M, et al. Lung diseases associated with occupational and environmental exposures subsume a wide spectrum of conditions. Clin Chest Med 2012;33(4):xi–xii.
2. Blackley DJ, Reynolds LE, Short C, et al. Progressive massive fibrosis in coal miners from 3 clinics in Virginia. JAMA 2018;319(5):500–1.
3. Rose C, Heinzerling A, Patel K, et al. Severe silicosis in engineered stone fabrication workers—California, Colorado, Texas, and Washington, 2017-2019. MMWR Morb Mortal Wkly Rep 2019;68(38):813–8.
4. Rice MB, Thurston GD, Balmes JR, et al. Climate change: a global threat to cardiopulmonary health. Am J Respir Crit Care Med 2014;189(5):512–9.
5. Qiu J. One world, one health: combating infectious diseases in the age of globalization. Natl Sci Rev 2017;4(3):493–9.
6. CDC COVID-19 Response Team. Characteristics of health care personnel with COVID-19—United States, February 12-April 9, 2020. MMWR Morb Mortal Wkly Rep 2020;69(15):477–81.
7. Wallace M, Hagan L, Curran KG, et al. COVID-19 in correctional and detention facilities—United States, February–April 2020. MMWR Morb Mortal Wkly Rep 2020;69(19):587–90.

8. Waltenburg MA, Victoroff T, Rose CE, et al. Update: COVID-19 among workers in meat and poultry processing facilities—United States, April-May 2020. MMWR Morb Mortal Wkly Rep 2020;69(27):887–92.
9. Blanc PD, Annesi-Maesano I, Balmes JR, et al. The occupational burden of nonmalignant respiratory diseases. An Official American Thoracic Society and European Respiratory Society statement. Am J Respir Crit Care Med 2019;199(11):1312–34.
10. Chang A, Schnall AH, Law R, et al. Cleaning and disinfectant chemical exposures and temporal associations with COVID-19—National Poison Data System, United States, January 1, 2020–March 31, 2020. MMWR Morb Mortal Wkly Rep 2020;69:496–8.

Master Clinician and Public Health Practitioner

Selected Occupational and Environmental Pulmonary Cases

Efia James, MD, MPH*, Brian Linde, MD, MPH, Carrie A. Redlich, MD, MPH

KEYWORDS

- Occupational lung diseases • Work-related asthma • Occupational history
- Environmental exposures • Indoor air quality

KEY POINTS

- An assessment of a patient's occupational and environmental exposures is an essential component of the clinical evaluation of all patients presenting with respiratory diseases.
- Clinicians who care for patients with respiratory diseases should be familiar with resources to assist patients with occupational and environmental lung disease.
- Clinicians who care for patients with respiratory diseases can play an important role in advocating for changes in the home environment or workplace of patients with exposure-related respiratory disease. Such actions can improve patient outcomes and also potentially provide broader public health benefits.

INTRODUCTION

As described in this issue of *Clinics in Chest Medicine*, occupational and environmental exposures can contribute to the full spectrum of respiratory disease yet continue to be greatly underrecognized by clinicians. It is important that clinicians who care for patients with respiratory diseases maintain a high index of suspicion for occupational and environmental contributing factors and, importantly, also know how to diagnose work and environmental respiratory conditions, because recognition and subsequent interventions can improve individual outcomes and also have an impact on public health. Mastering occupational and environmental medicine (OEM) clinical decision making requires specialized clinical skills. Central among these is obtaining an appropriate work and exposure history (**Boxes 1** and **2**) and then utilizing a basic framework to incorporate this information into OEM diagnostic clinical reasoning. Additionally, familiarity with readily available OEM resources (**Tables 1** and **2**) can greatly facilitate clinical evaluations and also provide clinicians with guidance for themselves and their patients on exposure reduction and managing workplace issues. The following 4 cases illustrate the key components in OEM clinical decision making, summarized in **Box 3**.

CASE 1

A 29-year-old man with a history of childhood asthma presents for evaluation of worsening shortness of breath and cough. His symptoms began approximately a year ago, after his family moved into a rental apartment. He states that prior to this move, he routinely experienced 1 to 2 mild asthma exacerbations per year triggered by seasonal changes but never required inpatient hospitalization or maintenance inhaler therapy. Two months after moving into his current apartment,

Department of Medicine, Yale Occupational and Environmental Medicine Program, Yale School of Medicine, 367 Cedar Street, ESHA 2nd Floor, New Haven, CT 06510, USA
* Corresponding author.
E-mail address: efia.james@yale.edu

Clin Chest Med 41 (2020) 567–580
https://doi.org/10.1016/j.ccm.2020.08.019
0272-5231/20/Published by Elsevier Inc.

Box 1
Key components of the occupational history

Job history[a]

Name of current and former employers and industry

Job title, daily duties, and tasks

Duration and years of employment

Workplace description

Work processes? Final products

The scale of operations

Inhalational exposures to dust, fumes, or specific substances

Ventilation

Is personal protective equipment used while working?

How many employees? Size of the workplace?

Any OSHA complaints, inspections, or citations?

Work-related symptoms or conditions

Did symptoms begin after starting work at the current employer?

Are symptoms better away from work (ie, after work, weekends, or vacation)?

Are there other employees with similar symptoms or conditions?

[a] Focus on the jobs of most concern based on the clinical condition (eg, for occupational asthma, focus on the job when asthma first began; for COPD, focus on longest-held jobs).

his symptoms escalated, requiring 7 visits to the emergency room in the past year. He now is prescribed daily budesonide/formoterol and montelukast, in addition to albuterol as needed. He reports improvement in symptoms when he was out of town for several days.

The patient is married with 3 children, all of whom also have experienced increased asthma symptoms over the past year and have had to miss school. He recently lost his job due to absenteeism secondary to his frequent asthma exacerbations.

He provides a copy of a recent property inspection, which documents a poorly maintained apartment in a multiunit building without air conditioning. The report notes water damage from roof and plumbing leaks, the presence of surface mold and pest infestation, and odors of tobacco smoke from adjacent apartments. He does not have any pets or hobbies. He is hoping his healthcare provider can help him find alternate housing.

Questions

1. What can you do to determine whether the patient's environment is exacerbating his asthma?
2. What is your role as a pulmonary or primary care clinician?
3. What resources are available to assist this patient?

Discussion

Asthma is a common respiratory disease, especially among working age adults, with the overall prevalence of asthma within the United States of approximately 8.0%, with the higher rates among minorities and people living below the poverty level.[1] As discussed in Brigham and colleagues' article, "Health Disparities in Environmental and Occupational Lung Disease," in this issue, socioeconomic factors and environmental and work exposures contribute substantially to asthma health disparities.[2] Because persons typically spend most of their time in their homes, it is important to identify and reduce home environmental exposures, especially in poorer urban areas.

Although it is common for clinicians to ask about pets, sick contacts, and travel, housing often is ignored. Subsidized housing has been associated with poor health outcomes, including higher rates of asthma.[3–7] Common contributing factors include inadequate maintenance, water intrusions, dampness, mold, pests, allergens, environmental tobacco smoke exposure, and outdoor air pollution, which typically are more prevalent in poor urban housing. Thus, key components of a thorough environmental history include questions regarding housing type, dampness, mold or pests, and smokers in the home (see **Box 2**).[8]

Questions

What can you do to determine if the patient's environment is exacerbating his asthma?

New-onset or worsening asthma should prompt a search for environmental and workplace triggers. This patient's asthma was well controlled before moving into his apartment, which is suggestive of a possible home source. His worsening asthma has been documented in his medical record with increased emergency room visits and use of inhalers. Spirometry with bronchodilator testing is helpful to confirm the diagnosis of asthma.

Box 2
Key questions in taking an environmental exposure history

Housing

- Where is housing located?
- What type of housing is it?
- When was the residence built?
- How many people live in the home?

Housing characteristics

- Any recent or current construction or remodeling?
- What type of heating and cooling is in the residence? Wood burning stoves or fireplaces?
- What type of flooring is in the residence (ie, hardwood, carpet, or area rugs)?
- Are there any current or recent issues with water incursion or dampness? Are there any signs of mold?
- Is there a basement? If so, is it finished? How much time is spent in the basement?

Exposures in the home

- Are there any issues with pests or rodents?
- Are there any pets in the home?
- Is there smoking in the home, adjacent units, or common areas?
- How often is the home cleaned, and what products are used to clean?
- Does the patient perform exterior yard work?

Hobbies and other sources of exposure

- What hobbies does patient and other members in the home participate in?
- Are there any hobbies that generate inhalational exposures?
- Are there environmental sources of air pollution, such as housing near major highways, industries, and construction?

Obtaining a detailed environmental history and documenting temporal associations of his symptoms with the apartment are essential to determining whether the home environment is exacerbating his asthma (see **Box 2**). Pertinent findings for the patient include residing in subsidized housing with multiple well-known environmental triggers, in this case documented in a home inspection report. Worsening asthma in his family members also is supportive. Other considerations could be work exposures, but his symptoms have persisted after he lost his job due to his asthma. His job loss and reduced income will make finding better housing more challenging.

What is your role as the health care provider?
There are several actions providers can take to help their patients access better housing. Providers should clearly describe the home exposures and document the temporal association in the medical record. Having the patient take pictures of the home can be informative. Clinicians also can help patients access social services to improve medical care coordination and employment difficulties and resolve housing issues.[9] If the patient requests, providers can provide a medical letter, which can prompt action on housing, while respecting patient privacy. For instance, clinicians can, with a patient's permission, recommend that landlords repair water leaks or other identified problems, such as implementing pest management services or enforcing a smoke-free policy in their properties.[10]

What resources are available to assist this patient?
Additional resources available to help patients, as provided in **Table 2**. For example, a qualitative home assessment, as was done by this patient's local health department, can be helpful in identifying and documenting specific home exposures or needed home repairs.[10]

The patient's apartment was eventually condemned by the local health department. The family received assistance in finding alternate housing. His asthma improved, as did his children's asthma. With his asthma better controlled, the patient also was able to find new employment.

CASE 2

A 51-year-old elementary school teacher with no prior history of asthma presents for evaluation of worsening respiratory symptoms while at work. Approximately 1 year ago, she began experiencing cough, shortness of breath, and chest tightness primarily at work. She is concerned about the conditions in her current classroom environment, which she describes as damp with musty odors, which are most noticeable after rainy or humid days. These conditions persist despite use of dehumidifiers. She notes that other teachers at her school also are experiencing respiratory and allergy-type symptoms. She also reports frequent use of cleaning products throughout the school but no direct use by her.

She is a lifetime nonsmoker and denies any significant exposures or symptoms in her home environment. Prior allergy testing was unremarkable.

Box 3
Key steps in occupational clinical decision making

1. Establish the patient's clinical diagnosis, such as asthma, COPD, or pulmonary fibrosis, using standard clinical diagnostic criteria.
2. Assess the patient's work exposures, including duration, timing and the magnitude of exposures (see **Box 1**).
3. Identify the types of work exposures, jobs, or industries (if any) have been associated with the patient's respiratory condition

   Perform a literature review (eg, PubMed, Google Scholar)

   - Examples of job/exposure—disease associations:

     Machinists → pulmonary fibrosis, asthma

     Asbestos → lung cancer, mesothelioma
4. Determine whether the temporal relationship (timing and duration of exposure) and the patient's exposure history are consistent with the disease process.
   - Examples

     Asbestosis typically presents 20 years to 30 years after initial exposure.

     Sensitizer-induced asthma usually develops months to years after repeated exposure to a sensitizing agent.
5. Evaluate the patient for other known risk factors for the disease, such as smoking, family history, other health conditions, and environmental exposures.
6. Based on the answers to the above questions, assess whether the patient's work exposures contributed to the patient's disease?
   - Consider the diagnostic certainty appropriate for the patient's situation, such as clinical management, research, workers' compensation, or exposure modification.
   - Is it more probable than not (>50%) that the exposure(s) is a substantial contributing factor? (This is most common standard for work-related diagnoses in the United States.)
7. Consider the impact of a work-related diagnosis on the patient's health, employment, socioeconomic situation, and available resources.

She is prescribed fluticasone propionate/salmeterol, montelukast and albuterol as needed.

Spirometry testing revealed mild airflow obstruction with a significant bronchodilator response.

She brings with her a report of an industrial hygiene evaluation which was performed in response to teacher complaints. The report notes that the school was built in the 1970s and has had longstanding problems related to its aging infrastructure, including water incursions, dampness, high humidity levels, and visible mold. Elevated carbon dioxide levels were noted in certain classrooms, indicative of inadequate ventilation. Air sampling performed in several classrooms revealed normal mold spore counts, below outdoor levels. The report also noted that only green cleaning products are used in the school.

Questions

1. How do you determine whether the teacher's asthma is secondary to work exposures and, if so, what type of work-related asthma (WRA) does she have?
2. How do you interpret the findings of an environmental investigative report?
3. How can a clinician assist a patient who wishes to continue working?
4. What can be done for others experiencing symptoms, and what are some of the resources for those experiencing work-related lung disease?

Discussion

WRA refers to asthma that is causally linked to work. WRA can be categorized further as either occupational asthma or work-exacerbated asthma. Occupational asthma is defined as the development of new-onset asthma due to workplace exposure(s), either irritants or allergens. Work-exacerbated asthma is defined as existing asthma that is worsened by workplace exposures.[11]

WRA occurs across numerous nonindustrial work settings, including schools, health care facilities, and office buildings as well as industrial settings. Cleaning products, dampness, mold, and microbial exposures, discussed in De Matteis and colleaguse' artcile, "Respiratory Health Effects of Exposure to Cleaning Products," and Molly Wolf and Peggy S. Lai's article, "Indoor Microbial Exposures and Chronic Lung Disease: From Microbial Toxins to the Microbiome,"in this issue, are commonly are associated with WRA as well as work-related upper-airway conditions, which can overlap with WRA (see Ambrose Lau and Susan M. Tarlo's article, "Work-Related Upper Airway Disorders," in this issue).[12]

Indoor air quality issues are an increasingly common problem due to the aging infrastructure of US public schools.[13] Approximately 32% of schools contain buildings described as being in fair to poor condition due to issues, such as plumbing, faulty heating/cooling systems, and damaged windows, leading to problems with mold, dampness, and pest infestation.[14] Such exposures are associated with upper respiratory symptoms, rhinitis, and asthma.[15–17]

WRA typically is diagnosed based on 3 steps: (1) confirming the diagnosis of asthma, (2) identify exposure(s) in the workplace that can cause or trigger asthma, and (3) determine association between asthma and work.[11,18]

Asthma commonly is diagnosed based on a typical clinical presentation and response to treatment. In the setting of decisions regarding work, however, it is particularly important to clarify the diagnosis of asthma.[11,18] Most commonly this is done by demonstrating reversible airflow obstruction on spirometry testing. Methacholine challenge and exercise testing also can be performed to document airway hyperresponsiveness. Corticosteroids can lead to false-negative tests. Conditions that commonly coexist with WRA should be considered, including rhinitis, conjunctivitis, vocal cord symptoms, discussed in see Ambrose Lau and Susan M. Tarlo's article, "Work-Related Upper Airway Disorders," in this issue.[12]

Identifying work exposures that can cause or trigger asthma is accomplished most commonly by a careful occupational history, which should focus primarily on the job when asthma symptoms started or worsened and include job title, industry, and a description of the workplace and daily tasks (see **Box 1**). Tasks, substances, or locations that trigger symptoms should be noted as well as any new processes. Several readily accessible resources (see **Table 1**) are available that can help obtain more information about workplace exposures, including jobs and exposures associated with WRA. For example, safety data sheets (SDSs) for products used in the work process can be helpful in identifying causative agents.[19]

The temporal association between work exposures and asthma is ascertained most commonly based on a careful history, including a history of prior asthma, the onset and timing of asthmatic symptoms in relationship to work, improvement away from work, and worse symptoms or greater use of inhalers when working. Serial peak expiratory flow measurements performed at and away from the workplace for several weeks on rare occasions can further establish a temporal relationship. Allergy testing can help identify environmental allergies and a few specific workplace allergens, but positive testing does not establish, nor negative testing rule out, a diagnosis of WRA.

Questions

How do you determine whether the teacher's asthma is secondary to her work exposures and, if so, what type of work-related asthma does she have?

In this case, considering the 3 criteria, discussed previously, and the 5 key steps in OEM clinical decision making (see **Box 3**), it can be concluded that this teacher's diagnosis is most consistent with WRA, specifically new-onset occupational asthma related to mold and dampness at her school. There are (1) diagnostic evidence of asthma (positive bronchodilator); (2) sufficient history of exposure to mold and dampness based on her history and the school environmental report (discussed later); (3) medical literature that supports the link between mold, dampness exposures, and asthma; (4) a consistent temporal relationship (onset and timing of symptoms related to school exposures); and (5) no other known risk factors. Thus, the diagnosis of occupational asthma related to school exposures can be made with substantial diagnostic certainty. It is not necessary to identify a single causative agent.

How do you interpret the findings of an environmental investigative report?

Environmental indoor air evaluations frequently are performed in response to concerns regarding indoor air quality, most commonly mold, although mold testing generally is NOT recommended, because mold is ubiquitous. These evaluations can be variable in quality and the findings represent a snapshot in time of select areas. Despite these limitations, indoor air evaluations frequently are performed, and thus it is important for clinicians to be familiar with these reports.

A proper environmental report should include the following information: qualifications of the inspector, statement of purpose, a description of what was done, a walk-through description of the workplace, interpretation of laboratory testing, and conclusions and recommendations.[20] Often, most helpful is the descriptive information, which can document hazards, such as visible mold, dampness, infrastructure problems, odors, and hazardous work processes or housekeeping practices. Elevated levels of carbon dioxide (produced by people in the room) can indicate ventilation problems. Elevated indoor compared with outdoor mold levels suggests mold growth inside the building. Carbon dioxide or mold results do not, however, rule out problems; visual inspection often finds signs of dampness and mold, despite negative mold testing.[20]

In this case, the environmental report confirmed long-standing problems with dampness and water incursions, conditions that promote mold growth. The high carbon dioxide levels confirmed inadequate ventilation. The normal mold results should not be interpreted as indicating a safe environment.

How can a clinician assist a patient with work-related asthma who wants or needs to continue working?

Early recognition of WRA can lead to better outcomes, including more stable employment, health benefits, and better asthma control.[21] Management of WRA is focused on exposure modification, patient education, and optimizing standard asthma medical therapy.[11,19] Several resources are available to assist clinicians and patients manage WRA, as shown in **Table 1**.

Briefly, workplace triggers should be reduced to the extent possible and standard asthma therapy optimized. With new-onset occupational asthma, removal is recommended if a specific workplace sensitizing agent (allergen) is identified. The need to step up asthma treatment should trigger further evaluation of possible work or environmental triggers.

Importantly, health care providers can play an important role in facilitating reasonable workplace accommodations for their patients. Accommodations to reduce or eliminate exposure can involve restriction from job tasks associated with the exposure or job transfer. Caution must be taken when recommending job restrictions because over-restricting can result in job loss, whereas under-restriction can subject the patient to ongoing exposure. Providers also should educate their patients about workers compensation and other available resources (see **Table 1**), such as the Family and Medical Leave Act.[22]

With this teacher, given problems with the school's infrastructure, the recommendation was made for the patient to move to another school facility until her building was remediated. Her asthmatic symptoms improved and she is teaching regularly in the new location.

What can be done for others experiencing symptoms?

It is not uncommon for additional coworkers to report similar symptoms. When several employees are exposed to the hazard, employees or the employer can request a workplace investigation by the National Institute for Occupational Safety and Health (NIOSH) Health Hazard Evaluation (HHE) Program.

The program evaluates work exposures and related health effects and provides free consultative services to identify and reduce hazards.[23] Other options are listed in **Table 1**.

In the case of this patient, a complaint had been filed with the Occupational Health and Safety Administration (OSHA) by an employee, which prompted a workplace investigation. In addition to investigating reported violations, OSHA offers free consultative services that provide on-site evaluations and recommendations. OSHA can be contacted by a health care provider, worker, or employer to perform an inspection.[24]

CASE 3

A 70-year old man with long-standing interstitial findings on imaging was referred to for evaluation of potential occupational causes of his lung disease. He was diagnosed with chronic obstructive pulmonary disease (COPD) disease 20 years earlier during a hospitalization for pneumonia.

The patient has been managed with inhaled corticosteroids, bronchodilators, and supplemental oxygen. Recent pulmonary function tests demonstrated mixed restrictive-obstructive deficits with moderative air flow obstruction and a diminished diffusing capacity for carbon monoxide. His CT scan shows extensive bilateral parenchymal changes more prominent in the upper lung zones with nodular densities, scarring, bronchiectasis, and focal masses, some with calcification. There are no pleural plaques. Review of prior films showed that his imaging findings have been relatively stable over the 20-year interval.

After high school, he worked as a material handler at an iron foundry for 10 years without any personal protective equipment. After this, he worked in a variety of construction jobs for the next 30 years, both new construction and demolition work. He does not remember doing any sandblasting, welding, or direct work with asbestos. He has been retired for 10 years and is a lifetime nonsmoker.

Questions

1. What are the most important elements of his exposure history?
2. How much occupational exposure did this patient have and was it enough to cause his disease?
3. What is his most likely diagnosis?
4. The foundry has been out of business for decades and he is retired. What is the point of now diagnosing his chronic lung disease as occupational?

Discussion

This never-smoker patient with mixed obstructive and restrictive lung disease had been diagnosed and treated as COPD for many years. His chest imaging shows chronic nodular fibrotic changes, some larger masses, and bronchiectasis. His occupational history of working in foundries and construction indicates years of exposure to dusts and fumes, including silica, asbestos, construction dusts, and diesel exhaust fumes. A recent America Thoracic Society–European Respiratory Society statement estimated that occupational exposures contribute to a substantial proportion of chronic respiratory disease, including 26% of idiopathic pulmonary fibrosis and 14% of COPD,[25] in addition to the well-defined pneumoconioses, such as asbestosis and silicosis, discussed further in Reynolds and colleagues' article, "Occupational Contributions to Interstitial Lung Disease," and Krefft and colleagues' article, "Silicosis – An Update and Guide for Clinicians," in this issue.[26,27] Thus several of this patient's work exposures could have contributed to his chronic fibrotic lung disease with mixed obstructive and restrictive physiology. The challenge for the clinician is to determine which (if any) of his exposures over 50 years of work in dusty environments contributed to his chronic lung disease.

Questions

What are the most important elements of this patient's exposure history?

Occupational exposures should be considered in all patients with interstitial lung disease (ILD). For patients with chronic lung disease, the best and most time-efficient approach is to obtain a chronologic work history beginning with the patient's first to most present job (see **Box 1**), focusing on dirty jobs with inhalational exposure.[28] Because most occupational ILDs have a long latency period, 10 years to 30 years or more after exposure, it is important to consider early jobs and work exposures, even if of shorter duration, because work exposures overall now are better controlled in most industries. Some notable exceptions related to silica, coal mining, and firefighter exposures, are discussed in Leonard H.T. Go and Robert A. Cohen's article, "Coal Workers Pneumoconiosis and Other Mining-Related Lung Disease: New Manifestations of Illness in an Age-Old Occupation,", Krefft and colleagues' article, "Silicosis – An Update and Guide for Clinicians," and Kathleen Navarro's article, "Working in Smoke: Wildfire Impacts on the Health of Firefighters and Outdoor Workers and Mitigation Strategies," in this issue.[27,29,30] For each job, key information that should be obtained includes job title, type of industry, and years employed (see **Box 1**). A description of the work tasks, processes, and materials used, including approximate proportion of time spent doing particular tasks, also is helpful in assessing the types and magnitude of work exposures.

Clinicians frequently are not familiar with the major hazardous exposures for different jobs and industries, especially historic ones. Several easily accessible online resources can help clinicians identify the main hazardous exposures for specific industries and jobs as well as lung diseases associated with these exposures, as noted in **Table 1**.

In this case, foundry work involved a metal casting process using molds with crystalline silica. Cleaning the silica off the metal castings can generate high levels of respirable crystalline silica, and silicosis is well known to occur in foundry workers.[31] Construction work also can involve exposure to crystalline silica as well as asbestos, diesel exhaust fumes, and other dusts and fumes.[32]

In addition to the work environment, it also is important to assess for exposures in the home environment, such as hobbies, pets, and wood stoves. Questionnaires and training materials are available to assist the clinician in obtaining a complete occupational and environmental history.[33]

How much occupational exposure did this patient have and was it enough to cause his disease?

Quantitative exposure data is rarely available for patients' workplaces, especially for past jobs. By far the best way to estimate the magnitude of exposure is from the occupational history (see **Box 1**). A description of the work processes, the scale of operations, dust control methods, and years and dates of relevant exposure can help quantify the magnitude and duration of exposure. Details, such as visible dust or mist in the air, dust on work clothes or in sputum, and usage of personal protective equipment, also are helpful in estimating past exposures.

In this case, the patient reported an open work floor plan in the foundry where, even though he did not clean the casts himself, he worked in close proximity to the casting work in a very dusty environment. He worked at the job full-time long hours for a decade and during a time period, in the 1950s to 1960s, when engineering controls and personal protective equipment were more limited. On this basis, it is reasonable to estimate that his past exposure to respirable silica at this foundry was substantial. His construction work, by description, involved a range of activities but predominately was a supervisory role. He did not directly sandblast, cut through cement or rocks, or work directly installing or removing asbestos. He worked around diesel exhaust vehicles and welding fumes only occasionally. Thus, crystalline silica from his years working in the foundry was his dominant inhalational exposure.

A quick review of the medical literature and the online resources provided (see **Table 1**) can help determine whether his 10 years of foundry work was sufficient silica exposure to cause his lung disease. Foundry work is well known to lead to silicosis, including in workers with less than 10 years employment.[34]

What is the most patient's most likely diagnosis?

The patient most likely has silicosis, based on his chest imaging, mixed obstructive restrictive physiology, and a history of substantial occupational exposure to crystalline silica dust. His COPD also likely is related to his silica exposure given he is a lifelong nonsmoker and silica exposure also is associated with COPD. As discussed previously, exposures related to his work in construction were relatively low compared with the foundry. The relatively slow progression of his disease is consistent with silicosis and occupational pneumoconioses in general. That he was misdiagnosed as COPD rather than silicosis for many years, despite abnormal chest imaging suggestive of silicosis, is not surprising, given the widespread under-recognition of occupational lung diseases. His diagnosis of silicosis is further supported by the well-established association between foundry work, respirable silica exposure, and silicosis in the medical literature.[31] Silicosis is one of the few occupational lung diseases with distinct chest imaging features, yet findings can overlap with nonoccupational lung diseases, such as sarcoidosis, as discussed in Lara Walkoff and Stephen Hobbs' article, "Chest Imaging in the Diagnosis of Occupational Lung Diseases," in this issue.[35]

Considering the key steps in OEM clinical decision making (see **Box 3**), there are (1) sufficient diagnostic evidence of disease (pulmonary fibrosis and silicosis) based on chest imaging and pulmonary function tests; (2) sufficient history of exposure to silica, (3) medical literature strongly supporting the link between the silica exposure, the industry he worked in and the disease; (4) consistent temporal relationship (onset many years after exposure); and (5) no other known major risk factors. Thus, the diagnosis of occupational silicosis related to his past foundry work can be made, in this case with substantial diagnostic certainty.

The foundry has been out of business for decades and he is retired. What is the point of now diagnosing his chronic lung disease as occupational?

Even though his disease has progressed slowly and his silica exposure was in the remote past, it remains important to establish the diagnosis of silicosis from a public health perspective and to optimize this patient's well-being. It is important to remember that occupational diseases are preventable. Clinician recognition and diagnosis of occupational lung diseases are essential to surveillance and prevention of future disease. Surveillance data, which can be based on sources, such as periodic workplace surveillance, insurance or workers compensation claims, death certificates, or mandatory governmental reporting, can identify disease clusters, track trends, estimate disease burden, and inform occupational safety and health practices, so as to prevent future disease.

In this case, the diagnosis of silicosis also may make the patient eligible for compensation and benefits to assist with medical expenses, his respiratory impairment, and lost wages.[36,37] There often are funds established to enable benefits when employers are no longer around. Available resources to assist patients and clinicians are provided in **Table 1**. An attorney knowledgeable in worker's compensation could help the patient navigate the system and become aware of what benefits are available.

CASE 4

A 62-year-old man former smoker with severe COPD and prior history working as a steam fitter and welder was referred for evaluation of occupational contributions to his lung disease. He retired at age 59, 3 years prior to the visit due to progressive worsening of his respiratory symptoms and inability to perform his job.

On evaluation, his exercise tolerance was 10 meters of walking, and he has difficulty performing activities of daily living, such as dressing. A recent pulmonary function test showed severe air flow obstruction with a forced expiratory volume in the first second of expiration of 27% and a severely reduced diffusion capacity. Chest computed tomography (CT) imaging showed marked emphysema. The patient uses a daily long-acting β_2-agonist and anticholinergic inhaler and an albuterol rescue inhaler approximately 4 times per day. He is a former smoker, having smoked a pack per day for 20 years before quitting 15 years ago in his mid-40s. There is no family history of lung disease.

The patient worked as a steam fitter and welder for 40 years across a variety of industrial sites, including his last 20 years at a small medical center. This job involved daily welding of galvanized steel and other metals for equipment repair and also construction of shelving. His welding was done in a basement mechanical room and in confined spaces where ventilation was very limited.

Review of his spirometry records showed a marked decline in lung function over the past 15 years, despite smoking cessation. The patient wants to know if his work exposures caused his COPD.

Questions

1. When should you suspect occupational exposure in a patient with COPD?
2. What are the important details of the exposure history in this case?
3. How does the physician account for multifactorial causation?
4. Can you make a diagnosis of occupational COPD in this patient?

Discussion

Although the development of COPD is associated primarily with smoking, numerous other important contributing work and environmental risk factors have been identified. Occupational COPD has been defined as "COPD where there has been a material contribution made to its development, or severity, by inhaled workplace agent(s)."[38] Occupational exposures account for about 14% of COPD and about 30% of COPD in nonsmokers, based on an extensive and consistent epidemiologic literature across multiple countries and populations.[25,38] Several causative exposures have been identified, including vapors, gases, dusts, and fumes; coal; cadmium; silica; and biomass.[25,38] Multiple occupations have been associated with increased risk of COPD, including welders, miners, construction workers, agricultural workers, and warehouse and dock workers.[39–41] Yet clinicians rarely consider nonsmoking causes for COPD and occupational COPD rarely is diagnosed.

Questions

When should you suspect occupational exposure in a patient with chronic obstructive pulmonary disease?

Given the substantial occupational burden of COPD and the wide range of occupations at increased risk of COPD, occupational COPD should be considered in all patients with COPD, even in those with extensive smoking history. Identification of occupational contributions is important for optimal patient management (eliminating further harmful exposures) as well as for occupational surveillance and developing better preventive measures.

What are the important details of the exposure history in this case?

Similar to evaluating patients with ILD, the best and most time-efficient approach is to obtain a chronologic work history beginning with the patient's first to most present job (see **Box 1**) and focusing on jobs with notable inhalational exposure and longer duration jobs.[28] Questions should focus on the types, magnitude, and duration of inhalational exposures, such as dusts, fumes, vapors, particulates, and agricultural exposures. Questions also should focus on the presence of engineering controls (such as enclosures and ventilation), administrative controls (worker training programs), and personal protective equipment, all of which can reduce the individual worker's level of exposure (see **Box 1**).

This patient reported regularly welding in poorly ventilated spaces with suboptimal respiratory protective equipment. He welded on a daily basis for more than 4 hours a day. Welding can generate various metal fumes, gases, oxides, combustion products, and particulates, with greater inhalational exposures in poorly ventilated areas and confined spaces.[42] His history thus supports significant exposures to welding fumes and gases during his 20 years working at the medical center. His initial 20 years as a union welder he reported better ventilation, respiratory protection, and regular medical surveillance, including spirometry.

Also important in this case are his other risk factors for COPD and the timing of exposures. He had a 20-pack-year smoking history and stopped smoking approximately 5 years into his job at the medical center, 15 years prior to his leaving work due to his severe COPD. He also should be asked about home and environmental exposures, such as a wood-burning fireplace, furnace, or stove, and hobbies, all of which were negative. He cooked infrequently on an electric stove. How does the physician account for multifactorial causation?

It is important for a clinician to be aware of the standards of causation in different settings and compensation systems. Although these vary, the question is not whether the exposure in question definitively and exclusively caused the illness. Rather, the typical standard is whether it is more probable than not that work exposures contributed to the patient's condition.[37] This standard takes into account that evidence rarely is definitive and that many diseases have multiple risk factors. Thus, the clinician determines whether work exposures contributed to disease onset, progression, and/or severity while also considering other known risk factors for the disease.

In this case, the patient had substantial exposures to welding fumes, as discussed previously, and also had a significant prior smoking history. Additional considerations that can help assess causality with multiple risk factors are the magnitude and timing of the different exposures, the timing of exposures relative to disease onset or progression, and the strength of the different risk factors. In this case, occupational exposures contribute to COPD even in heavy smokers.[38] His lung function declined rapidly after he stopped smoking, during the time he continued to have substantial welding exposures, whereas smoking cessation is known to limit further excessive decline in lung function.[43]

Can you make a diagnosis of occupational chronic obstructive lung disease in this patient? Using the key steps in OEM decision making (**see Box 3**), the clinician can make a diagnosis of occupational COPD in this patient. There is (1) sufficient diagnostic evidence of disease (COPD diagnosis is clear), (2) sufficient history of exposure to welding fumes, (3) medical literature that supports the link between welding-type exposures and COPD in both smokers and nonsmokers, (4) consistent temporal relationship (his lung function worsened during and after the time he was welding), and (5) other known risk factors, such as smoking, were considered.

Thus, the diagnosis of occupational COPD related to his prior welding can be made with substantial diagnostic certainty. His smoking also contributed to his COPD.

Regular medical surveillance and earlier recognition of his occupational COPD could have led to interventions to reduce work exposures, such as engineering controls and respiratory protection, and likely less severe COPD.

SUMMARY

The preceding 4 cases highlight an approach that clinicians can use when evaluating any patient with possible occupational and/or environmental lung disease. OEM clinical decision making requires a high level of suspicion and specialized skills, most important of which is taking a thorough work and exposure history and then utilizing a basic framework to incorporate this information in to the key steps involved in OEM clinical decision making. Although the processes and governmental systems related to occupational lung disease can be unfamiliar and daunting, the diagnostic approach and resources provided in this article should enable clinicians to gain confidence in diagnosing occupational and environmental lung diseases. The cases also highlight the need to increase awareness of occupational and environmental lung diseases among clinicians as well as the need for better surveillance and prevention of these diseases. The articles to follow in this volume provide up-to-date information on the spectrum of work and environmental lung disease.

DISCLOSURE

The authors have nothing to disclose.

Funding sources: none.

Table 1
Provider and patient selected occupational resources

Information about the workplace and exposures	
OSHA establishment search • Enables searching for a specific business to see if there is a history of complaints or citations regarding hazards in the workplace Safety and health topics • Provides information on several respiratory hazards	https://www.osha.gov/pls/imis/establishment.html https://www.osha.gov/SLTC/text_index.html
NIOSH • Workplace Health and Safety Topics—organized by hazards, exposures, industries, and occupations • Indoor air quality	https://www.cdc.gov/niosh/index.htm https://www.cdc.gov/niosh/topics/default.html https://www.cdc.gov/niosh/topics/indoorenv/mold.html

Safety Data Sheets	Employees can request SDSs on substances present in the workplace. The employer is required to provide this information.
Association for Occupational and Environmental Clinics asthmagen exposure data base	http://www.aoecdata.org/ online searchable database of workplace exposures that can cause asthma
Further workplace information, investigations, and filing a complaint	
NIOSH Health Hazard Evaluations • Used to determine if there are any health hazards in the workplace and give recommendations for remediation • There also is a search feature to determine if a business has had an HHE in the past.	https://www.cdc.gov/niosh/hhe/default.html https://www2a.cdc.gov/hhe/search.asp
OSHA—filing a complaint • Workers and providers can file complaints regarding unsafe or hazardous workplaces. • Complaints can be submitted online, via fax, email, mail, phone, or from the local OSHA office. • 1–800–321–6742	https://www.osha.gov/workers/file_complaint.html
Unions, states, and other governmental agencies, trade and professional organizations	Union representatives can be a valuable resource, as can local governments and relevant organizations
Resources to help manage the patient	
US Department of Labor, Office of Workers' Compensation Programs • Provides links to state workers' compensation programs for the private sector or state government employees	https://www.dol.gov/owcp/#
US Department of Labor Family and Medical Leave Act • Provides information regarding employee eligibility for family and medical leave, including general guidance, fact sheets, and forms.	https://www.dol.gov/agencies/whd/fmla
Job Accommodation Network • Provides information regarding the Americans with Disabilities Act and reasonable accommodations	https://askjan.org/index.cfm https://askjan.org/publications/individuals/employee-guide.cfm
Association for Occupational and Environmental Clinics	Network of over 60 clinics in the US where patients can be referred for further OEM evaluation http://www.aoec.org/directory.htm
Unions, state, and other governmental agencies, trade and professional organizations and attorneys	Union representatives can be a valuable resource, as can local governments, relevant organizations, and attorneys familiar with workers compensation and other benefit programs.

Table 2
Selected Resources for Evaluating and Managing Home and Environmental Exposures

Resource	Link
American Lung Association • Indoor and outdoor air pollutants and health	https://www.lung.org/clean-air/at-home http://www.stateoftheair.org/
US Environmental Protection Agency • Indoor Air Quality Tools in Schools • Environmental Protection Agency 10 steps to making your home asthma-friendly • Home environment checklist • Implementing an asthma home visit program	https://www.epa.gov/iaq-schools https://www.epa.gov/asthma/10-steps-making-your-home-asthma-friendly https://www.epa.gov/sites/production/files/2018-05/documents/asthma_home_environment_checklist.pdf https://www.epa.gov/sites/production/files/2013-08/documents/implementing_an_asthma_home_visit_program.pdf
Agency for Toxic Substances and Disease Registry • A comprehensive profile of toxic substances • Toxic substance portal—health effects of toxic substances	https://www.atsdr.cdc.gov/ https://www.atsdr.cdc.gov/toxprofiledocs/index.html https://www.atsdr.cdc.gov/substances/index.asp
State and local health department and other governmental agencies	Valuable resources for assistance addressing environmental hazards. Health department resources often are found on the department's Web page.
Association of Environmental and Occupational Medicine Clinics	Network of more than 60 clinics in the Untied States where patients can be referred for further OEM evaluation http://www.aoec.org/directory.htm

REFERENCES

1. CDC: most recent national asthma data. 2020. Available at: https://www.cdc.gov/asthma/most_recent_national_asthma_data.htm. Accessed February 1, 2020.
2. Brigham E, Allbright K, Harris D. Health disparities in environmental and occupational lung diseases. Clin Chest Med 2020. in press.
3. Mehta AJ, Dooley DP, Kane J, et al. Subsidized housing and adult asthma in Boston, 2010–2015. Am J Public Health 2018;108(8):1059–65.
4. Adamkiewicz G, Spengler JD, Harley AE, et al. Environmental conditions in low-income urban housing: clustering and associations with self-reported health. Am J Public Health 2014;104(9):1650–6.
5. Moses L, Morrissey K, Sharpe RA, et al. Exposure to indoor mouldy odour increases the risk of asthma in older adults living in social housing. Int J Environ Res Public Health 2019;16(14).
6. Rosenfeld L, Chew GL, Rudd R, et al. Are building-level characteristics associated with indoor allergens in the household? J Urban Health 2011;88(1):14–29.
7. Northridge J, Ramirez OF, Stingone JA, et al. The role of housing type and housing quality in urban children with asthma. J Urban Health 2010;87(2):211–24.
8. Redlich CA, Balmes J. Occupational and environmental lung disease. In: George RB, Light RW, Matthay MA, editors. Chest medicine. 4th edition. Baltimore (MD): Williams and Wilkins; 2000. p. 314–45.
9. McGregor J, Mercer SW, Harris FM. Health benefits of primary care social work for adults with complex health and social needs: a systematic review. Health Soc Care Community 2018;26(1):1–13.

10. Crocker DD, Kinyota S, Dumitru GG, et al. Effectiveness of home-based, multi-trigger, multicomponent interventions with an environmental focus for reducing asthma morbidity: a community guide systematic review. Am J Prev Med 2011;41(2 Suppl 1): S5–32.
11. Tarlo SM, Balmes J, Balkissoon R, et al. Diagnosis and management of work-related asthma: American College of Chest Physicians Consensus Statement. Chest 2008;134(3):1S–41S.
12. Lau A, Tarlo SM. Work-related upper airway disorders. Clin Chest Med 2020. in press.
13. Annesi-Maesano I, Baiz N, Banerjee S, et al. Indoor air quality and sources in schools and related health effects. J Toxicol Environ Health B Crit Rev 2013; 16(8):491–550.
14. Alexander D, Lewis L. Condition of America's public school facilities: 2012–13 (NCES 2014-022). U.S. Department of Education. Washington, DC: National Center for Education Statistics; 2014.
15. Fisk WJ, Lei-Gomez Q, Mendell MJ. Meta-analyses of the associations of respiratory health effects with dampness and mold in homes. Indoor Air 2007; 17(4):284–96.
16. Annesi-Maesano I, Hulin M, Lavaud F, et al. Poor air quality in classrooms related to asthma and rhinitis in primary schoolchildren of the French 6 Cities Study. Thorax 2012;67(8):682–8.
17. Dangman KH, Bracker AL, Storey E. Work-related asthma in teachers in Connecticut: association with chronic water damage and fungal growth in schools. Conn Med 2005;69(1):9–17.
18. Harber P, Redlich CA, Hines S, et al. Recommendations for a clinical decision support system for work-related asthma in primary care settings. J Occup Environ Med 2017;59(11):e231–5.
19. Vandenplas O, Suojalehto H, Cullinan P. Diagnosing occupational asthma. Clin Exp Allergy 2017;47(1): 6–18.
20. Horner WE, Barnes C, Codina R, et al. Guide for interpreting reports from inspections/investigations of indoor mold. J Allergy Clin Immunol 2008;121(3): 592–7.e7.
21. Tarlo SM, Lemiere C. Occupational asthma. N Engl J Med 2014;370(7):640–9.
22. U.S. Department of Labor: family and medical leave act. Available at: https://www.dol.gov/agencies/whd/fmla. Accessed February 1, 2020.
23. National Institute of Safety and Health: health hazard evaluations. Available at: https://www.cdc.gov/niosh/hhe/. Accessed February 1, 2020.
24. Occupational Safety and Health Administration: file a complaint. Available at: https://www.osha.gov/workers/file_complaint.html. Accessed February 1, 2020.
25. Blanc PD, Annesi-Maesano I, Balmes JR, et al. The occupational burden of nonmalignant respiratory diseases. An official American Thoracic Society and European Respiratory Society Statement. Am J Respir Crit Care Med 2019;199(11): 1312–34.
26. Reynolds C, Feary J, Cullinan P. Occupational contributions to interstitial lung disease. Clin Chest Med 2020. in press.
27. Krefft S, Wolff J, Rose CS. Silicosis - persistence of an old disease, old and new exposure settings and prevention. Clin Chest Med 2020. in press.
28. Glazer CS, Newman LS. Occupational interstitial lung disease. Clin Chest Med 2004;25(3):467–78, vi.
29. Navarro K. The changing nature of wildfires: update on the respiratory health of first responders. Clin Chest Med 2020. in press.
30. Cohen RA, Go LHT. Coal workers pneumoconiosis and other mining-related lung disease: the re-emergence of an old disease. Clin Chest Med 2020. in press.
31. Rosenman KD, Reilly MJ, Rice C, et al. Silicosis among foundry workers. Implication for the need to revise the OSHA standard. Am J Epidemiol 1996; 144(9):890–900.
32. Woskie SR, Kalil A, Bello D, et al. Exposures to quartz, diesel, dust, and welding fumes during heavy and highway construction. AIHA J (Fairfax, Va) 2002;63(4):447–57.
33. Agency for toxic substances & disease registry: taking an exposure history. Available at: https://www.atsdr.cdc.gov/csem/csem.asp?csem=33&po=0. Accessed February 1, 2020.
34. Reilly MJ, Timmer SJ, Rosenman KD. The burden of silicosis in Michigan: 1988-2016. Ann Am Thorac Soc 2018;15(12):1404–10.
35. Hobbs S, Walkoff L. Chest imaging in the diagnosis of occupational lung diseases. Clin Chest Med 2020. in press.
36. Sood A. Performing a lung disability evaluation: how, when, and why? J Occup Environ Med 2014; 56(Suppl 10):S23–9.
37. Taiwo OA, Cain HC. Pulmonary impairment and disability. Clin Chest Med 2002;23(4):841–51.
38. Fishwick D, Sen D, Barber C, et al. Occupational chronic obstructive pulmonary disease: a standard of care. Occup Med (Lond) 2015;65(4): 270–82.

39. Fishwick D, Barber CM, Darby AC. Chronic obstructive pulmonary disease and the workplace. Chron Respir Dis 2010;7(2):113–22.
40. Fishwick D, Darby A, Hnizdo E, et al. COPD causation and workplace exposures: an assessment of agreement among expert clinical raters. COPD 2013;10(2):172–9.
41. De Matteis S, Jarvis D, Darnton A, et al. The occupations at increased risk of COPD: analysis of lifetime job-histories in the population-based UK Biobank Cohort. Eur Respir J 2019;54(1).
42. Antonini JM. Health effects of welding. Crit Rev Toxicol 2003;33(1):61–103.
43. Willemse BW, Postma DS, Timens W, et al. The impact of smoking cessation on respiratory symptoms, lung function, airway hyperresponsiveness and inflammation. Eur Respir J 2004;23(3): 464–76.

Chest Imaging in the Diagnosis of Occupational Lung Diseases

Lara Walkoff, MD[a,*], Stephen Hobbs, MD[b]

KEYWORDS

- Pneumoconiosis • Asbestosis • Silicosis • Coal workers' pneumoconiosis • Imaging
- High-resolution computed tomography

KEY POINTS

- Despite the widespread use of chest radiographs in screening for pneumoconioses, high-resolution computed tomography (HRCT) is both more sensitive and more specific, particularly early in the disease course.
- Occupational and environmental lung diseases may manifest in a variety of HRCT patterns, including fibrosis, diffuse micronodules, diffuse opacities, air trapping, pleural disease, and lymphadenopathy.
- Many HRCT features of occupational and environmental lung diseases overlap with other disease processes; therefore, radiologists should always consider the possibility of occupational and environmental causes in the differential.
- In many cases, imaging alone is not sufficient for the diagnosis of a pneumoconiosis but is considered along with additional parameters including exposure history, physical examination, pulmonary function testing, laboratory findings, and histopathologic evaluation.
- As new technologies emerge and industrial practices evolve, so will the prevalence as well as the manifestations of occupational and environmental lung diseases on imaging.

INTRODUCTION

Occupational lung diseases (OLDs) result from the inhalation of organic or inorganic dusts, gases, or organisms. Pneumoconioses are a subset of OLDs caused by mineral dust inhalation. OLDs result in substantial morbidity and mortality worldwide, with an estimated 30,000 deaths annually related to asbestosis, silicosis, and coal workers' pneumoconiosis combined. Taking into account occupational asthma, the impact of OLDs is even larger.[1] Imaging plays a crucial role in the diagnosis and monitoring of these lung diseases; however, the sensitivity and specificity for detection and diagnosis vary greatly depending on the imaging modality used. High-resolution computed tomography (HRCT) has the greatest diagnostic accuracy for occupational and environmental lung diseases, although it is not routinely used in screening because of cost, availability, radiation exposure, and policies of regulatory agencies. OLDs may pose a diagnostic challenge for radiologists, because an exposure history is often unknown, and many entities unrelated to occupational and environmental exposures show similar imaging findings. As a result, even in the absence of a provided exposure history, radiologists should consider the possibility of an OLD when formulating a differential. Some of the more common OLDs encountered on imaging include the major pneumoconioses of asbestosis, silicosis, and coal workers' pneumoconiosis, as

[a] Divisions of Thoracic and Cardiovascular Radiology, Mayo Clinic College of Medicine, 200 First Street SW, Rochester, MN 55905, USA; [b] Radiology Informatics and Integrated Clinical Operations, Division of Cardiovascular and Thoracic Radiology, UK HealthCare Imaging Informatics, University of Kentucky, 800 Rose Street, HX 302, Lexington, KY 40536, USA
* Corresponding author.
E-mail address: walkoff.lara@mayo.edu

Clin Chest Med 41 (2020) 581–603
https://doi.org/10.1016/j.ccm.2020.08.007
0272-5231/20/

well as hypersensitivity pneumonitis. The prevalence, imaging manifestations, and causes of OLDs will continue to evolve as new lines of manufacturing emerge, existing materials are used in new manners, and workplace regulations change, requiring clinicians interpreting imaging to stay apprised of such transformations. In addition, as with other disease processes, imaging should not be interpreted in isolation, because the diagnosis of an OLD is often a multidisciplinary effort, taking into account a combination of exposure history, laboratory testing, pulmonary function testing, imaging, and histopathology.[2]

CHOICE OF IMAGING MODALITY

Despite the use of computed tomography (CT) in screening for entities other than pneumoconioses, such as lung cancer, radiographs remain the initial imaging test of choice across the world for pneumoconiosis screening.[2] However, numerous studies have shown radiographs to be both less sensitive and less specific than CT, particularly for the detection of early pneumoconioses. For example, in patients with coal workers pneumoconiosis (CWP), 23% to 40% of patients with chest radiographs categorized as negative had micronodules present on CT.[3,4] Multiple studies also found chest radiographs to be less sensitive in the detection of asbestos-related changes compared with CT.[5–7] Ground-glass opacities visible on CT, which may be a manifestation of hypersensitivity pneumonitis, are notoriously difficult to appreciate on radiograph. An additional challenge posed by radiographs is the nonspecific appearance of the abnormalities. Opacities identified on chest radiograph during the assessment for pneumoconiosis could be the result of myriad other diffuse lung diseases, such as cigarette smoking alone[8] or non–occupation-related bronchiectasis.[4] Furthermore, the boundary between normal and abnormal can be subjective and difficult to accurately delineate.[2] Despite their limitations, radiographs remain the initial test of choice for screening in the setting of occupational exposure[9] because of low cost, accessibility, and low radiation dose.[2]

Although HRCT is not a primary screening method, it may be obtained when a patient is symptomatic[9] or findings on radiograph are equivocal. CT findings may also be nonspecific and overlap with entities not related to OLDs. For example, there are well-known similarities in appearance between sarcoidosis, silicosis, berylliosis, and CWP. When protocoling HRCT in cases where pneumoconiosis is in the clinical differential, thin-section noncontrast supine inspiratory views should be performed, as well as expiratory and prone series. Expiratory imaging allows the assessment of air trapping, because regions of lung parenchyma with air trapping do not increase in attenuation with expiration. Prone views can be used to differentiate dependent atelectasis from fibrosis, because atelectasis should resolve in the prone position, whereas fibrosis persists.

Although MRI and fluorine-18-2-fluoro-2-deoxy-D-glucose (FDG) PET may have utility in the evaluation of malignancy, particularly mesothelioma, these modalities do not currently have a role in screening in the setting of occupational exposures.[9]

STANDARDIZED IMAGING CLASSIFICATION SYSTEMS FOR PNEUMOCONIOSES

The most widely used standardized classification system for the imaging assessment of pneumoconioses is the International Labor Office (ILO) classification, which is intended for the purposes of epidemiologic research, screening, and surveillance of individuals with occupations with dust exposure, although no specific diagnosis is assigned during image classification.[10] The ILO system of grading is based on findings on posterior-anterior (PA) projection chest radiograph, which is assessed for parenchymal and pleural abnormalities, with findings recorded on a standardized form. Small opacities are described by profusion (concentration), affected lung zones, shape, and size. Profusion is based on a 12-subcategory scale. Shape and size designations are denoted by p, q, and r for small round opacities of increasing size and s, t, and u for small irregular opacities of increasing size (<1.5 mm, 1.5–3 mm, and 3–10 mm, respectively). Large opacities (longest dimension >10 mm) are also assigned a category based on size. Pleural abnormalities include pleural plaques and diffuse pleural thickening, which are evaluated separately on the right and left sides. If plaques are present, the location, presence of calcification, extent, and costophrenic angle obliteration are noted. A series of 2 letter codes for additional abnormalities identified can also be noted on the standardized interpretation form. Appropriate designations are chosen based on written definitions and comparison with a set of 22 standard radiographs. These standards are available in both hard copy and, more recently, digitized formats, both of which have shown comparable classification results.[11] The National Institute for Occupational Safety and Health (NIOSH) offers a B-reader program to certify physicians to categorize studies using the ILO classification system. To become a B reader, clinicians must pass an initial standardized examination grading 125 chest radiographs, and must recertify with an abbreviated examination every 4 years to maintain B-reader status.[12] For individuals who are not B-reader certified, an A-reader certification may be obtained by either attending a specified seminar on pneumoconioses or submitting documentation of 6 correctly classified chest radiographs for review.

The primary critiques of the ILO classification system are largely related to inter-rater variability in scoring and poor sensitivity and specificity compared with CT. For example, in 1 study of coal workers, nearly one-quarter of patients classified as having a negative radiograph showed evidence of coal workers' pneumoconiosis by CT.[3] In contrast, in that same study, half of the patients graded as positive for evidence of CWP on radiograph had a normal chest CT scan.[3] In a separate study, CT showed micronodules in 40% of CWP patients graded as negative by the ILO classification system.[4] CT is also more sensitive than radiograph in detecting small opacity changes of early silicosis, with less inter-reader variability.[13] In a separate study of accelerated silicosis, HRCT was able to diagnose progressive massive fibrosis (PMF) in approximately one-third more cases than radiograph.[14] In addition, it is known that small irregular opacities on chest radiograph may be seen in cigarette smokers in the absence of a pneumoconiosis.[8]

Multiple CT scoring systems have been proposed to categorize pneumoconioses in a reproducible fashion, including 2 created specifically for asbestos-related findings.[5,15] The International Classification of High-resolution Computed Tomography for Occupational and Environmental Respiratory Diseases (ICOERD) scoring system was developed for the screening and diagnosis of OLDs in a manner similar to the ILO classification for radiographs[16] and correlates with the ILO system.[17] A study of dust-exposed workers showed good interobserver agreement for rounded opacities, irregular opacities, emphysema, and honeycombing, although less good agreement for pleural thickening using the ICOERD system.[18] In addition, although the use of ICOERD is superior to radiograph in the detection of early manifestations of pneumoconioses, it has not been shown to have improved correlation with pulmonary function, perhaps owing to HRCT's detection of less extensive parenchymal and pleural changes.[19]

None of these classification systems (ILO, ICOERD, or alternatives) are currently used in routine clinical practice; they are primarily used for medicolegal evaluations and research.

CLASSIFICATION OF OCCUPATIONAL LUNG DISEASES

The spectrum of OLDs may be classified in a variety of manners. For example, the entities may be broadly separated into having either fibrogenic (eg, asbestos, silica, coal, beryllium, talc, aluminum, hard metals) or nonfibrogenic (siderosis) effects. Alternatively, OLDs may be classified based on the typical HRCT patterns; for example, fibrosis, diffuse micronodules, diffuse opacities, or findings of small airways disease (centrilobular nodules, bronchial wall thickening, mosaic attenuation, and air trapping on expiratory imaging). The most common OLDs producing various HRCT findings are presented in **Table 1**. When fibrosis is present, features suggesting a non–usual interstitial pneumonia (UIP) diagnosis[20] or alternative diagnosis to UIP[21] including extensive consolidation or ground-glass opacities, mosaic attenuation with sharply defined air trapping on expiration, diffuse nodules or cysts, pleural plaques, pleural effusions, pleural thickening, or extensive lymph node enlargement should prompt consideration of an OLD. Although not as relevant to imaging appearance, OLDs are sometimes referred to as the major (asbestosis, silicosis, and CWP) and minor pneumoconioses (chronic beryllium disease, hard metal lung disease, aluminosis, talcosis, and siderosis), or categorized based on pathophysiologic response into immune-mediated (hypersensitivity pneumonitis, chronic beryllium disease, and hard metal lung disease) and non–immune-mediated entities.

ASBESTOS-RELATED DISEASE

Asbestos-related pulmonary parenchymal and pleural disease is caused by the inhalation of asbestos fibers. Exposure may occur during the mining of asbestos or in occupations where asbestos fibers are encountered, such as insulation, shipbuilding, and construction. **Table 2** lists the most common occupational conditions associated with various OLDs. Inhaled asbestos fibers have a fibrogenic effect on respiratory bronchioles and pleura.[22] Many imaging manifestations of asbestos exposure have a long latency period, with pleural effusions the earliest manifestation occurring approximately 10 years after exposure.[23] The most common indicator of asbestos exposure is pleural plaques, which have a latency period of around 20 to 30 years before they are visible on radiograph[22]; calcification of the pleural plaques is rarely evident before 20 years after exposure.[24] Diffuse pleural

Table 1
Occupational lung diseases and typically associated HRCT patterns

HRCT Pattern	Occupational or Environmental Lung Disease
Fibrosis	Asbestosis[22,31,38] Chronic silicosis[50] Coal workers' pneumoconiosis[50] Chronic hypersensitivity pneumonitis[64] Chronic beryllium disease[78] Aluminosis[85] Hard metal lung disease[81]
Diffuse Micronodules	
Centrilobular	Acute silicosis[45] Chronic silicosis[48,50] Coal workers' pneumoconiosis[50] Hypersensitivity pneumonitis[64] Siderosis[76] Aluminosis[85] Inhalational talcosis[88,92]
Perilymphatic	Chronic silicosis[48,50] Coal workers' pneumoconiosis[50] Chronic beryllium disease[78]
Diffuse Opacities	
Consolidation	Acute silicosis[45] Hypersensitivity pneumonitis[68]
Ground Glass	Acute silicosis[45] Hypersensitivity pneumonitis[64,68] Hard metal lung disease[81]
Crazy Paving	Acute silicosis[45]
Mass-like Opacities	
Conglomerate Masses	Chronic complicated silicosis[50] Chronic complicated coal workers' pneumoconiosis[3] Chronic beryllium disease[78] Inhalational talcosis[95]
Rounded Atelectasis	Asbestos exposure[22,23,31,38]
Cysts	Chronic hypersensitivity pneumonitis[72]
Air Trapping	Hypersensitivity pneumonitis[64] Occupational asthma[30]
Bronchial Wall Thickening	Chronic beryllium disease[78] Occupational asthma[30]
Pleural Disease	
Effusion	Asbestos exposure[22,23,31,38]
Plaques	Asbestos exposure[22,23,31,38] Chronic silicosis (pseudoplaques)[53–55] Coal workers' pneumoconiosis (pseudoplaques)[3] Chronic beryllium disease (pseudoplaques)[78]
Lymph Nodes	
Lymph Node Enlargement	Acute silicosis[45] Chronic silicosis[48] Coal workers' pneumoconiosis[3] Chronic beryllium disease[78]
Lymph Node Calcification	Chronic silicosis[48] Coal workers' pneumoconiosis[3] Chronic beryllium disease[88]

Table 2
Occupations associated with occupational and environmental lung diseases

Occupational or Environmental Lung Disease	Associated Occupation or Exposure
Asbestos – Related Lung Disease	Historic: shipyard workers, auto and railroad mechanics, asbestos miners[22] Current: asbestos abatement, building remodeling[38]
Silicosis	Mining, construction (tunneling, sandblasting, concrete work), glass manufacturing, ceramics, foundries, denim sandblasting, quartz manufacturing[43]
Coal Workers' Pneumoconiosis	Coal mining[43]
Hypersensitivity Pneumonitis	Farming, avian exposures, hot tubs, humidifiers, numerous[64]
Berylliosis	Historic: fluorescent lamp manufacturing[77] Current: aerospace workers, nuclear workers, electronics manufacturing, dentistry[76,77]
Hard Metal Lung Disease	Manufacturing hard metal cutting tools, oil well drilling, armor plating, and diamond polishing[80,81]
Aluminosis	Alumina abrasive manufacture, pyrotechnic manufacture[86]
Talcosis (inhalational)	Cosmetics manufacture, industrial manufacturing[30,91]

thickening has a variable latency period, typically in the range of 10 to 40 years after exposure,[38] whereas mesothelioma presents approximately 35 to 40 years after exposure.[25] Asbestosis has a latency period of approximately 20 years.[22] The typical latency periods of asbestos-related pleural and parenchymal changes are summarized in **Table 3**.

Table 3
Latency period of asbestos-related pleural and pulmonary parenchymal changes

Manifestation	Years After Asbestos Exposure
Pleural	
Effusion	10[23]
Diffuse Pleural Thickening	10–40[38]
Plaques	20–30[22]
Mesothelioma	35–40[25]
Parenchymal	
Asbestosis	20[22]

Benign pleural disease is the most common radiologic manifestation of prior asbestos exposure.[23] Benign pleural effusions are the earliest manifestation and may develop within 10 years of exposure.[26] The effusions are typically exudative and may persist, resolve, or recur over time.[27] Mesothelioma should be excluded in the setting of late-developing effusions.[23]

Pleural plaques are circumscribed, well-demarcated focal regions of pleural thickening or fibrosis, usually arising from the parietal pleura, separated from the underlying ribs and extrapleural soft tissues by a thin layer of extrapleural fat.[23] The typical distribution is the mid to lower posterolateral and lateral chest wall, paravertebral pleura, and dome of the diaphragm.[24] On radiograph, the appearance of noncalcified pleural plaques depends on location, but they may appear as focal pleural opacity or nodular opacity projected over the lung. When calcified, plaques may resemble a holly leaf when viewed en face. When present along the medial, lateral, and diaphragmatic pleural surfaces and viewed in profile, they appear as a linear focus of high attenuation (**Fig. 1**). Pleural plaques are usually present bilaterally, but may be asymmetric. CT is superior for the detection of pleural plaques; in 1 study, plaques were visible on 59% of radiographs compared with 95% of CT scans.[6] Plaques are most commonly located along the posterolateral and paraspinal regions of the pleura, with sparing of the apices and costophrenic angles.[23] Plaques located along the dome of the diaphragm are nearly pathognomonic for asbestos exposure.[23] Plaques may be calcified in approximately 10% to 15% of patients on radiograph[23]; however, the reported prevalence of calcification on CT is variable, with reports of calcification in up to 60% of patients.[28] Prominent extrapleural fat can mimic the appearance of a pleural plaque on radiograph but can be readily distinguished on CT because of attenuation differences. In isolation, pleural plaques are not associated with significant reductions in pulmonary function and are not precursors to mesothelioma.[29,30]

Diffuse pleural thickening (DPT) appears as a continuous sheet of soft tissue attenuation that, unlike pleural plaques, often involves the costophrenic angles and apices, and rarely calcifies.[31] Also in contrast with pleural plaques, DPT primarily affects the visceral pleura,[23] is substantially less common,[32] and is less specific for asbestos exposure. DPT can occur in the setting of prior infection, hemothorax, and connective tissue diseases.[23] Furthermore, DPT is likely dose related and has been shown to result in impairments of pulmonary function.[29] On radiograph, DPT is generally defined as a smooth, noninterrupted pleural density extending over at least one-fourth of the chest wall, with or without costophrenic angle obliteration,[33] although the ILO definition requires that it be in continuity with an obliterated costophrenic angle.[10] DPT is more ill-defined and irregular compared with discrete pleural

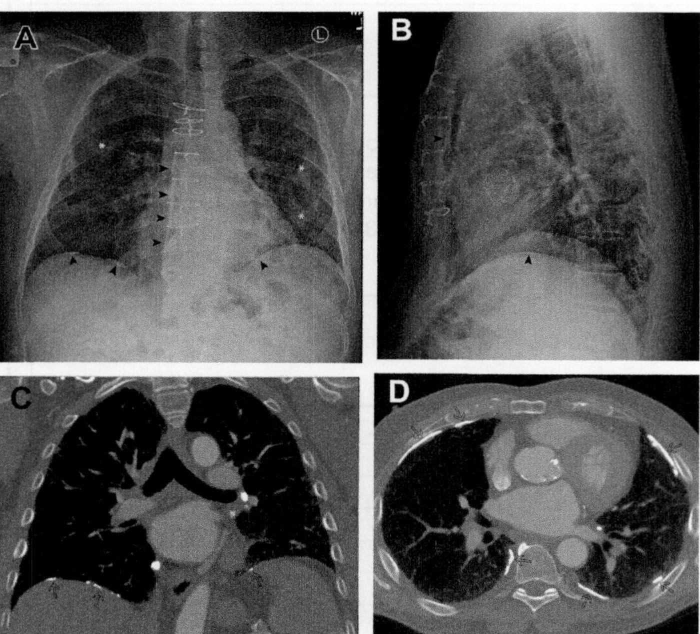

Fig. 1. Calcified pleural plaques in the setting of asbestos exposure. PA (*A*) and lateral (*B*) chest radiographs with calcified pleural plaques viewed face on (*asterisks*) and in profile (*arrowheads*). Coronal (*C*) and axial (*D*) CT images on bone window with corresponding calcified pleural plaques bilaterally (*open arrows*).

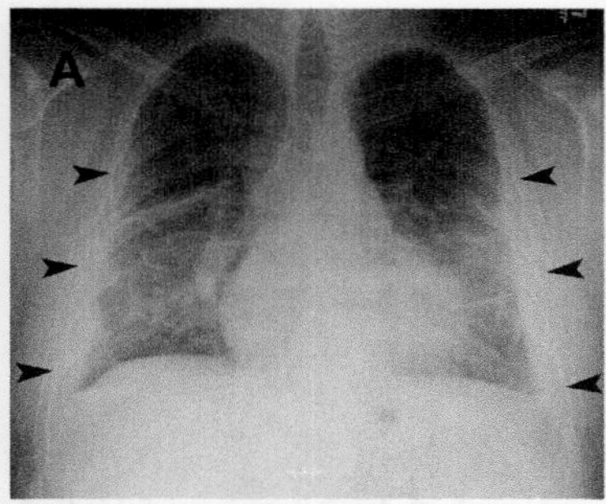

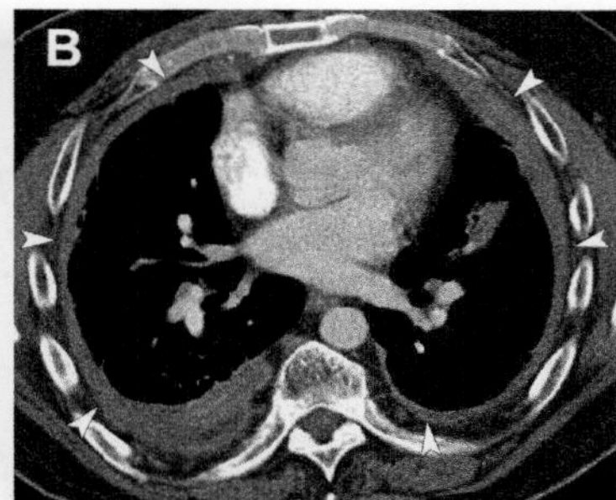

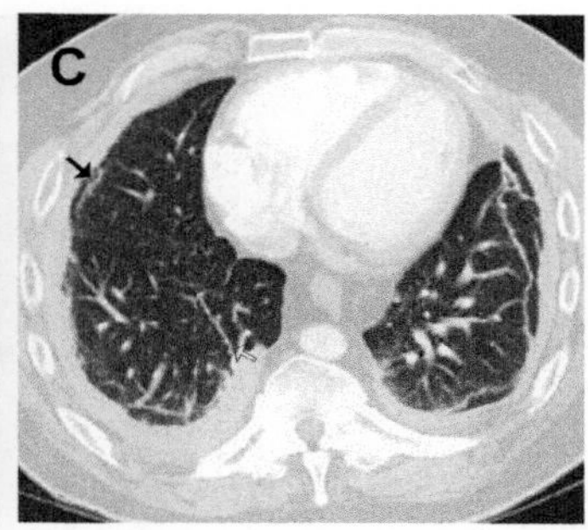

Fig. 2. Asbestos-related diffuse pleural thickening. PA chest radiograph (*A*) shows a linear opacity projecting over the lateral portions of both lungs, which is contiguous with blunted costophrenic angles, and involves greater than half of the length of the chest wall (*black arrowheads*). Multiple linear opacities are present throughout both mid and lower lungs. Mediastinal window axial CT (*B*) reveals diffuse soft tissue attenuation thickening of the bilateral anterior, lateral, and posterior pleural surfaces (*white arrowheads*), although the mediastinal pleura is spared. Lung window axial CT (*C*) shows parenchymal bands (*open arrows*) and subpleural curvilinear lines (*arrow*), in keeping with asbestos-related disease.

plaques.[24] On CT, it is defined as a continuous sheet of pleural thickening more than 5 cm wide, more than 8 cm in craniocaudal extent, and more than 3 mm thick[34] (**Fig. 2**). A benign pleural effusion often precedes the development of DPT.[23] DPT may be unilateral or bilateral. Compared with malignant pleural mesothelioma, mediastinal pleural thickening is less common in the setting of DPT. Other features favoring malignant pleural thickening over DPT include a pleural rind, pleural nodularity, and thickening measuring more than 1 cm.[35]

Parenchymal findings may manifest as asbestosis: interstitial fibrosis caused by asbestos exposure. Fibrosis begins surrounding the respiratory bronchioles in the lower lungs, where there tends to be greatest accumulation of asbestos fibers.[30] This condition manifests as small dotlike and branching subpleural opacities, which are the earliest asbestos-related parenchymal finding visible on CT.[36] Eventually progression to diffuse interstitial fibrosis may occur. On radiograph, this appears as lower lung zone predominant irregular linear (reticular) opacities with associated volume loss that may extend superiorly as disease progresses and result in honeycombing. On HRCT, findings are similar to a UIP pattern of fibrosis, with subpleural and lower lung zone predominant reticulations, evidence of volume loss, and traction bronchiectasis[31] (**Fig. 3**). When advanced, honeycombing may be present (**Fig. 4**). Most patients with asbestosis have either pleural plaques or DPT, suggesting the cause of asbestosis, and importantly not compatible with idiopathic pulmonary fibrosis (IPF). However, asbestosis can exist in the absence of pleural plaques[37] and the degree of fibrosis has a dose-dependent relationship with exposure.[38]

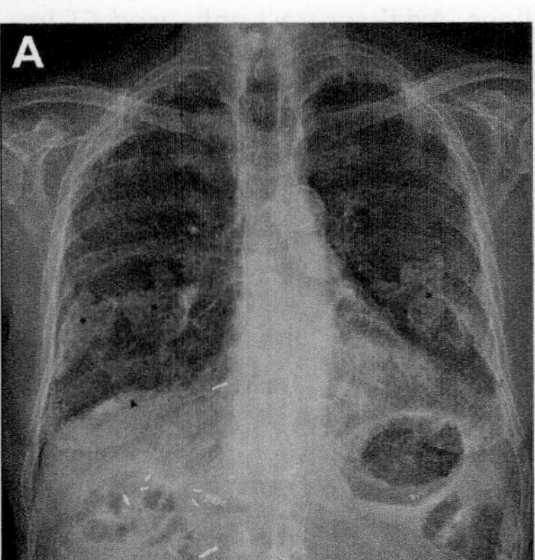

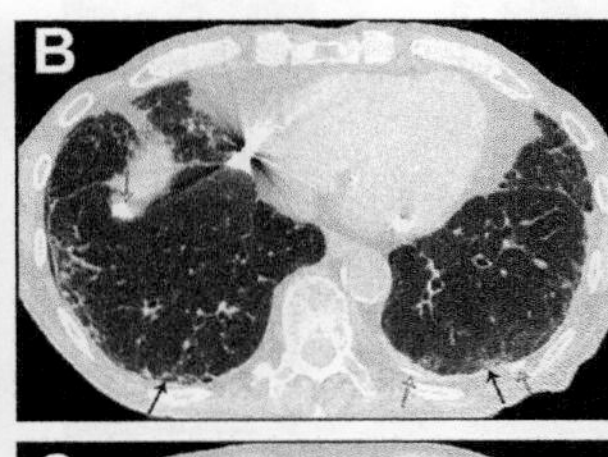

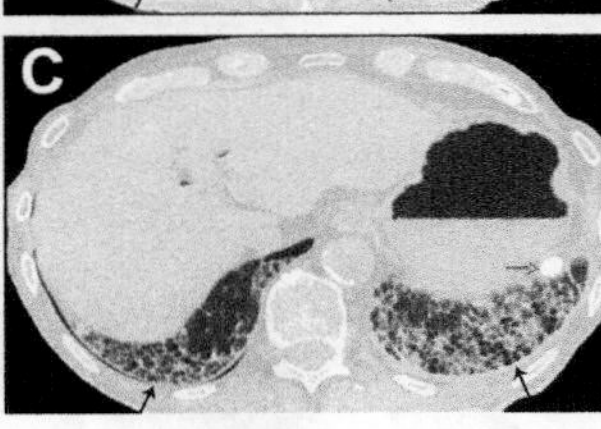

Fig. 3. Asbestosis. PA chest radiograph (*A*) shows bilateral calcified pleural plaques. When viewed en face the plaques have a holly-leaf morphology (*asterisks*). In profile, the plaques are linear (*solid arrowhead*). Increased interstitial markings are present, most conspicuous in the lower lungs (*open arrowheads*). Lung window axial CT images through the lung bases (*B*, *C*) show peripheral reticulations, architectural distortion, and traction bronchiectasis (*closed arrows*) consistent with fibrosis. Calcified plaques are present along the hemidiaphragms and posterior pleura (*open arrows*). A small right pneumothorax, vascular calcifications, pneumobilia, and upper abdominal surgical clips are incidentally present.

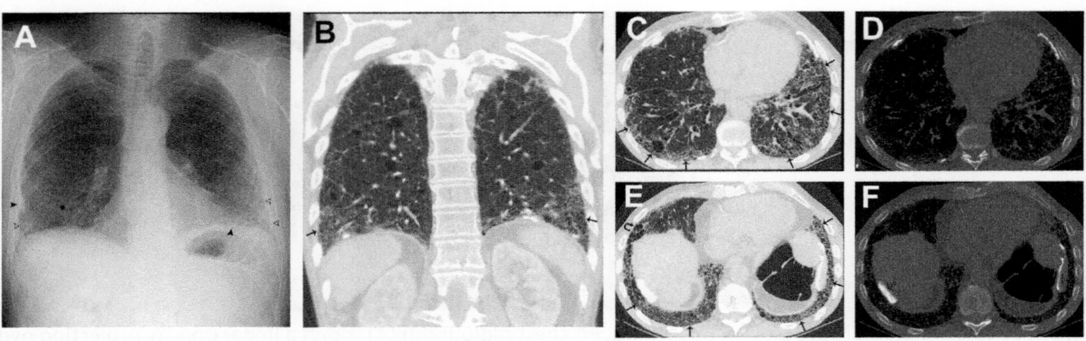

Fig. 4. Asbestosis with honeycombing. PA chest radiograph (*A*) shows increased interstitial markings throughout the bilateral lungs (*open arrowheads*) with pleural plaques viewed face on (*asterisk*) and in profile (*solid arrowheads*). Coronal (*B*) and axial (*C, E*) CT images on lung windows show lower lung predominant peripheral reticulations, volume loss, architectural distortion, and traction bronchiectasis (*closed arrows*), consistent with fibrosis. Small areas of honeycomb change (*curved arrow, E*) and scattered foci of emphysema are present (*B, C*). Bilateral calcified pleural plaques (*open arrows*) are visible on axial CT images at the corresponding levels on bone windows (*D, F*). The parenchymal pattern on CT is consistent with a UIP pattern of fibrosis; however, the presence of calcified pleural plaques make findings nearly diagnostic of asbestosis.

Other parenchymal manifestations of asbestos exposure include parenchymal bands and subpleural curvilinear lines (**Fig. 5**), both of which are more common in asbestosis than other causes of pulmonary fibrosis.[39] Parenchymal bands are defined as linear densities 2 to 5 cm in length running through the lung, often not in the direction of pulmonary blood vessels, and usually extending to the pleural surface; parenchymal bands are fixed and should not change with prone positioning.[37] Subpleural curvilinear lines are linear markings 5 to 10 cm in length occurring less than 1 cm from the inner chest wall.[39]

Rounded atelectasis develops as a result of an underling pleural abnormality, typically pleural effusion, plaque, or thickening. On radiograph, this appears as a rounded or oval subpleural opacity with associated volume loss. The region where rounded atelectasis abuts aerated lung is well defined, although the site of contact with the pleura tends to appear hazy or less well defined.[38] On CT, rounded atelectasis should show (1) a rounded or oval masslike appearance; (2) volume loss in the surrounding lung; (3) abutment of the pleural surface; and (4) curvilinear pulmonary vessels converging on the opacity, referred to as the comet tail sign[40] (**Fig. 6**). All 4 of these features should generally be present to make a confident diagnosis of rounded atelectasis. It can be located anywhere, although most commonly it is found in

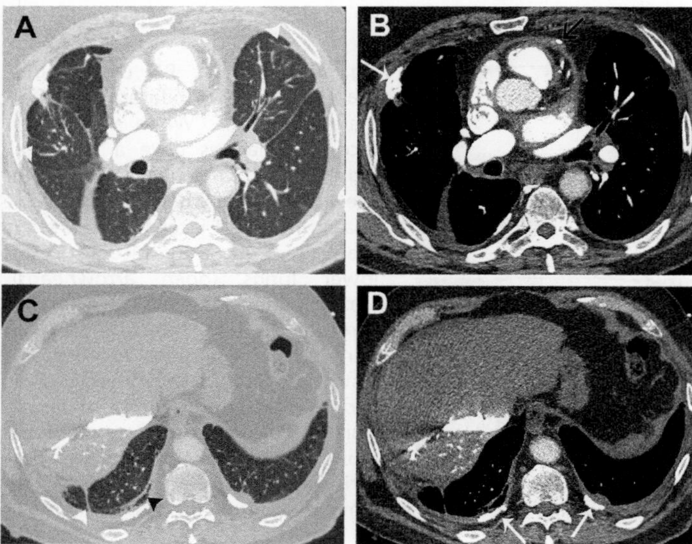

Fig. 5. Asbestosis with parenchymal bands and subpleural curvilinear lines. Axial contrast-enhanced CT images on lung windows in the at the mid and lower lungs (*A, C*) show parenchymal bands (*white arrowheads*) and subpleural curvilinear lines (*black arrowhead, C*). Calcified (*white arrows*) pleural plaques are visible on axial CT images on mediastinal window setting (*B, D*). Also present are diffuse pericardial thickening, focal pericardial calcification (*black arrow, B*) and reflux of contrast into the hepatic veins (*D*) consistent with constrictive pericarditis.

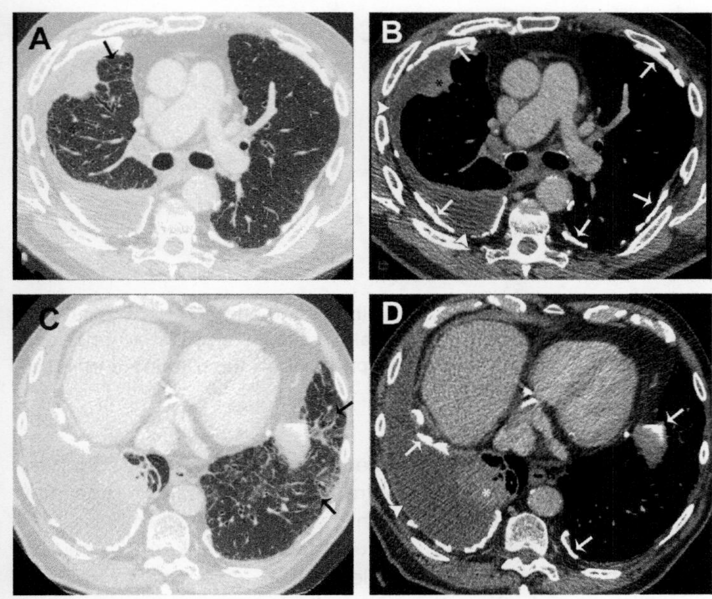

Fig. 6. Effusion and rounded atelectasis in the setting of asbestos exposure. Axial contrast-enhanced CT images on lung (*A, C*) and mediastinal (*B, D*) windows at corresponding levels. A moderate-sized right pleural effusion is partially loculated laterally (*white arrowheads*). Rounded opacity in the right lower lobe immediately adjacent to the effusion shows volume loss, comet-tailing of vessels, and homogeneous enhancement, consistent with rounded atelectasis (*white asterisk, D*). Another smaller focus of rounded atelectasis is present anteriorly (*black asterisk, B*). Calcified pleural plaques (*white arrows*) are consistent with history of prior asbestos exposure. Mild reticular and ground-glass opacities (*black arrows*), greatest in the left lower lobe, with mild bronchiolectasis, are compatible with asbestosis.

the posterior lower lungs.[40] Rounded atelectasis enhances uniformly after intravenous contrast administration but should not be metabolically active on FDG-PET/CT (at or less than blood pool activity).[41] When the appearance is atypical on CT, serial CT follow-up, PET/CT, and/or biopsy can be used to exclude malignancy.

SILICOSIS AND COAL WORKERS' PNEUMOCONIOSIS

Silicosis and CWP are 2 distinct entities with nearly indistinguishable imaging manifestations. In both entities, CT has been shown to be more sensitive for the evaluation of small nodule/opacity profusion.[3,42] Inhalation of silica dust (crystalline silica) occurs most commonly in individuals working in mining, construction, and quartz manufacturing.[43] There is evidence of a dose-response relationship between the length of exposure to silica dust and the prevalence of silicosis. In addition, the rate of silicosis was shown to be 50% higher in heavy smokers with at least 20 years of experience in a population of Dutch fine-ceramics workers.[44]

Subtypes of silicosis are based on the intensity and duration of exposure.[43] They are not mutually exclusive and more than 1 may be present at a given time.[42] The subtypes are (1) acute silicosis or silicoproteinosis, (2) chronic simple silicosis, (3) accelerated silicosis, and (4) chronic complicated silicosis or PMF.

Acute silicosis or silicoproteinosis occurs over a short period of time (ie, months to several years) in workers exposed to large amounts of silica dust and often results in death caused by respiratory failure.[45] Findings on radiograph include diffuse reticulonodular opacities and/or upper lung zone predominant perihilar airspace consolidation, with or without air bronchograms.[45,46] Mediastinal lymphadenopathy may also be visible.[46] On HRCT, acute silicosis may show poorly defined centrilobular nodular opacities, bilateral ground-glass opacities, and regions of consolidation[45] (**Fig. 7**). The classic manifestation is interlobular septal thickening and ground-glass opacities, referred to as a crazy-paving pattern, corresponding histologically with periodic acid–Schiff–positive proteinaceous alveolar exudate.[45,46] Although the crazy-paving pattern is commonly associated with pulmonary alveolar proteinosis, it is nonspecific, with multiple causes that include *Pneumocystis jiroveci* infection, bronchogenic adenocarcinoma, pulmonary hemorrhage, edema, organizing pneumonia, lipoid pneumonia, and toxic inhalation.[47] Acute silicosis sometimes includes poorly defined centrilobular nodules and dependent consolidation.[45] Hilar lymph node enlargement, which is not typically seen in idiopathic pulmonary alveolar proteinosis, may also be present.[45]

Chronic simple silicosis typically occurs 10 to 20 years after exposure and presents on radiograph as multiple small nodular opacities throughout both lungs, greatest in the upper and posterior lungs.[30] In a study of stone cutters, the most common chest radiograph findings in

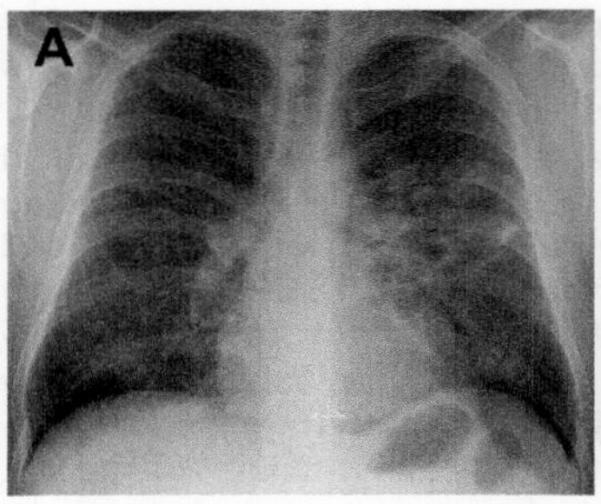

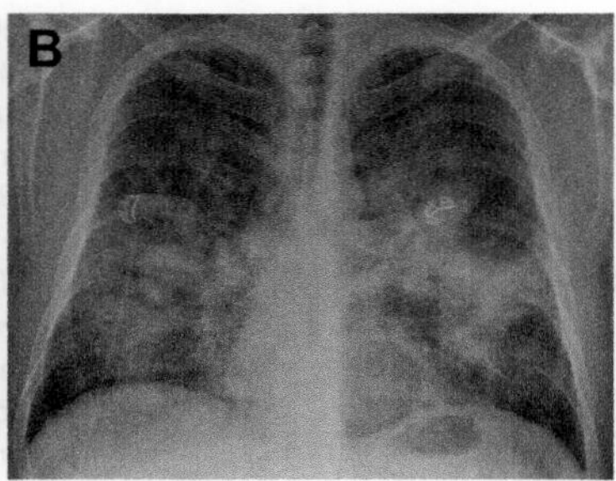

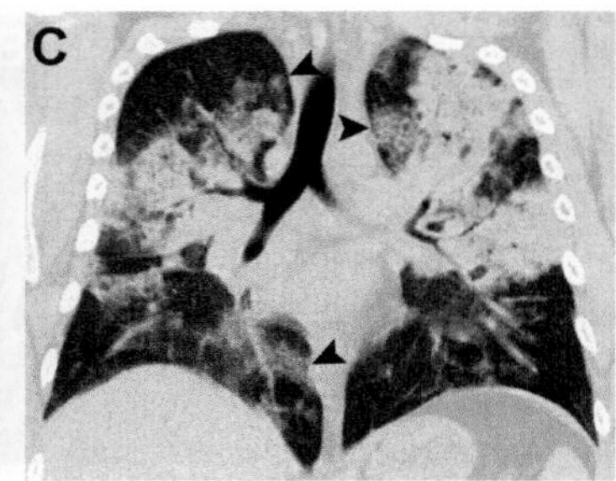

Fig. 7. Acute silicosis. PA chest radiographs taken 4 months apart (*A, B*) show increasing bilateral patchy perihilar consolidative opacities. Lung window coronal chest CT (*C*) shows multifocal perihilar consolidative opacities, greatest in the mid and upper lungs. Several less dense foci of ground-glass opacification superimposed on interlobular septal thickening (crazy paving) are also present (*arrowheads*).

patients with silicosis were small nodules with the ILO designation qp.[48] Nodule calcification may be visible in 20% of patients on chest radiograph.[43] On HRCT, chronic simple silicosis presents as multiple small bilateral and symmetric pulmonary nodules measuring 5 mm or less, with a predilection for the upper and posterior lung zones[48,49] (**Fig. 8**). This distribution is hypothesized to be caused by the poorer lymphatic clearance in these regions related to gravity, pulmonary arterial pressure, and decreased chest wall excursion.[22] Often branching centrilobular nodules are seen in addition to nodules along the subpleura, interlobular septa, and peribronchovascular interstitium.[48,50] Nodules may be branching, punctate, or ill-defined, with the ill-defined opacities corresponding histologically to irregular fibrosis surrounding a respiratory bronchiole.[51] Confluent nodules and interlobular septal thickening may also be present.[48] Mediastinal and hilar lymph nodes may be enlarged, most commonly in the low right paratracheal, subcarinal, and paraesophageal stations.[48] Mediastinal and hilar lymph nodes often calcify, although, despite the classic association of egg-shell peripheral lymph node calcification with silicosis,[50] several studies suggest punctate, diffuse, and central patterns of calcification may be more common.[48,52] Emphysema may be present in both smokers and nonsmokers.[48] Pseudoplaques, multiple small coalescent nodules abutting the visceral pleura, can be seen on HRCT in both chronic silicosis and CWP, and should be distinguished from true pleural plaques.[53–55]

Chronic simple silicosis and CWP may be challenging to differentiate from sarcoidosis, and should be considered in the differential. When present, paracicatricial emphysema is almost exclusively seen in pneumoconioses, and a peribronchovascular distribution of lesions is more suggestive of sarcoidosis[56]; however, in practice, tissue sampling may be required.

Chronic complicated silicosis, or PMF, occurs when the nodules of chronic simple silicosis coalesce. Radiographs show bilateral opacities measuring greater than 10 mm, which are usually symmetric and located in the upper lung zones.[50] On CT, the coalesced nodules appear as irregular soft tissue attenuation masses, often with associated calcification and volume loss in the adjacent

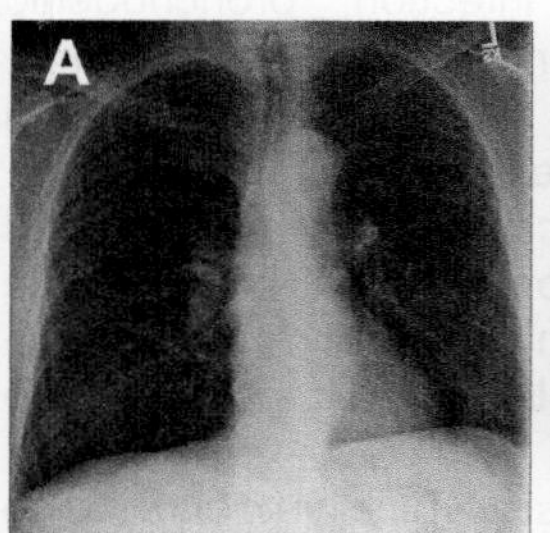

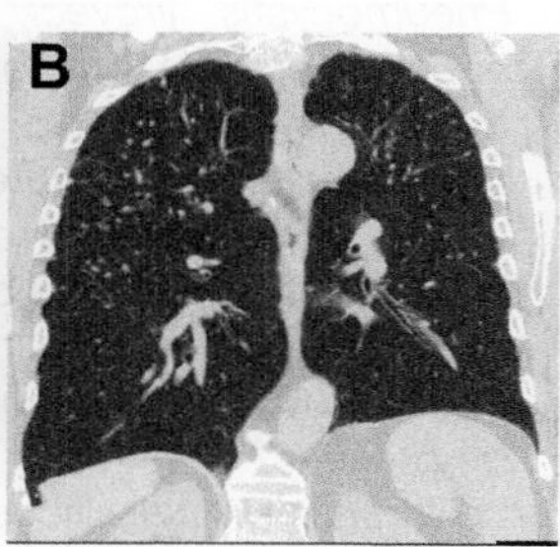

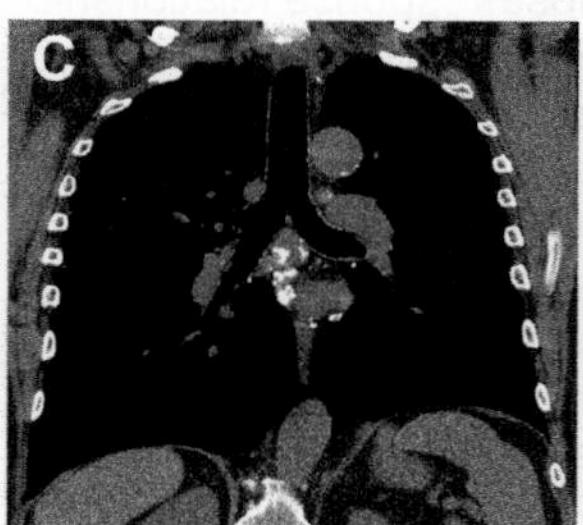

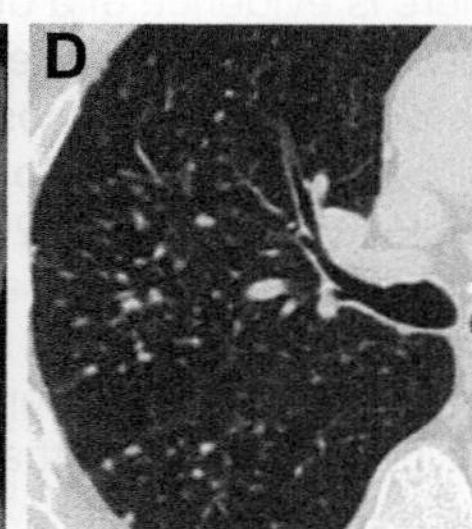

Fig. 8. Chronic simple silicosis. Multiple small round nodules with profusion greatest in the upper lungs are visible on PA radiograph (*A*). Coronal and magnified axial lung window CT images (*B, D*) show multiple small soft tissue attenuation pulmonary nodules in a perilymphatic distribution, primarily located in the upper and mid lungs. Mediastinal lymph nodes with eccentric and central calcifications are visible on coronal mediastinal window CT images (*C*).

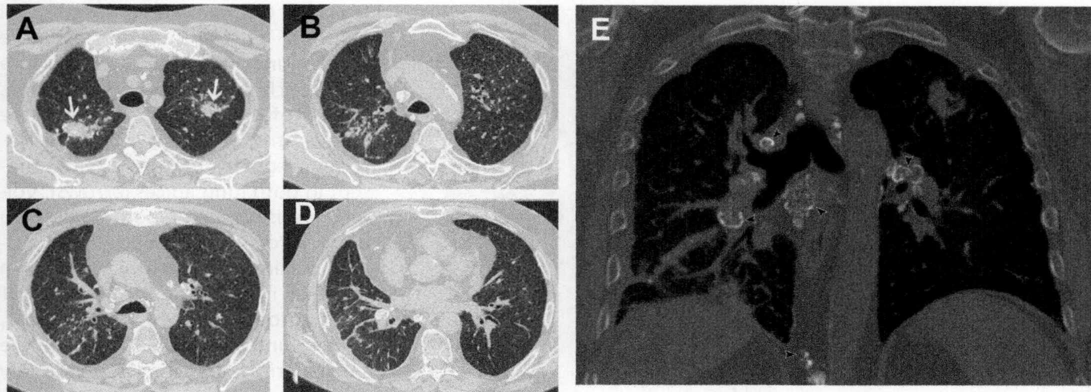

Fig. 9. Chronic complicated silicosis. Axial CT lung window images ordered from cranial to caudal (*A–D*) show innumerable tiny ground-glass, soft tissue attenuation, and calcified pulmonary nodules in a subpleural and peribronchovascular distribution, most concentrated in the upper lungs. Conglomerate nodular masses (PMF) containing small calcifications are present in the bilateral upper lobes (*white arrows, A*). Coronal bone window CT image (*E*) better shows enlarged and peripherally calcified (eggshell) hilar and mediastinal lymph nodes (*arrowheads*). Findings are consistent with chronic complicated silicosis. This patient also had seropositive rheumatoid arthritis, and therefore Caplan syndrome, the combination of rheumatoid arthritis and pneumoconiosis.

lung parenchyma[50] (**Fig. 9**). Findings usually progress over time, extending toward the hila, with increasing paracicatricial emphysema. PMF may be FDG avid on PET/CT, even in the absence of superimposed infection or malignancy, which substantially limits the utility of PET/CT for evaluation of suspected malignant nodules in this setting[57] (**Fig. 10**). As such, biopsy or continued imaging follow-up are frequently the only viable options for evaluation of suspected malignant masses in patients with PMF. PMF is associated with pulmonary functional impairment.[30]

Accelerated silicosis occurs in individuals with heavy dust exposure over a short period of time, typically developing 3 to 10 years after exposure, compared with 10 to 20 years after exposure in individuals with lower concentrations of silica dust.[45] Radiologically, accelerated silicosis may resemble both chronic simple and/or complicated silicosis, with small nodules and/or PMF and a predilection for the upper posterior lungs.[45,52]

CWP is caused by the inhalation of coal dust free of silica, primarily occurring in miners. The severity and prevalence of CWP are related to

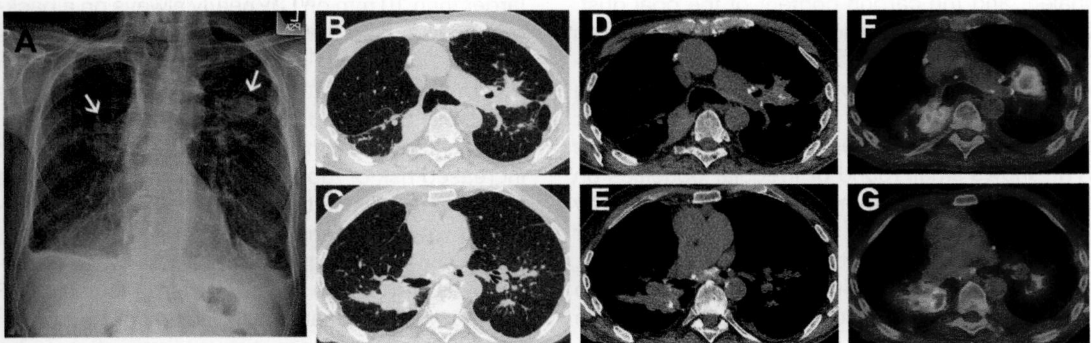

Fig. 10. Chronic complicated silicosis. PA chest radiograph (*A*) shows bilateral upper lung perihilar partially calcified masses (*arrows*) with associated regional architectural distortion and volume loss resulting in upward hilar retraction. Small bilateral pleural effusions are also present. Axial CT images at the level of the carina and right pulmonary artery on lung window (*B, C*) and mediastinal window (*D, E*) settings show partially calcified masses in the bilateral upper posterior lungs extending toward both hila with associated volume loss and architectural distortion. Multiple surrounding small perilymphatic nodules and partially calcified lymph nodes are also present. Axial fusion images from an FDG-PET/CT (*F, G*) reveal the bilateral perihilar masses to be FDG avid. Biopsy of the right mass was performed because of the progressive asymmetric rate of enlargement but did not reveal malignancy.

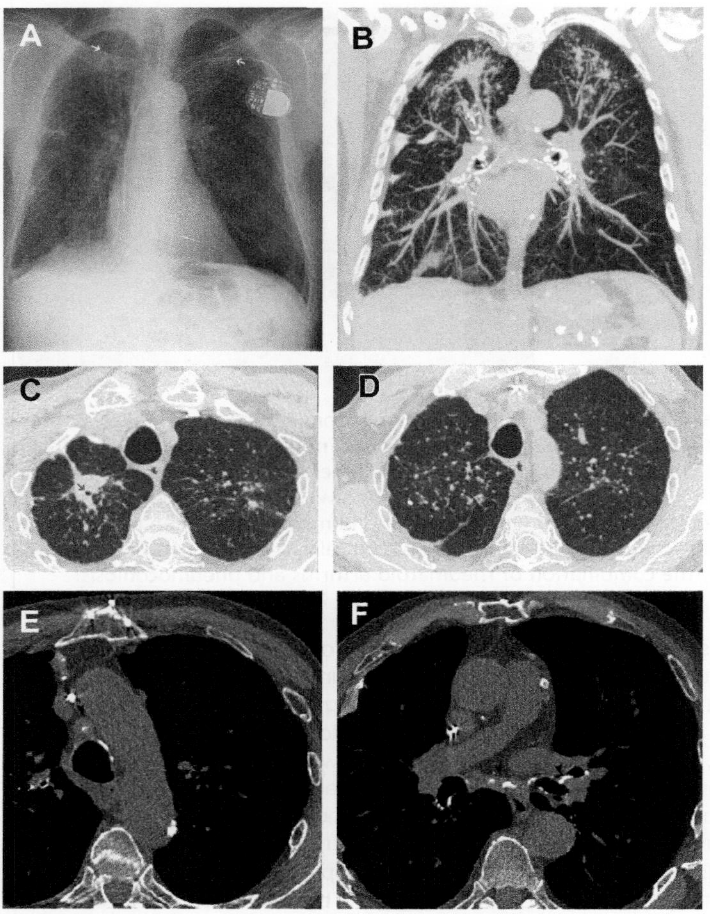

Fig. 11. Chronic complicated coal workers' pneumoconiosis. Multiple small round pulmonary nodules in a peribronchovascular distribution, most profuse in the upper lungs, are visible on PA chest radiograph (*A*). Small irregular opacities are also present in both lung apices (*arrows*). Volume loss is present in both lungs, with upward retraction of both hila. Coronal maximum intensity projection (MIP) CT image (*B*) and thin axial CT slices through both upper lobes (*C, D*) on lung window show multiple small perilymphatic solid pulmonary nodules, predominantly in the upper and mid lungs. Irregular solid conglomerate nodules and masses are present in the lung apices, with a dilated airway within the right apical conglomerate mass (*open arrow, C*). On mediastinal window axial CT slices at the level of the aortic arch and subcarinal region (*E, F*), mediastinal and hilar lymph nodes with central calcifications are present. Findings are consistent with chronic complicated coal workers' pneumoconiosis in this patient with a history of coal mining. Note that the imaging findings are indistinguishable from those present in silicosis. Cardiac pacemaker, sternotomy, and changes related to coronary artery bypass grafting are also visible.

the duration of exposure, amount of coal dust inhaled, and the carbon content of the coal dust, with higher concentrations associated with an increased risk of CWP.[43] CWP is nearly indistinguishable from silicosis on imaging, despite having distinct histopathologic findings.[50] The 2 major forms of CWP are simple and complicated. Simple CWP shows small round or irregular opacities on radiograph, most commonly types s, p, or q by the ILO classification,[58] typically with an upper lobe and posterior distribution. As in silicosis, these nodules may calcify,[50] although they do so more frequently in silicosis.[43] On CT there are diffuse small nodules in perilymphatic and sometimes centrilobular distributions with a predilection for the upper and posterior lungs[50] (**Fig. 11**). Hilar and mediastinal lymph node enlargement may be present.

Like chronic complicated silicosis, chronic complicated CWP also results in PMF. On chest radiograph, this appears as bilateral upper lung opacities with associated volume loss. These findings correspond with conglomerate nodules larger than 10 mm on CT, nearly always on a background of simple CWP,[3,58] with associated volume loss and commonly paracicatricial emphysema.[50] Pleural thickening at the costophrenic angles has also been described.[58]

Patients with both silicosis and CWP are at an increased risk of tuberculous and nontuberculous mycobacterial infections[59–61] (**Fig. 12**). Superimposed mycobacterial infections may cavitate, which can be a diagnostic challenge when malignancy is also in the differential. In addition, PMF may cavitate because of ischemic necrosis[50] and, in these instances, tissue diagnosis may be required.

HYPERSENSITIVITY PNEUMONITIS

Hypersensitivity pneumonitis (HP), also known as extrinsic allergic alveolitis, is caused by an immune-mediated response to the inhalation of organic antigens.[62] On histology, HP results in

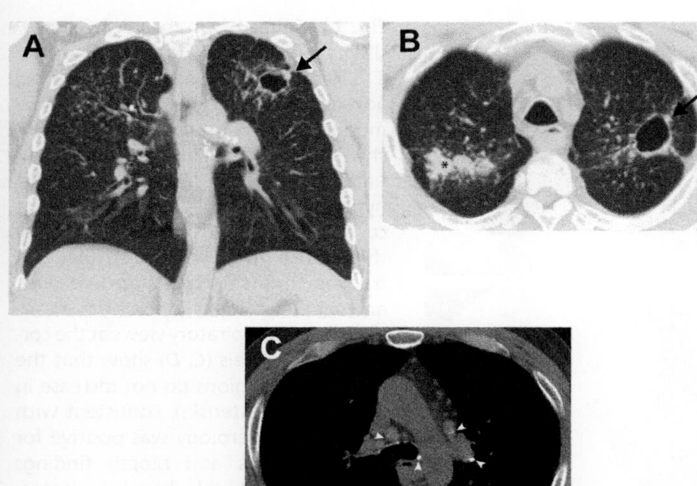

Fig. 12. Silicotuberculosis. Lung window coronal (*A*) and axial (*B*) CT images show numerous small perilymphatic nodules in both upper lobes and a conglomerate nodular mass in the right upper lobe (*asterisk*, *B*). A cavitary lesion is present in the left upper lobe (*arrows*), consistent with known superimposed tuberculosis. Multiple partially calcified hilar and mediastinal lymph nodes (*arrowheads*) can be seen on mediastinal window axial CT (*C*).

cellular bronchiolitis, diffuse interstitial infiltrates of chronic inflammatory cells, and noncaseating granulomas with a predilection for the peribronchiolar region.[63] Numerous exposures have been implicated, including *Aspergillus* and thermophilic *Actinomyces* in agriculture (so-called farmer's lung), nontuberculous mycobacteria in hot tubs (hot-tub lung), avian antigens (bird fancier's lung), and low-molecular-weight chemicals that combine with human proteins to form antigens.[64] A study of patients presenting to a tertiary care center in the United States found avian antigens to be the most common cause, followed by hot tub–related *Mycobacterium avium* complex.[65] No single finding is diagnostic for HP, but patient symptoms, physical examination findings, imaging studies, laboratory analysis, and histopathology should be considered when making the diagnosis.[66] An exposure history is helpful, when present, but a causative agent is never identified in a substantial proportion of cases.[65,66] As with other OLDs, CT is more sensitive for detection of findings compared with radiograph.[64,67] CT findings depend on the chronicity of the illness, with stages conventionally categorized as acute, subacute, or chronic, although there may be overlap, with acute-on-chronic presentations occurring.

The acute stage of HP begins hours after exposure in individuals that have been previously sensitized to the antigen, and quickly resolves, although it may recur with subsequent exposures.[62] Imaging findings in the acute phase of HP are less well documented, which may be because of the abrupt onset and resolution and/or the challenging diagnosis.[62] HRCT findings resemble pulmonary edema, with multifocal ground-glass opacities and/or consolidation.[68]

In the subacute phase, typically occurring days after exposure, chest radiograph findings are nonspecific and may even be normal.[69] HRCT shows patchy or diffuse bilateral ground-glass opacities and poorly defined small ground-glass centrilobular nodules measuring less than 5 mm.[64,69] Findings are distributed throughout both lungs but may have a mid or lower lung predominance.[64] Mosaic attenuation on inspiratory images correlating with air trapping on expiratory views is common[68] (**Fig. 13**). The head-cheese sign described in subacute HP reflects a combination of ground-glass opacities, regions of normal attenuation lung, and hyperlucent lung caused by air trapping,[70] resembling the processed meat product. Airspace consolidation, interlobular septal thickening, and pleural thickening are atypical findings.[69]

In chronic HP, the primary manifestation is fibrosis, with reticular opacities with associated regions of ground glass, volume loss, and traction bronchiectasis in a peribronchovascular, patchy, or subpleural distribution. Fibrosis in the setting of chronic HP may have a predilection for the upper or mid zones or no zonal predication, although the costophrenic sulci and apices may be spared.[64,71,72] Honeycombing is common, observed in 50% of bird fanciers with chronic HP,[69] although it was less prevalent in other

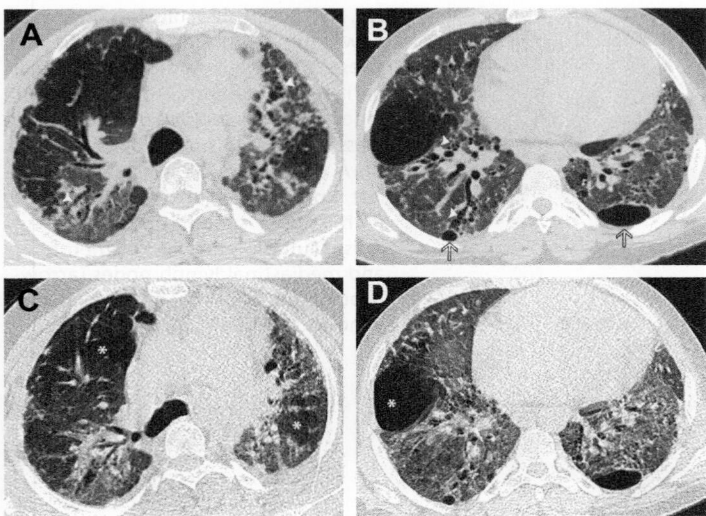

Fig. 13. Subacute on chronic hypersensitivity pneumonitis. Lung window axial CT slices in inspiration at the level of the aortic arch (*A*) and lower lobes (*B*) show mosaic attenuation of the lung parenchyma with areas of ground-glass attenuation and other regions of relative hyperlucency. Small nodular foci of consolidation, mild interlobular septal thickening, peripheral reticulations, traction bronchiectasis (*arrowheads*), and subpleural cysts (*open arrows*) are also present. Expiratory views at the corresponding levels (*C, D*) show that the hyperlucent regions do not increase in attenuation (*asterisks*), consistent with air trapping. Serology was positive for avian antigens and biopsy findings were consistent with chronic hypersensitivity pneumonitis in this bird enthusiast who had kept more than 100 birds before diagnosis.

causes, present in 37% of all studied HP cases in Japan.[73] Honeycombing may be present throughout both lungs, often without an apical-basal predilection.[69] This pattern is in contrast with IPF, where the greatest distribution is typically in the lower lung zones.[72] Emphysema has been shown in nonsmokers at high rates in studies of farmers and bird fanciers with chronic HP.[69,74] Cysts are present within regions of ground glass in nearly 40% of cases of chronic HP.[72] Air trapping on expiratory images is also common.[68] In both subacute and chronic forms, the ground-glass opacities tend to resolve after exposure to the offending antigen is removed.[69] Although the aforementioned findings are typical, multiple atypical appearances have been documented and can mimic other causes of interstitial lung disease.

CHRONIC BERYLLIUM DISEASE

Chronic beryllium disease is caused by exposure to beryllium or its salts in the form of fumes, dusts, or aerosols, resulting in a noncaseating granulomatous HP in genetically predisposed individuals and affecting multiple organ systems.[75] CBD is most commonly encountered in individuals working in nuclear industry, aerospace engineering, ceramics, dentistry, and electronics manufacture.[76] Acute berylliosis had been nearly entirely eliminated because of industrial regulations.[2,75] CBD is diagnosed based on history, imaging findings, and the beryllium lymphocyte proliferation test, which can be used because of the immune-mediated nature of beryllium disease. The beryllium lymphocyte proliferation test is quite specific and useful in distinguishing berylliosis from other potential mimics, such as sarcoidosis.

On radiograph, most patients with abnormal findings have small round or irregular opacities, which are typically symmetric and involve all lung zones.[75] Upward hilar retraction with architectural distortion, linear scars, upper lobe conglomerate masses, emphysema, pleural thickening, and hilar lymph node enlargement may also be observed.[75] In a small study of patients with biopsy-proven beryllium disease, only 54% had an abnormal chest radiograph.[77] CT findings include small nodules along bronchovascular bundles or interlobular septa, often associated with interlobular septal thickening.[77,78] Patchy ground-glass opacities, conglomerate masses, bronchial wall thickening, and pleural irregularity may also be observed.[77,78] Hilar and mediastinal lymphadenopathy is common.[77] In the later stages of disease, fibrosis may manifest as peripheral reticulations, traction bronchiectasis, and occasionally honeycomb change[78] (**Fig. 14**). Because of the overlap in imaging appearance, chronic beryllium disease should be considered in the differential for all patients with findings suggestive of sarcoidosis.[79]

HARD METAL LUNG DISEASE

Alloys of tungsten carbide, cobalt, and small amounts of other elements are combined to produce a hard and heat-resistant material.[80] Manufacturing of this alloy results in the release of dusts and vapors containing cobalt, the primary culprit in hard metal lung disease (HMLD).[80,81] This condition is encountered in industries where there

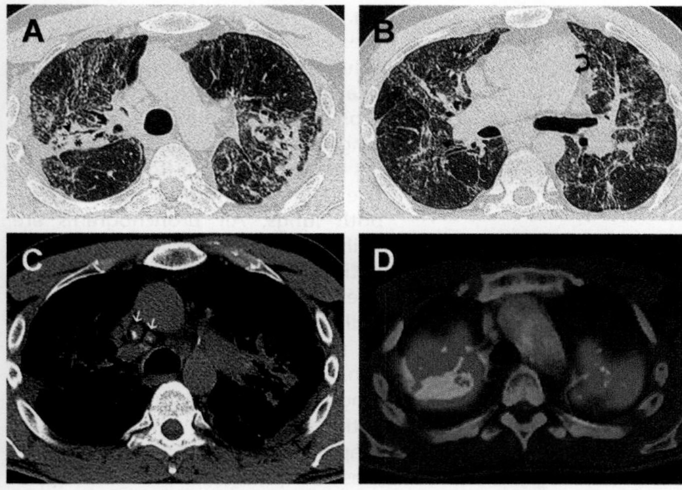

Fig. 14. Chronic beryllium disease. Axial lung window CT images at the level of the aortic arch (*A*) and right pulmonary artery (*B*) show extensive perilymphatic nodularity, interlobular septal thickening, patchy ground-glass attenuation, and conglomerate masses (*asterisk*) in the bilateral upper lungs with associated volume loss, traction bronchiectasis (*arrowheads*), and architectural distortion. Soft tissue window axial CT slice (*C*) shows partially calcified lymph nodes in the low right paratracheal region (*white arrows*) and focal pleural thickening and/or fluid (*black arrows*). Note the dilated main pulmonary artery (*curved arrow, B*), which may indicate pulmonary hypertension. Increased FDG activity within these conglomerate masses is present on axial FDG-PET/CT fusion image (*D*) and was unchanged in size over serial studies and consistent with changes related to chronic beryllium disease rather than malignancy. Histopathologic evaluation of the bilateral explanted lungs at time of transplant showed diffuse granulomatous pneumonitis consistent with the patient's history of occupational beryllium exposure.

is grinding of hard metal cutting tools, oil-well drilling, armor plating, and diamond polishing.[80] Diagnosis is based on an exposure history, clinical features, radiologic findings, histopathology showing giant cell interstitial pneumonia or interstitial lung disease, and/or evidence of metals within lung parenchyma on scanning electron microscopy. Pulmonary findings may manifest as asthma, HP, or interstitial fibrosis.[81,82] The presence of giant cell interstitial pneumonia at histopathology is nearly pathognomonic, and bizarre multinucleated giant cells are also highly suggestive when present in bronchoalveolar lavage fluid.[81,83]

Chest radiographs in HMLD may be normal or show a nonspecific interstitial process with small irregular linear, nodular opacities, and fibrosis.[81,82] On HRCT, HMLD can have variable appearances with findings resembling sarcoidosis, NSIP, or UIP.[81] Reports describe multilobular consolidations, ground-glass opacities with parenchymal distortion, traction bronchiolectasis, and dilated air bronchograms within areas of consolidation[84] (**Fig. 15**). Peripheral reticulation and peripheral cystic spaces may also occur.[81,82]

ALUMINOSIS

Aluminosis is caused by inhalation of aluminum powder and aluminum oxide,[85] with exposures including alumina abrasive manufacture and bar metal stamping to produce powder used in pyrotechnic manufacture.[86] Chest radiographs may be normal or show nonspecific small rounded and irregular opacities, more pronounced in the upper or mid lungs.[76,85] In the early stages, HRCT may show upper lung predominant small rounded ill-defined centrilobular opacities measuring 3 mm or less, which can resemble silicosis, HP, or respiratory bronchiolitis.[76,85] Upper lung predominant reticular and nodular interstitial fibrosis with subpleural bullous emphysema may be shown on HRCT in more advanced stages.[51,85] Fibrosis associated with aluminosis carries the risk of increased spontaneous pneumothorax.[76,85] Increased attenuation mediastinal and hilar lymph nodes have also been reported.[87]

SIDEROSIS

Siderosis results from the accumulation of iron oxide within pulmonary macrophages and is most commonly documented in welders exposed to metal fumes, hence the name electric arc welder's lung or welder's pneumoconiosis.[50] Chest radiograph may reveal fine nodules that are most conspicuous in the mid or lower lungs[76] On HRCT, the most frequently encountered findings are small centrilobular nodules (thought to reflect the deposition of macrophages containing iron oxide particles distributed along the perivascular and peribronchial lymphatics)[84,88] and branching linear centrilobular structures with a slight upper lung predominance. In some cases, small ground-glass opacities are also present,[51,89] and findings can resemble HP. Emphysema has been reported, but may be confounded by concurrent smoking.[84] Siderosis is not typically associated with fibrosis;

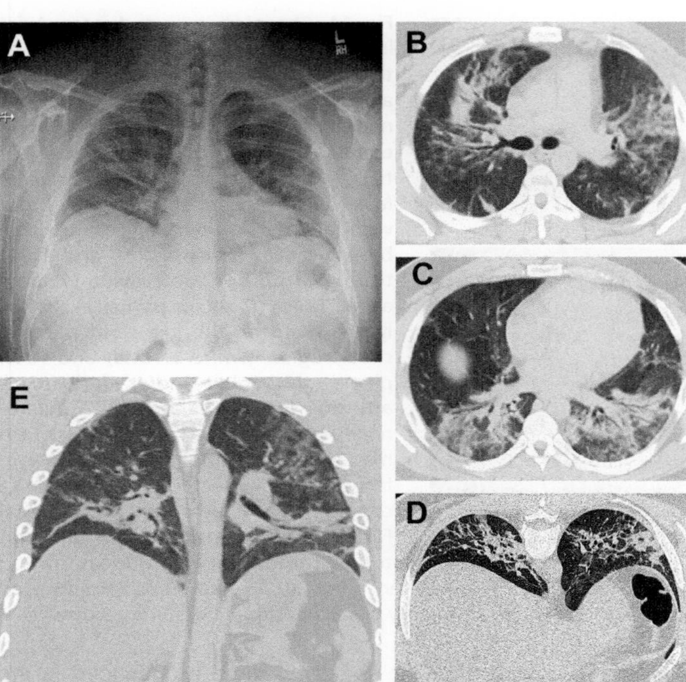

Fig. 15. Hard metal lung disease. PA chest radiograph (*A*) shows low lung volumes with bilateral perihilar linear opacities and increased interstitial prominence in the mid and lower lungs. Lung window axial chest CT slices (*B, C*) reveal multifocal consolidative and ground-glass opacities in both lungs. Air bronchograms are visible within the regions of consolidation. Findings persist on prone images (*D*), which are helpful to exclude basilar atelectasis as a cause of the opacities. Linear regions of consolidation in the mid to lower lungs on coronal CT (*E*) correspond with the findings on chest radiograph. Additional ground-glass opacities are present in the left upper lobe, which are not clearly visible on radiograph.

however, in some cases, the iron is mixed with silica, producing silicosiderosis, which may result in fibrosis.[88,90] Accumulation of iron can cause hilar and mediastinal lymph nodes to have increased attenuation (**Fig. 16**).

TALCOSIS

Pure talc in mineral form as crystalline magnesium silicate is used in cosmetics and as a lubricant in consumer goods and industrial processes.[91] The 3 forms of inhalational talc-related pulmonary disease are (1) talcosilicosis, (2) talcoasbestosis, and (3) pure talcosis. A fourth form of talcosis is related to intravenous injection of crushed oral talc-containing medication tablets.[92] All types result in a foreign body granulomatous inflammation leading to progressive fibrosis. History and imaging findings can point to the diagnosis; however, definitive diagnosis may require tissue sampling.[93]

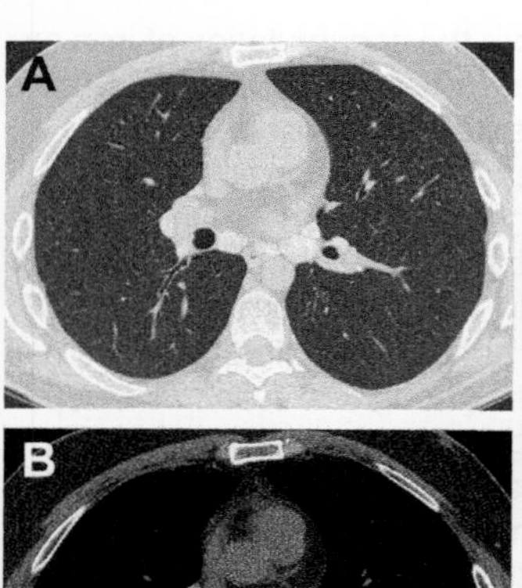

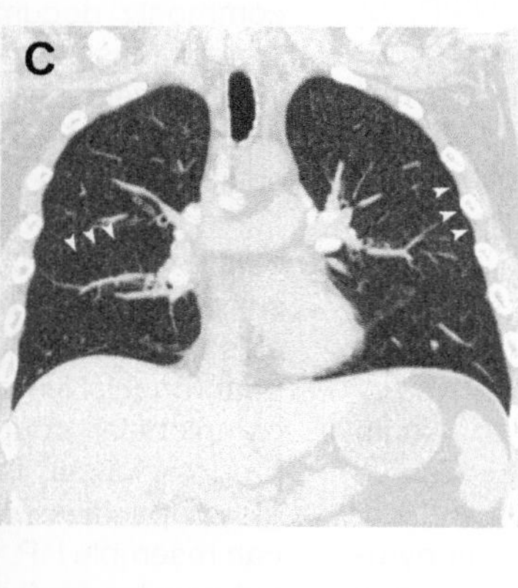

Fig. 16. Siderosis in a welder. Innumerable centrilobular micronodules are present on axial thin-section lung window CT image (*A*). Coronal MIP image (*C*) increases the conspicuity of the nodules, which are slightly more profuse in the upper lungs relative to the bases. Note the immediate subpleural and fissural sparing (*arrowheads*). Diffusely hyperattenuating hilar and mediastinal lymph nodes (*arrows*) are visible on axial mediastinal window CT image (*B*), as a result of iron deposition.

Talcosilicosis and talcoasbestosis affect individuals exposed to impure talc dust also containing silica or asbestos fibers, respectively.[93] Imaging manifestations are similar to those produced by the inhalation of silica and asbestos fibers alone.[91] Radiograph findings of pure inhalational talcosis show small nodules and irregular opacities with either a lower lung or diffuse distribution.[91] HRCT findings suggestive of talcosis are small centrilobular and subpleural nodules measuring up to 1 mm in diameter,[94] which in the later stages may be associated with diffuse interstitial thickening[91] and conglomerate masses containing areas of high attenuation, similar in appearance to PMF or sarcoidosis.[95] High-attenuation mediastinal lymph nodes may also be present.[76] In the inhalational forms, emphysema may be seen in a centrilobular or apical distribution; however, panlobular emphysema in the lower lobes is associated with intravenous talcosis.[92] In intravenous talcosis, talc particles are often larger compared with the inhalational form, and may be visible in other organs on microscopy.[91] On HRCT, small nodules, including sometimes tree-in-bud nodules and high-attenuation conglomerate masses, may be seen.[94]

WORK-RELATED ASTHMA

Work-related asthma includes occupational asthma (asthma caused by workplace exposures) and workplace-exacerbated asthma (preexisting asthma worsened by workplace exposures) and is one of the most common OLDs, with hundreds of reported causes.[30] Hyperinflation manifesting as flattening of the hemidiaphragms, as well as bronchial wall thickening, may be present on radiograph.[30] HRCT shows findings of small airways disease, which cannot be differentiated from nonoccupational causes, and include bronchial wall thickening, mosaic attenuation, and air trapping on expiratory imaging.[30]

NEWER AND EMERGING OCCUPATIONAL LUNG DISEASES

Radiology plays a critical role in the screening and surveillance of OLDs and will continue to be central in the understanding of the presentation and natural history of emerging and evolving entities. In recent years, not only have new OLDs appeared but the established major pneumoconioses have manifested in new workplace environments.[96]

A systematic review on artificial stone–associated silicosis, predominantly associated with manufacturing, finishing, and installation of countertops, noted cases in Australia, Israel, and Spain over the past 20 years.[97] More recently, in the United States between 2017 and 2019, 18 silicosis cases were reported among individuals in the engineered stone fabrication industry, which exposes workers to dusts from a quartz-based composite material containing crystalline silica, commonly used in countertops.[98] Of these 18 cases, 2 were fatal, the first associated fatalities reported in the United States. The most common chest CT manifestations included ground-glass opacities, solid micronodules in both centrilobular and perilymphatic distributions (13 of 18 with an upper lung predominance), and mediastinal lymphadenopathy.[98] Additional cases of artificial stone–associated silicosis in other countries are emerging, included 2 reported in the past year in Belgium.[99]

World Trade Center–related lung disease is thought to be the result of complex mixture of airborne contaminants released during the terrorist attack on the World Trade Center in New York on September 11, 2001, manifesting primarily in first responders.[100] A sarcoidosislike constellation of findings has been described with bilateral perilymphatic nodules, coalescent nodularity with a predilection for the upper lung zones, and hilar and mediastinal lymphadenopathy.[101] Airway wall thickening associated with air flow decline has also been described.[102] It is likely that many of the clinical and imaging sequelae will be elucidated in the coming years.

Additional examples of more recently reported OLDs include:

- Accelerated silicosis in 44 workers involved in denim sandblasting was reported as a novel cause in Turkey in 2010.[52]
- Indium lung, caused by indium tin oxide, a component of the transparent coating of liquid crystal display and plasma televisions, has gained attention over the past 2 decades, with HRCT features including pulmonary alveolar proteinosis pattern, nodules,[103] and interstitial fibrosis.[104]
- Flavor workers' lung was described in 2002 in 8 individuals who were exposed to the ketone diacetyl used in the production of butter flavoring in a microwave popcorn production facility, resulting in bronchiolitis obliterans.[105] HRCT findings included mosaic attenuation, air trapping on expiratory imaging, and bronchial wall thickening,[106] with constrictive bronchiolitis on histopathology.[107]
- Flock workers' lung has been reported in individuals involved in the production of thin nylon fibers caused by inhalation, with CT showing diffuse micronodules, patchy ground-glass

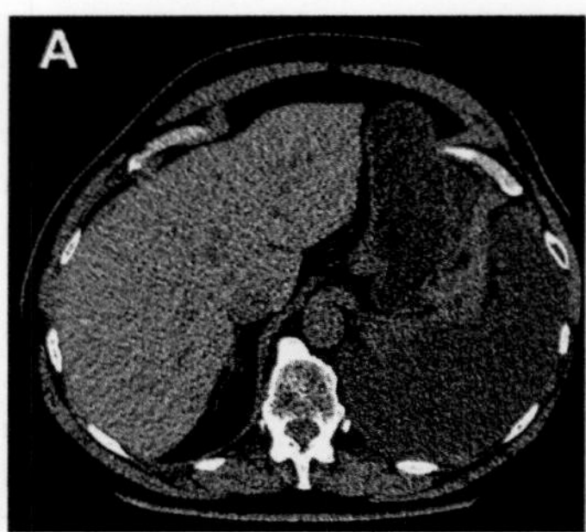

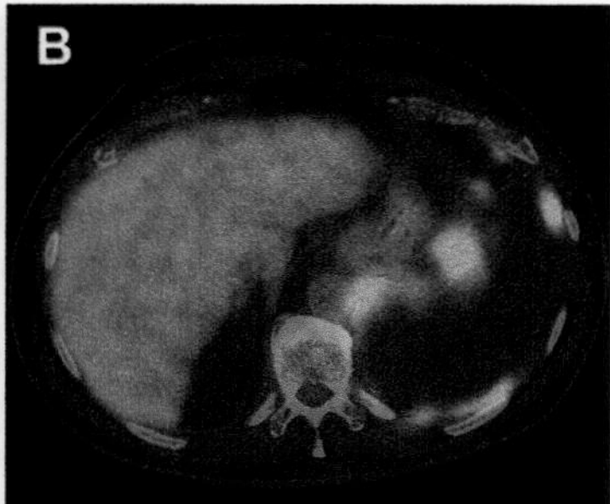

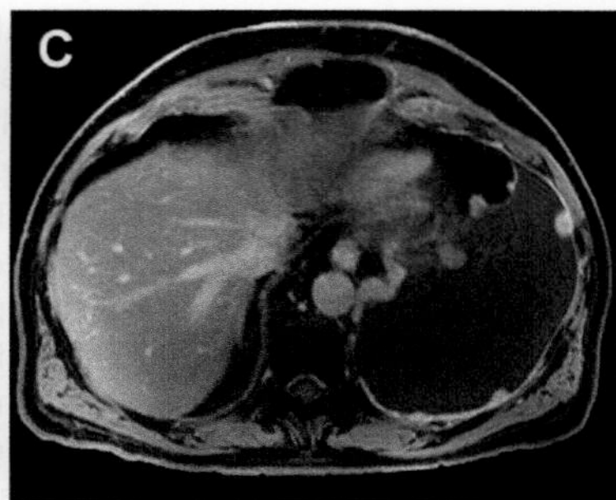

Fig. 17. Epithelioid mesothelioma in a patient with prior asbestos exposure. Axial noncontrast enhanced CT images through the lung bases and upper abdomen demonstrates an at least moderate sized left pleural effusion (*A*). FDG PET/CT fusion images reveal multiple hypermetabolic nodular foci along the medial, lateral, and posterior aspects of the pleura (*B*). Pleural thickening and multiple enhancing pleural nodules are visible on T1 weighted, fat-suppressed, post-contrast MRI (*C*), corresponding with the foci of increased FDG activity on PET/CT. Note the increased conspicuity of the pleural nodules on both PET/CT and MRI relative to noncontrast enhanced CT.

opacities, consolidation, and honeycomb change.[108]

- A component of aerosolized paint, Acramin FWN, inhaled by Spanish textile workers, resulting in HRCT patterns including patchy subpleural airspace resembling idiopathic organizing pneumonia, interstitial fibrosis, and multiple micronodules.[88,109]

IMAGING MALIGNANCY IN THE SETTING OF OCCUPATIONAL LUNG DISEASES

Malignancy poses an additional imaging challenge in the setting of OLDs, because several pneumoconioses are associated with an increased risk of malignancy in addition to having HRCT findings that can mimic malignancy. The increased risk of lung cancer caused by asbestosis and silicosis has been well established.[110–112] Rounded atelectasis in the case of asbestosis and conglomerate masses in the case of silicosis can have an appearance on HRCT that can be difficult to differentiate from malignancy. Exposure to asbestos is associated with an increased risk of both bronchogenic carcinoma and malignant pleural mesothelioma. Bronchogenic carcinoma is the most common thoracic malignancy associated with prior asbestos exposure. As in the general population, adenocarcinoma is the most common subtype, comprising 46% of bronchogenic carcinoma in 1 study of asbestos-exposed individuals.[113] Some analyses indicate smoking and asbestos exposure have a synergistic effect on the risk of lung cancer development, whereas others have shown evidence to the contrary.[114,115] When the characteristic features of rounded atelectasis are present, it can be confidently diagnosed without further work-up; however, when not present, it has the potential to mimic malignancy. In these instances, FDG-PET/CT can be helpful because rounded atelectasis should not be metabolically active, in contrast with malignancy.[41]

Malignant pleural mesothelioma also has a well-established relationship with asbestos exposure, although, compared with the benign manifestations of asbestos-related pleural disease, it has a much longer latency period of approximately 40 years.[116] CT is the diagnostic standard for the initial evaluation of mesothelioma; however, overlap in imaging findings of benign asbestos-related pleural disease, such as pleural effusions and DPT, may confound the diagnosis (**Fig. 17**). A pleural rind, pleural nodularity, pleural thickening greater than 1 cm, and mediastinal pleural involvement are more commonly seen in the setting of mesothelioma than DPT.[35] FDG-PET/CT may be helpful in these cases, with FDG uptake shown to be significantly higher in mesothelioma.[117] FDG-PET can also help with selection of a biopsy target when mesothelioma is suspected on a background of benign pleural changes and can evaluate for extrapleural disease.[117] At present, MRI is not routinely used for the detection and evaluation of mesothelioma, because CT and MRI have nearly equivalent diagnostic accuracy in staging, although CT is usually more readily accessible and less costly. Although MRI is superior to CT for showing focal chest wall invasion, endothoracic fascia involvement, and diaphragmatic invasion, these features do not typically affect surgical management.[118]

Differentiating PMF from malignancy in patients with silicosis may also pose a diagnostic challenge. Both lesions may appear masslike, cavitate, and show increased FDG activity along with increased uptake in hilar and mediastinal lymph nodes.[50] A small case series of patients with CWP and PMF showed a range of maximal standardized uptake values (SUVmax) on FDG-PET, with none of the lesions attributable to malignancy.[119] A separate study of patients with PMF undergoing FDG-PET showed a significantly higher SUVmax in malignant lesions compared with PMF, although the diagnostic accuracy was only 77%.[120] There is evidence that MRI may be helpful in differentiating the 2 entities, with PMF tending to show low signal intensity relative to skeletal muscle on T2-weighted sequences because of the presence of fibrotic tissue, compared with malignancy, which is intermediate to high signal intensity on T2-weighted sequences; however, this finding is also not entirely specific.[121]

The National Lung Screening Trial (NLST) showed the benefit of low-dose CT scans in decreasing the mortality from lung cancer in high-risk individuals.[122] In its recommendations, the United States Preventive Service Task Force (USPSTF) notes that occupational exposures should be taken into account during the risk assessment for lung cancer; however, occupational exposures are not included in the recommendations for lung cancer screening using low-dose CT.[123] The American Association for Thoracic Surgery (AATS) and National Comprehensive Cancer Network (NCCN) do include recommendations for potential screening of individuals with occupational exposures. One of the groups in the AATS screening recommendations for low-dose CT is "younger patients (aged 50 years) with a 20-pack-year smoking history [...] if they have an additional risk factor that produces a 5% risk of developing a lung cancer over the next 5 years."[124] NCCN recommends low-dose CT screening in individuals meeting criteria similar to those proposed by the USPSTF, in addition to those with a 20-pack-year smoking history and 1 additional risk factor, which includes occupational exposure, specifically mentioning asbestos, silica, coal smoke, and beryllium.[125] A meta-analysis of low-dose chest CT screening for lung cancer in individuals with asbestos exposure showed that the rate of detection of lung cancer was at least equal to that of heavy smokers in the NLST (approximately 1%) and had a similar proportion of stage I diagnoses.[126] A low-dose CT screening program implemented in US nuclear weapons workers also had a similar screening yield and lung cancer stage distribution to the NLST,[127] which argues for the utility of including patients with high-risk occupational exposures in screening recommendations.

SUMMARY

Imaging plays a critical role in the diagnosis and monitoring of OLDs. Although chest radiographs are the standard for screening and surveillance and likely will be for the foreseeable future, HRCT has shown increased sensitivity and specificity for the diagnosis and monitoring of OLDs. Despite the well-described HRCT patterns for multiple OLDs, substantial overlap with other entities and atypical presentations exist. Physicians interpreting imaging should always consider the possibility of an OLD when formulating a differential. As new entities continue to emerge with evolving industrial practices, imaging will remain a key component of the diagnostic evaluation and monitoring for complications.

REFERENCES

1. Driscoll T, Nelson DI, Steenland K, et al. The global burden of non malignant respiratory disease due to occupational airborne exposures. Am J Ind Med 2005;48(6):432–45.
2. Cox C, Rose C, Lynch D. State of the art: imaging of occupational lung disease. Radiology 2014; 270(3):681–96.
3. Remy-Jardin M, Degreef JM, Beuscart R, et al. Coal worker's pneumoconiosis: CT assessment in exposed workers and correlation with radiographic findings. Radiology 1990;177(2):363–71.
4. Gevenois PA, Pichot E, Dargent F, et al. Low grade coal worker's pneumoconiosis. Comparison of CT and chest radiography. Acta Radiol 1994;35(4): 351–6. Available at: http://www.ncbi.nlm.nih.gov/pubmed/8011384.
5. Huuskonen O, Kivisaari L, Zitting A, et al. High-resolution computed tomography classification of lung fibrosis for patients with asbestos-related disease. Scand J Work Environ Health 2001;27(2):106–12.
6. Al Jarad N, Poulakis N, Pearson MC, et al. Assessment of asbestos-induced pleural disease by computed tomography — correlation with chest radiograph and lung function. Respir Med 1991; 85(3):203–8.
7. Aberle DR, Gamsu G, Ray CS. High-resolution CT of benign asbestos-related diseases: clinical and radiographic correlation. Am J Roentgenol 1988; 151(5):883–91.
8. Weiss W. Cigarette smoke, asbestos, and small irregular opacities. Am Rev Respir Dis 1984; 130(2):293–301.
9. American College of Radiology. ACR appropriateness criteria occupational lung diseases. 2019. Available at: https://acsearch.acr.org/docs/3091680/Narrative/. Accessed December 10, 2019.

10. Guidelines for the use of the ILO international classification of radiographs of pneumoconioses. 2011th edition. Geneva (Switzerland): International Labour Office; 2011. Available at: https://www.ilo.org/wcmsp5/groups/public/—ed_protect/—protrav/—safework/documents/publication/wcms_168260.pdf.
11. Halldin CN, Petsonk EL, Laney AS. Validation of the international labour Office digitized standard images for recognition and classification of radiographs of pneumoconiosis. Acad Radiol 2014;21(3):305–11.
12. Wagner GR, Attfield MD, Kennedy RD, et al. The NIOSH B reader certification program. An update report. J Occup Med 1992;34(9):879–84. Available at: http://www.ncbi.nlm.nih.gov/pubmed/1447592.
13. Bégin R, Ostiguy G, Fillion R, et al. Computed tomography scan in the early detection of silicosis. Am Rev Respir Dis 1991;144(3_pt_1):697–705.
14. Lopes AJ, Mogami R, Capone D, et al. High-resolution computed tomography in silicosis: correlation with chest radiography and pulmonary function tests* Tomografia Computadorizada de Alta Resolução Na Silicose: Correlação Com Radiografia e Testes de Função Pulmonar. vol. 34.; 2008.
15. Al Jarad N, Wilkinson P, Pearson MC, et al. A new high resolution computed tomography scoring system for pulmonary fibrosis, pleural disease, and emphysema in patients with asbestos related disease. Br J Ind Med 1992;49(2):73–84.
16. Kusaka Y, Hering KG, Parker JE, editors. International classification of HRCT for occupational and environmental respiratory diseases. Tokyo: Springer-Verlag; 2005. https://doi.org/10.1007/4-431-27512-6.
17. Tamura T, Suganuma N, Hering KG, et al. Relationships (I) of international classification of high-resolution computed tomography for occupational and environmental respiratory diseases with the ilo international classification of radiographs of pneumoconioses for parenchymal abnormalities. Ind Health 2015;53(3):260–70.
18. Suganuma N, Kusaka Y, Hering KG, et al. Selection of reference films based on reliability assessment of a classification of high-resolution computed tomography for pneumoconioses. Int Arch Occup Environ Health 2006;79(6):472–6.
19. Şener MU, Şimsek C, Özkara Ş, et al. Comparison of the international classification of high-resolution computed tomography for occupational and environmental respiratory diseases with the International Labor Organization international classification of radiographs of pneumoconiosis. Ind Health 2019;57(4):495–502.
20. Lynch DA, Sverzellati N, Travis WD, et al. Diagnostic criteria for idiopathic pulmonary fibrosis: a Fleischner Society white paper. Lancet Respir Med 2018;6(2):138–53.
21. Raghu G, Remy-Jardin M, Myers JL, et al. Diagnosis of idiopathic pulmonary fibrosis an Official ATS/ERS/JRS/ALAT Clinical practice guideline. Am J Respir Crit Care Med 2018;198(5):e44–68.
22. Kim K-I, Kim CW, Lee MK, et al. Imaging of occupational lung disease. Radiographics 2001;21(6):1371–91.
23. Peacock C, Copley SJ, Hansell DM. Asbestos-related benign pleural disease. Clin Radiol 2000;55(6):422–32.
24. Fletcher DE, Edge JR. The early radiological changes in pulmonary and pleural asbestosis. Clin Radiol 1970;21(4):355–65.
25. Miller BH, Rosado-de-Christenson ML, Mason AC, et al. From the archives of the AFIP. Malignant pleural mesothelioma: radiologic-pathologic correlation. Radiographics 1996;16(3):613–44.
26. Kim EA, Kyung, Lee S, et al. Radiographic and CT findings in complications following pulmonary resection. Radiographics 2002;22:67–86.
27. Hillerdal G, Ozesmi M. Benign asbestos pleural effusion: 73 exudates in 60 patients. Eur J Respir Dis 1987;71(2):113–21. Available at: http://www.ncbi.nlm.nih.gov/pubmed/3622660.
28. Rabinowitz JG, Efremidis SC, Cohen B, et al. A comparative study of mesothelioma and asbestosis using computed tomography and conventional chest radiography. Radiology 1982;144(3):453–60.
29. Jones RN, McLoud T, Rockoff SD. The radiographic pleural abnormalities in asbestos exposure. J Thorac Imaging 1988;3(4):57–66.
30. Champlin J, Edwards R, Pipavath S. Imaging of occupational lung disease. Radiol Clin North Am 2016;54(6):1077–96.
31. Roach HD, Davies GJ, Attanoos R, et al. Asbestos: when the dust settles - an imaging review of asbestos-related disease. Radiographics 2002;22(SPEC. ISS):167–84.
32. Bourbeau J, Ernst P, Chrome J, et al. The relationship between respiratory impairment and asbestos-related pleural abnormality in an active work force. Am Rev Respir Dis 1990;142(4):837–42.
33. McLoud TC, Woods BO, Carrington CB, et al. Diffuse pleural thickening in an asbestos-exposed population: prevalence and causes. Am J Roentgenol 1985;144(1):9–18.
34. Lynch DA, Gamsu G, Aberle DR. Conventional and high resolution computed tomography in the diagnosis of asbestos-related diseases. Radiographics 1989;9(3):523–51.
35. Leung AN, Muller NL, Miller RR. CT in differential diagnosis of diffuse pleural disease. Am J Roentgenol 1990;154(3):487–92.

36. Akira M, Yokoyama K, Yamamoto S, et al. Early asbestosis: evaluation with high-resolution CT. Radiology 1991;178(2):409–16.
37. Gamsu G, Aberle DR, Lynch D. Computed tomography in the diagnosis of asbestos-related thoracic disease. J Thorac Imaging 1989;4(1):61–7.
38. Hobbs S. Asbestos-related disease. In: Walker C, Chung J, Hobbs S, et al, editors. Müller's imaging of the chest. 2nd ed. Philadelphia: Elsevier Health Sciences; 2019. p. 775–92. Expert Radiology.
39. Yoshimura H, Hatakeyama M, Otsuji H, et al. Pulmonary asbestosis: CT study of subpleural curvilinear shadow. Work in progress. Radiology 1986; 158(3):653–8.
40. Batra P, Brown K, Hayashi K, et al. Rounded atelectasis. J Thorac Imaging 1996;11(3). Available at: https://journals.lww.com/thoracicimaging/Fulltext/1996/22000/Rounded_Atelectasis.3.aspx.
41. McAdams HP, Erasums JJ, Patz EF, et al. Evaluation of patients with round atelectasis using 2-[18F]-fluoro-2-deoxy-D-glucose PET. J Comput Assist Tomogr 1998;22(4):601–4.
42. Vallyathan VGF. Pathologic responses to inhaled silica. In: V C, V, WE W, editors. Silica and silica-induced lung diseases. Boca Raton (FL): CRC Press; 1995. p. 39–59. Available at: https://www.cdc.gov/niosh/nioshtic-2/20037000.html.
43. Hobbs S. Silicosis and coal workers' pneumoconiosis. In: Walker C, Chung J, Hobbs S, et al, editors. Müller's imaging of the chest. 2nd ed. Philadelphia: Elsevier Health Sciences; 2019. p. 793–808.
44. Swaen GMH, Passier PECA, van Attekum AMNG. Prevalence of silicosis in the Dutch fine-ceramic industry. Int Arch Occup Environ Health 1988;60(1): 71–4.
45. Marchiori E, Ferreira A, Müller NL. Silicoproteinosis: high-resolution CT and histologic findings. J Thorac Imaging 2001;16(2):127–9.
46. Dee P, Suratt P, Winn W. The radiographic findings in acute silicosis. Radiology 1978;126(2): 359–63.
47. Rossi SE, Erasmus JJ, Volpacchio M, et al. "Crazy-paving" pattern at thin-section CT of the lungs: radiologic- pathologic overview. Radiographics 2003;1509–19.
48. Dos Santos Antao VC, Pinheiro GA, Terra-Filho M, et al. High-resolution CT in silicosis: correlation with radiographic findings and functional impairment. J Comput Assist Tomogr 2005;29(3): 350–6.
49. Stark P, Jacobson F, Shaffer K. Standard imaging in silicosis and coal worker's pneumoconiosis. Radiol Clin North Am 1992;30(6):1147–54. Available at: http://www.ncbi.nlm.nih.gov/pubmed/1410305.
50. Chong S, Lee KS, Chung MJ, et al. Pneumoconiosis: comparison of imaging and pathologic findings. Radiographics 2006;26(1):59–77.
51. Akira M, Higashihara T, Yokoyama K, et al. Radiographic type p pneumoconiosis: high-resolution CT. Radiology 1989;171(1):117–23.
52. Ozmen CA, Nazaroglu H, Yildiz T, et al. MDCT findings of Denim-Sandblasting-induced silicosis: a cross-sectional study. Environ Health 2010. https://doi.org/10.1186/1476-069X-9-17.
53. Remy-Jardin M, Beuscart R, Sault MC, et al. Subpleural micronodules in diffuse infiltrative lung diseases: evaluation with thin-section CT scans. Radiology 1990;177(1):133–9.
54. Hansell DM, Bankier AA, MacMahon H, et al. Fleischner Society: glossary of terms for thoracic imaging. Radiology 2008;246(3):697–722.
55. Alfudhili KM, Lynch DA, Laurent F, et al. Focal pleural thickening mimicking pleural plaques on chest computed tomography: tips and tricks. Br J Radiol 2016;89(1057):20150792.
56. Di Nicola E, De Filippis F, Mereu M, et al. Can HRCT distinguish between sarcoidosis and pneumoconiosis presenting with hilar/perihilar masses? In: European Congress of Radiology. March 01 - 05, 2012; Vienna, Austria. https://doi.org/10.1594/ecr2012/C-2466.
57. Chung SY, Lee JH, Kim TH, et al. 18F-FDG PET imaging of progressive massive fibrosis. Ann Nucl Med 2010;24(1):21–7.
58. Young RC, Rachal RE, Carr PG, et al. Patterns of coal workers' pneumoconiosis in Appalachian former coal miners. J Natl Med Assoc 1992;84(1): 41–8. Available at: http://www.ncbi.nlm.nih.gov/pubmed/1602501.
59. Hayton C, Hoyle J. P221 Silicosis and mycobacterium disease: is it a problem in the UK?. In: Danger at work: occupational lung disease and asthma. BMJ Publishing Group Ltd and British Thoracic Society; 2017. p. A203.2–205. https://doi.org/10.1136/thoraxjnl-2017-210983.363.
60. Shafiei M, Ghasemian A, Eslami M, et al. Risk factors and control strategies for silicotuberculosis as an occupational disease. New Microbes New Infect 2019;27:75–7.
61. Chenik F. Diagnostic features of silicosis and silicotuberculosis. Dis Chest 1938;4(1):18–20.
62. Matar LD, McAdams HP, Sporn TA. Hypersensitivity pneumonitis. Am J Roentgenol 2000;174(4): 1061–6.
63. Coleman A, Colby TV. Histologic diagnosis of extrinsic allergic alveolitis. Am J Surg Pathol 1988;12(7):514–8.
64. Glazer CS, Rose CS, Lynch DA. Clinical and radiologic manifestations of hypersensitivity pneumonitis. J Thorac Imaging 2002;17(4):261–72.
65. Hanak V, Golbin JM, Ryu JH. Causes and presenting features in 85 consecutive patients with hypersensitivity pneumonitis. Mayo Clin Proc 2007;82(7): 812–6.

66. Lacasse Y, Selman M, Costabel U, et al. Clinical diagnosis of hypersensitivity pneumonitis. Am J Respir Crit Care Med 2003;168(8):952–8.
67. Silver SF, Muller NL, Miller RR, et al. Hypersensitivity pneumonitis: evaluation with CT. Radiology 1989;173(2):441–5.
68. Silva CIS, Churg A, Müller NL. Hypersensitivity pneumonitis: spectrum of high-resolution CT and pathologic findings. Am J Roentgenol 2007;188(2):334–44.
69. Remy-Jardin M, Remy J, Wallaert B, et al. Subacute and chronic bird breeder hypersensitivity pneumonitis: sequential evaluation with CT and correlation with lung function tests and bronchoalveolar lavage. Radiology 1993;189(1):111–8.
70. Torres PPTe S, Moreira MAR, Silva DGST, et al. High-resolution computed tomography and histopathological findings in hypersensitivity pneumonitis: a pictorial essay. Radiol Bras 2016;49(2):112–6.
71. Adler BD, Padley SP, Müller NL, et al. Chronic hypersensitivity pneumonitis: high-resolution CT and radiographic features in 16 patients. Radiology 1992;185(1):91–5.
72. Silva CIS, Müller NL, Lynch DA, et al. Chronic hypersensitivity pneumonitis: differentiation from idiopathic pulmonary fibrosis and nonspecific interstitial pneumonia by using thin-section CT. Radiology 2008;246(1):288–97.
73. Yoshizawa Y, Ohtani Y, Hayakawa H, et al. Chronic hypersensitivity pneumonitis in Japan: a nationwide epidemiologic survey. J Allergy Clin Immunol 1999;103(2):315–20.
74. Rkinjuntti-Pekkanen R, Rytkonen H, Kokkarinen J, et al. Long-term risk of emphysema in patients with farmer's lung and matched control farmers. Am J Respir Crit Care Med 1998;158(2):662–5.
75. Aronchick JM, Rossman MD, Miller WT. Chronic beryllium disease: diagnosis, radiographic findings, and correlation with pulmonary function tests. Radiology 1987;163(3):677–82.
76. Hobbs S. Uncommon pneumoconioses. In: Walker C, Chung J, Hobbs S, et al, eds. Müller's imaging of the chest. 2nd edition Philadelphia: Elsevier; 2019: 809–21.
77. Newman LS, Buschman DL, Newell JD, et al. Beryllium disease: assessment with CT. Radiology 1994; 190(3):835–40.
78. Sharma N, Patel J, Mohammed T-LH. Chronic beryllium disease. J Comput Assist Tomogr 2010; 34(6):945–8.
79. Muller-Quernheim J, Gaede K, Fireman E, et al. Diagnoses of chronic beryllium disease within cohorts of sarcoidosis patients. Eur Respir J 2006; 27(6):1190–5.
80. Cugell DW. The hard metal diseases. Clin Chest Med 1992;13(2):269–79. Available at: http://www.ncbi.nlm.nih.gov/pubmed/1511554. Accessed December 12, 2019.
81. Gotway MB, Golden JA, Warnock M, et al. Hard metal interstitial lung disease: high-resolution computed tomography appearance. J Thorac Imaging 2002;17(4):314–8.
82. Dunlop P, Müller NL, Wilson J, et al. Hard metal lung disease. J Thorac Imaging 2005;20(4): 301–4.
83. Ohori NP, Sciurba FC, Owens GR, et al. Giant-cell interstitial pneumonia and hard-metal pneumoconiosis. Am J Surg Pathol 1989;13(7):581–7.
84. Akira M. Uncommon pneumoconioses: CT and pathologic findings. Radiology 1995;197(2):403–9.
85. Kraus T, Schaller KH, Angerer J, et al. Aluminosis - detection of an almost forgotten disease with HRCT. J Occup Med Toxicol 2006;1(1):1–9.
86. Guidotti TL. Pulmonary aluminosis—a review. Toxicol Pathol 1975;3(16):16–8.
87. Vahlensieck M, Overlack A, Müller K-M. Computed tomographic high-attenuation mediastinal lymph nodes after aluminum exposition. Eur Radiol 2000;10(12):1945–6.
88. Flors L, Domingo ML, Leiva-Salinas C, et al. Uncommon occupational lung diseases: high-resolution CT findings. Am J Roentgenol 2010; 194(1):W20–6.
89. Han D, Goo JM, Im J, et al. Thin-section CT findings of arc-welders' pneumoconiosis. Korean J Radiol 2000;1(2):79.
90. Billings CG, Howard P. Occupational siderosis and welders' lung: a review. Monaldi Arch Chest Dis 1993;48(4):304–14. Available at: http://www.ncbi.nlm.nih.gov/pubmed/8257971.
91. Feigin D. Talc: understanding its manifestations in the chest. Am J Roentgenol 1986;146(2):295–301.
92. Marchiori E, Lourenço S, Gasparetto TD, et al. Pulmonary talcosis: imaging findings. Lung 2010; 188(2):165–71.
93. Verlynde G, Agneessens E, Dargent J-L. Pulmonary talcosis due to daily inhalation of talc powder. J Belg Soc Radiol 2018;102(1). https://doi.org/10.5334/jbsr.1384.
94. Padley SPG, Adler BD, Staples CA, et al. Pulmonary talcosis: CT findings in three cases. Radiology 1993;186(1):125–7.
95. Paré JP, Cote G, Fraser RS. Long-term follow-up of drug abusers with intravenous talcosis. Am Rev Respir Dis 1989;139(1):233–41.
96. Cox CW, Lynch DA. Medical imaging in occupational and environmental lung disease. Curr Opin Pulm Med 2015;21(2):163–70.
97. Leso V, Fontana L, Romano R, et al. Artificial stone associated silicosis: a systematic review. Int J Environ Res Public Health 2019;16(4):1–17.
98. Rose C, Heinzerling A, Patel K, et al. Severe silicosis in engineered stone fabrication workers — California, Colorado, Texas, and Washington, 2017–2019. MMWR Morb Mortal Wkly Rep 2019;

68(38):813–8. Available at: https://www.cdc.gov/mmwr/cme/conted_info.html#weekly.

99. Ronsmans S, Decoster L, Keirsbilck S, et al. Artificial stone-associated silicosis in Belgium. Occup Environ Med 2019;76(2):133–4.
100. Banauch GI, Dhala A, Prezant DJ. Pulmonary disease in rescue workers at the World Trade Center site. Curr Opin Pulm Med 2005;11(2):160–8.
101. Girvin F, Zeig-Owens R, Gupta D, et al. Radiologic features of world trade center-related sarcoidosis in exposed NYC fire department rescue workers. J Thorac Imaging 2016;31(5):296–303.
102. de la Hoz RE, Liu X, Doucette JT, et al. Increased airway wall thickness is associated with adverse longitudinal first–second forced expiratory volume trajectories of former world trade center workers. Lung 2018;196(4):481–9.
103. Cummings KJ, Donat WE, Ettensohn DB, et al. Pulmonary alveolar proteinosis in workers at an indium processing facility. Am J Respir Crit Care Med 2010;181(5):458–64.
104. Cummings KJ, Nakano M, Omae K, et al. Indium lung disease. Chest 2012;141(6):1512–21.
105. Kreiss K, Gomaa A, Kullman G, et al. Clinical bronchiolitis obliterans in workers at a microwave-popcorn plant. N Engl J Med 2002;347(5):330–8.
106. Van Rooy FGBGJ, Rooyackers JM, Prokop M, et al. Bronchiolitis obliterans syndrome in chemical workers producing diacetyl for food flavorings. Am J Respir Crit Care Med 2007;176(5):498–504.
107. Ahuja J, Kanne JP, Meyer CA. Occupational lung disease. Semin Roentgenol 2015;50(1):40–51.
108. Sauler M, Gulati M. Newly recognized occupational and environmental causes of chronic terminal airways and parenchymal lung disease. Clin Chest Med 2012;33(4):667–80.
109. Romero S, Hernández L, Gil J, et al. Organizing pneumonia in textile printing workers: a clinical description. Eur Respir J 1998;11(2):265–71.
110. Archontogeorgis K, Steiropoulos P, Tzouvelekis A, et al. Lung cancer and interstitial lung diseases: a systematic review. Pulm Med 2012;2012:1–11.
111. Weiss W. Asbestosis: a marker for the increased risk of lung cancer among workers exposed to asbestos. Chest 1999;115(2):536–49.
112. Smith AH, Lopipero PA, Barroga VR. Meta-analysis of studies of lung cancer among silicotics. Epidemiology 1995;6(6):617–24.
113. Uguen M, Dewitte J-D, Marcorelles P, et al. Asbestos-related lung cancers: a retrospective clinical and pathological study. Mol Clin Oncol 2017;7(1):135–9.
114. Samet JM, Epler GR, Gaensler EA, et al. Absence of synergism between exposure to asbestos and cigarette smoking in asbestosis. Am Rev Respir Dis 1979;120(1):75–82.
115. Ngamwong Y, Tangamornsuksan W, Lohitnavy O, et al. Additive synergism between asbestos and smoking in lung cancer risk: a systematic review and meta-analysis. Langevin SM. PLoS One 2015;10(8):e0135798.
116. Yates DH, Corrin B, Stidolph PN, et al. Malignant mesothelioma in south east England: clinicopathological experience of 272 cases. Thorax 1997;52(6):507–12.
117. Yildirim H, Metintas M, Entok E, et al. Clinical value of fluorodeoxyglucose-positron emission tomography/computed tomography in differentiation of malignant mesothelioma from asbestos-related benign pleural disease: an observational pilot study. J Thorac Oncol 2009;4(12):1480–4.
118. Heelan RT, Rusch VW, Begg CB, et al. Staging of malignant pleural mesothelioma: comparison of CT and MR imaging. Am J Roentgenol 1999;172(4):1039–47.
119. Reichert M, Bensadoun ES. PET imaging in patients with coal workers pneumoconiosis and suspected malignancy. J Thorac Oncol 2009;4(5):649–51.
120. Choi EK, Park HL, Yoo IR, et al. The clinical value of F-18 FDG PET/CT in differentiating malignant from benign lesions in pneumoconiosis patients. Eur Radiol 2019. https://doi.org/10.1007/s00330-019-06342-1.
121. Ogihara Y, Ashizawa K, Hayashi H, et al. Progressive massive fibrosis in patients with pneumoconiosis: utility of MRI in differentiating from lung cancer. Acta Radiol 2018;59(1):72–80.
122. The National Lung Screening Trial Research Team. Reduced lung-cancer mortality with low-dose computed tomographic screening. N Engl J Med 2011;365(5):395–409.
123. Moyer VA. Screening for lung cancer: U.S. Preventive services Task force recommendation statement. Ann Intern Med 2014;160(5):330–8.
124. Jaklitsch MT, Jacobson FL, Austin JHM, et al. The American Association for Thoracic Surgery guidelines for lung cancer screening using low-dose computed tomography scans for lung cancer survivors and other high-risk groups. J Thorac Cardiovasc Surg 2012;144(1):33–8.
125. Wood DE, Kazerooni EA, Baum SL, et al. Lung cancer screening, version 3.2018, NCCN Clinical Practice Guidelines in Oncology. J Natl Compr Canc Netw 2018;16(4):412–41.
126. Ollier M, Chamoux A, Naughton G, et al. Chest CT scan screening for lung cancer in asbestos occupational exposure: a systematic review and meta-analysis. Chest 2014;145(6):1339–46.
127. Markowitz SB, Manowitz A, Miller JA, et al. Yield of low-dose computerized tomography screening for lung cancer in high-risk workers: the case of 7189 US Nuclear Weapons Workers. Am J Public Health 2018;108(10):1296–302.

Informatics Approaches for Recognition, Management, and Prevention of Occupational Respiratory Disease

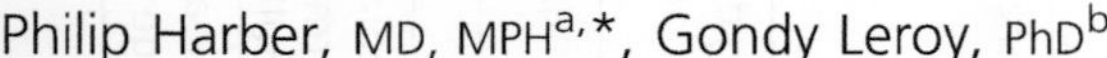

Philip Harber, MD, MPH[a,*], Gondy Leroy, PhD[b]

KEYWORDS

- Occupational lung disease • Asthma • Informatics • Computer systems
- Occupational health surveillance • Natural language processing • Machine learning • Ontology

KEY POINTS

- Computer and information systems improve the efficiency and scope of data sharing among workers, patients, exposure assessors, public health systems, and researchers.
- Information resources are available for primary care providers, specialists, workers, and patients; many have a limited workplace focus.
- Improved methods to classify relevant occupation, industry, exposure, and health data are urgently needed.
- Potentially transformative approaches include machine learning, natural language processing, and ontology development.
- Occupational respiratory disease professionals should use computer and information systems to incrementally improve traditional approaches and modify fundamental paradigms.

INTRODUCTION

Occupational–respiratory medicine has many computer and information science needs posed by the uniquely wide range of information, but applications are currently less well-developed than in other areas of respiratory medicine. Nevertheless, some applications are currently available and contribute significantly. This article provides an overview organized by class of user, including several examples (**Table 1**), followed by an introduction to emerging transformative tools.

PATIENTS AND WORKERS

Many patient-oriented allergy and respiratory disorder applications are available, ranging from smartphones to specialized devices and personal computers. However, the majority emphasize asthma with little description of other obstructive disease or pneumoconioses.

Education is provided via websites and in apps. **Table 2** lists examples for patients and other users. Some include information about work-related asthma or commingle workplace and community-based exposures such as air pollution.

[a] Mel and Enid Zuckerman College of Public Health, University of Arizona, Medical Research Building, Room 112, 1656 East Mabel Steet, Tucson, AZ 85724, USA; [b] Eller College of Management, University of Arizona, McClelland Hall, 1130 East Helen Street, Tucosn, AZ 85721, USA
* Corresponding author.
E-mail address: pharber@arizona.edu

Clin Chest Med 41 (2020) 605–621
https://doi.org/10.1016/j.ccm.2020.08.008

chestmed.theclinics.com

Table 1
Classes of computer information system by main beneficiaries

User	Purpose	Typical Limitations	Examples
Patient/worker	Provide general information related to the specific job or illness.	Oriented to patients, not workers.	Websites of governmental agencies, professional organizations
Primary care provider	Overcome potential limits of specific knowledge	Requires a priori motivation; many are difficult to use	National of Library of Medicine toxicology resources, Wikipedia, NIOSH, Occupational Safety and Health Administration, industry organizations
Specialist clinician	Meet narrow specific needs.	Standalone, not well-integrated; incompatible with many computer systems; require specialized knowledge	BViewer (radiology); SPIROLA (spirometry); workers compensation treatment guidelines
Clinical service systems managers	Facilitate workflow; systematize documentation and information sharing; guide and improve health services	Current EHRs for occupational respiratory disease are limited. Few effective and validated clinical decision support systems	Electronic health records; clinical decision support systems
Public health professionals	Support surveillance systems	Most current computer systems simply make traditional surveillance methods more efficient rather than introduce new categories of analysis (eg, they use only limited data fields)	Autocoders; electronic reporting
Clinicians and others assessing exposure	Provide exposure data for individuals and groups	Broader inputs have been more widely implemented in air pollution than occupational studies	Streaming data; citizen science; satellite images; online maps
Researchers	Create new knowledge	Many occupational health studies still focus on a small number of agents.	Autocoding; data models
Additional applications			
Information sharing	Support multidirectional information sharing	Limited implementation	Social media (eg, Twitter); text transformation—simplification and audio bulleting
Evolving tools	Potentially transformative	Require more development and validation	Machine learning algorithms; natural language processing; ontologies

Table 2
Examples of educational resources

American Academy of Allergy Asthma and Immunology	https://www.aaaai.org/conditions-and-treatments/library/asthma-library/occupational-asthma
American Lung Association	https://www.lung.org/lung-health-and-diseases/lung-disease-lookup/asthma/living-with-asthma/creating-asthma-friendly-environments/guide-to-controlling-asthma-at-work.html
American Thoracic Society	https://www.thoracic.org/patients/patient-resources/breathing-in-america/resources/chapter-13-occupational-lung-diseases.pdf https://www.thoracic.org/patients/patient-resources/resources/occupational-lung-disease.pdf
American College of Allergy and Immunology	https://acaai.org/search/site/Occupational
National Institute for Occupational Safety and Health (many resources)	Diseases: https://www.cdc.gov/niosh/respiratory/default.html Respirators: https://www.cdc.gov/niosh/topics/respirators/default.html
Canadian resources	https://www.ccohs.ca/oshanswers/diseases/asthma.html https://lungontario.ca/a-to-z/work-related-asthma-symptoms
National Heart, Lung, and Blood Institute (NHLBI) "Employers, employees, and worksites"	https://www.nhlbi.nih.gov/health-pro/resources/lung/naci/audiences/work.htm
National Library of Medicine	https://pubchem.ncbi.nlm.nih.gov/
United Kingdom Asthma UK	https://www.asthma.org.uk/advice/understanding-asthma/types/occupational-asthma/ Occupational asthma.org http://www.occupationalasthma.com/

These websites help to motivate workers to consider workplace factors affecting their health status, which in turn may empower patients to encourage their treating clinicians to pay attention to these matters.

Some apps support interaction with health care providers, monitoring, and management of asthma.[1] For example, spirometry using a flow sensor attached to a personal phone has been demonstrated to be technically accurate.[2] Such a system may prove useful for work related-asthma to overcome limitations of peak flow recording.

There are, however, significant limitations with many of these resources: (a) Most professional organizations aim at "patients" rather than "workers" and therefore will be viewed only by persons who have a diagnosed pulmonary condition. (b) Professional organizations encourage contacting the personal health care provider. Yet, some providers have inadequate time, knowledge, or incentive to provide the necessary follow-up.[3] (c) Much information is available only in English, whereas many of the most vulnerable workers speak other languages. (d) Some freestanding focused sites are difficult for workers and patients to find. (e) Many patient-oriented sites do not address occupational lung disease per se. Ramsey and associates[4] reviewed asthma related websites and found they emphasized pharmaceuticals, and none were noted to deal with workplace exposures. Kagen and Garland's review[1] of apps, including physician–patient communication and monitoring methods, reported none related to workplace factors; clinicians felt that air pollution was important, but they did not mention workplace. Harber and Leroy[5] found that Twitter posts pointing to asthma or chronic obstructive pulmonary disease (COPD) sites rarely include workplace references. (f) Nearly all the sources are set up to broadcast from "experts" to laypersons, without meaningful opportunity for workers to share their insights. (g) As with other patient-focused websites, the principle of *caveat emptor* (aka, "buyer beware") applies here. There is no standardized rating of the quality of information provided. Thus, although useful for selected patients, many of the educational sites do not meet the needs of workers.

PRIMARY CARE AND PULMONARY CLINICIANS

Similar to resources for patients, resources for primary care clinicians emphasize diagnostic criteria and medication treatment, with limited information relevant to workplace aspects. Some worker-patients will find these resources useful despite the technical terminology. Some allow entry of information, although many are primarily for information dissemination. Few have easy search operations so that a busy clinician can identify specific information relevant to exposures of an individual worker-patient. Quickly consulting widely available web resources such as Wikipedia or a Google/Bing query can help health care providers to understand the nature and terminology for specific jobs and industries. In addition, several resources have been created specifically for occupational health purposes:

The US National Library of Medicine (NLM) has offered helpful online resources to identify chemicals or other agents affecting respiratory health.[6] Although NLM recently eliminated the centralized toxicology resource, many other resources are available and their locations are listed at https://www.nlm.nih.gov/toxnet/index.html. Several NLM examples are provided here.

Haz-Map is particularly convenient because it automatically links information from distinct domains. It allows accessing information from different starting points, for example, job, agent, task, work process, industry, nonoccupational activity disease, sign or symptoms. For example, specifying "painting-pigments" and "asthma" points to 70 agents for which more detailed information is provided.

Haz-Map also illustrates limitations. (a) It does not include many chemicals, agents, and processes. (b) It uses a "controlled vocabulary" in which terms used by workers are not included. (c) There is no systematic process for assessing the validity of linkages. Most decisions are from the dedicated occupational physician developer. For example, "dyspnea-exertional" links to pleural plaques. (d) It is difficult to update because it relies on manual ad hoc methods.[7] (e) Relationships are binary (yes/no) without consideration of dose or strength of association. (f) Temporal relations are not represented; for example, irritant-induced asthma may develop soon after a single exposure, whereas chronic beryllium disease always has significant latency. (g) It only suggests possibilities rather than leading to a definitive diagnosis. Clinicians must be cautious about not establish a diagnosis solely from this resource. (h) The NLM has "retired" Haz-Map, but it is still available elsewhere (https://haz-map.com/).

The NLM Hazardous Substances Data Bank is more comprehensive, containing information on 5929 chemical agents with more than 150 fields of information. The Hazardous Substances Data Bank has been incorporated within PubChem (https://pubchem.ncbi.nlm.nih.gov/). Comprehensiveness and search capacity are major strengths. Search is facilitated by allowing either text or a chemical formula. Unlike Haz-Map, the Hazardous Substances Data Bank used a formal process for curation, with careful systematic review of entries. However, finding relevant information is a needle in a haystack problem, making this difficult for clinicians who are time constrained or unfamiliar with technical toxicology characterizations. For example, "diacetyl," a well-known cause of bronchiolitis obliterans, links to more than 13,000 distinct compounds and 3151 literature references. Even restricting the inquiry to "diacetyl lung" yields 128 references.

SPECIALIST OCCUPATIONAL CLINICIANS

Other clinically oriented systems assist pulmonary, allergy, and occupational medicine physicians whose practices emphasize occupational respiratory disorders. They have a narrow scope and assume relevant expertise. Two products available without charge from the National Institute for Occupational Safety and Health (NIOSH) and worker's compensation treatment guidelines illustrate strengths and weaknesses.

Spirometry Longitudinal Data Analysis was developed to help monitor lung function in the occupational health setting.[8] Applied to individual workers, the software graphs and quantifies the rate of decline in lung function over time and can facilitate the early identification of those with an excessive decline in lung function. Applied to groups of workers, it facilitates identifying individual outliers and subgroups with accelerated decreases in lung function possibly related to exposure. The software also provides feedback concerning the overall quality of a workplace spirometry surveillance program. It operates as a standalone system and is an option in several commercially available spirometers. It works well with many commercially available database systems, However, it may be incompatible with 64 bit personal computers.

The NIOSH's BViewer software assists clinicians interpret digital chest radiographs for pneumoconioses. Chest plain film images may be imported as Digital Imaging and Communications in Medicine files and displayed in a consistent fashion, decreasing the variability of visual display characteristics (eg, contrast) among digital radiographic image viewers. It work wells with the International Labor Organization system for classifying chest radiographs regarding pneumoconioses. It functions as a standalone program and may be incompatible with the image viewing systems commonly used in medical centers (Picture Archiving and Communication System). Because it is standalone and requires prior installation as well as a learning curve for its proper use, its usefulness is limited to physicians with a major practice commitment to recognizing pneumoconioses and/or workplace radiographic surveillance. This may be found at: https://www.cdc.gov/niosh/topics/chestradiography/digital-images.html.

Several practice guidelines for workers compensation are provided in online interactive systems, such as MDGuidelines, which typically require paid subscriptions with private vendors.[9,10] For example, American College of Occupational and Environmental Medicine has published guidelines on the diagnosis and management of work-related asthma and interstitial lung disease,[11,12] with more detailed interactive versions available in online formats.[9,10] Because these guidelines are referenced in several state workers' compensation regulations and are workplace focused, they are most useful for physicians specializing in workers compensation care.

These products share several characteristics. (a) They generally are not useful for primary care clinicians, who may be unfamiliar with the International Labor Organization pneumoconiosis radiography scheme or workplace spirometry surveillance. (b) They are primarily useful for pulmonary and occupational medicine subspecialists whose practices focus on occupational lung diseases. (c) The NIOSH software is incompatible with some widely used clinical information systems, and the workers' compensation guidelines require financial commitment. (d) It appears that they will not be regularly updated for compliance with existing standards such as Logical Observation Identifiers Names and Codes and Health Level 7.[13]

CLINICAL SERVICE SYSTEMS MANAGERS

Information technology systems to support clinical practice are widely used throughout health care and exemplified by electronic health record (EHR) systems. The HITECH Act in the United States required most health care providers to migrate to EHRs.[13] These systems go well beyond simply replacing paper records. Properly used, they provide interoperability, standardization, quality monitoring and improvement, and foster discovering new knowledge.

Clinical decision support (CDS) systems range from advisory statements to mandating a response. Unlike general guidelines, the CDS output is generally patient specific and prescriptive (e.g.," You should do this" rather than "clinician should consider..."). **Fig. 1** shows a general approach: information from several sources is integrated with general knowledge from a "library" to create specific strongly recommended actions following a series of "If... Then" rules. Additional information such as input from the patient or laboratory tests is then added, making additional recommendations. The system automatically monitors whether the recommended actions have been taken and generates a prompt to the provider if they have not occurred. In addition, the data may be (confidentially) integrated into a larger database, useful for public health surveillance or fostering future machine learning pattern recognition approaches to supplant the "if... Then rules". An example is provided by a joint American Thoracic Society (ATS)/NIOSH working group for recognizing work-related asthma (WRA) in primary care settings.[14] New onset asthma or change in medications creates a prompt to ask the patient several simple questions and/or confirm that spirometry had been conducted. Based upon the responses, the system makes additional case-specific recommendations such as referral for consultation or workplace changes.

The ATS/NIOSH example (14) provides alerts to consider work-related asthma. The alerts focus upon narrowly defined issues such as agents relevant to the specific patient to reduce alerts that are irrelevant to the specific patient. This recommended CDS system triggers automatically based on information in standard EHRs. Presenting relevant causes of work-related asthma provides both the patient and clinician specific information upon which they should focus. The system also supports performance monitoring (eg, proportion of patients with asthma diagnosis who have supporting spirometry, percentage of recommended follow-up visits accomplished).

Balancing sensitivity and comprehensiveness with feasibility and acceptability requires compromises. (a) The list of causative exposures is incomplete, targeted to the most frequent ones. (b) Full implementation requires that the EHR integrate

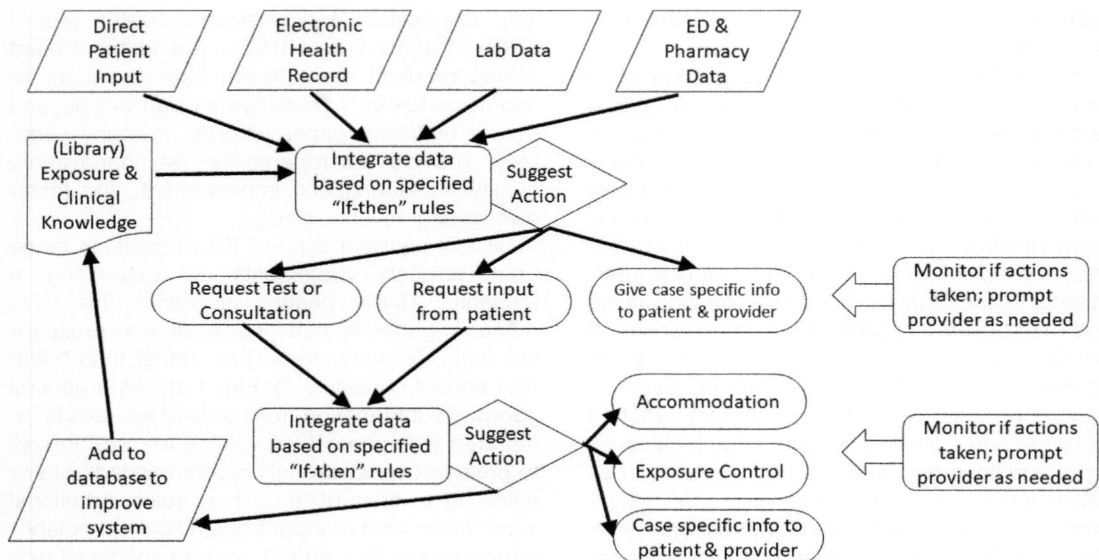

Fig. 1. Clinical Decision Support Paradigm System. The figure illustrates a paradigm for integrating information from multiple sources (e.g., patient input, electronic health record, pulmonary function laboratory) to generate actionable recommendations. As acquired, additional information generates additional specific recommendations. The system monitors whether recommendations have been implemented and provides prompts to the clinician as needed. Data may also be contributed to a database for support a future machine learning or public health surveillance. (*Adapted from* Harber P, Redlich CA, Hines S, et al. Recommendations for a Clinical Decision Support System for Work-Related Asthma in Primary Care Settings. J Occup Environ Med 2017; 59: e231-e235; with permission.)

data from multiple clinics, pharmacy, and laboratory testing. (c) The primary clinician may have inadequate access to occupational lung disease specialists in their region. (d) The system has not been validated in a trial. Indeed, use of the 3 questions to trigger consideration of work-related asthma was unsuccessful in a simple Canadian trial, probably because it required clinicians to exit the main EHR and manually log into an entirely separate system.[15]

PUBLIC HEALTH PRACTICE

Public health practice systematically collects and analyzes health and exposure data.[16] Increasing electronic reporting bypasses delays of paper forms. Computer methods can change the scope and velocity of collection, real-time analysis, and dissemination of information. Reporting could be encouraged if clinicians saw immediate patient benefit for entering data.[16] Surveillance systems no longer need to be constrained by limiting the number and types of data fields such as *International Classification of Diseases* diagnosis, industry code, and job code (see the section on Ontologies).

Traditional methods convert industry, occupation, and disease from text to numerical codes from standard classification schemes (**Table 3**). Replacing manual coders with autocoding systems reduces the time and expertise needed. Autocoders are discussed in the Researcher section.

The Internet further facilitates dissemination of information from public health agencies to the public and health care providers. Social media can reach large numbers of persons efficiently but need evaluation of impact. The NIOSH "Science Blog" with 22,000 persons subscribed was evaluated in a user survey.[17] Nearly all considered it useful. Respondents were predominantly occupational health and safety professionals (24%) or health care professionals (21%). None represented employers or unions. Few came from high-risk industries such as manufacturing, agriculture, forestry, and fishing.

In Web 2.0, information exchange is bidirectional, and monitoring social media can estimate the public's interest in particular topics. Web 2.0 refers to the use of the Internet for bidirectional information exchange, whereby information providers and consumers can interact. Social media is an example of such Web 2.0 technology; monitoring these interactions can estimate the public's interests and concerns. An analysis of Twitter

Table 3
Standard classification systems

System	Purpose	Structure	Location	Owner
Standard Occupational Classification	Occupation with 23 major groups and 867 detailed occupations	Hierarchy	https://www.bls.gov/soc/2018/major_groups.htm	US Bureau of Labor Statistics
North American Industry Classification System	Industry (production processes) with 1057 specific items grouped into 20 sectors	Hierarchy	https://www.census.gov/eos/www/naics/index.html	US Census Bureau
International Classification of Diseases–Clinical Modification	Disease classifications, primarily used for billing purposes	Hierarchy plus special modifiers	https://www.cms.gov/Medicare/Coding/ICD10	US Centers for Medicare and Medicaid services, derived from World Health Organization
CAS Registry	Standardized method of identifying chemicals	Sequentially listed	https://www.cas.org/support/documentation/chemical-substances/faqs	American Chemical Society
Globally Harmonized System of Classification and Labeling of Chemicals	Specific classifications are provided for respiratory sensitization.	Broad categories, non-numerical	http://www.unece.org/fileadmin/DAM/trans/danger/publi/ghs/ghs_rev08/ST-SG-AC10-30-Rev8e.pdf	United Nations
O'Net	Data for 974 jobs, including description of potential exposures and 4 categories of physical requirements[59] Limited detail, but helpful to provide basic information	Multiple cross-links among domains	https://www.onetcenter.org/overview.html	North Carolina Department of Commerce (federally supported)
Health Level Seven	Widely accepted standard for storing and interoperability of health information	Extensively documented relationship structure.	https://www.hl7.org/about/index.cfm?ref=nav	Health Level Seven International

(*continued on next page*)

Table 3
(continued)

System	Purpose	Structure	Location	Owner
Logical Observation Identifiers Names and Codes	Standard codes for laboratory tests and observations	Coding structure includes details, where each digit implies a characteristic	https://loinc.org/	Regenstrief Institute
SNOMED CT	Standardized collection of medical terms with clear definitions	Include cross-linking internally and to external standards Multiple language versions	http://www.snomed.org/	SNOMED International[60]

activity about asthma or COPD found there were few tweets about occupational aspects, whereas community air pollution received considerable attention.[5] This finding underscores the need for enhanced outreach on the importance of workplace exposures in contributing to asthma and COPD.

Monitoring Internet use can provide information about trends in respiratory disease, but it is necessary to understand the source. In Twitter, original personal communications are less common than repetitive transmission (retweets) of the same content or from institutional sources.[18] Trending search engine keywords can potentially identify influenza epidemics earlier than traditional methods used by the Centers for Disease Control and Prevention.[19,20] Wearable devices can provide additional data to monitor respiratory illnesses such as influenza; for example, heart rate data from FitBit users may be more accurate than queries because they reflect actual physiologic responses rather than just reflecting interest among many persons who may not actually be ill.[21] Several location tracking apps have been widely implemented to facilitate contact tracing during the coronavirus disease-19 pandemic; evaluation of their effectiveness is likely to be reported over the next few years.

CLINICIANS AND OTHERS ASSESSING EXPOSURE

Assessing the exposures of individuals and populations is central to recognition and prevention of occupational and environmental lung diseases. Data linkage methods are facilitating greater specificity than using only generic terms such as vapor, gas, dust, and fume.

Readily available interactive maps such as Google Maps are useful for gaining insight into physical aspects affecting exposures. Viewing street or satellite views of manufacturing plants, transportation facilities, mining operations, and other facilities helps clinicians and patients to understand potential exposures. Questions such as the size of the facility, location of the loading dock relative to the patient's work location, and proximity of the patient's work location to the area of a chemical spill can easily be seen. In addition, for many locations, historic images are available on the websites, helping to better understand past work exposures. Images can also show whether air handlers and exhaust systems such as roof cyclones for carpentry shops are present. The Environmental Protection Agency had provided community exposure maps to show geospatial distribution of exposures.[22]

In the past, occupational exposure assessment focused on 1 or a small number of exposure agents. The need to consider the totality of an individual's exposures is increasingly recognized. Multiple exposures may be concurrently determined by interlinking information sources for more complete assessment of the exposome of each individual. The exposome "is composed of every exposure to which an individual is subjected from conception to death."[23] Integrating many sources requires systematic standardized exposure metrics accepted by the multiple providers of data. Although medicine is moving toward defined standards, exposure scientists have not yet meaningfully standardized metrics and terms. An alternative approach is to develop comprehensive ontologies and algorithms to meaningfully combine information from diverse sources without a priori universal agreement. Ontologies are discussed in more detail elsewhere in this article.

The scale of available exposure data ranges from broad geographic areas to worker–task–time specific data. As exposure data informatics linkages evolve, methods to overcome differences in available detail (granularity) are needed. The integration of area industrial hygiene air measurements, available personal sampling, task or activity-based industrial hygiene data, with personnel records, and geospatial modeling will maximize the exposure information available for each person (even if granularity differs).

In addition to generic applications, sensors can provide more detailed and specific information. Simple sensors may be produced economically and communicate with smartphones. Personal sensors for exposure, activity, and location can provide more detailed information to estimate individual exposures. It should no longer be necessary to assume that everyone spends the same amount of time indoors and outdoors. Inhalation dose generally depends on personal ventilatory volumes, which in turn depend on exertion level. Personal exertion sensors (mobile phone-based or dedicated devices such as Fitbit) are ubiquitous and can continuously provide both exertion and geospatial data for the individual. Loh and colleagues[24] summarized many of the opportunities already available.

The information density of images is frequently much greater than that of discrete digital numerical data. Related fields such as self-driving cars will continue to improve technology for viewing still images or video for exposure assessment. Weichenthal and associates[25] summarize opportunities for analyzing complex geospatial pictorial data. This promising approach is not ready for widespread use. In addition to local, on-the-ground tracking, satellite images show promise for exposure assessment.[26] Although currently used primarily for air pollution, significant opportunities also exist in occupational health, particularly as spatial resolution improves. Increasingly simple and economical environmental sensors, ease of logging and transmission data, and the ability to use aerial and satellite imagery will have great impact on exposure assessment in low-income, resource-limited countries. It should no longer be necessary to have well-trained professionals using expensive and difficult to maintain equipment to measure exposure.[27] Currently available methods include sensors for specific chemicals, activity monitors, and barcode readers to identify products in use.[24,28,29]

Such new methods enable "citizen science" to measure and share information systematically. Although widely used in air pollution than occupational health studies, several workplace-oriented applications are presented in a recent article.[30] This work expands the number of sources of exposure data, no longer relying on professional exposure scientists for data collection. Although promising, these approaches require attention to data quality and potential biases. Cellphone images of workplaces spills are already used for exposure reconstruction.

Clinicians may search the gray literature for information for a specific case. The gray literature is defined as the extensive material that is not part of the formal scientific literature such as peer-reviewed journal publications or textbooks. For example, NIOSH publishes exposure assessments in its Health Hazard Evaluation program. Publicly accessible databases of the Occupational Safety and Health Administration and the Mine Safety and Health Administration sites show inspections and incident reports, but they are not user friendly (https://www.osha.gov/enforcement/toppenalties).

The Site Exposure Matrix of the Department of Labor exemplifies detailed workplace exposure information that is occasionally available (www.sem.dol.gov). This web-based resource for workers associated with the Department of Energy nuclear programs provides information on toxic workplace exposures from a variety of sources, including workers, industrial hygienists, and historic documents. Exposure information ranges from broad categories such as the presence of beryllium-containing materials in a specific Department of Energy facility to highly specific descriptions (eg, beryllium materials in the trash in 1961 in the West San Fernando Valley of Los Angeles). Limitations include the paucity of quantitative information.[31]

RESEARCHERS

Knowledge discovery is usually a 2-phase process: First, someone suspects a new hazard–disease causal association or case cluster in a segment of an industry. This is often an ad hoc process (eg, Bis(chloromethyl)ether–associated small cell lung carcinoma and diacetyl lung disease were initially suspected by pulmonary and occupational medicine community clinicians. In the second phase, formal epidemiologic studies quantitatively explore specific hypotheses.[32–34] Ad hoc recognition of a small number of cases of silicosis among workers manufacturing engineered countertops subsequently led to more systematic approaches.[35,36] Currently, it is unlikely that health surveillance of broad aggregate groups such as "All Other Nonmetallic Mineral Product Manufacturing" would have identified this problem. However, future application machine learning (ML) systems may help to automatically identify unusual patterns. Computer and information systems facilitate current research methods by automatically assigning standardized numerical codes to industry and occupation (autocoders), acquiring interview and other data efficiently, and improving exposure assessment as discussed elsewhere in this article. More fundamental changes are discussed elsewhere in this article.

Social media foster inclusion of new sources for collecting new data, gauging public concerns,[37,38] or for evaluating and tagging newly created data. One such platform created an infrastructure for this effort. Amazon Mechanical Turk accesses several hundred thousand geographically dispersed "workers" who can rapidly complete questionnaires and evaluate or label a variety of inputs. For example, participants with asthma who are actively employed completed questionnaires about 4 factors—asthma caused by work, asthma worsened by work, asthma affecting work, and accommodations to improve personal work ability.[39] Recruitment can be accomplished efficiently, and web-based methods may avoid implicit selection biases owing to recruitment from a limited institution or geographic area. However, it is difficult to assess whether the participants are representative of the target population. Although diverse, Amazon Mechanical Turk workers are not fully representative of the American workers.

Several studies have evaluated autoencoders (not to be confused with the new deep learning autoencoder neural networks). The accuracy of the NIOSH NIOCCS is good, but is decreased if the system tries to assign very specific job codes or minimize the number of entries for which a code cannot be assigned.[40,41] One assessment of autocoding to 23 broad groups or 840 more specific groups found good performance only when industry title was manually entered (kappa agreement scores about 65% and 40% for broad and specific titles).[40]

In the UK, a particularly promising technique was implemented as OSCAR (Occupational Self-Coding Automatic Recording) for the UK Biobank study.[42] More than 100,000 study participants used an online decision tree approach to enter their lifetime occupational history. Starting with broader categories, OSCAR then presented more narrow choices, each of which was linked to a standard UK occupational code. Agreement with manual coding in a subsample had kappa of 0.62 for 25 broad-level categories and 0.45 for 353 specific groups. Unlike most of the other autocoders, participants iteratively select the best job and linked code rather than fill out a traditional form with no interaction.

Regardless of the coding approach, several distinct systems are being used to represent occupational health–relevant information. Each consists of a set of narrowly defined fields (eg, job title), and only specific values may be entered within each. In contrast with the single domain systems (eg, for job title only), NIOSH developed the Occupational Data for Health (ODH), which the developers suggest encapsulates the necessary information. The ODH includes the present/most recent job and the usual job occupation and industry, but does not systematically capture information about the nature of work, tasks, protective measures, and so on. It is nevertheless an important step by providing specific occupational health data for inclusion in EHRs (http://hl7.org/fhir/us/odh/index.html). Rajamani and colleagues[43] examined the ability to map fields from 20 resources to the ODH. Areas such as employer, exposures, and work-related illness or injury could be mapped to the ODH content, but required establishing a cross-index matrix and specific definitions. Overall, evaluations found that ODH could cross-map with most of the other traditional data models but noted limitations in granularity (detail) and temporality (time course).[41]

Lindemann and coworkers[44] extended the NIOSH ODH approach to include temporal relationships (such as "prior job"), thereby overcoming the ODH constraint of looking at only 2 epochs of work (current and most frequent job). Aldekhyyel and associates[45] developed a different characterization scheme using employment status, name of occupation, occupation, industry, workplace, job duty, employer name, and equipment. They analyzed 3.5 million health records from the University of Minnesota and found that 2336 unique entries free text occupational entries covered 87% of the overall data set.

TRANSFORMATIVE APPROACHES

In contrast with incrementally improving methods, new paradigms for occupational health are emerging. Three example technologies that can be leveraged for this are ML, natural language processing (NLP), and ontology optimization. Combined, they can significantly change how and how much new knowledge is gained, especially when leveraging efficient data-gathering techniques.

Machine Learning

ML algorithms assist in automatically discovering new patterns and learning new knowledge. ML has wide potential applicability for occupational lung diseases, although use to date is more limited than other areas of respiratory medicine. ML algorithms can be grouped into 3 broad groups according to their purpose. Clustering algorithms are unsupervised learning algorithms that group data items using the data features. Classification and prediction algorithms assign labels (eg, diagnoses) to data. These processes require representative training data with labels assumed to be correct. By building an internal model, ML learns to assign the labels to new, unseen examples. Other ML vary in their purpose. For example, optimization is a frequent use and different approaches exist. Some algorithms are standalone algorithms, whereas others are components in more comprehensive systems. Other purposes are simpler and have broad appeal. For example, finding unknown associations between different types of data items through association rule mining is an early use of algorithms with simple and useful outcomes (eg, early examples of such use can be found in marketing with product placement such as placing commonly purchased products together).

A new direction in ML is the use of deep learning algorithms. These algorithms are much more powerful than regular neural networks because they comprise more layers of neurons, and the neurons and connections between them leverage more advanced functions. Cheap computing power and large storage through cloud computing have recently increased their use. Open source libraries for deep and other ML algorithms encourage use by researchers (for example, PyTorch[46]).

A particular strength of ML for data mining is independence of a priori assumptions and explicit hypotheses. Thus, the systems may identify relationships that would otherwise not have been anticipated by experts. Clustering algorithms are frequent in biomedicine. For example, genetic analyses are often conducted without a priori hypotheses, but may subsequently point investigators to unsuspected functional roles of genes based on other genes with which they are grouped. Further, ML can develop classifiers and predictors using a very large number of features, many more than human experts would consider. Conversely, some consider ML to be a "black box" technique, accomplishing a task without providing any insight into underlying mechanisms.

ML can perform complex pattern recognition tasks currently conducted by human experts. Pneumoconiosis surveillance depends on standardized interpretation of radiographs by expert physicians certified to use the International Labor Organization Classification scheme. A combination of automated pneumoconiosis interpretation and overview for other problems by general chest radiologists may represent a long-term solution to the worsening shortage of certified B-readers.[47] Pneumoconiosis classification may be particularly amenable to automated systems because there is only a limited range of findings to assess. Preliminary studies have investigated automated pneumoconiosis interpretation.[48–52] ML has phenotypically characterized asthma from complex medical records.[53] This strategy should be applied to automatically detect unrecognized occupational lung diseases from systematically monitoring EHRs. Specific diseases may be easily found within very large bodies of data; for example, we used simple filters to identify asthma and COPD among the mass of Twitter posts.[5,18]

Natural Language Processing

NLP algorithms are useful when information is contained in unstructured free text. Free text is the natural form of communication for patients, workers, and health professionals. It contains much information that is often ignored in traditional data mining. Reducing the full information to a few codes is a 1-way process; the unused information is often ignored or even removed and not available if new interests develop in the future. When full, free text is available and retained, additional information can be extracted. NLP expands the range of potential inputs, incorporating everything from worker statements to clinical notes. **Fig. 2** shows a patient history, clinic note, and corresponding codes. In addition to loss of information content, translation among the 3 languages—namely, patient history, medical note jargon, and standard codes—is needed and could be automated.

Two broad approaches to NLP are used—rule-based and statistical algorithms. In rule-based algorithms, a large series of designated rules are specified and applied. Statistical approaches rely on ML algorithms for many of their underlying components. Typical NLP tasks to be completed before any advanced analysis is done are tokenization (ie, recognizing individual words), sentence splitting, parts-of-speech tagging (ie, recognizing nouns and verbs), followed by applying parsers that can recognize shallow or very advanced grammatical structures using a variety of types (eg, shallow parsers, syntax parsers, and dependency parsers). Excellent open source tools for most of these steps exist. Once these steps have been completed, additional functionality that is project specific is required.

Entity extraction (also called named entity recognition) is particularly relevant. This process entails recognizing and labeling a variety of terms. It requires first applying the basic NLP steps and is often combined with ontology lookup (see the section on Ontologies). For example, scanning large corpora for key terms indicating entities of interest, such as di-isocyanate, when found in conjunction with an asthma diagnosis can suggest an important relationship. Recognizing individual terms can be done with rule-based approaches. In this case, patterns are defined that may combine a variety of specifications, such as individually specified terms, broad categories (eg, sports activities), and terms matching specific sections of an ontology (eg, lung diseases). When training data exist, such as large sets of examples of terms for different entities, ML algorithms are more commonly used.

When no specific information is predefined as being of interest, a broad simple analysis can provide insight in the content of free text. Such analysis is easily conducted by frequency counts of common nouns, verbs, and phrases. These can be recognized by applying the basic NLP steps. Often, lists based solely on frequency are long and several formulas may assign more or less weight to terms depending on how well they represent the content of a document or EHR (eg, term-frequency–inverse document frequency based formula) or a category of EHR (eg, point mutual information formula). For example, we extracted frequent terms from 86,000 mining industry free text incident reports to identify key exposures and injuries.[54]

Currently, information from patients must be shared with a clinician, who then must enter it, and then the record must be coded. NLP can enable input directly from workers, patients, and safety officers by efficiently processing the text

PATIENT	"Ever since the car hit the back of my shuttle while I was loading a suitcase into my shuttle at the Delta terminal, my back and right leg hurt. The shots improve it a little bit, but not totally. I like the physical therapist, but she made me work too hard. I think I'm getting better slowly, but I can't go back to lifting suitcases into my van..."	
Clinic Note	30 yo wf c 8 mos LBP post MVA . On WC. TTD PE: NAD VS WNL BMI 32 DTR 2+Bilat SLR-R/+L ROM F45 E 5 Lat 10/10 Tx NSAID, PT, s/p ESI x 2 TTD x 1 mo, Rec RTC 2 wks RTW 1 mo. NSAID PT x 6 Not MMI	
Codes	SOC 53-3053	shuttle driver and chauffeur
	NAICS 485999	airport limousine services
	ICD S39.012	low back strain
	CPT 97110	Therapeutic exercise
	NDC 68084-703-01	Ibuprofen
	HL 7 SCTID: 2415007	Lumbosacral radiculopathy (disorder)

Fig. 2. Three languages. This figure illustrates the 3 distinct jargons used by patients, clinicians, and standard coders and information content loss.

and presenting it in a format useful for further analysis without the bottleneck and content loss of coding. A study using Amazon Mechanical Turk found that persons with asthma had considerable interest in ways to modify their workplace (personal accommodation),[39] whereas this typically receives low priority from clinicians and many researchers.

Ontologies

Systematically representing information is central to advancing information science for occupational respiratory disease. An ontology consists of a systematic representation of entities and the relationships among them. Ontologies have existed as early as Aristotle, but are now particularly key because they make information and knowledge accessible to computer and information systems.

A good ontology should be exhaustive (incorporate all necessary information), scalable, flexible, and consistent. The main components are the entities, some approach to grouping these, and the relationships between them. An ontology for occupational respiratory issues is particularly needed because of the unusually wide variety of necessary information. For example, the NLM's Unified Medical Language System (UMLS)[55] combines ontologies from different domains. It contains different vocabularies (forming the Metathesaurus) and groups these by concept (all terms are assigned to a concept) and higher level semantic types (eg, sign and symptoms, organic chemical). Full occupational health ontologies are rare, but commonly used taxonomies for job and industry (Standard Occupational Classification, North American Industry Classification System) are available (see **Table 3**).

Vocabularies can be created top-down or bottom-up. Top-down vocabularies are defined and limited. Several organizations have processes for consensus-based creation of standardized vocabularies and concept definitions. These include FHIR (Fast Healthcare Interoperability Resources), Health Level 7 standards, SNOMED, and Logical Observation Identifiers Names and Codes. Health Level 7 initially had concerns about the NIOSH proposal to require industry and occupation because of concerns about difficulty using the controlled vocabularies in Standard Occupational Classification and North American Industry Classification System. (Fortunately, this is moving ahead on a trial basis.[56]) Bottom-up approaches allow unrestricted vocabularies, reflecting how real-life workers, patients, clinicians, and others actually represent and organize their knowledge. Top-down approaches can be optimized for combination with other systems, but bottom-up approaches are broader and representative of all stakeholders (**Box 1**). The UMLS has inadequate occupational health vocabularies. For example, among 80,000 mining health incident reports, many exposure terms were not contained in the UMLS.[54] The vocabulary used by 5000 participants with early COPD who were asked to describe their work linked very poorly with the terminology used by experts.[54,57]

A method of expressing relationships among terms is also necessary. Some dictionaries contain a variety of parent–child relationships. For

Box 1
Key stakeholders

- Patients
- Workers
- Employers
- Community members
- Insurers and other payers
- Primary care health care providers
- Pulmonary and allergy/immunology specialists
- Occupational physicians and nurses
- Public health agencies (eg, local and state health departments)
- Regulatory agencies, such as Occupational Safety and Health Administration and the Environmental Protection Agency
- Researchers
- Worker advocates
- Research agencies such as the Centers for Disease Control and Prevention-NIOSH and the National Institutes of Health

example, WordNet (https://wordnet.princeton.edu/, a general English dictionary) contains hypernym (a concept with broader meaning) and hyponym (a concept with narrower meaning) relationships and groups terms with the same semantic meaning. In addition to these Isa relationships, the UMLS contains a variety of broader relationships among its semantic types (referred to as the Sematic Network).

Commonly used systems such as Standard Occupational Classification and *International Classification of Diseases—Clinical Modification* use a limited model with parent–child relationships. These classifications each operate within a single domain such as occupation, disease, or chemical, and do not represent essential relationships among domains, such as between industry and disease. These hierarchies support applying information associated with a broader term to more narrow subterms. Implying relationships solely from numerical proximity is inadequate; although physicians and correctional officers have increased risk of tuberculosis, their codes are far apart. An empirical EHR study found that 19% of entries for occupation included acronyms that were difficult to automatically disambiguate.[45] Developers of the UK OSCAR system, described elsewhere in this article, incorporated 2 methods to overcome inherent limitations in the standard classification system used in the UK.[42] First, the language in the UK standard classifications was technical and needed more understandable corresponding terminology for use by participants. Second, the 3-level decision tree they produced did not directly follow the hierarchical education/economic space structure, but rather was hardwired to be logical to participants (eg, engineer and engineering technician are close together, although in the standard hierarchical codes, they are far apart because of differences in education level).

Existing systems for relationships have several shortcomings. The UMLS uses more extensive relationships and contains a semantic network with 54 relationship categories. However, these relationships do not necessarily hold at the term level. Haz-Map includes interclass relationships, but its ad hoc manual creation and limited extent constrain scalability. Real-life thinkers use many more relationship types. In a simple study of associations, Harber and associates[58] asked industrial hygienists, occupational physicians, respiratory physicians what they associate with the terms wood, wheeze, and weld. Notably, most of the associations were across categories. Computer methods are needed to facilitate identifying factors seen by other related professional disciplines. Even simple generic additions such as "is a synonym for" and "is associated with" would greatly enhance its usefulness.

SUMMARY

Modern information science, computer algorithms, and web applications can assist current approaches to occupational respiratory diseases and may lead to fundamental changes in recognizing occupational lung disease in both individual patients and population groups. Some methods are immediately useful to patients, workers, clinicians, and others whereas others are in more developmental stages. Overcoming resistance to fundamental conceptual changes as well as disseminating effective practical tools will greatly aid the field.

CLINICS CARE POINTS

- Clinicians should seek expsoure information from sites listed in Table 1.
- Characteristics of many jobs areshownin the O'Net website.

DISCLOSURE

The authors have no conflict of interest, nor specific funding for this work.

REFERENCES

1. Kagen S, Garland A. Asthma and allergy mobile apps in 2018. Curr Allergy Asthma Rep 2019;19:6.
2. Zhou P, Yang L, Huang YX. A smart phone based handheld wireless spirometer with functions and precision comparable to laboratory spirometers. Sensors (Basel) 2019;19:2487.
3. Harber P, Merz B. Time and knowledge barriers to recognizing occupational disease. J Occup Environ Med 2001;43:285–8.
4. Ramsey RR, Caromody JK, Voorhees SE, et al. A systematic evaluation of asthma management apps examining behavior change techniques. J Allergy Clin Immunol In Pract 2019;7:2583–91.
5. Harber P, Leroy G. Insights from twitter about public perceptions of asthma, COPD, and exposures. J Occup Environ Med 2019;61:484–90.
6. Downs JW, Hakkinen PJ. What online toxicology resources are available at No cost from the (US) National Library of Medicine to assist practicing OEM physicians? J Occup Environ Med 2015;57:e85–90.
7. Brown J, Michie S, Geraghty AW, et al. Internet-based intervention for smoking cessation (StopAdvisor) in people with low and high socioeconomic status: a randomised controlled trial. Lancet Respir Med 2014;2:997–1006.
8. National Institute for Occupational Safety and Health. SPIROLA. Spirometry longitudinal data analysis version 3.0.3. Morgantown (WV): Centers for Disease Control and Prevention; 2016.
9. ReedGroup MDGuidelines. MDGuidelines. 2020. Available at: https://www.mdguidelines.com/. Accessed February 4, 2020.
10. ODG MCG. Industry-leading medical treatment & return to work guidelines. 2020. Available at: https://www.mcg.com/odg/about-odg/. Accessed December 4, 2020.
11. Jolly AT, Klees JE, Pacheco KA, et al. Work-related asthma. J Occup Environ Med 2015;57:e121–9.
12. Litow FK, Petsonk EL, Bohnker BK, et al. Occupational interstitial lung diseases. J Occup Environ Med 2015;57:1250–4.
13. Dept. of Health and Human Services. HITECH Act enforcement interim final rule. 2017. Available at: https://www.hhs.gov/hipaa/for-professionals/special-topics/hitech-act-enforcement-interim-final-rule/index.html. Accessed August 19, 2020.
14. Harber P, Redlich CA, Hines S, et al. Recommendations for a clinical decision support system for work-related asthma in primary care settings. J Occup Environ Med 2017;59:e231–5.
15. Killorn KR, Dostaler SM, Groome PA, et al. The use of a work-related asthma screening questionnaire in a primary care asthma program: an intervention trial. J Asthma 2015;52:398–406.
16. Harber P, Ha J, Roach M. Arizona hospital discharge and emergency department database: implications for occupational health surveillance. J Occup Environ Med 2017;59:417–23.
17. Sublet V, Spring C, Howard J, National Institute for Occupational Safety and Health. Does social media improve communication? Evaluating the NIOSH science blog. Am J Ind Med 2011;54:384–94.
18. Leroy G, Harber P, Revere D. Public sharing of medical advice using social media: an analysis of a Twitter. Seventeenth International Conference on Grey Literature. Amsterdam, the Netherlands, December 1-2, 2015.
19. Alessa A, Faezipour M. A review of influenza detection and prediction through social networking sites. Theor Biol Med Model 2018;15:2.
20. Baltrusaitis K, Brownstein JS, Scarpino SV, et al. Comparison of crowd-sourced, electronic health records based, and traditional health-care based influenza-tracking systems at multiple spatial resolutions in the United States of America. BMC Infect Dis 2018;18:403.
21. Vibound C, Snatillna A. Fitbit-informed influenza forecasts. Lancet Digital Health 2020;2:e54–5. Available at: https://www.thelancet.com/action/showPdf?pii=S2589-7500%2819%2930241-9.
22. Environmental Protection Agency. EnviroAtlas. Available at: https://www.epa.gov/enviroatlas. Accessed February 4, 2020.
23. Wild CP. The exposome: from concept to utility. Int J Epidemiol 2012;41:24–32.
24. Loh M, Sarigiannis D, Gotti A, et al. How sensors might help define the external exposome. Int J Environ Res Public Health 2017;14:434.
25. Weichenthal S, Hatzopoulou M, Brauer M. A picture tells a thousand...exposures: opportunities and challenges of deep learning image analyses in exposure science and environmental epidemiology. Environ Int 2019;122:3–10.
26. Environmental Protection Agency. Satellite – based air quality observing systems. Available at: https://www3.epa.gov/ttn/amtic/files/ambient/pm25/cenr/sat051506.pdf. Accessed February 4, 2020.
27. Cromar KR, Duncan BN, Bartonova A, et al. Air pollution monitoring for health research and patient care. An Official American Thoracic Society Workshop Report. Ann Am Thorac Soc 2019;16:1207–14.
28. Gaskins AJ, Hart JE. The use of personal and indoor air pollution monitors in reproductive epidemiology studies. Paediatr Perinat Epidemiol 2020;34(5):513–21.
29. Qin X, Wu T, Zhu Y, et al. A paper based milli-cantilever sensor for detecting hydrocarbon gases via smartphone camera. Anal Chem 2020;92:8480–6.

30. Moore AC, Anderson AA, Long M, et al. The power of the crowd: prospects and pitfalls for citizen science in occupational health. J Occup Environ Hyg 2019;16:191–8.
31. Institute of Medicine. Review of the Department of Labor's Site Exposure Matrix Database. Washington, DC: The National Academies Press; 2013. https://doi.org/10.17226/18266.
32. Weiss W. Epidemic curve of respiratory cancer due to chloromethyl ethers. J Natl Cancer Inst 1982;69: 1265–70.
33. Kreiss K, Gomaa A, Kullman G, et al. Clinical bronchiolitis obliterans in workers at a microwave-popcorn plant. N Engl J Med 2002; 347:330–8.
34. Parmet AJ. Bronchiolitis in popcorn-factory workers. N Engl J Med 2002;347:1980–2 [author reply: 1980–2; discussion 1980–2].
35. Friedman GK, Harrison R, Bojes H, et al, Centers for Disease Control and Prevention (CDC). Notes from the field: silicosis in a countertop fabricator - Texas, 2014. MMWR Morb Mortal Wkly Rep 2015;64: 129–30.
36. Rose C, Heinzerling A, Patel K, et al. Severe silicosis in engineered stone fabrication workers - California, Colorado, Texas, and Washington, 2017-2019. MMWR Morb Mortal Wkly Rep 2019;68:813–8.
37. Harber P, Leroy G. Social media use for occupational lung disease. Curr Opin Allergy Clin Immunol 2017;17:72–7.
38. Sinnenberg L, Buttenheim A, Kevin Padrez K, et al. Twitter as a tool for health research: a systematic review. Am J Public Health 2017;107(1): e1–8.
39. Harber P, Leroy G. Assessing work-asthma interaction with Amazon Mechanical Turk. J Occup Environ Med 2015;57:381–5.
40. Buckner-Petty S, Dale AM, Evanoff BA. Efficiency of autocoding programs for converting job descriptors into standard occupational classification (SOC) codes. Am J Ind Med 2019;62:59–68.
41. Schmitz M, Forst L. Industry and occupation in the electronic health record: an investigation of the National Institute for Occupational Safety and Health Industry and Occupation computerized coding system. JMIR Med Inform 2016;4:e5.
42. De Matteis S, Jarvis D, Young H, et al. Occupational self-coding and automatic recording (OSCAR): a novel web-based tool to collect and code lifetime job histories in large population-based studies. Scand J Work Environ Health 2017;43:181–6.
43. Rajamani S, Chen ES, Lindemann E, et al. Representation of occupational information across resources and validation of the occupational data for health model. J Am Med Inform Assoc 2018;25: 197–205.
44. Lindemann EA, Chen ES, Rajamani S, et al. Assessing the representation of occupation information in free-text clinical documents across multiple sources. Stud Health Technol Inform 2017;245: 486–90.
45. Aldekhyyel R, Chen ES, Rajamani S, et al. Content and quality of free-text occupation documentation in the electronic health record. AMIA Annu Symp Proc 2017;2016:1708–16.
46. PyTorch. PyTorch: from research to production. 2020. Available at: https://pytorch.org/. Accessed August 1, 2020.
47. Halldin CN, Hale JM, Weissman DN, et al. The National Institute for occupational safety and health B reader certification program-an update report (1987 to 2018) and future directions. J Occup Environ Med 2019;61: 1045–51.
48. Okumura E, Kawashita I, Ishida T. Computerized analysis of pneumoconiosis in digital chest radiography: effect of artificial neural network trained with power spectra. J Digit Imaging 2011;24: 1126–32.
49. Okumura E, Kawashita I, Ishida T. Computerized classification of pneumoconiosis on digital chest radiography artificial neural network with three stages. J Digit Imaging 2017;30: 413–26.
50. Zhu B, Chen H, Chen B, et al. Support vector machine model for diagnosing pneumoconiosis based on wavelet texture features of digital chest radiographs. J Digit Imaging 2014;27: 90–7.
51. Zhu B, Luo W, Li B, et al. The development and evaluation of a computerized diagnosis scheme for pneumoconiosis on digital chest radiographs. Biomed Eng Online 2014; 13:141.
52. Zhu L, Zheng R, Jin H, et al. Automatic detection and recognition of silicosis in chest radiograph. Biomed Mater Eng 2014;24:3389–95.
53. Ross MK, Yoon J, van der Schaar A, et al. Discovering pediatric asthma phenotypes on the basis of response to controller medication using machine learning. Ann Am Thorac Soc 2018;15: 49–58.
54. Harber P, Leroy G. Feasibility and utility of Lexical analysis for occupational health text. J Occup Environ Med 2017;59:578–87.
55. Humphreys BL, Lindberg DA. The UMLS project: making the conceptual connection between users and the information they need. Bull Med Libr Assoc 1993;81:170–7.
56. Health Level Seven International (HL7). HL7 FHIR profile: occupational data for health (ODH), release 1.1. 2019. Available at: http://hl7.org/fhir/us/odh/STU1/. Accessed February 1, 2020.

57. Harber P, Crawford L, Liu K, et al. Working words: real-life lexicon of North American workers. J Occup Environ Med 2005;47:859–64.
58. Harber P, Miller G, Smitherman J. Work coding: beyond SIC and SOC, BOC and DOT. J Occup Med 1991;33:1274–80.
59. National Center for O*NET Development. The O*NET® content model. 2019. Available at: https://www.onetcenter.org/content.html. Accessed January 22, 2020.
60. SNOMED Inetrnational. SNOMED CT browser. 2020. Available at: https://browser.ihtsdotools.org/?perspective=full&conceptId1=404684003&edition=MAIN/SNOMEDCT-US/2019-09-01&release=&languages=en. Accessed January 20, 2020.

Health Disparities in Environmental and Occupational Lung Disease

Emily Brigham, MD, MHS[a], Kassandra Allbright, MD[b], Drew Harris, MD[c,*]

KEYWORDS

• Health disparities • Health equity • Social determinants of health • Environmental health
• Occupational health

KEY POINTS

- Health disparities exist in many chronic lung diseases between different ages, races, the sexes, and geographic regions.
- Modifiable risk factors for pulmonary disparities are highlighted and include occupational and environmental exposures, psychosocial stressors, health behaviors, health literacy, health care provider bias, and health care access.
- Strategies to address the upstream risk factors and decrease existing disparities require multidisciplinary and multilevel approaches.

INTRODUCTION

The respiratory system provides a large surface area for direct contact with airborne environmental and occupational exposures. As such, pulmonary disease is a significant outcome of interest in public health efforts to decrease the impact of these exposures. Targeted strategies are informed by a focus on vulnerable and disadvantaged populations, defined by disparities in exposure, susceptibility to disease, and resources to manage morbidity. The US Office of Disease Prevention and Health Promotion provides guidance on health disparities within the *Healthy People 2020* initiative, noting these populations as:

> *groups of people who have systematically experienced greater obstacles to health based on their racial or ethnic group; religion; socioeconomic status; gender; age; mental health; cognitive, sensory, or physical disability; sexual orientation or gender identity; geographic location; or other characteristics historically linked to discrimination or exclusion.*[1]

A similar policy statement was published by a joint effort between 2 leading professional societies, namely, the American Thoracic Society and the European Respiratory Society.[2] Recognition of disparities and associated social determinants of health[3] provides opportunity to reduce disparities and improve respiratory health at both the individual and population levels.

Diseases evaluated in this article include asthma, chronic obstructive pulmonary disease (COPD), pneumoconiosis, and lung cancer. Guided by the focus on disparities, sections are purposively organized by the characteristic in which disparity occurs, with evidence for individual diagnoses presented within each section. Importantly, although presented separately, factors often overlap or synergize to heighten risk

[a] Division of Pulmonary and Critical Care, Johns Hopkins University, 1830 East Monument Street 5th Floor, Baltimore, MD 21287, USA; [b] Department of Medicine, Johns Hopkins University, 1830 East Monument Street 5th Floor, Baltimore, MD 21287, USA; [c] Division of Pulmonary and Critical Care and Public Health Sciences, University of Virginia, Pulmonary Clinic 2nd Floor, 1221 Lee Street, Charlottesville, VA 22903, USA
* Corresponding author.
E-mail address: DH3MX@hscmail.mcc.virginia.edu
Twitter: @emily_brigham (E.B.)

Clin Chest Med 41 (2020) 623–639
https://doi.org/10.1016/j.ccm.2020.08.009

(**Fig. 1**).[4] For concision, evidence summation is primarily focused on evidence from developed nations, and is followed by a discussion of potential or proven interventions within this context to provide equal health opportunity.

AGE

Age carries implications for likelihood of disease, likelihood of detection of disease, and treatments offered. The concept and defining of windows of susceptibility is applicable to all exposures, although for few has this been completely explored owing to infeasibility or a focus on alternate priorities. For others, exposures are more limited to an isolated time range, and so individual susceptibility plays a greater role in a usual age range of exposure. Diseases uncommon in childhood are perhaps less likely to be detected when present or detected at a delayed rate, whereas common diseases may be misdiagnosed or overdiagnosed, usually among adults and the elderly. Further, most treatment trials occur in adult populations, with the effect extrapolated or only later examined in pediatric populations.[5] This can lead to delays in approval or insurance coverage of potentially helpful medications in children, and the off-label use of medications that do not have substantial safety data outside of adult use. The United States has updated research and marketing regulations to reduce these biases,[6–9] but lags in pediatric trials persist. At the opposite end of the age spectrum, treatments may again become limited either by comorbidities or age restrictions (ie, lung transplantation).

Asthma

With the exception of the first few years, asthma is ubiquitous across all life stages. Caution in diagnosis is warranted under age 6, given the broad differential for wheeze, dyspnea, and cough in combination with difficulty in obtaining reliable spirometry.[10] In support of this, although nearly 50% of children will experience at least 1 wheezing episode by the age of 6,[11] a majority of these children will not have asthma.[12]

Pediatric populations have a higher prevalence of asthma than adult populations (8.4% vs 7.7% in the United States, respectively).[13] Environmental risk factors contributing to pediatric asthma disparities are unique from those of adults, and include prenatal factors (maternal exposures to tobacco smoke) and postnatal factors (severe respiratory syncytial virus infection, indoor exposure to mold/fungi and other allergens, outdoor air pollution). Obesity may also predispose to childhood asthma.[14] Remission rates of childhood

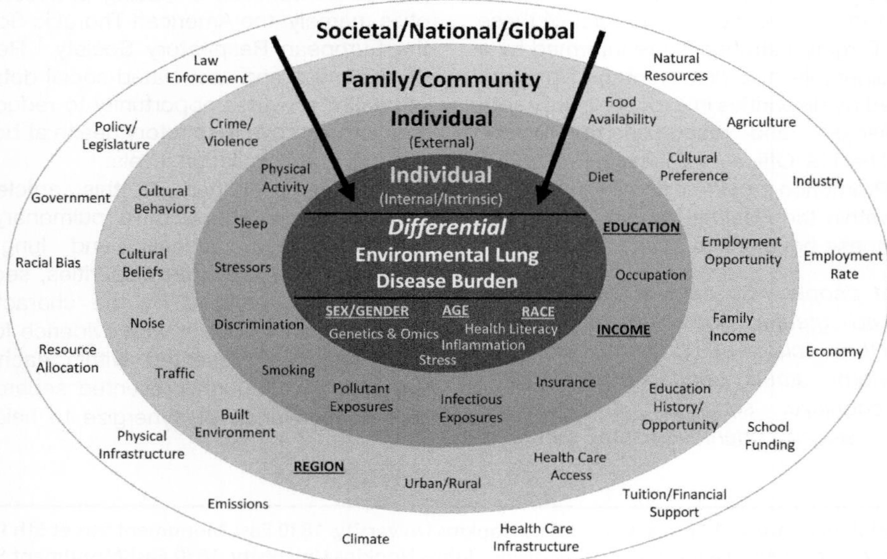

Fig. 1. Spheres of influence. Factors contributing to environmental respiratory disease disparities are complex and diverse. A proposed framework for consideration is presented, with examples of influential factors represented by level of impact and organization. Factors may associate within or across levels, increasing complexity and reinforcing the need for interdisciplinary research and potential multi-layer interventions to address health disparities in environmental respiratory disease. Section titles are capitalized and bolded within the figure for emphasis, and represent high concentration of evidence related to health disparities.

asthma range up to 65% and may be inversely related to severity.[15–17]

Adult-onset asthma is common; one-half of middle-aged individuals with asthma report an adult onset, and with advancing age this proportion increases.[18,19] Risk factors for adult asthma include a history of childhood asthma, obesity, and tobacco smoke exposure. Occupational exposures, including chemicals, aerosols, and other inhalable products, may account for 10% to 25% of adult-onset asthma cases.[20] Obesity and chronic rhinitis may also play a role in adult-onset disease.[21–24] Adult asthma remission is rare.

In terms of morbidity, although health care use is higher in the United States among children than adults with asthma, mortality rates are higher among adults (13.4 vs 2.5 deaths per million).[13] Factors contributing to greater health care use among children with asthma include the frequency of viral infections, less personal control over environmental exposures (eg, environmental tobacco smoke), difficulties in symptom reporting and objective monitoring (eg, unable to accurately report symptoms or perform peak flow); children are largely protected from occupational exposures until late adolescence. Adults have a higher risk of accompanying comorbidities, which may complicate asthma presentations. Limited patient understanding, late recognition by providers, underappreciation of severity, or financial pressure to continue employment may lead to delayed presentation and/or continued exposure to occupational triggers.

Chronic Obstructive Pulmonary Disease

COPD, the combined result of genetic predisposition, early life exposures precluding achievement of maximum lung function, and cumulative exposures, is primarily a disease of adulthood. The diagnosis is predicated on the development of fixed airway obstruction in the setting of symptoms consistent with the disease and environmental exposures. The Global Obstructive Lung Disease guidelines advocate for use of a fixed forced expiratory volume in 1 second/forced vital capacity ratio (<0.70) to confirm the disease.[25] Notably, because the forced expiratory volume in 1 second/forced vital capacity ratio decreases with age, the use of this definition favors diagnosis in older populations and underdiagnoses younger populations. The use of alternate definitions (such as the lower limit of normal equations personalized to height, race, sex, and age[26,27]) has been proposed, although the diagnosis is rarely made under the age of 40 years.

Factors that preclude achievement of peak lung function in early life may predispose individuals to COPD development, and plausibly at an earlier age, include prematurity, uncontrolled asthma, and primary and secondhand tobacco smoke exposure. These factors and others often coalesce in lower socioeconomic circumstances and may predispose affected populations to COPD at earlier time points.

Perceived health and health-related quality of life is important, because COPD has no cure and is accelerated by ongoing exposure. Of note, for the same severity of dyspnea, younger individuals report lower health-related quality of life,[28] suggesting that early development of COPD may be particularly impactful. COPD outcomes with aging are complicated by the development of comorbidities (such as cardiac disease or lung cancer), which are often related to the causative exposure for lung disease.

Pneumoconiosis

The literature regarding age-related disparities in pneumoconiosis are sparse. Because disease development occurs in response to occupational dust exposures, pneumoconiosis is largely a disease of adults. The likelihood of disease is largely related to cumulative exposure, often on the orders of years or decades with or without a latent period. For silicosis, however, younger age may be a risk factor for radiographic progression,[29] and a mortality owing to silicosis has been reported in a 19-year-old patient in the United States.[30] Acute, large-volume exposures can notably produce symptoms on the order of weeks.

Lung Cancer

Lung cancers in pediatric populations are rare, but include carcinoid, inflammatory myofibroblastic tumor, and plueropulmonary blastoma. Even more rarely seen tumors include small cell carcinoma and adenocarcinoma.[31] Pediatric lung cancer is rarely related to environmental history; rather genetic predisposition is common. The exception to this is exposure to radon,[32] a naturally occurring radioactive gas that can be found in many areas in the United States. The risk of lung cancer in children exposed to radon is twice as high as adults; if coexposed to tobacco smoke, lung cancer risk increases by a factor of 20.[32] Survival of pediatric lung cancer is difficult to calculate based on low rates of occurrence, and varies by disease.

Although lung cancers in adult populations may also be related to genetic predisposition, there is an enhanced link with environmental exposures;

most prominently primary tobacco smoke. Smoking is thought to account for 90% of lung cancer cases in the United States,[33] and is strongly linked with the development of nonsmall cell carcinoma, the most common form of primary lung cancer. Other predisposing environmental factors include ambient air pollution, occupational exposures (notably, the presence of pneumoconiosis is associated with an increased risk of lung carcinoma), and radon gas.[33] As cumulative exposure increases risk, the risk of incident lung cancer increases with time and intensity of exposure, often associated with advancing age. The average age of diagnosis in the United States is 70 years,[34] and advanced age is associated with lower survival,[35] likely owing to factors including comorbidities, anticipated versus actual tolerance of therapy,[36] and treatment allocation.

RACE

Disentangling the direct effects of race in epidemiologic studies is challenging. In developed countries, race is often deeply intertwined with socioeconomic status (SES) and complicated by historical and contemporary sociopolitical conflict. Causal factors that may contribute to known racial disparities in pulmonary health include the impact of racial differences in poverty, health care access,[37] health behaviors,[38] exposure to environmental and occupational hazards,[39,40] regional and neighborhood segregation,[41] implicit bias in health care,[42] and genetic variation.[43] Additionally, race may mitigate or augment the impact of these factors, increasing the complexity of the association. For example, health gains from protective factors (eg, higher SES) may not be experienced equally across racial groups—the concept of minorities' diminished returns.[44,45]

Asthma

Racial disparities in asthma are well-documented, with disproportionate prevalence and impact in minority populations.[46] The US adult asthma prevalence is 8% in non-Hispanic whites, as compared with 10% in non-Hispanic blacks. Although Hispanic populations overall have a lower rate (6%) of asthma, Puerto Rican populations have a disproportionately high (13%) asthma prevalence.[13] Blacks have more than double the mortality rate of whites (23% vs 8%),[13] and are also more likely to have severe or poorly controlled asthma and decreased asthma related quality of life metrics as compared with their non-Hispanic white peers.[47]

Although genetic susceptibility seems to play a role,[48] differential exposures are a likely contributing factor.[49] Racial minorities are more likely to reside in urban, industrial-adjacent neighborhoods and to have homes near major roadways,[50] which increases exposure to air pollution. Higher air pollutant concentrations, both indoor and ambient, associate with a negative impact on pulmonary function and asthma morbidity.[51,52] Early childhood exposures to air pollution may also increase lifetime risk of asthma development and severity.[53] In addition to air pollution, disparities in tobacco smoke exposure are important to consider; African American children and adults are more likely to be exposed to second-hand smoke than any other racial or ethnic group in the United States.[54] The lifetime risk of asthma is increased with tobacco exposure, including prenatal exposure.[55] Environmental exposures linked to asthma development and severity also include psychosocial stress at any life stage. Maternal distress has been linked to childhood asthma[56] in minority communities, as has the psychosocial stresses of neighborhood violence[57] and the experience of racial discrimination itself.[58] Covarying SES disparities (ie, income, education) in minority groups are additionally likely to contribute to differential asthma morbidity outcomes.[49]

Chronic Obstructive Pulmonary Disease

Currently, 4% of adult Hispanics in the United States, 6.1% of African Americans, and 6.3% of non-Hispanic whites have COPD.[59] Although in developed countries COPD is often the result of tobacco smoking, there are differences in COPD prevalence between racial groups that do not correlate with historical rates of tobacco use.[60] Although racial differences in susceptibility to tobacco smoke are not yet fully understood, some studies suggest that African Americans have increased loss of lung function per pack-year of smoking.[61] As is also the case in asthma, genetic predisposition may contribute to racial disparities in COPD prevalence and morbidity.[48,62,63] Despite similar overall COPD prevalence and lower smoking rates in African Americans compared with non-Hispanic whites,[64] the burden of early-onset COPD is highest in African Americans.[65,66]

Many of the same environmental and occupational exposures that are known to worsen asthma are also implicated in COPD and are likely to contribute to racial disparities through differential exposure.[67] Additionally, minority patients have diminishing returns on positive SES modifiers in COPD; higher educational status in blacks does not, on average, provide the same degree of protection from COPD as it does in non-Hispanic whites.[44]

Pneumoconiosis

The literature regarding racial disparities in pneumoconiosis is scant. The majority of the US coal mining workforce is white (88%),[68] and coal workers pneumoconiosis is therefore largely represented in this racial group.[69] A report of severe silicosis in several US states and related to stone fabrication was noted mainly in Hispanic workers.[70] A second descriptive study of silicosis cases in Michigan over the previous 2 decades describes an increase risk to African Americans versus non-Hispanic whites in both prevalence and severity, but is unable to offer other insights into this racial disparity.[71]

Lung Cancer

The lung cancer incidence rate in African Americans is higher than incidence rate in non-Hispanic whites.[72,73] In addition, African Americans with lung cancer have worse morbidity and higher age-adjusted mortality than other racial groups.[74] There are many factors contributing to these disparities. African Americans are more likely to present with advanced stage disease.[75] One recent study suggests that of those who are eligible for lung cancer screening computed tomography scans, African Americans are significantly less likely to have been screened than non-Hispanic whites.[76] This finding is particularly important to consider given that a decrease in lung cancer-specific mortality caused by lung cancer screening computed tomography scan was more pronounced in African Americans than in non-Hispanic whites.[77]

There are also important racial differences in lung cancer treatment. Among National Lung Screening Trial participants who had early stage lung cancers and who were considered fit to undergo surgical resection, African American men were significantly less likely than non-Hispanic white men to undergo potentially curative surgery.[78] Other studies have shown that African Americans are less likely to receive timely surgery, chemotherapy, or radiation for later stage disease relative to non-Hispanic white patients.[79]

In addition, other explanations for racial differences in lung cancer mortality maybe secondary to distrust, limited access to care and health beliefs regarding lung cancer and its treatment.[80,81] In addition, occupational exposures correlated with lung cancer[82] have also been found to have racially disparate risks. Studies of oven workers have found increased lung cancer mortality risk in African American and non-white workers compared with white workers.[83,84] Investigators have suggested a link between proximity to potential carcinogens with increased cancer mortality and, further, found that significant racial differences existed in exposure risk, with African American and non-white workers disproportionately in the highest risk sites (eg, "topside").

SEX

There is growing evidence that disparities in lung diseases exist between the sexes. It is widely known that some rare lung diseases occur almost entirely in women (eg, lymphangioleiomyomatosis and pleural or parenchymal endometriosis). Less attention has been directed toward differences between genders in more common lung diseases including asthma, COPD, pneumoconiosis and lung cancer.

Asthma

Sex differences in asthma prevalence, morbidity, and mortality are widely reported in epidemiologic studies. Boys have a higher prevalence of asthma compared with girls, with this difference most pronounced in early childhood.[85] Boys under the age of 15 have a higher rate of hospitalizations owing to asthma than do girls of similar age.[86] After puberty, asthma prevalence, severity, and morbidity disproportionately impacts women.[85] Women above the age of 15 are more likely than men to be hospitalized for asthma. Women with asthma have an increased risk for life-threatening asthma and emergency room visitations for asthma exacerbations, and in the United States, asthma mortality rates are significantly higher in females than males.[87,88]

Biological sex differences as well as differences in sociocultural, behavioral, and environmental factors should all be considered in explaining sex disparities in asthma. Higher estrogen and progesterone levels can influence immune function and resident lung cells that may render women more susceptible to asthma and asthma morbidity.[89,90] Conversely, higher testosterone levels have been associated with better lung function and can modulate the inflammatory process in asthma.[91,92] Multiple studies further suggest a higher incidence of work-related asthma in women.[93–95] Although the gender distribution of work-related asthma may reflect the gender distribution of adult asthma, other potential contributing factors include differences in job tasks, inadequate fit testing in females who use respirators, and sex differences in lung size and structure impacting lung deposition of toxic inhaled agents.[93]

Sexual minority women (including those who identify as lesbian or bisexual) are more likely than heterosexual women to be diagnosed with asthma.[96] This may be due to higher rates of psychosocial stress and cigarette smoking, in addition to higher rates of obesity seen in same-sex partnered women96 (women are at heightened risk for obesity-related asthma). Other factors, including deficiencies in cultural competency among providers of sexual minority women, can lead to health care avoidance and worsened health outcomes, in part owing to sexual orientation.[97]

Chronic Obstructive Pulmonary Disease

Although age-adjusted mortality rates for COPD are higher for men than women, this mortality gap has decreased sharply over the past few decades. Gender differences in smoking rates partially explain current COPD gender disparities. Smoking prevalence in US women has decreased at a slower rate than in US men over the last 50 years.[98] Lung function decline in women is greater than the decline seen in men when adjusted for the amount of tobacco smoked.[99] However, many other factors are important to consider including genetic differences between the sexes and the social, cultural, and environmental context of COPD in women.[97] Women living in poverty, especially in developing countries, have higher exposure to household air pollution, which is associated with higher COPD prevalence among women.[100] Occupational risk factors unique to women are additionally important factors to consider: women employed in protective service, food preparation and serving, production, and transportation and material moving demonstrate prevalence estimates of COPD that were 2 to 4 times higher than males.[101] Further, primary care providers maybe more likely to underdiagnose COPD in women than in men.[102] Women may have more difficulty quitting smoking than men, although smoking cessation medications may help to attenuate this difference.[103]

Pneumoconiosis

There are limited data examining the prevalence, severity, or causation of sex disparities in pneumoconiosis. Diagnoses are largely seen in men owing to cultural norms within at-risk occupations. In recent descriptions, nearly 100% of those with advanced coal worker's pneumoconiosis are men.[104,105] Similarly, in large epidemiologic surveillance programs for silicosis across multiple states in the United States, more than 95% of cases occurred in men,[106] including in the recent resurgence of silicosis in artificial stone manufacturing.[70] Although asbestos exposures can occur owing to both occupational and nonoccupational exposures, asbestosis predominantly impacts males, which is largely due to the occupational risk factors. Construction work was the most frequently recorded industry on death certificates with asbestosis as the cause of death,[107] and women comprise less than 10% of the United States construction workforce.[68]

Lung Cancer

The age-adjusted incidence and mortality rates associated with lung cancer remain lower in women than in men, largely owing to lower historical rates of smoking among women.[108] However, among those born since the mid 1960s, the incidence rates of lung cancer have become higher among young women than among young men.[109] Additional causative factors outside smoking and susceptibility to tobacco smoke are unclear.[109–112] Other possible explanations for sex disparities in lung cancer incidence include a decrease in occupational and environmental carcinogens (eg, asbestos) in recent decades that has resulted in a decrease in lung cancers in males (and not females) owing to gender differences within occupations associated with increased exposures.[113]

Compared with men, women are (1) more likely to be diagnosed with lung cancer at an early age,[114] (2) more likely to be diagnosed at earlier stages,[115] and (3) more likely to be diagnosed with lung cancer if a nonsmoker.[116] Despite these differences, many studies have shown more favorable survival for women with lung cancer regardless of age, histologic subtype, or stage of disease at presentation.[115,117] Long term-survival benefits for women are in part related to women having better postoperative outcomes in lung cancer surgery with subsequent expedited ability to begin adjuvant therapy in a timely manner.[118]

SOCIOECONOMIC STATUS

SES is a measure of social standing, represented by a combination of education, income, and occupation.[119] These 3 variables are intricately linked,[120] and indeed several studies demonstrate associations between aggregate measures combining income and education (with or without occupation and other indicators) and environmental lung diseases.[121,122] However, in epidemiologic research, income or education are often used as individually representative of SES.[123] Because income and education represent unique points of potential intervention to reduce disparities, we consider the concepts separately while acknowledging interrelatedness.

Socioeconomic Status: as Represented by Education

Education is usually completed in early adulthood, and is strongly influenced by parental attributes. As such, it is often applied as a measure of early life SES.[124,125] Parental education is frequently used as an indicator of child SES. In other cases, where individuals decline to report income, education may be the most convenient and representative variable.

Educational attainment has far-reaching implications for disease development and morbidity. It reflects the presence of or access to resources, both material and intellectual, by both parents and the patient from an early age. It also captures a degree of cognitive functioning, which carries implications for health literacy, capacity for communication with health resources, and health behaviors. Finally, education is a determinant of employment status, type of employment, and income.[124–126] This factor not only influences likelihood of exposure to respiratory hazards via occupation, but also has direct implications for financial resources.

Asthma

Ample evidence supports an inverse relationship between education level and asthma diagnosis. In pediatric populations, higher parental education is associated with protection against incident asthma,[127] and is linked with better home environmental control behaviors and less exposure to tobacco smoke.[122] The association is consistent within adult populations, even when accounting for occupational exposures.[128] Educational attainment has also been linked to asthma morbidity. Lower parental health literacy is related to worse asthma control in children,[129] and likewise lower educational attainment is linked to worse asthma control in adults with asthma.[130]

Chronic obstructive pulmonary disease

Lower educational attainment has been linked to increased COPD morbidity, including lower lung function, greater disease severity, more physical limitations, a higher risk of hospitalization for COPD, and worse radiographic emphysema.[131–133] In 1 cross-sectional study, the association between educational attainment was modified by income, and most consistent among medium- and high-income groups (>$20,000 annual household income, Northern California).[132] Low health literacy may represent an additional risk factor for poor COPD outcomes, independent of education.[134]

Pneumoconiosis

In developed countries, pneumoconiosis primarily occurs in the occupational setting via exposure to coal, silica, or asbestos during mining.[135] For an underground mining worker, although a high school degree may be requested or required, with additional coursework or apprenticeship, experience may be used to replace formal educational requirements. Silicosis and asbestosis also occur in the context of construction, masonry, and manufacturing. Shipyard and power plant workers are at risk of asbestosis as well. Although not exclusively, these positions are largely filled by individuals without advanced degrees. Therefore, individuals with educational attainment just above, at, or below the high school education level may be disproportionately represented in populations with pneumoconiosis. At least one study outside of the United States also demonstrates that lower educational attainment is associated with a lesser awareness (knowledge of the disease and protective factors) for silicosis, which could plausibly translate to higher disease burden in those with less formal education.[136]

Lung cancer

Lower educational attainment is consistently associated with a higher risk of lung cancer, independent of smoking exposures and despite adjustment for occupational histories when available.[137–142] Although some individual studies report increased mortality rates in groups with lower educational attainment,[143] a large meta-analysis found no difference in survival by education.[144] Within the context of a pooled clinical trial population, educational attainment was not predictive of lung cancer survival.[145] A smaller study of patients with advanced nonsmall cell populations enrolled in clinical trials demonstrated that higher education was associated with longer survival despite similar treatments.[146] The cause of these disparate results are unknown, bear additional investigation, and may suggest that lung cancer subgroups have unique susceptibilities to educational attainment or associated variables in regards to clinical outcomes.

Socioeconomic Status: as Represented by Income

Income is most often captured by self-report, and presented either at the individual or family/household level by independent epidemiologic investigations or in aggregate, summarized form through community or census resources. Income provides a means to access resources for health, education, and environmental change. The latter may present as residence in a neighborhood with lower pollutant levels, access to healthful foods, higher resourced schools, and lower violence. Alternatively, a higher income may provide the opportunity for home indoor environmental modifications important for maximizing respiratory health among susceptible individuals (ie, pest abatement, mold remediation, or even relocation). Additionally, a higher income may be related to skilled work and demand, providing a decreased risk for occupational exposures and job flexibility if removal from the workplace is required. This relationship is neither absolute nor linear, because some higher risk occupations do provide compensation commensurate with risk, and reverse causality requires consideration, because job loss and income reduction may occur in the setting of occupational lung disease.[147,148] Finally, income level is negatively associated with smoking, a constant and important confounder in all investigations relating income to environmentally mediated lung disease,[149] and also a potent opportunity for intervention to decrease disparity.

Asthma

Lower parental or household income has been associated with incident asthma in childhood and adolescence,[150] adult-onset asthma,[151] and with pediatric asthma prevalence in cross-sectional analyses.[152] However, contradictory evidence exists; a longitudinal study of adolescents in Canada reported no significant association between household income and incident asthma,[153] and an additional Canadian study reports no difference in asthma prevalence by neighborhood household income up to age 35; thereafter, income was negatively associated with asthma prevalence.[154] Regarding morbidity, higher income has been associated with more favorable immune regulation and sensitivity to glucocorticoid therapy in pediatric populations with asthma,[122] as well as better asthma control and a lower exacerbation rates.[155,156]

Chronic Obstructive Pulmonary Disease

COPD incidence and prevalence has been inversely linked to income.[157,158] Low income may additionally confer vulnerability to poor outcomes. Low income is an independent predictor of lung function decline in smokers.[159] Lower household income has also been associated with greater COPD disease severity, worse lung function, and greater physical limitation.[132,160]

Pneumoconiosis

Published associations between income and disparities in pneumoconiosis are lacking, likely owing to the direct occupational links and therefore presumed relative homogeneity of income among those at highest risk. The national average annual salary for an underground coal miner is approximately $49,000.[161] Front-line construction and manufacturing worker salaries tend to lie closer to minimum wage (approximately $30,000 annually), whereas masonry workers have the capacity to expand beyond this income. Thus, this income range will have an inevitably higher prevalence of this disease manifestation.

Lung cancer

Several studies and the results of a meta-analysis demonstrate that income is inversely associated with lung cancer risk.[137,140] Furthermore, a 2018 meta-analysis summarizing current literature demonstrates worse survival for low-income versus high-income individuals.[144] Given the complexities of factors affecting and affected by income, the translation of this finding into a meaningful intervention warrants further consideration.

GEOGRAPHIC DISPARITIES

Location plays a primary role in determining both exposures and access to resources relevant to pulmonary health. Geographic differences in climate, leading to differences in health factors such as air pollution, pollen and allergen exposures, and vector-borne diseases are also important to consider in understanding regional disparities in health.[162] Regional and community location determines access to resources, including affordable housing, quality education, public safety, foods availability, health services, public transportation, and occupational opportunity. These resources are subject to change and may interact; for example, a decrease in employment opportunity increases unemployment, impacting population insurance status and functionally decreasing health services availability and housing affordability.[163] Housing location is a further key factor in personal indoor and outdoor exposures, as well as accessibility to community and regional resources. In addition, politics and public health policies specific to a geographic region can impact many important determinants of health ranging from access to care to differences in tobacco regulation.

Although there is no consensus unit of geography on which health and health care is measured, differences between countries, regions (eg, Appalachia or the Pacific Northwest), states, counties, cities, ZIP codes, and neighborhoods are all important units to consider to target and provide resources to improve respiratory disparities.

Asthma

Within the United States, there are wide regional differences in asthma prevalence, morbidity and mortality. Asthma prevalence is highest in the Northeast (New Hampshire 13.2%, Massachusetts 11.5%), Central Appalachia (West Virginia 12.7%, Kentucky 10.7%), and Puerto Rico (12.1%), compared with the national average of 9.4%.[13] Among those who have asthma, asthma control also varies by state, but does not follow a specific geographic pattern. Rates of uncontrolled asthma in adults with asthma ranges from 52% in Massachusetts to 73% in Missouri.[13] A recent study comparing asthma mortality in every US county found that counties along the southern half of the Mississippi River (including counties within Mississippi, Arkansas, and Louisiana), as well as in counties within Georgia and South Carolina, to have the highest mortality.[164]

Regardless of state or geographic region, a higher asthma prevalence and increased asthma morbidity is seen in poor, urban areas throughout the United States.[165,166] Explanatory factors include differences in racial composition, poor health literacy,[167] inadequate access to care, increased indoor pollutants, increased tobacco smoke exposure,[168] and higher exposure to indoor allergens,[169] violence, and psychosocial stress.[170] In contrast, rural geographic regions have lower rates of atopy and asthma compared with the general population.[171–173] Exposure to inhaled or ingested microbial pathogens with subsequent effects on immune function is widely hypothesized for the protective effect of living in rural areas, especially within farming communities.[174]

Chronic Obstructive Pulmonary Disease

COPD prevalence has wide geographic variability. Increased rates of COPD are found in Appalachia (Kentucky 10.1%, West Virginia 8.8%) and in the Southern United States (Alabama 9.9%, Mississippi 8.6%) as compared with national averages (6.5%).[175] Higher rates of COPD are seen in nonmetropolitan areas; age-adjusted rates of COPD ranged from 4.7% of those living in large metropolitan areas to 8.2% in rural areas.[176] COPD morbidity and mortality follows similar geographic trends, with a disproportionate burden in rural areas.[176,177]

Geographic disparities in COPD prevalence and morbidity can be attributed to regionally shared economic, environmental, and behavioral risk factors. As an example, counties in Appalachia have higher rates of poverty (16.3%) compared with the United States average (14.6%),[178] and low SES is a known risk factor for COPD incidence.[179] In addition, in Appalachian counties 22.5% of adults report being cigarette smokers compared with 16.3% at the national level.[180] Other environmental etiologies relevant in Appalachian communities, such as dust in coal mines, are known to cause COPD even in the absence of smoking.[181] COPD morbidity in Appalachia, designated as an underserved area, is driven in part by inadequate access to care owing to geographic isolation.

Pneumoconiosis

Increased rates of diagnosis and mortality from coal workers' pneumoconiosis are almost entirely concentrated in central Appalachia.[164] The largest cluster of progressive massive fibrosis the most advanced stage of coal workers' pneumoconiosis, ever reported was recently described in Appalachia.[105] The highest rates of deaths from coal workers' pneumoconiosis were found in counties in Appalachia (42.5 deaths per 100,000); in comparison, more than 90% of counties in the United States had a coal workers' pneumoconiosis death rate of less than 1 per 100,000. Changes in mining technology, inadequate dust monitoring in slope mines, and increased cutting of rock owing to mining of smaller coal seams common in Appalachia (with subsequent exposure to toxic levels of silica) are all factors that are likely contributing factors.[182]

The highest concentrations of silicosis-related deaths seem to occur in areas associated with mining industries.[183] Age-standardized mortality from silicosis is significantly higher in the Southwestern United States.[164] Data describing the geographic differences in the prevalence or morbidity of asbestosis are limited; however, county-level mortality rates from asbestosis shows several geographic clusters,[164] including Libby, Montana (where asbestos-containing vermiculite was mined and milled from the 1920s to 1990), and counties bordering the gulf coast within Texas, Mississippi, and Alabama (owing to asbestos exposures within oil refineries and shipyards).

Lung Cancer

In the United States, higher rates of lung cancer are seen in the South and Midwest, and lower rates are seen in the West.[72] Lung cancer rates are the highest in rural regions of the country[184]; the most rural counties have an annual lung cancer incidence of almost twice that of the largest

Box 1
Approaches to health disparity reduction

1. Promote disparity awareness.
2. Empower health professionals with knowledge and tools.
3. Engage vulnerable populations in research.
4. Shape responsive research agendas.
5. Advance precision/personalized medicine.
6. Encourage and achieve workforce equity.
7. Develop and advocate for relevant policy.

Data from Refs.[43,194]

metropolitan areas (97.57 per 100,000 population vs 56.56 per 100,000 population).[185] Smoking rates parallel lung cancer prevalence in counties throughout the United States[186]; regional differences in tobacco control and tobacco policy may affect smoking rates and impact rates of lung cancer.[187] Differences in environmental exposures (such as indoor radon exposure and air pollution),[188,189] as well as socioeconomic factors are also important to consider when accounting for geographic lung cancer disparities.

Lung cancer mortality rates also vary by geographic region. The lowest mortality rates are along the United States border with Mexico, Utah, Colorado, and parts of Arizona, New Mexico, and Idaho, and the largest geographic cluster of high lung cancer mortality rates is centered in central Appalachia (>100 deaths per 100,000).[190] A recent analysis has shown that, when compared with large metropolitan areas, residents of rural counties are more likely to present with late stage lung cancer and have a higher death rate from lung cancer.[184] There are numerous factors that drive increased lung cancer mortality in rural regions including high rates of poverty, inadequate health care access, decreased availability of lung cancer screening programs, and a decreased supply of subspecialist physicians, including disparities in access to potentially curative resections for early stage lung cancers.[185,191–193]

SUMMARY

To achieve respiratory health equality, understanding, and addressing the causes of existing pulmonary health disparities is essential. With many complex and inter-related health determinants contributing to existing respiratory health disparities, strategies to decrease existing disparities require multidisciplinary and multilevel approaches. Many modifiable risk factors for pulmonary disparities are highlighted in this article and include occupational and environmental exposures, psychosocial stressors, health behaviors, health literacy, health care provider bias, and health care access. The American Thoracic Society has endorsed a multidisciplinary approach to decrease health disparities (**Box 1**) that includes (1) increasing health disparity awareness, (2) empowering health professionals with knowledge and tools to address disparities, (3) engaging vulnerable populations in research studies for greater representation, (4) shaping research agendas to focus on root causes, to identify modifiable targets and promote innovative approaches to reduce disparities, (5) advancing the fields of precision or personalized medicine to optimize individualization of treatment, (6) achieving equity in the pulmonary and critical care workforce, and (7) developing and advocating for health-related policy aimed at improving the respiratory health of disadvantaged and vulnerable populations.[43,194]

DISCLOSURE

The authors have nothing to disclose.

REFERENCES

1. DHHS. HealthyPeople.gov [Internet]. Disparities. Available at: https://www.healthypeople.gov/2020/about/foundation-health-measures/Disparities. Accessed January 20, 2020.
2. Schraufnagel DE, Blasi F, Kraft M, et al. An official American Thoracic Society/European Respiratory Society policy statement: disparities in respiratory health. Am J Respir Crit Care Med 2013;188(7):865–71.
3. Social determinants of health | CDC [Internet]. 2019. Available at: https://www.cdc.gov/socialdeterminants/index.htm. Accessed January 20, 2020.
4. Braveman P, Gottlieb L. The social determinants of health: it's time to consider the causes of the causes. Public Health Rep 2014;129(Suppl 2):19–31.
5. Bavdekar SB. Pediatric clinical trials. Perspect Clin Res 2013;4(1):89–99.
6. Commissioner O of the. Food and Drug Administration Modernization Act (FDAMA) of 1997 [Internet]. FDA. 2018. Available at: http://www.fda.gov/regulatory-information/selected-amendments-fdc-act/food-and-drug-administration-modernization-act-fdama-1997. Accessed January 20, 2020.
7. NIH Guide: NIH policy and guidelines on the inclusion of children as participants in research involving human subjects [Internet]. Available at:

https://grants.nih.gov/grants/guide/notice-files/not98-024.html. Accessed 2020 Jan 20.

8. Best Pharmaceuticals for Children Act - BPCA [Internet]. Available at: https://www.nichd.nih.gov/ https://www.nichd.nih.gov/research/supported/bpca. Accessed January 20, 2020.
9. DeWine M. S.650 - 108th Congress (2003-2004): Pediatric Research Equity Act of 2003 [Internet]. 2003. Available from: https://www.congress.gov/bill/108th-congress/senate-bill/650. Accessed January 20, 2020.
10. 2019 GINA main report [Internet]. Global Initiative for Asthma - GINA. Available at: https://ginasthma.org/gina-reports/. Accessed January 20, 2020.
11. Martinez FD, Wright AL, Taussig LM, et al. Asthma and wheezing in the first six years of life. The Group Health Medical Associates. N Engl J Med 1995; 332(3):133–8.
12. Taussig LM, Wright AL, Holberg CJ, et al. Tucson Children's respiratory study: 1980 to present. J Allergy Clin Immunol 2003;111(4):661–75 [quiz: 676].
13. CDC. Asthma's effect on the nation. [Internet]. Centers for Disease Control and Prevention. 2019. Available at: https://www.cdc.gov/asthma/asthmadata.htm. Accessed January 20, 2020.
14. Castro-Rodriguez JA, Forno E, Rodriguez-Martinez CE, et al. Risk and protective factors for childhood asthma: what is the evidence? J Allergy Clin Immunol Pract 2016;4(6):1111–22.
15. Burgess JA, Matheson MC, Gurrin LC, et al. Factors influencing asthma remission: a longitudinal study from childhood to middle age. Thorax 2011; 66(6):508–13.
16. Tai A, Tran H, Roberts M, et al. Outcomes of childhood asthma to the age of 50 years. J Allergy Clin Immunol 2014;133(6):1572–8.e3.
17. Sears MR, Greene JM, Willan AR, et al. A longitudinal, population-based, cohort study of childhood asthma followed to adulthood. N Engl J Med 2003;349(15):1414–22.
18. Sood A, Qualls C, Schuyler M, et al. Adult-onset asthma becomes the dominant phenotype among women by age 40 years. the longitudinal CARDIA study. Ann Am Thorac Soc 2013;10(3):188–97.
19. Tan DJ, Walters EH, Perret JL, et al. Clinical and functional differences between early-onset and late-onset adult asthma: a population-based Tasmanian Longitudinal Health Study. Thorax 2016; 71(11):981–7.
20. Kogevinas M, Zock J-P, Jarvis D, et al. Exposure to substances in the workplace and new-onset asthma: an international prospective population-based study (ECRHS-II). Lancet 2007;370(9584):336–41.
21. Shaaban R, Zureik M, Soussan D, et al. Rhinitis and onset of asthma: a longitudinal population-based study. Lancet 2008;372(9643):1049–57.
22. Camargo CA, Weiss ST, Zhang S, et al. Prospective study of body mass index, weight change, and risk of adult-onset asthma in women. Arch Intern Med 1999;159(21):2582–8.
23. Shore SA, Fredberg JJ. Obesity, smooth muscle, and airway hyperresponsiveness. J Allergy Clin Immunol 2005;115(5):925–7.
24. Beuther DA, Sutherland ER. Overweight, obesity, and incident asthma: a meta-analysis of prospective epidemiologic studies. Am J Respir Crit Care Med 2007;175(7):661–6.
25. Global initiative for chronic obstructive lung disease [Internet]. Global initiative for chronic obstructive lung disease - GOLD. Available at: https://goldcopd.org/. Accessed January 20, 2020.
26. Hankinson JL, Odencrantz JR, Fedan KB. Spirometric reference values from a sample of the general U.S. population. Am J Respir Crit Care Med 1999;159(1):179–87.
27. Quanjer PH, Stanojevic S, Cole TJ, et al. Multi-ethnic reference values for spirometry for the 3-95-yr age range: the global lung function 2012 equations. Eur Respir J 2012;40(6):1324–43.
28. Martinez CH, Diaz AA, Parulekar AD, et al. Age-related differences in health-related quality of life in COPD: an analysis of the COPDGene and SPIROMICS Cohorts. Chest 2016;149(4):927–35.
29. Akgun M, Araz O, Ucar EY, et al. Silicosis appears inevitable among former Denim Sandblasters: a 4-year follow-up study. Chest 2015;148(3):647–54.
30. Bang KM, Mazurek JM, Wood JM, et al. Silicosis mortality trends and new exposures to respirable crystalline silica - United States, 2001-2010. MMWR Morb Mortal Wkly Rep 2015;64(5):117–20.
31. Yu DC, Grabowski MJ, Kozakewich HP, et al. Primary lung tumors in children and adolescents: a 90-year experience. J Pediatr Surg 2010;45(6): 1090–5.
32. ATSDR. Radon Toxicity case study: who is at risk of radon exposure? | ATSDR - environmental medicine & environmental health education - CSEM [Internet]. Available at: https://www.atsdr.cdc.gov/csem/csem.asp?csem=8&po=7. Accessed January 20, 2020.
33. American Lung Association. Lung Cancer Fact Sheet [Internet]. Available at: https://www.lung.org/lung-health-and-diseases/lung-disease-lookup/lung-cancer/resource-library/lung-cancer-fact-sheet.html.
34. Lung Cancer Statistics | How common is lung cancer [Internet]. Available at: https://www.cancer.org/cancer/lung-cancer/about/key-statistics.html. Accessed January 20, 2020.
35. Tas F, Ciftci R, Kilic L, et al. Age is a prognostic factor affecting survival in lung cancer patients. Oncol Lett 2013;6(5):1507–13.

36. Booton R, Jones M, Thatcher N. Lung cancer 7: management of lung cancer in elderly patients. Thorax 2003;58(8):711–20.
37. Manuel JI. Racial/ethnic and gender disparities in health care use and access. Health Serv Res 2018;53(3):1407–29.
38. Bolen JC, Rhodes L, Powell-Griner EE, et al. State-specific prevalence of selected health behaviors, by race and ethnicity–Behavioral Risk Factor Surveillance System, 1997. MMWR CDC Surveill Summ 2000;49(2):1–60.
39. Jacobs DE. Environmental health disparities in housing. Am J Public Health 2011;101(Suppl 1): S115–22.
40. Mikati I, Benson AF, Luben TJ, et al. Disparities in distribution of particulate matter emission sources by race and poverty status. Am J Public Health 2018;108(4):480–5.
41. Bailey ZD, Krieger N, Agénor M, et al. Structural racism and health inequities in the USA: evidence and interventions. Lancet 2017;389(10077): 1453–63.
42. Dehon E, Weiss N, Jones J, et al. A systematic review of the impact of physician implicit racial bias on clinical decision making. Acad Emerg Med 2017;24(8):895–904.
43. Celedón JC, Burchard EG, Schraufnagel D, et al. An American Thoracic Society/National Heart, Lung, and Blood Institute Workshop report: addressing respiratory health equality in the United States. Ann Am Thorac Soc 2017;14(5):814–26.
44. Assari S, Chalian H, Bazargan M. High education level protects European Americans but not African Americans against chronic obstructive pulmonary disease: National Health Interview survey. Int J Biomed Eng Clin Sci 2019;5(2):16–23.
45. Assari S. Health disparities due to diminished return among Black Americans: public policy solutions. Soc Issues Policy Rev 2018;12(1): 112–45.
46. Forno E, Celedón JC. Health disparities in asthma. Am J Respir Crit Care Med 2012;185(10):1033–5.
47. Guilbert T, Zeiger RS, Haselkorn T, et al. Racial disparities in asthma-related health outcomes in children with severe/difficult-to-treat asthma. J Allergy Clin Immunol Pract 2019;7(2):568–77.
48. Torgerson DG, Ampleford EJ, Chiu GY, et al. Meta-analysis of genome-wide association studies of asthma in ethnically diverse North American populations. Nat Genet 2011;43(9):887–92.
49. Fitzpatrick AM, Gillespie SE, Mauger DT, et al. Racial disparities in asthma-related health care use in the National Heart, Lung, and Blood Institute's severe asthma research program. J Allergy Clin Immunol 2019;143(6):2052–61.
50. Boehmer TK, Foster SL, Henry JR, et al, Centers for Disease Control and Prevention (CDC). Residential proximity to major highways - United States, 2010. MMWR Suppl 2013;62(3):46–50.
51. Guarnieri M, Balmes JR. Outdoor air pollution and asthma. Lancet 2014;383(9928):1581–92.
52. Breysse PN, Diette GB, Matsui EC, et al. Indoor air pollution and asthma in children. Proc Am Thorac Soc 2010;7(2):102–6.
53. Kravitz-Wirtz N, Teixeira S, Hajat A, et al. Early-life air pollution exposure, neighborhood poverty, and childhood asthma in the United States, 1990–2014. Int J Environ Res Public Health 2018;15(6):1–14. Available at: https://www.ncbi.nlm.nih.gov/pmc/articles/PMC6025399/.
54. Tsai J, Homa DM, Gentzke AS, et al. Exposure to secondhand smoke among Nonsmokers - United States, 1988-2014. MMWR Morb Mortal Wkly Rep 2018;67(48):1342–6.
55. Gilliland FD, Li YF, Peters JM. Effects of maternal smoking during pregnancy and environmental tobacco smoke on asthma and wheezing in children. Am J Respir Crit Care Med 2001;163(2):429–36.
56. Kozyrskyj AL, Mai XM, McGrath P, et al. Continued exposure to maternal distress in early life is associated with an increased risk of childhood asthma. - PubMed - NCBI [Internet]. Am J Respir Crit Care Med 2008;177(2):142–7. Available at: https://www.ncbi.nlm.nih.gov/pubmed/17932381.
57. Bellin M, Osteen P, Collins K, et al. The influence of community violence and protective factors on asthma morbidity and healthcare utilization in high-risk children. Bull N Y Acad Med 2014;91(4): 677–89.
58. Barnthouse M, Jones BL. The impact of environmental chronic and toxic stress on asthma. Clin Rev Allergy Immunol 2019;57(3):427–38.
59. Centers for Disease Control and Prevention (CDC). Chronic obstructive pulmonary disease among adults–United States, 2011. MMWR Morb Mortal Wkly Rep 2012;61(46):938–43.
60. Celedón JC. Achieving respiratory health equality: a United States perspective. Humana Press; 2016. p. 210.
61. Dransfield MT, Davis JJ, Gerald LB, et al. Racial and gender differences in susceptibility to tobacco smoke among patients with chronic obstructive pulmonary disease. Respir Med 2006;100(6): 1110–6.
62. Wang X, Li W, Huang K, et al. Genetic variants in ADAM33 are associated with airway inflammation and lung function in COPD. BMC Pulm Med 2014;14:173.
63. Aldrich MC, Kumar R, Colangelo LA, et al. Genetic ancestry-smoking interactions and lung function in African Americans: a cohort study. PLoS One 2012; 7(6):e39541.
64. Jamal A, Dube SR, King BA. Tobacco use screening and counseling during hospital

outpatient visits among US adults, 2005-2010. Prev Chronic Dis 2015;12:E132.

65. Foreman MG, Zhang L, Murphy J, et al. Early-onset chronic obstructive pulmonary disease is associated with female sex, maternal factors, and African American race in the COPDGene study. Am J Respir Crit Care Med 2011;184(4):414–20.
66. Kamil F, Pinzon I, Foreman MG. Sex and race factors in early-onset COPD. Curr Opin Pulm Med 2013;19(2):140–4.
67. Pleasants RA, Riley IL, Mannino DM. Defining and targeting health disparities in chronic obstructive pulmonary disease. Int J Chron Obstruct Pulmon Dis 2016;11:2475–96.
68. Employed persons by detailed industry, sex, race, and Hispanic or Latino ethnicity [Internet]. Available at: https://www.bls.gov/cps/cpsaat18.htm. Accessed January 20, 2020.
69. Mazurek JM. Coal workers' pneumoconiosis–attributable years of potential life lost to life expectancy and potential life lost before age 65 Years — United States, 1999–2016. MMWR Morb Mortal Wkly Rep 2018;67:819–24. Available at: https://www.cdc.gov/mmwr/volumes/67/wr/mm6730a3.htm.
70. Rose C, Heinzerling A, Patel K, et al. Severe silicosis in engineered stone fabrication workers - California, Colorado, Texas, and Washington, 2017-2019. MMWR Morb Mortal Wkly Rep 2019;68(38):813–8.
71. Reilly MJ, Timmer SJ, Rosenman KD. The burden of silicosis in Michigan: 1988–2016. Ann Am Thorac Soc 2018;15(12):1404–10.
72. Centers for Disease Control and Prevention (CDC). Racial/Ethnic disparities and geographic differences in lung cancer incidence — 38 States and the District of Columbia, 1998-2006. MMWR Morb Mortal Wkly Rep 2010;59(44):1434–8.
73. Gadgeel SM, Kalemkerian GP. Racial differences in lung cancer. Cancer Metastasis Rev 2003;22(1):39–46.
74. QuickStats. Age-adjusted death rates* from lung cancer,† by race/ethnicity - National Vital Statistics System, United States, 2001-2016. MMWR Morb Mortal Wkly Rep 2018;67(30):840.
75. Varlotto JM, Voland R, McKie K, et al. Population-based differences in the outcome and presentation of lung cancer patients based upon racial, histologic, and economic factors in all lung patients and those with metastatic disease. Cancer Med 2018;7(4):1211–20.
76. Japuntich SJ, Krieger NH, Salvas AL, et al. Racial disparities in lung cancer screening: an exploratory investigation. J Natl Med Assoc 2018;110(5):424–7.
77. Tanner NT, Gebregziabher M, Hughes Halbert C, et al. Racial differences in outcomes within the national lung screening trial. Implications for widespread implementation. Am J Respir Crit Care Med 2015;192(2):200–8.
78. Balekian AA, Wisnivesky JP, Gould MK. Surgical disparities among patients with stage I lung cancer in the national lung screening trial. Chest 2019;155(1):44–52.
79. Shugarman LR, Mack K, Sorbero MES, et al. Race and sex differences in the receipt of timely and appropriate lung cancer treatment. Med Care 2009;47(7):774–81.
80. Farjah F, Wood DE, Yanez ND, et al. Racial disparities among patients with lung cancer who were recommended operative therapy. Arch Surg 2009;144(1):14–8.
81. Ruparel M, Navani N. Fulfilling the dream. Toward reducing inequalities in lung cancer screening. Am J Respir Crit Care Med 2015;192(2):125–7.
82. De Matteis S, Consonni D, Bertazzi PA. Exposure to occupational carcinogens and lung cancer risk. Evolution of epidemiological estimates of attributable fraction. Acta Biomed 2008;79(Suppl 1):34–42.
83. Birdsey J, Alterman T, Petersen MR. Race, occupation, and lung cancer: detecting disparities with death certificate data. J Occup Environ Med 2007;49(11):1257–63.
84. Lloyd JW. Long-term mortality study of steelworkers. V. Respiratory cancer in coke plant workers. J Occup Med 1971;13(2):53–68.
85. de Marco R, Locatelli F, Sunyer J, et al. Differences in incidence of reported asthma related to age in men and women. A retrospective analysis of the data of the European Respiratory Health Survey. Am J Respir Crit Care Med 2000;162(1):68–74.
86. Chen Y, Stewart P, Johansen H, et al. Sex difference in hospitalization due to asthma in relation to age. J Clin Epidemiol 2003;56(2):180–7.
87. van der Merwe L, de Klerk A, Kidd M, et al. Case-control study of severe life threatening asthma (SLTA) in a developing community. Thorax 2006;61(9):756–60.
88. Kodadhala V, Obi J, Wessly P, et al. Asthma-related mortality in the United States, 1999 to 2015: a multiple causes of death analysis. Ann Allergy Asthma Immunol 2018;120(6):614–9.
89. Melgert BN, Ray A, Hylkema MN, et al. Are there reasons why adult asthma is more common in females? Curr Allergy Asthma Rep 2007;7(2):143–50.
90. Yung JA, Fuseini H, Newcomb DC. Hormones, sex, and asthma. Ann Allergy Asthma Immunol 2018;120(5):488–94.
91. Mohan SS, Knuiman MW, Divitini ML, et al. Higher serum testosterone and dihydrotestosterone, but not oestradiol, are independently associated with favourable indices of lung function in community-

dwelling men. Clin Endocrinol (Oxf) 2015;83(2): 268–76.

92. Cephus J-Y, Stier MT, Fuseini H, et al. Testosterone attenuates group 2 innate lymphoid cell-mediated airway inflammation. Cell Rep 2017 28;21(9): 2487–99.
93. White GE, Seaman C, Filios MS, et al. Gender differences in work-related asthma: surveillance data from California, Massachusetts, Michigan, and New Jersey, 1993-2008. J Asthma 2014; 51(7):691–702.
94. Anderson NJ, Reeb-Whitaker CK, Bonauto DK, et al. Work-related asthma in Washington state. J Asthma 2011;48(8):773–82.
95. Fletcher AM, London MA, Gelberg KH, et al. Characteristics of patients with work-related asthma seen in the New York state occupational health clinics. J Occup Environ Med 2006;48(11): 1203–11.
96. Blosnich JR, Lee JGL, Bossarte R, et al. Asthma disparities and within-group differences in a national, probability sample of same-sex partnered adults. Am J Public Health 2013;103(9):e83–7.
97. Pinkerton KE, Harbaugh M, Han MK, et al. Women and lung disease. Sex differences and global health disparities. Am J Respir Crit Care Med 2015;192(1):11–6.
98. United States Surgeon General. The health consequences of smoking - 50 Years of progress: a report of the Surgeon general: (510072014-001) [Internet]. American Psychological Association. 2014. Available at: http://doi.apa.org/get-pe-doi.cfm?doi=10.1037/e510072014-001. Accessed January 20, 2020.
99. Gan WQ, Man SFP, Postma DS, et al. Female smokers beyond the perimenopausal period are at increased risk of chronic obstructive pulmonary disease: a systematic review and meta-analysis. Respir Res 2006;7:52.
100. Siddharthan T, Grigsby MR, Goodman D, et al. Association between household air pollution exposure and chronic obstructive pulmonary disease outcomes in 13 low- and middle-income country settings. Am J Respir Crit Care Med 2018 01;197(5): 611–20.
101. Doney B, Hnizdo E, Syamlal G, et al. Prevalence of chronic obstructive pulmonary disease among US working adults aged 40 to 70 years. National Health Interview Survey data 2004 to 2011. J Occup Environ Med 2014;56(10):1088–93.
102. Chapman KR, Tashkin DP, Pye DJ. Gender bias in the diagnosis of COPD. Chest 2001;119(6):1691–5.
103. Smith PH, Kasza KA, Hyland A, et al. Gender differences in medication use and cigarette smoking cessation: results from the International Tobacco Control Four Country Survey. Nicotine Tob Res 2015;17(4):463–72.
104. Laney AS, Blackley DJ, Halldin CN. Radiographic disease progression in contemporary US coal miners with progressive massive fibrosis. Occup Environ Med 2017;74(7):517–20.
105. Blackley DJ, Reynolds LE, Short C, et al. Progressive massive fibrosis in coal miners from 3 Clinics in Virginia. JAMA 2018;319(5):500–1.
106. Maxfield R, Alo C, Reilly MJ, et al. Surveillance for silicosis, 1993–Illinois, Michigan, New Jersey, North Carolina, Ohio, Texas, and Wisconsin. MMWR CDC Surveill Summ 1997;46(1):13–28.
107. Asbestosis [Internet]. Available at: https://wwwn.cdc.gov/eWorld/Grouping/Asbestosis/92. Accessed January 20, 2020.
108. Holford TR, Levy DT, McKay LA, et al. Patterns of birth cohort-specific smoking histories, 1965-2009. Am J Prev Med 2014;46(2):e31–7.
109. Jemal A, Miller KD, Ma J, et al. Higher lung cancer incidence in young women than young men in the United States. N Engl J Med 2018;378(21): 1999–2009.
110. Risch HA, Howe GR, Jain M, et al. Are female smokers at higher risk for lung cancer than male smokers? A case-control analysis by histologic type. Am J Epidemiol 1993;138(5): 281–93.
111. Ramchandran K, Patel JD. Sex differences in susceptibility to carcinogens. Semin Oncol 2009; 36(6):516–23.
112. Mollerup S, Berge G, Baera R, et al. Sex differences in risk of lung cancer: expression of genes in the PAH bioactivation pathway in relation to smoking and bulky DNA adducts. Int J Cancer 2006;119(4):741–4.
113. Hellyer JA, Patel MI. Sex disparities in lung cancer incidence: validation of a long-observed trend. Transl Lung Cancer Res 2019;8(4):543–5.
114. Harichand-Herdt S, Ramalingam SS. Gender-associated differences in lung cancer: clinical characteristics and treatment outcomes in women. Semin Oncol 2009;36(6):572–80.
115. Sagerup CMT, Småstuen M, Johannesen TB, et al. Sex-specific trends in lung cancer incidence and survival: a population study of 40,118 cases. Thorax 2011;66(4):301–7.
116. Wakelee HA, Chang ET, Gomez SL, et al. Lung cancer incidence in never smokers. J Clin Oncol 2007;25(5):472–8.
117. Fu JB, Kau TY, Severson RK, et al. Lung cancer in women: analysis of the national Surveillance, Epidemiology, and End Results database. Chest 2005;127(3):768–77.
118. Tong BC, Kosinski AS, Burfeind WR, et al. Sex differences in early outcomes after lung cancer resection: analysis of the Society of Thoracic Surgeons General Thoracic Database. J Thorac Cardiovasc Surg 2014;148(1):13–8.

119. Socioeconomic status [Internet]. Available at: https://www.apa.org https://www.apa.org/topics/socioeconomic-status/index. Accessed January 20, 2020.
120. Bureau UC. Personal income: PINC-04 [Internet]. The United States Census Bureau. Available at: https://www.census.gov/data/tables/time-series/demo/income-poverty/cps-pinc/pinc-04.html. Accessed January 20, 2020.
121. Hovanec J, Siemiatycki J, Conway DI, et al. Lung cancer and socioeconomic status in a pooled analysis of case-control studies. PLoS One 2018;13(2):e0192999.
122. Chen E, Shalowitz MU, Story RE, et al. Dimensions of socioeconomic status and childhood asthma outcomes: evidence for distinct behavioral and biological associations. Psychosom Med 2016;78(9):1043–52.
123. Uphoff E, Cabieses B, Pinart M, et al. A systematic review of socioeconomic position in relation to asthma and allergic diseases. Eur Respir J 2015;46(2):364–74.
124. Galobardes B, Shaw M, Lawlor DA, et al. Indicators of socioeconomic position (part 1). J Epidemiol Community Health 2006;60(1):7–12.
125. Davey Smith G, Hart C, Hole D, et al. Education and occupational social class: which is the more important indicator of mortality risk? J Epidemiol Community Health 1998;52(3):153–60.
126. Socioeconomic position [Internet]. Available at: https://deepblue.lib.umich.edu/handle/2027.42/51520?show=full. Accessed January 20, 2020.
127. Gong T, Lundholm C, Rejnö G, et al. Parental socioeconomic status, childhood asthma and medication use–a population-based study. PLoS One 2014;9(9):e106579.
128. Eagan TML, Gulsvik A, Eide GE, et al. The effect of educational level on the incidence of asthma and respiratory symptoms. Respir Med 2004;98(8):730–6.
129. Harrington KF, Zhang B, Magruder T, et al. The impact of parent's health literacy on pediatric asthma outcomes. Pediatr Allergy Immunol Pulmonol 2015;28(1):20–6.
130. Emilio CC, Mingotti CFB, Fiorin PR, et al. Is a low level of education a limiting factor for asthma control in a population with access to pulmonologists and to treatment? J Bras Pneumol 2019;45(1):e20180052.
131. Prescott E, Lange P, Vestbo J. Socioeconomic status, lung function and admission to hospital for COPD: results from the Copenhagen City Heart Study. Eur Respir J 1999;13(5):1109–14.
132. Eisner MD, Blanc PD, Omachi TA, et al. Socioeconomic status, race and COPD health outcomes. J Epidemiol Community Health 2011;65(1):26–34.
133. Gjerdevik M, Grydeland TB, Washko GR, et al. The relationship of educational attainment with pulmonary emphysema and airway wall thickness. Ann Am Thorac Soc 2015;12(6):813–20.
134. Omachi TA, Sarkar U, Yelin EH, et al. Lower health literacy is associated with poorer health status and outcomes in chronic obstructive pulmonary disease. J Gen Intern Med 2013;28(1):74–81.
135. Wagner GR. Asbestosis and silicosis. Lancet 1997;349(9061):1311–5.
136. Nandi S, Burnase N, Barapatre A, et al. Assessment of silicosis awareness among stone mine workers of Rajasthan state. Indian J Occup Environ Med 2018;22(2):97–100.
137. Mao Y, Hu J, Ugnat AM, et al, Canadian Cancer Registries Epidemiology Research Group. Socioeconomic status and lung cancer risk in Canada. Int J Epidemiol 2001;30(4):809–17.
138. Mitra D, Shaw A, Tjepkema M, et al. Social determinants of lung cancer incidence in Canada: a 13-year prospective study. Health Rep 2015;26(6):12–20.
139. Aldrich MC, Selvin S, Wrensch MR, et al. Socioeconomic status and lung cancer: unraveling the contribution of genetic admixture. Am J Public Health 2013;103(10):e73–80.
140. Sidorchuk A, Agardh EE, Aremu O, et al. Socioeconomic differences in lung cancer incidence: a systematic review and meta-analysis. Cancer Causes Control CCC 2009;20(4):459–71.
141. Mouw T, Koster A, Wright ME, et al. Education and risk of cancer in a large cohort of men and women in the United States. PLoS One 2008;3(11):e3639.
142. van Loon AJ, Goldbohm RA, van den Brandt PA. Lung cancer: is there an association with socioeconomic status in The Netherlands? J Epidemiol Community Health 1995;49(1):65–9.
143. Albano JD, Ward E, Jemal A, et al. Cancer mortality in the United States by education level and race. J Natl Cancer Inst 2007;99(18):1384–94.
144. Finke I, Behrens G, Weisser L, et al. Socioeconomic differences and lung cancer survival-systematic review and meta-analysis. Front Oncol 2018;8:536.
145. Herndon JE, Kornblith AB, Holland JC, et al. Patient education level as a predictor of survival in lung cancer clinical trials. J Clin Oncol 2008;26(25):4116–23.
146. Di Maio M, Signoriello S, Morabito A, et al. Prognostic impact of education level of patients with advanced non-small cell lung cancer enrolled in clinical trials. Lung Cancer 2012;76(3):457–64.
147. Ameille J, Pairon JC, Bayeux MC, et al. Consequences of occupational asthma on employment and financial status: a follow-up study. Eur Respir J 1997;10(1):55–8.
148. Bracker A, Blumberg J, Hodgson M, et al. Industrial hygiene recommendations as interventions: a

collaborative model within occupational medicine. Appl Occup Environ Hyg 1999;14(2):85–96.
149. Smoking rates still high among low-income Americans: disparities ongoing | the Nation's Health [Internet]. Available at: http://thenationshealth.aphapublications.org/content/47/8/1.2. Accessed January 20, 2020.
150. Grabenhenrich LB, Gough H, Reich A, et al. Early-life determinants of asthma from birth to age 20 years: a German birth cohort study. J Allergy Clin Immunol 2014;133(4):979–88.
151. McWhorter WP, Polis MA, Kaslow RA. Occurrence, predictors, and consequences of adult asthma in NHANESI and follow-up survey. Am Rev Respir Dis 1989;139(3):721–4.
152. Litonjua AA, Carey VJ, Weiss ST, et al. Race, socioeconomic factors, and area of residence are associated with asthma prevalence. Pediatr Pulmonol 1999;28(6):394–401.
153. Lawson JA, Janssen I, Bruner MW, et al. Asthma incidence and risk factors in a national longitudinal sample of adolescent Canadians: a prospective cohort study. BMC Pulm Med 2014;14:51.
154. Erzen D, Carriere KC, Dik N, et al. Income level and asthma prevalence and care patterns. Am J Respir Crit Care Med 1997;155(3):1060–5.
155. Cope SF, Ungar WJ, Glazier RH. Socioeconomic factors and asthma control in children. Pediatr Pulmonol 2008;43(8):745–52.
156. Ungar WJ, Paterson JM, Gomes T, et al. Relationship of asthma management, socioeconomic status, and medication insurance characteristics to exacerbation frequency in children with asthma. Ann Allergy Asthma Immunol 2011;106(1):17–23.
157. Borné Y, Ashraf W, Zaigham S, et al. Socioeconomic circumstances and incidence of chronic obstructive pulmonary disease (COPD) in an urban population in Sweden. COPD 2019;16(1):51–7.
158. Jamie Sullivan MPH, Pravosud V, David M, et al. National and state estimates of COPD morbidity and mortality — United States, 2014-2015. Chronic Obstr Pulm Dis 2018;5(4):324–33.
159. Lowe KE, Make BJ, Crapo JD, et al. Association of low income with pulmonary disease progression in smokers with and without chronic obstructive pulmonary disease. ERJ Open Res 2018;4(4).
160. Porta AS, Lam N, Novotny P, et al, NETT Research Group. Low income as a determinant of exercise capacity in COPD. Chron Respir Dis 2019;16. 1479972318809491.
161. Job Search - Millions of Jobs Hiring Near You [Internet]. ZipRecruiter. Available at: https://www.ziprecruiter.com/. Accessed January 20, 2020.
162. Haines A, Kovats RS, Campbell-Lendrum D, et al. Climate change and human health: impacts, vulnerability, and mitigation. Lancet 2006; 367(9528):2101–9.
163. Souza K, Steege AL, Baron SL. Surveillance of occupational health disparities: challenges and opportunities. Am J Ind Med 2010;53(2):84–94.
164. Dwyer-Lindgren L, Bertozzi-Villa A, Stubbs RW, et al. Trends and patterns of differences in chronic respiratory disease mortality among US counties, 1980-2014. JAMA 2017;318(12):1136–49.
165. Mak H, Johnston P, Abbey H, et al. Prevalence of asthma and health service utilization of asthmatic children in an inner city. J Allergy Clin Immunol 1982;70(5):367–72.
166. Busse WW. The National Institutes of Allergy and Infectious Diseases networks on asthma in inner-city children: an approach to improved care. J Allergy Clin Immunol 2010;125(3):529–37 [quiz: 538–9].
167. Halm EA, Mora P, Leventhal H. No symptoms, no asthma: the acute episodic disease belief is associated with poor self-management among inner-city adults with persistent asthma. Chest 2006; 129(3):573–80.
168. Poowuttikul P, Saini S, Seth D. Inner-City asthma in children. Clin Rev Allergy Immunol 2019;56(2): 248–68.
169. Rosenstreich DL, Eggleston P, Kattan M, et al. The role of cockroach allergy and exposure to cockroach allergen in causing morbidity among inner-city children with asthma. N Engl J Med 1997; 336(19):1356–63.
170. Landeo-Gutierrez J, Forno E, Miller GE, et al. Exposure to violence, psychosocial stress, and asthma. Am J Respir Crit Care Med 2020;201(8):917–22.
171. Riedler J, Braun-Fahrländer C, Eder W, et al. Exposure to farming in early life and development of asthma and allergy: a cross-sectional survey. Lancet 2001;358(9288):1129–33.
172. Ernst P, Cormier Y. Relative scarcity of asthma and atopy among rural adolescents raised on a farm. Am J Respir Crit Care Med 2000; 161(5):1563–6.
173. Braun-Fahrländer C, Gassner M, Grize L, et al. Prevalence of hay fever and allergic sensitization in farmer's children and their peers living in the same rural community. SCARPOL team. Swiss Study on Childhood Allergy and Respiratory Symptoms with Respect to Air Pollution. Clin Exp Allergy 1999;29(1):28–34.
174. Douwes J, Pearce N. Asthma and the westernization "package. Int J Epidemiol 2002;31(6): 1098–102.
175. Ford ES, Croft JB, Mannino DM, et al. COPD surveillance–United States, 1999-2011. Chest 2013; 144(1):284–305.
176. Croft JB, Wheaton AG, Liu Y, et al. Urban-rural county and state differences in chronic obstructive pulmonary disease - United States, 2015. MMWR Morb Mortal Wkly Rep 2018;67(7):205–11.

177. Holt JB, Zhang X, Presley-Cantrell L, et al. Geographic disparities in chronic obstructive pulmonary disease (COPD) hospitalization among Medicare beneficiaries in the United States. Int J Chron Obstruct Pulmon Dis 2011;6:321–8.
178. The Appalachian Region: a data overview from the 2013-2017 American Community Survey - Appalachian Regional Commission [Internet]. Available at: https://www.arc.gov/research/researchreportdetails.asp?REPORT_ID=159. Accessed January 20, 2020.
179. Kanervisto M, Vasankari T, Laitinen T, et al. Low socioeconomic status is associated with chronic obstructive airway diseases. Respir Med 2011; 105(8):1140–6.
180. Health Disparities in Appalachia - Appalachian Regional Commission [Internet]. Available at: https://www.arc.gov/research/researchreportdetails.asp?REPORT_ID=138. Accessed January 20, 2020.
181. Laney AS, Weissman DN. Respiratory diseases caused by coal mine dust. J Occup Environ Med 2014;56(Suppl 10):S18–22.
182. Cohen RA, Petsonk EL, Rose C, et al. Lung pathology in U.S. coal workers with rapidly progressive pneumoconiosis implicates silica and silicates. Am J Respir Crit Care Med 2016;193(6):673–80.
183. Thomas CR, Kelley TR. A brief review of silicosis in the United States. Environ Health Insights 2010;4: 21–6.
184. Henley SJ, Anderson RN, Thomas CC, et al. Invasive cancer incidence, 2004-2013, and deaths, 2006-2015, in nonmetropolitan and metropolitan counties - United States. Morb Mortal Wkly Rep Surveill Summ 2017;66(14):1–13.
185. Atkins GT, Kim T, Munson J. Residence in rural areas of the United States and lung cancer mortality. Disease incidence, treatment disparities, and stage-specific survival. Ann Am Thorac Soc 2017;14(3):403–11.
186. Alberg AJ, Samet JM. Epidemiology of lung cancer. Chest 2003;123(1 Suppl):21S–49S.
187. Hahn EJ, Rayens MK, Wiggins AT, et al. Lung cancer incidence and the strength of municipal smoke-free ordinances. Cancer 2018;124(2):374–80.
188. US EPA O. Find Information about Local Radon Zones and State Contact Information [Internet]. US EPA. 2014. Available at: https://www.epa.gov/radon/find-information-about-local-radon-zones-and-state-contact-information. Accessed January 20, 2020.
189. Cohen AJ. Outdoor air pollution and lung cancer. Environ Health Perspect 2000;108(Suppl 4): 743–50.
190. Mokdad AH, Dwyer-Lindgren L, Fitzmaurice C, et al. Trends and patterns of disparities in cancer mortality among US counties, 1980-2014. JAMA 2017;317(4):388–406.
191. Shugarman LR, Sorbero MES, Tian H, et al. An exploration of urban and rural differences in lung cancer survival among Medicare beneficiaries. Am J Public Health 2008;98(7):1280–7.
192. Jenkins WD, Matthews AK, Bailey A, et al. Rural areas are disproportionately impacted by smoking and lung cancer. Prev Med Rep 2018;10:200–3.
193. Martin AN, Hassinger TE, Kozower BD, et al. Disparities in lung cancer screening availability: lessons from Southwest Virginia. Ann Thorac Surg 2019;108(2):412–6.
194. Thakur N, McGarry ME, Oh SS, et al. The lung corps' approach to reducing health disparities in respiratory disease. Ann Am Thorac Soc 2014; 11(4):655–60.

Respiratory Health Effects of Exposure to Cleaning Products

Sara De Matteis, MD, MPH, PhD[a,b,*], Steven Ronsmans, MD[c,d,1], Benoit Nemery, MD, PhD[d,1]

KEYWORDS

• Cleaning • Respiratory health • Occupational health • Epidemiology • Toxicology

KEY POINTS

- Cleaning-related respiratory health effects are an important occupational and public health issue.
- A wide variety of respiratory symptoms and conditions have been reported as linked to use of cleaning products.
- Cleaning agents have hazardous properties, which may lead to health effects via several underlying mechanisms.
- Preventive measures to avoid the cleaning-related respiratory health burden are warranted.

INTRODUCTION: WHY IS THIS AN IMPORTANT PUBLIC HEALTH ISSUE?

There is consistent and growing evidence of an epidemic of "asthma-like" symptoms among professional cleaners. Important questions remain unanswered: How big is this problem worldwide? Which cleaning agents are dangerous and how do they affect the lungs? And, is it really asthma?

This issue is important to clinical and public health, given the large and increasing number of professional cleaners (about 4 million in Europe),[1] many from vulnerable groups, such as women, immigrants, and those of low socioeconomic status. Such figures are likely an underestimation given that many in this job sector are self-employed and others may not be legal residents.

There are significant public health costs arising from:

a .Cleaners who leave work because of ill health, and

b .Cleaners who develop chronic respiratory effects that persist, even if they avoid further exposure.

In addition, there are potentially important health implications for all end-users of cleaning products during domestic housekeeping. The public health impact may be higher still if there are effects from passive, bystander exposure, including vulnerable subjects such as children. In this article, we address these issues using the available evidence on this topic, from epidemiology to toxicology, to give a broad but concise overview on what it known to

Funding sources: S. Ronsmans is supported by the Fund Van Mulders-Moonens managed by the King Baudouin Foundation (2018-J3812960–209723) and by KU Leuven C2 project funding (C24/18/085).

[a] Department of Medical Sciences and Public Health, University of Cagliari, Cagliari, Italy; [b] NHLI, Imperial College London, London, United Kingdom; [c] Clinic for Occupational and Environmental Medicine, Department of Pulmonary Medicine, University Hospitals Leuven, Leuven, Belgium; [d] Centre for Environment and Health, Department of Public Health and Primary Care, KU Leuven, Leuven, Belgium

[1] Herestraat 49, box 706, B-3000 Leuven, Belgium.

* Corresponding author. Cittadella Universitaria di Monserrato, Asse Didattico Medicina, Blocco I, Piano 0, Stanza 18, Cagliari 09042, Italy.

E-mail addresses: sara.dem@unica.it; s.de-matteis@imperial.ac.uk

Twitter: @SaraOccEpi (S.D.M.)

Clin Chest Med 41 (2020) 641–650

https://doi.org/10.1016/j.ccm.2020.08.010

date and how to prevent the burden of cleaning-associated respiratory disorders.

IS THERE A GLOBAL "ASTHMA" EPIDEMIC AMONG PROFESSIONAL CLEANERS?

A number of population and workforce based studies worldwide have reported an increased prevalence and incidence of asthma-like symptoms among professional cleaners, mostly in the developed countries (Europe, the United States).[2,3] Recently a meta-analysis[4] of 16 high-quality epidemiologic studies addressing asthma-like symptoms in professional cleaners was performed (**Fig. 1**). Cleaning health issues have been reported mainly in female professional cleaners, with no specific age or ethnical patterns. Neither atopy nor smoking habit seem to be related to an increased risk. Most of the evidence comes from epidemiologic population-based studies[4] (see **Fig. 1**). This finding is not surprising, given the nature of the cleaning sector, which is mostly based on part-time and self-employed workers, thus making it difficult to recruit and conduct traditional occupational cohort studies.

Most cohort studies have involved hospital nurses with cleaning tasks, thus limiting external generalizability because of exposure to peculiar cleaning agents used to disinfect or sterilize medical instruments or inpatients units, summarized in **Fig. 1**. The majority of the cohort studies have a cross-sectional design, are thus may be affected by the healthy worker survivor effect bias; that is, the underestimation of the true prevalence of a health condition in a workforce owing to the negative selection of the workers who become ill or unfit and so leave their job and, vice versa, the retention of the healthiest and fittest workers. Also, occupational exposure to cleaning agents is mostly retrospectively self-reported, so may be affected by the so-called recall bias (ie, systematic error in reporting past exposure or conditions). Cleaners who are affected by significant respiratory symptoms or are ill may be more likely than asymptomatic or healthy ones to report previous exposure to cleaning agents, especially to those with pungent odor, such as bleach, so possibly producing differential misclassification of exposure and spurious causal associations with these types of substances. Understandably, none of the studies were able to measure quantitatively exposure to cleaning agents and dose-responses, which would further strengthen the validity of the associations.

In relation to the health outcome definitions, most of the epidemiology studies have defined asthma as self-reported by cleaners. Only a few used a spirometry-based definition, and so misclassification of the outcome and an overestimation of the true asthma prevalence in this workforce is possible. In contrast, the fact that this epidemic of respiratory disease has been reported only in cleaners and not others job categories, and

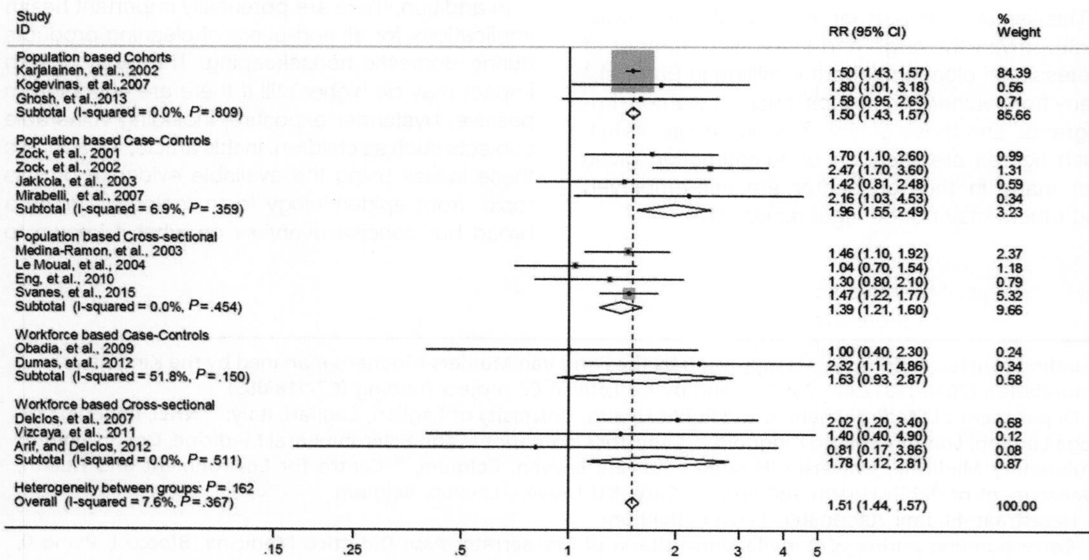

Fig. 1. Meta-analysis of 16 studies evaluating the association between professional cleaning exposure and asthma risk (relative risk [RR] and 95% confidence interval [CI]). (*From* Archangelidi O, De Matteis S, Jarvis D. P146 Cleaning products and respiratory health outcomes in professional cleaners: a systematic review and meta-analysis. *Thorax*. 2018;73(Suppl 4):A181-A182. With permission.)

consistently in time and space across several countries, supports the validity of these epidemiologic findings. A further issue is related to the challenge of defining occupational asthma (ie, adult new-onset asthma caused by respiratory hazards at work) and to differentiate it from work-exacerbated asthma (ie, preexisting asthma triggered or aggravated by respiratory hazards at work).

Given these caveats, this recent meta-analysis, which pooled 16 high-quality epidemiologic studies that similarly defined occupational asthma among cleaners, estimated a pooled substantially increased relative risk of occupational asthma of 1.51 (95% confidence interval, 1.44–1.57) among cleaners (see **Fig. 1**).[4]

IS IT REALLY ASTHMA?

As reported elsewhere in this article, the definition of occupational asthma among cleaners in most previous epidemiologic studies is self-reported, and so potentially affected by disease misclassification. The gold standard for diagnosing sensitizer-induced allergic asthma (ie, positive specific inhalation challenge test with the suspected causal cleaning agent) has been reported in a few case report or case series studies only.[5,6] This result is not surprising, given the complexity and the costs associated with specific inhalation challenge testing, including a sealed inhalation chamber, the ability to generate and monitor the exposure, trained staff, and close monitoring in a hospital setting. Such testing is rarely accessible or feasible in most countries. Moreover, for irritant-induced asthma there is no such gold standard test, making the attribution of asthma to a specific irritant exposure difficult on an individual level.

Importantly the presentation of asthma among cleaners has been atypical, including less association with atopy, inflammatory biomarkers and eosinophilia, and limited bronchial reversibility.[7] This finding has generated scientific and clinical interest in evaluating a broader range of alternative cleaning-related respiratory health effects, including chronic obstructive pulmonary disease (COPD) and vocal cord dysfunction.

Among other respiratory outcomes presenting with asthma-like symptoms, the risk of COPD has been investigated in several epidemiologic studies. A significant association of cleaning job with spirometrically defined COPD (ie, forced expiratory volume in 1 second/forced vital capacity, with a forced vital capacity of less than the lower limit of normal) was found in a recent large population-based cross-sectional analysis of 228,614 people in the UK Biobank study. A 43% risk increase (prevalence ratio, 1.43; 95% confidence interval, 1.28–1.59) was found for cleaning occupation, which was also seen in analyses restricted to never smokers, and nonasthmatics.[8]

Two workforce-based studies found an increased risk of COPD in cleaners and hospital nurses. A cross-sectional study of 13,499 Northern European cleaners reported an increased risk of self-reported COPD (odds ratio, 1.69; 95% confidence interval, 1.29–2.20).[9] Of note, a recent US cohort study among hospital nurses found that regular use of chemical disinfectants increased the incidence of COPD by about 30%, with positive response trends for frequency and duration of exposure.[10] These findings support the hypothesis, discussed in detail elsewhere in this article, that exposure to noxious chemicals in cleaning products is able to produce not only acute but also chronic airways obstruction.

Also, a population-based cross-sectional study found a significant increase in phlegm and dyspnea prevalence suggestive for chronic bronchitis among cleaners compared with office workers used as controls, taking into account tobacco smoking as potential confounder.[11] Another population-based case-control study found a similar result among domestic cleaners only when chronic bronchitis symptoms were combined with asthma symptoms as an outcome.[12]

Of note, some authors have suggested, based on case series, that upper airway conditions that mimic asthma symptoms, such as vocal cord dysfunction (ie, paradoxic laryngeal movement resulting in inappropriate adduction of the vocal cords), may be associated with exposure to cleaning agents and be mediated by irritative mechanisms.[13]

WHAT ARE CLEANING PRODUCTS?

Cleaning products are complex chemical mixtures used to facilitate dust and dirt removal (**Fig. 2**), to disinfect, and to maintain surfaces. Household users and professional cleaners use a broad range of products: all-purpose cleaners, specialty cleaners (eg, for floor, bathroom, oven), surface care products, decalcifiers, laundry products, dishwashing agents, drain cleaners, and so on. The patterns of use of domestic cleaning products—such as sprays, household bleach, and ammonia—differ substantially across different countries.[14]

In health care settings, products for cleaning medical instruments (eg, endoscopes) and disinfection, in addition to common cleaning agents, are regularly used.[15] Special cleaning products

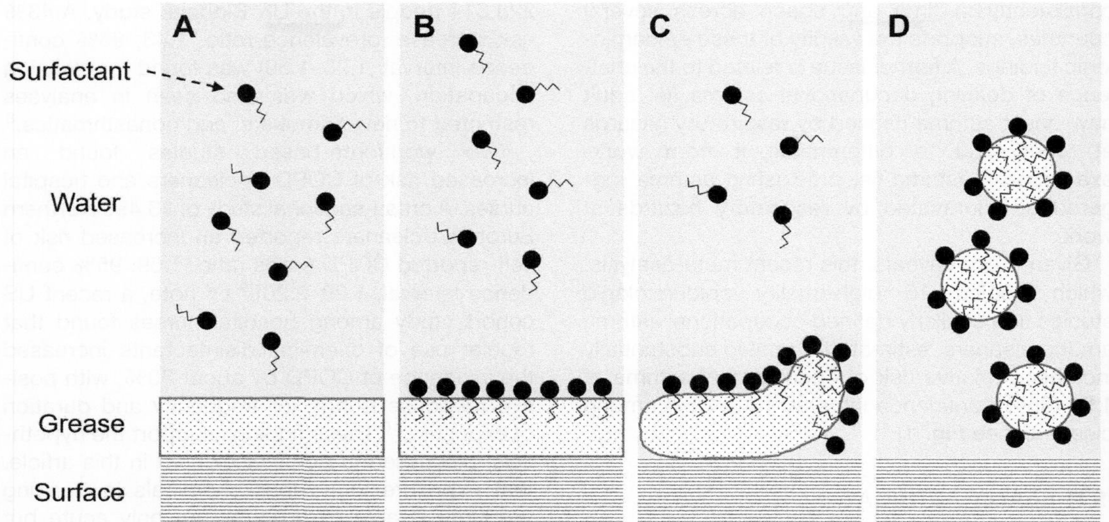

Fig. 2. Mechanism of action of soaps and detergents on dirt. (*A*) Detergent or soap dissolves in water. (*B*) Hydrophilic head and lipophilic tail of surfactant ions orientate themselves in water and grease. (*C*) Grease separated from surface. (*D*) Clean surface.

are also used in food preparation, agriculture and intensive animal farming, façade cleaning, graffiti removal, and industrial cleaning. Disinfectants are included in a wide range of cleaning products—including common household products—to destroy microbial life through different mechanisms, or combinations of mechanisms, such as damage to microbial cell walls, damage to microbial DNA, and protein denaturation.[16] Commonly used disinfectants are chlorine-releasing compounds, such as hypochlorite (household bleach) and chloramine-T, alcohols (ethanol, isopropanol), aldehydes (formaldehyde, glutaraldehyde, orthophthalaldehyde), quaternary ammonium compounds (benzalkonium chloride), oxygen-releasing compounds (hydrogen peroxide, peracetic acid), biguanides (chlorhexidine), and enzymes (see **Fig. 2**)

Cleaning products are an ever-changing technology. In the 1960s, proteolytic enzymes were introduced to improve the efficacy of washing powders, leading to high rates of asthma among detergent production workers,[17] and some evidence for IgE-associated allergy among domestic users.[18] Encapsulation of enzymes and engineering controls in the detergent factories led to decreases in the occurrence of asthma. In recent decades, a number of new enzymes (proteases, amylases, lipases, cellulases) have been introduced in several types of cleaning products[19]—many now known to be potent respiratory sensitizers. More recently, cleaning products containing living microorganisms or spores—such as *Bacillus* spores[20]—as active ingredients have been introduced on the market. The respiratory health effects of these microbial-based cleaning products are poorly studied. Nevertheless, it is reasonable to consider them as possible respiratory sensitizers.[21]

PRODUCTION AND RESPIRATORY UPTAKE OF CLEANING-RELATED GASES AND PARTICLES

When using cleaning products ingredients can become airborne in gaseous form (volatile compounds) or as an aerosol (volatile and nonvolatile compounds). The site where airborne compounds are deposited in the airways is an important determinant of where and whether respiratory effects will occur.

Volatile constituents or reaction products of the cleaning products can enter the gas phase during or after use. Air concentrations of volatilized compounds depend on the cleaning task, amount of product used, boiling point, surface tension, size of the surface (air–liquid interface), concentration of the compound, water temperature, and room size, humidity, temperature and ventilation.[22] Even normal use—that is, without mixing or using abnormally high amounts—of hypochlorite- and ammonia-containing products can produce air concentrations of chlorine and ammonia exceeding recommended occupational short-term exposure limits.[12,23]

A major concern associated with the use of hypochlorite (ClO^-) is that mixing with ammonia-based products, or even with urine, results in the formation of highly irritating chloramines ($NH_2Cl \rightarrow NHCl_2 \rightarrow NCl_3$), whereas mixing with acid-containing products creates chlorine gas (Cl_2). Mixing such cleaning products has been associated with irritant-induced asthma in cleaners.[3] Even without mixing, commercially available hypochlorite-containing products can emit substantial amounts of halogenated volatile compounds—mainly chloroform and carbon tetrachloride—owing to the reaction of hypochlorite with organic molecules, such as surfactants and fragrances.[24]

The site where an inhaled gas is deposited in the respiratory tract is mainly determined by its water solubility.[25] Highly water-soluble irritant gases, such as ammonia and hydrogen chloride, are mainly deposited in the upper airways, causing acute irritation while sparing the lower respiratory tract. Less soluble gases, such as ozone and several solvents, penetrate into the lower airway. They often cause no immediate symptoms but can cause irritant effects in the bronchi, terminal bronchioles, and alveoli. Gases of intermediate solubility, such as chlorine, may exert irritant effects widely throughout the respiratory tract.

Nonvolatile ingredients such as surfactants, acids and bases, quaternary ammonium compounds, preservatives, and enzymes can become airborne when droplets are produced by using sprays and, to a lesser extent, by splashing or pouring of liquid products or by secondary resuspension of particles from surfaces. The concentration and droplet size distribution of the aerosol generated by spraying depends largely on the spray nozzle and dispersion mechanism used (pump vs propellant spray).[26] An experimental study showed that using a low-pressure nozzle could decrease the inhalable and thoracic fraction by up to 92%.[27]

MECHANISMS OF ADVERSE RESPIRATORY EFFECTS

The wide range of compounds that can reach the airways at various sites, combined with the variable frequency and duration of exposure, result in a broad spectrum of potential respiratory health effects.[28] Cleaning products may contain well-established sensitizers or irritants, chemicals with poorly characterized respiratory effects, or mixtures of all 3 agents.

Sensitizer-Induced (Allergic) Rhinitis and Asthma

Some cleaning agents can induce sensitization by an immunologic mechanism and cause allergic rhinitis or asthma. Positive bronchial and nasal provocation tests have been reported for chloramine-T,[29,30] quaternary ammonium salts,[31,32] triclosan,[33] amines,[34] glutaraldehyde,[6] ortho-phthalaldehyde,[35] fragrances,[36] and enzymes.[37,38] An IgE-mediated mechanism has been suggested for very few compounds, such as chloramine-T,[39] ortho-phthalaldehyde,[40] and enzymes.[37] Most sensitizers in cleaning products probably act via immunologic non–IgE-mediated mechanisms. For ethylenediaminetetra-acetic acid, a pharmacologic mechanism—linked to its calcium-chelating activity—has been suggested by both experimental and clinical data.[41]

Interestingly, animal experiments have shown that the initial sensitization leading to the development of asthma does not necessarily occur in the airways, but might also occur via the skin.[42,43] Låstbom and colleagues[44] showed that guinea pigs that were first skin sensitized to 3-carene—a commonly used fragrance component and a potent skin-sensitizer—had an increased airway responsiveness after subsequent inhalation of 3-carene, when compared with non–skin-sensitized animals. This finding could be relevant for professional cleaners in whom allergic contact dermatitis is highly prevalent. Allergic contact dermatitis and asthmatic symptoms have been shown to be associated in this population.[45]

Irritant-Induced Respiratory Disorders

The respiratory health effects of cleaning products frequently are nonallergic, that is, they do not involve a specific recognition by the adaptive immune system. Rather they cause irritation by direct action on neurons or other cells. Such irritant responses can range from simple, transient discomfort to persistent conjunctivitis, rhinitis, sinusitis, pharyngitis, vocal cord dysfunction or inducible larynx obstruction,[46] asthma, bronchitis, COPD,[47] and rarely pneumonitis.[48,49] Irritants can induce new-onset asthma after a single, high-level exposure (known as reactive airways dysfunction syndrome), as well as after chronic exposure to moderate levels of irritants. Also, preexisting asthma can be exacerbated by irritant exposures (work-exacerbated asthma).[50] Cases of toxic pneumonitis have been reported owing to waterproofing agents[48] and mixing of household ammonia and bleach.[49]

According to the Globally Harmonized System of Classification and Labeling of Chemicals respiratory irritants are labeled with the hazard statement H335 ("May cause respiratory irritation"). The term respiratory tract irritation can be used to indicate either or both of 2 different but interlinked toxicologic effects: sensory and tissue irritation.[51]

Sensory irritation

Sensory irritation occurs through stimulation of receptors in the afferent trigeminal or vagal nerves that innervate the airway (and ocular) mucosae. Two key transient receptor potential (TRP) channels are present in the afferent nerve endings in the airways: TRPV1 and TRPA1. These nonselective cation channels can be directly stimulated by a variety of inhaled agents and mediate sensory irritation as part of a physiologic response to make the subject aware of the presence of chemicals by inducing pain, nasal pungency, eye irritation, and defensive reflex responses, such as cough, sneezing, mucus hypersecretion, and bronchoconstriction.[52] Upon activation of the sensory nerves, various neuropeptides are released locally. These neuropeptides trigger an airway neurogenic inflammation[50] that reflects the transition from pure sensory, reversible effects to a general and inflammatory defense mechanism.

Animal experiments have shown that TRPA1 is essential for irritant-induced airway responses.[53,54] Hox and colleagues[55] demonstrated that the induction of airway hyperreactivity by inhalation of hypochlorite depends on TRPA1 stimulation. A rapid and concentration-dependent decline in respiratory rate in mice, is considered an important toxicologic parameter, because the RD_{50}—the irritant concentration inducing a 50% decrease in respiratory rate in mice (known as the Alarie animal bioassay)—correlates well with subjective complaints of sensory irritation in humans.[56]

Thus, it has been proposed that chronic irritant stimulation of TRPA1 and TRPV1 can lead to long-lasting neurogenic inflammation, contributing to tissue damage and the development of airway disease and to prolonged airway hyperreactivity to multiple irritants, clinically similar to irritant-induced asthma.[51,52] However, this sequence remains to be proven in humans.

Tissue irritation

Tissue irritation is characterized by direct epithelial damage of the airways induced by an irritant agent.[57] There is no clear correlation between exposure concentrations leading to sensory irritation—as measured with the Alarie animal bioassay—and those inducing tissue irritation in the respiratory tract after single or repeated exposure.[58] Some compounds may cause tissue irritation and injury without exhibiting much sensory warning (eg, hydrogen fluoride). However, the 2 mechanisms are interlinked, because injured epithelium can lead to exposure of nerve endings and induce neurogenic inflammation.[57] Also, damaged epithelial cells release signaling molecules, acting as warning signals to the nearby tissues, and initiating and modulating an inflammatory response, which in turn can modulate the sensitivity and expression of sensory neuronal TRP receptors.[52]

Human bronchial biopsies taken shortly after an acute exposure to chlorine showed considerable epithelial desquamation with an inflammatory exudate and swelling of the subepithelial space.[59] Experimental animal studies have confirmed the importance of airway barrier damage in the context of irritant-induced asthma.[60] Studies looking at long-term pathologic consequences of acute high-level irritant exposures followed by asthmatic symptoms (reactive airways dysfunction syndrome) showed significant neutrophilic and/or eosinophilic inflammatory changes in the bronchial wall and remodeling similar to allergic asthma in many aspects.[61]

Interactions Between Irritation and Sensitization

Several sensitizers also have irritant properties, including disinfectants (glutaraldehyde, quaternary ammonium salts, chloramine-T, isothiazolinone), ethanolamine and enzymes. Moreover, exposure to irritants and enzymes can increase the risk of sensitization[62] and may increase specific bronchial responsiveness to an allergen to which the subject has been previously sensitized.[63] Irritants can also disrupt the epithelial barrier and facilitate the crossing of allergens.[62] Moreover, airway epithelial cells express pattern recognition receptors that detect irritants and damage-associated molecular patterns released upon tissue damage. The activation of epithelial pattern recognition receptors leads to the release of endogenous danger signals that attract and activate innate and adaptive immune cells.[64] Interactions between allergenic and irritant exposures are particularly relevant to cleaners, given that cleaning products commonly contain multiple different agents and the use of multiple different cleaning products.

FUTURE STEPS AND CONCLUSIONS

Potential Preventive Strategies (Cleaning Agent Types, Formulations, and Respiratory Health Surveillance)

In the occupational health field, prevention is hierarchically classified into primary, secondary, and tertiary. The best practice is primary prevention, which aims to eliminate or at least minimize exposure to occupational hazards at work to avoid the consequent health effects among exposed workers. If this is unachievable, secondary prevention can be implemented via periodic occupational health surveillance of exposed workers for early detection of any adverse health effects or symptoms, and thus to prevent disease onset. When these interventions fail, tertiary prevention aims to diagnose and manage occupational disease that has already occurred. The last intervention should be considered a failure of an occupational health preventive strategy, both for the individual (worker's disease, potential job loss), and also for society (occupational disease medical costs, compensation costs).

In relation to the prevention of cleaning-related respiratory health effects, a primary preventive approach would focus on the identification and removal of cleaning agents capable of damaging the respiratory system. This approach is challenging for multiple reasons, including the increasing demand for cleaning and disinfecting products, manufacturer protections by industrial trade secrets (ie, not all ingredients must be disclosed in products labels), and more limited testing of the many agents in cleaning products for potential respiratory health effects. Under current international occupational health and safety regulations, manufacturers are now required to test (in vitro and in vivo) new agents for potential health effects, and for those already on the market, Globally Harmonized System of Classification and Labeling of Chemicals standardized risk phrases must be provided in the safety data sheets. In addition, occupational exposures can be regulated or restricted by national occupational health and safety regulations. However, occupational exposure limits have not been established for the majority of the more than 300 agents that have been reported as asthmagens or respiratory hazards.[65]

As knowledge about the respiratory health effects of cleaning products expands, manufacturers should avoid more hazardous ingredients (eg, quaternary ammonium compounds) and/or substitute less harmful formulations (eg, less volatile ortho-phthalaldehyde instead of glutaraldehyde). A growing number of green cleaning products are now available on the market, although it remains unclear how safe these green products are if inhaled. A recent cross-sectional study of 329 custodians found a lower prevalence of upper and lower respiratory symptoms in users of environmentally preferable cleaning products compared with traditional cleaning products.[2]

Another important primary preventive intervention is to decrease cleaning exposures through better education and training of cleaners about the risks of cleaning products and safer work practices, such as incorrect mixing of products or modification of specific job tasks. Inhalation accidents in cleaners, such as mixing bleach and ammonia in small, poorly ventilated areas, have led to irritant-induced occupational asthma and work-exacerbated asthma.[3] Specific job tasks, such as kitchen cleaning, furniture polishing, cleaning windows, washing dishes, mopping/waxing floors, spot cleaning carpets, and cleaning tiles and grout, have been identified as causing or exacerbating asthma, and can be targeted for preventive interventions.[12,66–68] General work practice guidance, such as limiting the use of spray products, avoiding excessive product usage and improving indoor ventilation, can decrease individual worker exposures. Personal respiratory protective equipment is considered the last resort, and there is no evidence or agreement on the efficacy of specific respirator type to protect against cleaning-related respiratory health effects.

In many countries, domestic cleaners are primarily used in the informal sector and/or in conditions characterized by low wages, limited worker organizations, few legal protections, and a limited ability to select the products they use. Preventive approaches based on participation and empowerment of cleaners have had success in identifying hazards and changing work practices.[69]

The substantial challenges in primary and secondary prevention supports implementation of occupational respiratory health surveillance programs among cleaners. For example, periodic questionnaires can be administered to cleaners as a screening tool to detect work-related respiratory symptoms and new or increased use of respiratory medications, and prompt referral for further medical evaluation, including spirometry and other diagnostic testing. A careful occupational and medical history, review of cleaning products and practices, and safety data sheets can help identify potential causative agents and support a diagnosis of work-related asthma. Peak flow diaries may identify work-related changes and further support a diagnosis of work-related asthma. Reduction or avoidance of exposure to the suspected hazardous cleaning agent(s) is recommended, along with standard medical treatment. Unfortunately, the high turnover and job instability of this type of workforce, combined with the reluctancy of workers to report symptoms for fear of losing their job, make respiratory health surveillance, clinical recognition, and preventive interventions challenging.

Ideally, respiratory health conditions suspected to be work-related among cleaners should be evaluated as early as possible to optimize management and limit further exposures to the potential causal agent(s) at work. Cleaners should be advised about available job options and compensation programs. In addition, cases of cleaning-related respiratory disease should be reported to available surveillance systems for occupational diseases, such as MODERNET in Europe,[70] to estimate the public health burden and incidence trends, identify new causal agents, and characterize associated respiratory phenotypes.

In conclusion, cleaning-related respiratory health effects are preventable by using an integrated multi-step approach focused on primary prevention to reduce cleaning exposures, as well as respiratory surveillance of cleaners and early diagnosis.

Research Gaps to Address

A collaborative effort with a multidisciplinary translational approach involving also cutting-edge molecular methods, and improved exposure assessment, could help to fill the knowledge gap on this important topic. Ideally, large prospective cohorts of professional cleaners should be followed longitudinally with quantitative and qualitative exposure assessment techniques, including personal air monitoring and task-based approaches. Such approaches can help to identify higher risk cleaning tasks and products, as well as dose–response relationships, which can support causal associations and better preventive strategies. There is also a need to better phenotype cleaning-associated respiratory health effects, including host characteristics, respiratory and non-respiratory health effects. Another important challenge is that cleaners commonly are exposed to multiple cleaning products, each one typically a mixture of substances, including irritants and/or allergens, which can interact with each other, and also differentially impact underlying pathogenic mechanisms. Further characterization of such exposures is needed to better understand cleaning-related respiratory conditions and protect exposed workers, a challenging black box.[71]

Given the large numbers of cleaners and cleaning and disinfectant products in use worldwide, and the expanding literature documenting increased risk of asthma, COPD, and other respiratory health effects in cleaners, it is also critical to increase awareness of cleaning-related respiratory disease among pulmonary and primary care providers.

DISCLOSURE

The authors have nothing to disclose.

REFERENCES

1. EU-OSHA – European Agency for Safety and Health at Work. The occupational safety and health of cleaning workers - Literature review. Luxembourg (Europe), 2009.
2. Folletti I, Siracusa A, Paolocci G. Update on asthma and cleaning agents. Curr Opin Allergy Clin Immunol 2017;17(2):90–5.
3. Siracusa A, De Blay F, Folletti I, et al. Asthma and exposure to cleaning products - a European academy of allergy and clinical immunology task force consensus statement. Allergy 2013;68(12):1532–45.
4. Archangelidi O, De Matteis S, Jarvis D. P146 Cleaning products and respiratory health outcomes in professional cleaners: a systematic review and meta-analysis. Thorax 2018;73(Suppl 4):A181–2.
5. Sastre J, Madero MF, Fernández-Nieto M, et al. Airway response to chlorine inhalation (bleach) among cleaning workers with and without bronchial hyperresponsiveness. Am J Ind Med 2011;54(4):293–9.
6. Vandenplas O, D'Alpaos V, Evrard G, et al. Asthma related to cleaning agents: a clinical insight. BMJ Open 2013;3(9):e003568.
7. Vizcaya D, Mirabelli MC, Orriols R, et al. Functional and biological characteristics of asthma in cleaning workers. Respir Med 2013;107(5):673–83.
8. De Matteis S, Jarvis D, Hutchings S, et al. Occupations associated with COPD risk in the large population-based UK Biobank cohort study. Occup Environ Med 2016;73(6):378–84. oemed-2015-103406.
9. Ø Svanes, Bertelsen RJ, Lygre SH, et al. Cleaning at home and at work in relation to lung function decline and airway obstruction. Am J Respir Crit Care Med 2018. https://doi.org/10.1164/rccm.201706-1311OC.
10. Dumas O, Varraso R, Boggs KM, et al. Association of occupational exposure to disinfectants with incidence of chronic obstructive pulmonary disease among us female nurses. JAMA Netw Open 2019;2(10):e1913563.
11. Karadzinska-Bislimovska J, Minov J, Risteska-Kuc S, et al. Bronchial hyperresponsiveness in women cooks and cleaners. Arh Hig Rada Toksikol 2007;58(2):223–31.
12. Medina-Ramón M, Zock JP, Kogevinas M, et al. Asthma, chronic bronchitis, and exposure to irritant agents in occupational domestic cleaning: a nested case-control study. Occup Environ Med 2005;62(9):598–606.
13. Perkner JJ, Fennelly KP, Balkissoon R, et al. Irritant-associated vocal cord dysfunction. J Occup Environ Med 1998;40(2):136.
14. Zock J, Plana E, Jarvis D, et al. The use of household cleaning sprays and adult asthma. Am J Respir Crit Care Med 2007;176(8):735–41.
15. Dumas O, Wiley AS, Henneberger PK, et al. Determinants of disinfectant use among nurses in U.S.

healthcare facilities. Am J Ind Med 2017;60(1): 131–40.

16. McDonnell G, Russell AD. Antiseptics and disinfectants: activity, action, and resistance. Clin Microbiol Rev 1999;12(1):147–79.
17. Flindt ML. Pulmonary disease due to inhalation of derivatives of Bacillus subtilis containing proteolytic enzyme. Lancet 1969;1(7607):1177–81.
18. Belin L, Hoborn J, Falsen E, et al. Enzyme sensitisation in consumers of enzyme-containing washing powder. Lancet 1970;2(7684):1153–7.
19. Budnik LT, Scheer E, Burge PS, et al. Sensitising effects of genetically modified enzymes used in flavour, fragrance, detergence and pharmaceutical production: cross-sectional study. Occup Environ Med 2017;74(1):39–45.
20. Berg NW, Evans MR, Sedivy J, et al. Safety assessment of the use of Bacillus-based cleaning products. Food Chem Toxicol 2018;116:42–52.
21. Bernstein L, Bernstein JA, Miller M, et al. Immune responses in farm workers after exposure to Bacillus thuringiensis pesticides. Environ Health Perspect 1999;107(7):8.
22. Bello A, Quinn MM, Perry MJ, et al. Quantitative assessment of airborne exposures generated during common cleaning tasks: a pilot study. Environ Health 2010;9:76.
23. Fedoruk MJ, Bronstein R, Kerger BD. Ammonia exposure and hazard assessment for selected household cleaning product uses. J Expo Sci Environ Epidemiol 2005;15(6):534–44.
24. Odabasi M. Halogenated volatile organic compounds from the use of chlorine-bleach-containing household products. Environ Sci Technol 2008; 42(5):1445–51.
25. Nemery B. Inhalation injury, chemical. In: Laurent GJ, Shapiro SD, editors. Encyclopedia of respiratory medicine. Oxford (United Kingdom): Academic Press; 2006. p. 208–16.
26. Schwarz K, Koch W. Thoracic and respirable aerosol fractions of spray products containing non-volatile compounds. J Occup Environ Hyg 2017;14(10):831–8.
27. Olsen R, Pedersen I, Berlinger B, et al. Rengjøringsmidler i Sprayform – Frigir de Helseskadelige Stoffer Til Arbeidsatmosfæren Som Kan Inhaleres Til Lungene?. Oslo (Norway): STAMI; 2017.
28. Cummings KJ, Virji MA. The long-term effects of cleaning on the lungs. Am J Respir Crit Care Med 2018;197(9):1099–101.
29. Kujala VM, Reijula KE, Ruotsalainen EM, et al. Occupational asthma due to chloramine-T solution. Respir Med 1995;89(10):693–5.
30. Mäkelä R, Kauppi P, Suuronen K, et al. Occupational asthma in professional cleaning work: a clinical study. Occup Med 2011;61(2):121–6.
31. Purohit A, Kopferschmitt-Kubler MC, Moreau C, et al. Quaternary ammonium compounds and occupational asthma. Int Arch Occup Environ Health 2000;73(6):423–7.
32. Burge PS, Richardson MN. Occupational asthma due to indirect exposure to lauryl dimethyl benzyl ammonium chloride used in a floor cleaner. Thorax 1994;49(8):842–3.
33. Walters GI, Robertson AS, Moore VC, et al. Occupational asthma caused by sensitization to a cleaning product containing triclosan. Ann Allergy Asthma Immunol 2017;118(3):370–1.
34. Savonius B, Keskinen H, Tuppurainen M, et al. Occupational asthma caused by ethanolamines. Allergy 1994;49(10):877–81.
35. Robitaille C, Boulet L-P. Occupational asthma after exposure to ortho-phthalaldehyde (OPA). Occup Environ Med 2015;72(5):381.
36. López-Sáez MP, Carrillo P, Huertas AJ, et al. Occupational asthma and dermatitis induced by eugenol in a cleaner. J Investig Allergol Clin Immunol 2015; 25(1):64–5.
37. Hole AM, Draper A, Jolliffe G, et al. Occupational asthma caused by bacillary amylase used in the detergent industry. Occup Environ Med 2000; 57(12):840–2.
38. Brant A, Hole A, Cannon J, et al. Occupational asthma caused by cellulase and lipase in the detergent industry. Occup Environ Med 2004;61(9): 793–5.
39. Kramps JA, van Toorenenbergen AW, Vooren PH, et al. Occupational asthma due to inhalation of chloramine-T. II. Demonstration of specific IgE antibodies. Int Arch Allergy Appl Immunol 1981;64(4): 428–38.
40. Suzukawa M, Komiya A, Koketsu R, et al. Three cases of ortho-phthalaldehyde-induced anaphylaxis after laryngoscopy: detection of specific IgE in serum. Allergol Int 2007;56(3):313–6.
41. Laborde-Castérot H, Villa AF, Rosenberg N, et al. Occupational rhinitis and asthma due to EDTA-containing detergents or disinfectants. Am J Ind Med 2012;55(8):677–82.
42. Pollaris L, Van Den Broucke S, Decaesteker T, et al. Dermal exposure determines the outcome of repeated airway exposure in a long-term chemical-induced asthma-like mouse model. Toxicology 2019;421:84–92.
43. Tsui H-C, Ronsmans S, Sadeleer LD, et al. Low-molecular weight agents inducing airway sensitization via skin exposure: a systematic review of experimental models. Eur Respir J 2019;54(suppl 63). https://doi.org/10.1183/13993003.congress-2019.PA5240.
44. Låstbom L, Boman A, Johnsson S, et al. Increased airway responsiveness of a common fragrance component, 3-carene, after skin sensitisation—a study in isolated Guinea pig lungs. Toxicol Lett 2003;145(2):189–96.

45. Lynde CB, Obadia M, Liss GM, et al. Cutaneous and respiratory symptoms among professional cleaners. Occup Med 2009;59(4):249–54.
46. Halvorsen T, Walsted ES, Bucca C, et al. Inducible laryngeal obstruction: an official joint European Respiratory Society and European Laryngological Society statement. Eur Respir J 2017;50(3):1602221.
47. Van den Borre L, Deboosere P. Health risks in the cleaning industry: a Belgian census-linked mortality study (1991–2011). Int Arch Occup Environ Health 2018;91(1):13–21.
48. Vernez D, Bruzzi R, Kupferschmidt H, et al. Acute respiratory syndrome after inhalation of waterproofing sprays: a posteriori exposure-response assessment in 102 cases. J Occup Environ Hyg 2006;3(5):250–61.
49. Reisz GR, Gammon RS. Toxic pneumonitis from mixing household cleaners. Chest 1986;89(1):49–52.
50. Vandenplas O, Wiszniewska M, Raulf M, et al. EAACI position paper: irritant-induced asthma. Allergy 2014;69(9):1141–53.
51. Brüning T, Bartsch R, Bolt HM, et al. Sensory irritation as a basis for setting occupational exposure limits. Arch Toxicol 2014;88(10):1855–79.
52. Bessac BF, Jordt S-E. Sensory detection and responses to toxic gases: mechanisms, health effects, and countermeasures. Proc Am Thorac Soc 2010; 7(4):269–77.
53. Bessac BF, Sivula M, von Hehn CA, et al. Transient receptor potential ankyrin 1 antagonists block the noxious effects of toxic industrial isocyanates and tear gases. FASEB J 2009;23(4):1102–14.
54. Taylor-Clark TE, Kiros F, Carr MJ, et al. Transient receptor potential ankyrin 1 mediates toluene diisocyanate-evoked respiratory irritation. Am J Respir Cell Mol Biol 2009;40(6):756–62.
55. Hox V, Vanoirbeek JA, Alpizar YA, et al. Crucial role of transient receptor potential ankyrin 1 and mast cells in induction of nonallergic airway hyperreactivity in mice. Am J Respir Crit Care Med 2013;187(5): 486–93.
56. Nielsen GD, Wolkoff P. Evaluation of airborne sensory irritants for setting exposure limits or guidelines: a systematic approach. Regul Toxicol Pharmacol 2017;90:308–17.
57. Maestrelli P, Boschetto P, Fabbri LM, et al. Mechanisms of occupational asthma. J Allergy Clin Immunol 2009;123(3):531–42 [quiz: 543–44].
58. Bos PMJ, Busschers M, Arts JHE. Evaluation of the sensory irritation test (Alarie test) for the assessment of respiratory tract irritation. J Occup Environ Med 2002;44(10):968–76.
59. Lemière C, Malo JL, Boutet M. Reactive airways dysfunction syndrome due to chlorine: sequential bronchial biopsies and functional assessment. Eur Respir J 1997;10(1):241–4.
60. Van Den Broucke S, Pollaris L, Vande Velde G, et al. Irritant-induced asthma to hypochlorite in mice due to impairment of the airway barrier. Arch Toxicol 2018;92(4):1551–61.
61. Takeda N, Maghni K, Daigle S, et al. Long-term pathologic consequences of acute irritant-induced asthma. J Allergy Clin Immunol 2009;124(5): 975–81.e1.
62. Biagini RE, Moorman WJ, Lewis TR, et al. Ozone enhancement of platinum asthma in a primate model. Am Rev Respir Dis 1986;134(4):719–25.
63. Molfino NA, Wright SC, Katz I, et al. Effect of low concentrations of ozone on inhaled allergen responses in asthmatic subjects. Lancet 1991; 338(8761):199–203.
64. Lambrecht BN, Hammad H. The airway epithelium in asthma. Nat Med 2012;18(5):684–92.
65. De Matteis S, Heederik D, Burdorf A, et al. Current and new challenges in occupational lung diseases. Eur Respir Rev 2017;26(146):170080.
66. Zock JP, Kogevinas M, Sunyer J, et al. Asthma risk, cleaning activities and use of specific cleaning products among Spanish indoor cleaners. Scand J Work Environ Health 2001;27(1):76–81.
67. Obadia M, Liss GM, Lou W, et al. Relationships between asthma and work exposures among non-domestic cleaners in Ontario. Am J Ind Med 2009; 52(9):716–23.
68. Rosenman K, Reilly MJ, Pechter E, et al. Cleaning Products and work-related asthma, 10 year update. J Occup Environ Med 2019. https://doi.org/10.1097/JOM.0000000000001771.
69. Flum M, Eduardo Siqueira C, DeCaro A, et al. Photovoice in the workplace: a participatory method to give voice to workers to identify health and safety hazards and promote workplace change—a study of university custodians. Am J Ind Med 2011; 53(11):1150–8.
70. Carder M, Seed MJ, Money A, et al. Occupational and work-related respiratory disease attributed to cleaning products. Occup Environ Med 2019. https://doi.org/10.1136/oemed-2018-105646. oemed-2018-105646.
71. De Matteis S, Cullinan P. Occupational asthma in cleaners: a challenging black box. Occup Environ Med 2015;72(11):755–6.

Work-Related Upper-Airway Disorders

Ambrose Lau, MD[a], Susan M. Tarlo, MB BS[b,*]

KEYWORDS

• Occupational • Allergic rhinitis • Rhinitis • Irritable larynx • Inducible laryngeal disorder
• Laryngeal cough

KEY POINTS

- Occupational exposures may cause or exacerbate rhinitis and often co-exist with occupational asthma.
- Occupational rhinitis can have a significant impact on quality of life and work productivity, especially "presenteeism."
- Laryngeal syndromes can mimic or accompany work-related asthma and can also lead to absenteeism.
- Chronic cough from laryngeal causes can be exacerbated by stimuli at work or outside the workplace that normally would not cause a cough, such as scented products, bleach, voice use, exercise, and cold air.
- Laryngoscopy with provocation and speech language therapy are important components of diagnosis and management of laryngeal syndromes.

INTRODUCTION

The upper airway refers to the portion of the airway above the vocal cords and includes the nasal cavities, pharynx, and larynx. This area is richly innervated with sensory fibers and reflex pathways that can stimulate cough, sneezing, secretions, and nasal obstruction. The passage of air through the nose helps to filter and condition the air before it enters the lower-respiratory tract. Mucous membranes in the upper airway are routinely exposed to environmental irritants and infectious organisms. In the workplace, the nose is often the primary target of vapors, gases, dusts, and fumes. The larynx serves 2 primary functions of protecting the lower-respiratory tract by occluding the airway and the modulation of the pitch and volume of sound generated.

The most common occupational upper-airway conditions are work-related rhinitis (WRR) and work-related laryngeal syndromes and are the subject of this review. Less common conditions, such as olfactory dysfunction and sinonasal neoplasms, also occur, but are not covered.

WORK-RELATED RHINITIS AND ASSOCIATION WITH WORK-RELATED ASTHMA

Rhinitis is a common condition affecting most individuals at some point in their lifetime. Symptoms are characterized by nasal congestion, discharge, itching, and sneezing. Prevalence of chronic allergic rhinitis has been reported to range from 15% to 30% in adults[1] and contributes significantly to reduced productivity in the workplace, reduced sleep adequacy, and poorer quality of life.[2]

Occupational rhinitis (OR) has been defined as "an inflammatory disease of the nose, which is characterized by intermittent or persistent

[a] Department of Medicine, Toronto Western Hospital, St Michael's Hospital, 399 Bathurst Street, Toronto, Ontario M5T 2S8, Canada; [b] Department of Medicine, Dalla Lana School of Public Health, University of Toronto, Toronto Western Hospital, St Michael's Hospital, EW7-449, 399 Bathurst Street, Toronto, Ontario M5T 2S8, Canada
* Corresponding author.
E-mail address: susan.tarlo@utoronto.ca

Clin Chest Med 41 (2020) 651–660
https://doi.org/10.1016/j.ccm.2020.08.001
0272-5231/20/

symptoms (ie, nasal obstruction, sneezing, rhinorrhea, itching) and/or variable nasal airflow limitation and/or hypersecretion arising out of causes and conditions attributable to a particular work environment and not to stimuli encountered outside the workplace."[3] Work-exacerbated rhinitis (WER) is preexisting or concurrent rhinitis that is made worse by the workplace. The more global term of WRR is used to describe both OR and WER. Paralleling the classification system for occupational asthma, OR can be further classified as allergic with a history of sensitization to a substance in the workplace, or irritant induced (**Fig. 1**). Although allergic OR is thought to require a period of latency, irritant-induced OR can occur with or without latency. When it occurs without latency, this is called reactive upper-airways dysfunction syndrome (RUDS).[4] The most severe form of RUDS is corrosive OR caused by exposure to a high concentration of an irritant chemical gas resulting in permanent nasal mucosal injury and breakdown with ulceration and occasionally septal perforation.[5]

Sensitizers for occupational asthma are thought to be also sensitizers for the upper airway. These sensitizers can be divided into high-molecular-weight (HMW) compounds or low-molecular-weight (LMW) compounds. Although for most HMW compounds an immunoglobulin E (IgE)-dependent mechanism has been suggested or demonstrated, hapten-protein conjugate targets for IgE have only been identified in a small number of cases involving LMW compounds.[6] The occupations with the highest risk of OR include animal workers, bakers, and food processing workers.[7] WER can be triggered by a wide variety of conditions in the workplace, which may include irritant gases, but also physical factors, such as temperature and humidity, odors including perfumes, and workplace stress.

The exact prevalence of WRR is unknown, but it is thought to be common. Significant underreporting is expected because WRR has often been seen as a relatively minor condition, and workers may choose not to report their symptoms. The lack of recognition of the condition as a compensable illness by workers' compensation boards may also contribute to the low rates of reporting. Last, the healthy worker effect may bias studies of prevalence because those individuals who remain in an occupation at risk for WRR are likely to be those without disease or with fewer symptoms.[8] Siracusa and colleagues[6] reviewed cross-sectional studies done in a variety of occupational settings and reported that the prevalence of OR ranged widely depending on the setting and method used to identify OR. In high-risk occupations, such as laboratory animal workers and bakers, the prevalence ranged from 9% to 45%. In a case series of patients being assessed for occupational asthma in a specialized occupational clinic setting, 58% of patients had positive nasal responses by specific inhalational challenge using acoustic rhinometry and nasal lavage.[9] Much like work-related asthma, it is expected that WER is a significant contributor and might account for most cases of WRR. However, definite data supporting this are lacking. The recognition of atopy and preexisting allergic rhinitis as being a risk factor for the development of WRR suggests that at least in some cases this represents WER, although sensitization and true OR on top of preexisting allergic rhinitis can also occur.

The close association of asthma and rhinitis has given rise to the United Airways Disease model. In this model of nose and lung interaction, the development of allergic rhinitis precedes and contributes to development of asthma through a variety of possible mechanisms, including (a) increased oral breathing and subsequent exposure of the lower airways to cold air and allergens, (b)

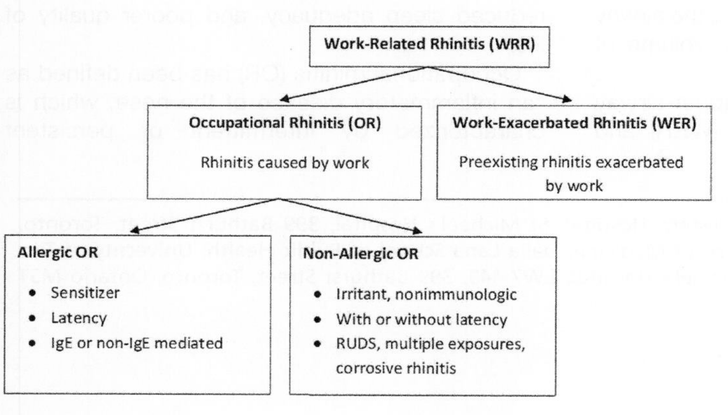

Fig. 1. Classification of WRR. (*Adapted from* Moscato G, Vandenplas O, Van Wijk RG, et al. EAACI position paper on occupational rhinitis. Respir Res. 2009;10:16; with permission.)

propagation of inflammation from the upper airway to the lower airway through postnasal drip or a shared systemic circulation, and (c) triggering of nasobronchial neural reflexes.[10] The crucial question of whether OR precedes occupational asthma was recently studied by Balogun and colleagues[11] in a systematic review. They identified 15 studies with sufficient data on both rhinitis and asthma and concluded that 9 of 15 demonstrated a statistically significant association between the diagnosis of asthma and rhinitis in individual workers. The temporal relationship between the two was not adequately addressed in the literature with only 4 of the 15 explicitly examining temporality. From these, 20% to 56% of patients had nasal symptoms or a diagnosis of OR before diagnosis with occupational asthma.[12–15] In 2 studies,[9,13] the association of OR with occupational asthma was higher in those individuals exposed to HMW sensitizers when compared with LMW agents, although this has not been consistently reported in the literature.[16]

Diagnosis and Management of Work-Related Rhinitis

The diagnosis of WRR begins with a detailed medical and occupational history with a particular focus on timing of nasal symptoms as they related to workplace exposures. History taking should also include a detailed review of the work process, workplace environment, protective equipment used, safety data sheets, and occurrence of symptoms in coworkers. Patient diaries for recording daily symptoms can be used to help identify work relatedness. Symptoms of OR are similar to those of non-OR and include rhinorrhea, sneezing, nasal blockage, and itchy nose. To date, no validated questionnaire for the diagnosis of OR exists. Physical examination may reveal swollen nasal turbinates, increased secretions, or nasal crusting. Nasal septal perforation is not common and suggests corrosive OR.[17]

Immunologic testing to demonstrate IgE sensitization to occupational agents by skin prick testing or immunoassay is useful in confirming a diagnosis of OR. This testing is usually limited to only HMW agents. Although some well-recognized LMW sensitizers, such as isocyanates, have commercially available test, most of these have not been validated. When commercial tests are not available, improvised skin-prick testing with materials brought from the workplace can be attempted but should be interpreted with caution, especially for chemicals because they are often skin irritants. False negative testing could occur because of a variety of factors, including the quality and validity of the extract. Local allergic rhinitis has more recently been identified as a new variant of allergic rhinitis whereby systemic IgE sensitization is not detected, but the patient displays a specific response during nasal allergen provocation testing. It is thought that the local production of IgE within the nasal tissue itself is the cause of symptoms and may affect a significant number of individuals diagnosed as having chronic nonallergic rhinitis.[18] In cases of workers with symptoms suggestive of OR, immunologic testing may be negative, prompting consideration of more detailed investigations with nasal provocation testing.

Objective measures of nasal patency or inflammation can be done in several ways, although may not be readily available outside of specialist clinics. Peak nasal inspiratory flow (PNIF) is the simplest way and measures the air flow through the nasal cavity during a forced inspiratory effort (**Fig. 2**). It is correlated well with symptoms and has been validated in clinical trials and nasal provocation challenges[19] but is very subject effort dependent. Similar to peak expiratory flow measurements in occupational asthma, PNIF has the advantage of being portable and allows for the use in the workplace, permitting serial self-measurements during a workplace challenge. Rhinomanometry determines nasal airway resistance by measuring pressure and flow during inspiration and expiration through the nose. Acoustic rhinometry (**Fig. 3**) measures nasal patency by using an applied acoustic pulse and measuring the reflected sound through a microphone.[20–22] All 3 methods have high interindividual variability; thus, comparison to values in healthy individuals is not possible. However, demonstrated individual reproducibility makes their use during nasal provocation testing and serial follow-up useful.[3]

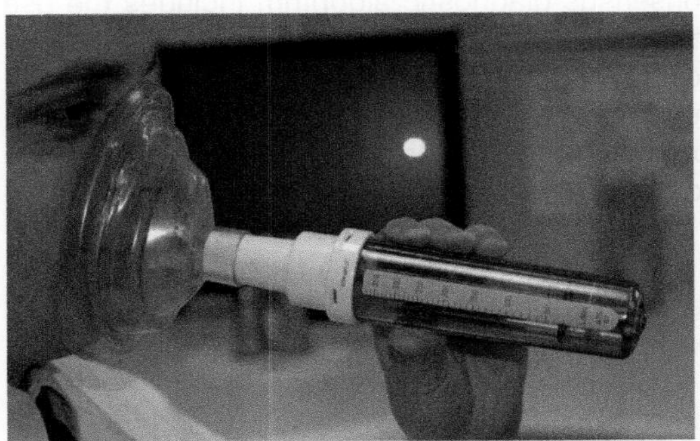

Fig. 2. Peak inspiratory nasal flow measurement. (*From* Scadding G, Hellings P, Alobid I, et al. Diagnostic tools in Rhinology EAACI position paper. Clin Transl Allergy. 2011;1(1):2; with permission.)

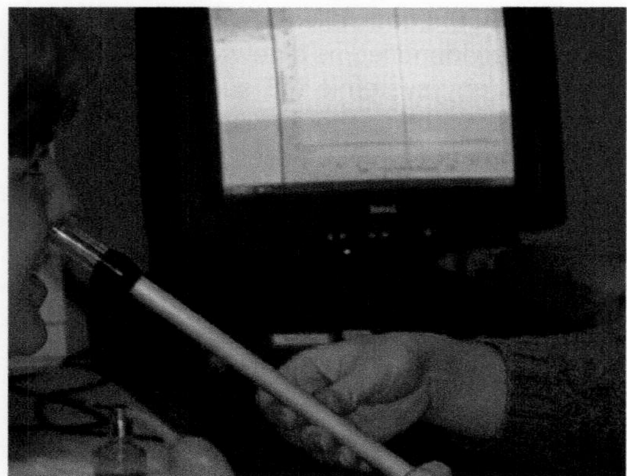

Fig. 3. Acoustic rhinometry. (*From* Scadding G, Hellings P, Alobid I, et al. Diagnostic tools in Rhinology EAACI position paper. Clin Transl Allergy. 2011;1(1):2; with permission.)

Analysis of nasal secretions for inflammatory markers and nasal cytology is an area of increasing interest in the assessment of OR,[23] and several investigators have studied this in a variety of populations with demonstration of differences between exposed and unexposed workers[24,25] as well as between HMW and LMW agents.[26] Use in clinical practice is variable with only nasal cytology being more accessible.

Nasal provocation tests remain the gold standard for confirming the diagnosis of OR, and this was reviewed recently by Ronsmans and colleagues.[27] Following exposure with a specific occupational agent or simulated work task, changes in symptoms, nasal patency, and nasal secretions can be assessed. Lack of standardization and validated comparison between methods makes this largely restricted to research and specialized occupational clinic settings.[28] Although the European Academy of Allergy Asthma and Clinical Immunology (EAACI) consensus diagnostic algorithm includes the use of nasal provocation testing[3] for a definitive diagnosis, its use even in specialist settings is variable. In a large French registry of workers investigated for occupational asthma and OR through occupational disease consultation centers, only 12% had a specific nasal provocation challenge test.[13] Conversely, a Finnish study reported 93% of patients had a confirmed diagnosis of OR by challenge test.[29]

The management of WRR and OR is focused on reducing or eliminating exposure to the causative agent or environment. For some workers, this may have a significant socioeconomic impact and professional change. Although occupational asthma is widely recognized as a work-related illness with commensurate compensation, compensation for OR varies widely from country to country.[3] Several studies have described improved quality of life in workers with cessation of exposure to workplace antigens when compared with workers with continued exposure.[29,30] It is likely that many workers continuing to work with exposure suffer "presenteeism" and reduced work productivity.[31] When complete avoidance is not possible, reduction in exposure through the use of environmental controls and ventilation systems, personal protective equipment, and exposure time reduction through scheduling can be used.[32] The effectiveness of these strategies is anecdotal, and it is recognized that individuals with rhinitis are more likely to leave their jobs.[33]

The pharmacologic management of WRR and OR is the same as for non-OR and includes nasal glucocorticoids, anticholinergic nasal sprays, antihistamines, leukotriene receptor antagonists, and nasal saline irrigation. Most studies of effectiveness have been described in nonoccupational allergic rhinitis. If the OR is due to exposure to a nonallergic response to irritants, these remedies may not be very effective. In the setting of continued exposure, pharmacotherapy may improve symptoms, but workers may continue to experience reduced quality of life. To date, no studies have described the efficacy of anti-IgE or anti-interleukin-5 monoclonal antibody therapy in OR. The frequent cooccurrence of occupational asthma with OR may complicate the management of both diseases because uncontrolled OR is likely to worsen asthma control.

Prevention of OR represents an important opportunity to reduce morbidity in a common illness. Screening workers before employment for atopy is unlikely to be effective given the high prevalence of atopy in the general population and would dramatically reduce the number of potential employees. Primary prevention strategies are likely to be more effective when focused on reducing the level of exposure, which has been identified in epidemiologic studies as the most important determinant of sensitization.[3] Modification of programs for preventing occupational asthma to also include OR would be sensible given the considerable overlap between the 2 conditions.

WORK-RELATED LARYNGEAL SYNDROMES INCLUDING LARYNGEAL CAUSES OF COUGH

Acute, transient laryngitis is common as a component of upper-respiratory viral infections and may be more common in those working with young children, such as in daycare or teachers. More prolonged or recurrent laryngeal syndromes are relatively common as a cause for asthmalike symptoms attributed to work exposures. In addition to being an important differential diagnosis, these syndromes can also coexist with asthma and can confound the diagnosis of work-related asthma.

The best recognized laryngeal syndromes that can present as being work related are those of (a) inducible laryngeal obstruction (ILO; formerly known as paradoxic vocal cord dysfunction [VCD]), (b) irritable larynx syndrome, (c) muscle tension dysphonia, and (d) laryngeal hypersensitivity cough syndrome.

Inducible Laryngeal Obstruction, Muscle Tension Dysphonia, and Irritable Larynx Syndrome

ILO,[34] formerly known as paradoxic VCD, has been described with increasing frequency since the early 1980s[35] and was initially suggested to be a form of conversion disorder.[36] There is paradoxic movement of the laryngeal muscles with respiration causing closing of the vocal cords during inspiration, resulting in a sensation of tightness in the neck, dyspnea with predominant difficulty on inspiration, dysphonia, and at times inspiratory wheezing or stridor. Without a detailed history of the symptoms, especially the history of neck tightness rather than midchest tightness, inspiratory rather than expiratory difficulty, and inspiratory rather than expiratory wheezes as well as the history of dysphonia, the patient may be incorrectly given a presumptive diagnosis of asthma. Indeed, early reports among patients assessed with VCD investigated at the specialty center in National Jewish Hospital, Denver, Colorado, who were predominantly young women, found that asthma had been misdiagnosed for an average of 4.8 years in 42 of the total 95 patients with VCD.[37] Those misdiagnosed with asthma had been receiving an average of 29 mg per day of prednisone regularly, for the incorrect assumption that symptoms were due to severe asthma. A more recent report of 40 patients with this syndrome identified a component of concurrent asthma in 29 of the patients.[38] Not surprisingly, those patients who do not have concurrent asthma, and even many who have both a laryngeal syndrome and concurrent asthma, will not have a satisfactory response to treatment with asthma medications. They may report an atypical improvement in symptoms with use of short-acting bronchodilators starting after the expected pharmacologic action, and likely unrelated to the bronchodilator effect, because the laryngeal component to symptoms will usually spontaneously improve shortly after leaving the provoking environment. VCD was renamed by a 2013 European and North American Consensus Conference as the term "inducible laryngeal obstruction."[39]

Triggers for ILO commonly include scented products, gasoline fumes, and tobacco smoke, usually associated with symptoms with low levels of exposure and occurring almost immediately, often clearing quickly on leaving the area. However, symptoms can be more prolonged and can be severe enough to lead to emergency visits, frequently resulting in treatment of presumed asthma or of possible anaphylaxis with presumed laryngeal edema.

Some patients have this syndrome solely triggered by exercise, and not by environmental exposures, typically young, otherwise healthy individuals who often have symptoms provoked by a combination of high stress and extreme physical exertion. In the occupational setting, this may especially be relevant for elite athletes or those in the military.[40]

Definitive diagnosis of ILO requires laryngoscopy and observation of paradoxic vocal cord movement with respiration (**Fig. 4**),[41] sometimes associated with a posterior vocal cord chink. These findings are best demonstrated at a time when symptoms are present, such as during an emergency visit. If the patient is assessed when acute symptoms are not present, then laryngoscopy may be normal. In that event, laryngoscopic evaluation in the clinic immediately after provocation by exposure to a reported trigger, such as a scented product, may facilitate the diagnosis. Stroboscopy can also be helpful in the evaluation to more clearly demonstrate paradoxic movement. Other local abnormalities may be seen, such as inflammatory changes reflecting gastroesophageal reflux (GERD), which may be an underlying precipitating factor, or structural vocal cord abnormalities, such as vocal cord polyps, which may contribute to symptoms or may be the sole cause of dysphonia.

Despite typical symptoms of ILO, in a subset of patients, the larynx appears normal on examination even at a time when symptoms are provoked. There may be extralaryngeal muscle tension, evident on palpation of the neck, that likely accounts for dysphonia and other symptoms in those patients, a condition termed "muscle tension dysphonia." In other patients with no abnormalities on physical examination but typical laryngeal symptoms on exposure to low-level irritants, a diagnosis of "irritable larynx syndrome" may be made to explain the constellation of symptoms, as a diagnosis of exclusion. This diagnosis is

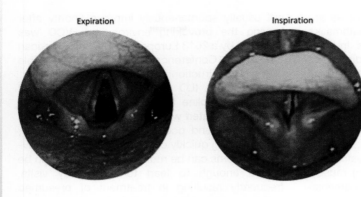

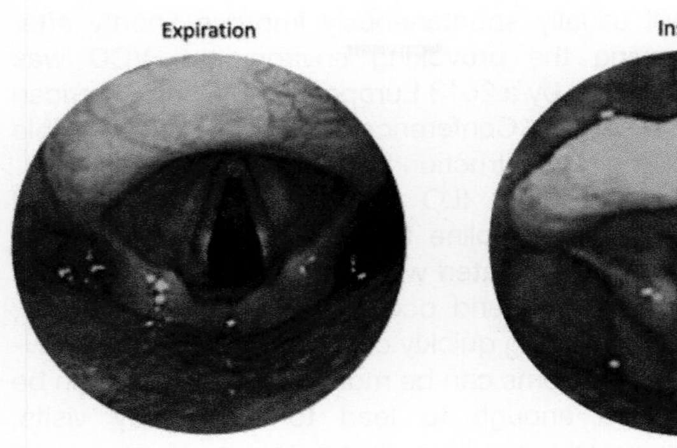

Fig. 4. Paradoxic vocal cord movement on inspiration. (*From* Cummings KJ, Fink JN, Vasudev M, Piacitelli C, Kreiss K. Vocal cord dysfunction related to water-damaged buildings. J Allergy Clin Immunol Pract. 2013;1(1):46-50; with permission.)

hypothesized to be a result of enhanced vagal sensory nerve activity in the larynx, possibly via transient receptor potential (TRP) channels, with a central nervous component magnifying the response and resulting in a sensation of laryngeal irritation with a secondary component of muscle dysfunction.

Associated conditions, such as GERD or rhinosinusitis with upper-airway inflammation, can underlie these disorders, and management of these may contribute to control of symptoms. Emotional stress and poor voice control (shouting, strained voice) can also worsen symptoms.

These laryngeal disorders are not specific to the workplace, but patients with these syndromes have commonly reported that symptoms occur mainly at work as recently reviewed,[42] especially among workers exposed to scented products, including cleaning agents, gasoline fumes, and second-hand smoke. Occupational groups commonly described include health care workers, for example, those using chlorinated disinfecting wipes, teachers, and office workers.

The diagnosis is suspected from a careful history and recognition that these conditions may occur alone or with asthma that may or may not be work related. The Newcastle laryngeal hypersensitivity questionnaire may be used to assist in diagnosis and assessment of response to management of a laryngeal syndrome.[43] Occupational exposures may exacerbate the laryngeal syndrome, and there may also be a component of work-related asthma, either occupational asthma or work-exacerbated asthma. As an example, a patient may have initially had a high-level irritant exposure at work, for example, from mixing ammonia and bleach with the development of irritant-induced occupational asthma, but on later return to work, they may have laryngeal symptoms from low exposures to cleaning products without objective evidence of asthma exacerbations. Rhinitis, both occupational and nonoccupational, may also exacerbate the syndrome through increased mouth breathing and postnasal drip.

Physical examination between episodes is typically normal, but when the patient is symptomatic, there is dysphonia, and there may be increased use of neck muscles on inspiration, and/or audible stridor.

It is important not to overlook any concurrent asthma or other pulmonary disease, and usual investigations include chest radiograph, pulmonary function testing with bronchodilator response, and where appropriate, methacholine challenge. These tests are usually normal if the patient does not have concurrent asthma and is asymptomatic at the time of testing. However, at the time of symptoms, spirometry may show reduced inspiratory flow rates. In some patients, the methacholine test can trigger symptoms, and there may be a need to stop the test before completion, but at that time there may be findings of inspiratory flow limitation on spirometry (**Fig. 5**).[41]

Otolaryngology assessment is most helpful when performed by an otolaryngologist specializing in the larynx, and working in conjunction with a speech language pathologist. Visualization of the larynx and assessment of extralaryngeal muscles, especially at the time of spontaneous or provoked symptoms, can provide the diagnosis.

Management focuses on (a) patient education as to the causes of their symptoms, and if appropriate, reassurance that symptoms are not due to lower-respiratory disease and are likely to improve with further management, (b) reducing exposure to triggers at work and outside the workplace when feasible, at least initially, as well as (c) reducing the response to triggers by managing any underlying conditions such as GERD, rhinosinusitis, and by stress management techniques, and (d) speech therapy techniques are often very

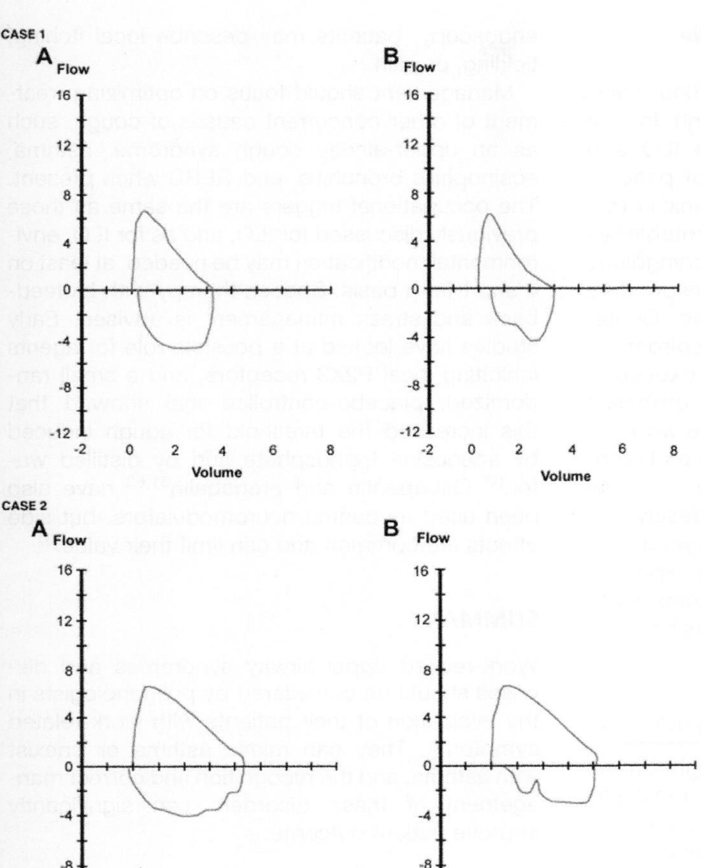

Fig. 5. Flow-volume loops in upper-airway obstruction induced by methacholine challenge. (*From* Cummings KJ, Fink JN, Vasudev M, Piacitelli C, Kreiss K. Vocal cord dysfunction related to water-damaged buildings. J Allergy Clin Immunol Pract. 2013;1(1):46-50; with permission.)

helpful and include optimizing voice use, ensuring adequate hydration, and use of exercises with biofeedback to reduce inappropriate laryngeal and neck muscle contraction. Any concurrent asthma is treated as appropriate.

Work accommodation may be needed, at least on a temporary basis. For some patients, provision of a scent-free environment as far as reasonable (eg, for a teacher or office worker) may be sufficient, but it is recognized that this is often difficult to enforce at work. Other workers, such as hospital workers, may be able to avoid areas with use of chlorinated disinfectants and other triggers. However, some may need to transfer to other duties away from clinical environments to avoid these exposures.

Although the above management strategies are often sufficient to allow workers to continue to work, or return to work, some patients do not have adequate control of their symptoms and may need additional measures. Medications that have been considered based on reports of response in laryngeal cough include anticholinergic agents, gabapentin, and potentially medications targeting TRP receptors, but there are currently no reported studies assessing these in irritable larynx syndromes. The contribution of the workplace to irritable larynx syndromes is currently based mainly on history because there are no objective tests to assess laryngeal changes at work versus off work. If symptoms have started after an accidental high-level irritant at work, with or without associated development of asthma, then it may be presumed to have an occupational cause. In other situations, it may be assumed to be work exacerbated. Workers' compensation claims for patients who need to miss work because of these syndromes are usually decided on a case-by-case basis.

Epidemiology of work-related irritable syndromes

There are relatively few studies reporting work-related irritable larynx syndromes, and few of these include differentiation between ILO and other laryngeal syndromes. A study of patients seen in an occupational lung disease clinic in Toronto[44] reported 9% with work-related irritable larynx syndrome as supported by otolaryngology assessment. Among follow-up of first responders and volunteers at the World Trade Center collapse, inspiratory flattening on spirometry was reported in 19%.[45] As may be expected, dysphonia and self-perceived voice problems are more common among those whose work requires greater use of their voice, such as teachers, service providers, and vocal performers.[46–48] There are a few descriptive studies of exercise-induced laryngeal symptoms, eg, in military personnel in whom 52% who had symptoms related them to high stress/anxiety.[49] The occurrence of inspiratory stridor has been reported in 5% of elite athletes.[50]

Laryngeal Hypersensitivity Cough Syndrome

There are many causes of chronic cough, but an etiologic diagnosis can be reached in most patients following a diagnostic algorithm, such as advised by the American College of Chest Physicians.[51,52] Occupational exposures can cause or be a contributing factor for many of the causes of chronic cough, as previously reviewed, and should be considered in all patients with chronic cough.[53,54] Laryngeal hypersensitivity cough syndrome is a term that was introduced in 2014 to consider after treatment or exclusion of other causes of chronic refractory cough,[55] with or without other features of ILO or muscle tension dysphonia (which have been reported in up to 85% of these patients).[56,57] A laryngeal cough hypersensitivity syndrome has been reported to occur in 40% or more of patients in a specialist cough clinic,[58,59] with features of chronic refractory cough triggered by low levels of thermal, chemical, or mechanical stimulation.[60]

The concept of laryngeal hypersensitivity cough syndrome is that there is a triggering of laryngeal airway mucosal vagal afferent nerve receptors and cation channels, for example, via TRP channels, that are relayed to the brainstem and are modulated by cortical influences. Cough may then be triggered by stimuli at work or outside the workplace that normally would not cause a cough, such as scented products, bleach, voice use, exercise, and cold air.[61] Despite a normal appearance to the laryngopharyngeal mucosa on endoscopy, patients may describe local itching, tickling, or pain.

Management should focus on optimizing treatment of other concurrent causes of cough, such as an upper-airway cough syndrome, asthma, eosinophilic bronchitis, and GERD when present. The occupational triggers are the same as those previously discussed for ILO, and as for ILO, environmental modification may be needed, at least on a short-term basis. Speech therapy with biofeedback and stress management is advised. Early studies have looked at a possible role for agents inhibiting local P2X3 receptors, and a small randomized, placebo-controlled trial showed that this increased the threshold for cough induced by adenosine triphosphate and by distilled water.[62] Gabapentin and pregabalin[61,63] have also been used as central neuromodulators, but side effects are common and can limit their value.[61]

SUMMARY

Work-related upper-airway syndromes and diseases should be considered by pulmonologists in the evaluation of their patients with work-related symptoms. They can mimic asthma or coexist with asthma, and the recognition and correct management of these disorders can significantly improve patient outcome.

DISCLOSURE

The authors have nothing to disclose.

REFERENCES

1. Wheatley LM, Togias A. Clinical practice. Allergic rhinitis. N Engl J Med 2015;372(5):456–63.
2. Meltzer EO, Nathan R, Derebery J, et al. Sleep, quality of life, and productivity impact of nasal symptoms in the United States: findings from the Burden of Rhinitis in America survey. Allergy Asthma Proc 2009;30(3):244–54.
3. Moscato G, Vandenplas O, Van Wijk RG, et al. EAACI position paper on occupational rhinitis. Respir Res 2009;10:16.
4. Meggs WJ. RADS and RUDS–the toxic induction of asthma and rhinitis. J Toxicol Clin Toxicol 1994; 32(5):487–501.
5. Castano R, Theriault G. Defining and classifying occupational rhinitis. J Laryngol Otol 2006;120(10): 812–7.
6. Siracusa A, Desrosiers M, Marabini A. Epidemiology of occupational rhinitis: prevalence, aetiology and determinants. Clin Exp Allergy 2000;30(11): 1519–34.

7. Hytonen M, Kanerva L, Malmberg H, et al. The risk of occupational rhinitis. Int Arch Occup Environ Health 1997;69(6):487–90.
8. Le Moual N, Kauffmann F, Eisen EA, et al. The healthy worker effect in asthma: work may cause asthma, but asthma may also influence work. Am J Respir Crit Care Med 2008;177(1):4–10.
9. Castano R, Gautrin D, Theriault G, et al. Occupational rhinitis in workers investigated for occupational asthma. Thorax 2009;64(1):50–4.
10. Giavina-Bianchi P, Aun MV, Takejima P, et al. United airway disease: current perspectives. J Asthma Allergy 2016;9:93–100.
11. Balogun RA, Siracusa A, Shusterman D. Occupational rhinitis and occupational asthma: association or progression? Am J Ind Med 2018;61(4):293–307.
12. Miedinger D, Gautrin D, Castano R. Upper airway symptoms among workers with work-related respiratory complaints. Occup Med (Lond) 2012;62(6): 427–34.
13. Ameille J, Hamelin K, Andujar P, et al. Occupational asthma and occupational rhinitis: the United Airways Disease Model revisited. Occup Environ Med 2013; 70(7):471–5.
14. Karjalainen A, Martikainen R, Klaukka T, et al. Risk of asthma among Finnish patients with occupational rhinitis. Chest 2003;123(1):283–8.
15. Walusiak J, Hanke W, Gorski P, et al. Respiratory allergy in apprentice bakers: do occupational allergies follow the allergic march? Allergy 2004; 59(4):442–50.
16. Malo JL, Lemiere C, Desjardins A, et al. Prevalence and intensity of rhinoconjunctivitis in subjects with occupational asthma. Eur Respir J 1997;10(7): 1513–5.
17. Castano R, Theriault G, Gautrin D. Categorizing nasal septal perforations of occupational origin as cases of corrosive rhinitis. Am J Ind Med 2007; 50(2):150–3.
18. Gomez F, Rondon C, Salas M, et al. Local allergic rhinitis: mechanisms, diagnosis and relevance for occupational rhinitis. Curr Opin Allergy Clin Immunol 2015;15(2):111–6.
19. Scadding G, Hellings P, Alobid I, et al. Diagnostic tools in rhinology EAACI position paper. Clin Transl Allergy 2011;1(1):2.
20. Clement PA, Gordts F. Standardisation committee on objective assessment of the nasal airway IRS, ERS. Consensus report on acoustic rhinometry and rhinomanometry. Rhinology 2005;43(3):169–79.
21. Castano R, Theriault G, Gautrin D, et al. Reproducibility of acoustic rhinometry in the investigation of occupational rhinitis. Am J Rhinol 2007;21(4): 474–7.
22. Castano R, Trudeau C, Ghezzo H. Correlation between acoustic rhinometry and subjective nasal patency during nasal challenge test in subjects with suspected occupational rhinitis; a prospective controlled study. Clin Otolaryngol 2010;35(6):462–7.
23. Quirce S, Lemiere C, de Blay F, et al. Noninvasive methods for assessment of airway inflammation in occupational settings. Allergy 2010;65(4): 445–58.
24. Castano R, Theriault G, Maghni K, et al. Reproducibility of nasal lavage in the context of the inhalation challenge investigation of occupational rhinitis. Am J Rhinol 2008;22(3):271–5.
25. Staffieri C, Lovato A, Aielli F, et al. Investigating nasal cytology as a potential tool for diagnosing occupational rhinitis in woodworkers. Int Forum Allergy Rhinol 2015;5(9):814–9.
26. Castano R, Yucesoy B, Johnson VJ, et al. Inflammatory proteins in nasal lavage of workers exposed to occupational agents. Clin Exp Allergy 2017;47(12): 1566–73.
27. Ronsmans S, Steelant B, Backaert W, et al. Diagnostic approach to occupational rhinitis: the role of nasal provocation tests. Curr Opin Allergy Clin Immunol 2019;20(2):122–30.
28. Moscato G, Rolla G, Siracusa A. Occupational rhinitis: consensus on diagnosis and medicolegal implications. Curr Opin Otolaryngol Head Neck Surg 2011;19(1):36–42.
29. Airaksinen LK, Luukkonen RA, Lindstrom I, et al. Long-term exposure and health-related quality of life among patients with occupational rhinitis. J Occup Environ Med 2009;51(11):1288–97.
30. Castano R, Trudeau C, Castellanos L, et al. Prospective outcome assessment of occupational rhinitis after removal from exposure. J Occup Environ Med 2013;55(5):579–85.
31. Maoua M, Maalel OE, Kacem I, et al. Quality of life and work productivity impairment of patients with allergic occupational rhinitis. Tanaffos 2019;18(1): 58–65.
32. Hellgren J, Karlsson G, Toren K. The dilemma of occupational rhinitis: management options. Am J Respir Med 2003;2(4):333–41.
33. Gerth van Wijk R, Patiwael JA, de Jong NW, et al. Occupational rhinitis in bell pepper greenhouse workers: determinants of leaving work and the effects of subsequent allergen avoidance on health-related quality of life. Allergy 2011;66(7):903–8.
34. Halvorsen T, Walsted ES, Bucca C, et al. Inducible laryngeal obstruction: an official joint European Respiratory Society and European Laryngological Society statement. Eur Respir J 2017;50(3): 1602221.
35. Kellman RM, Leopold DA. Paradoxical vocal cord motion: an important cause of stridor. Laryngoscope 1982;92(1):58–60.
36. Christopher KL, Wood RP 2nd, Eckert RC, et al. Vocal-cord dysfunction presenting as asthma. N Engl J Med 1983;308(26):1566–70.

37. Newman KB, Mason UG 3rd, Schmaling KB. Clinical features of vocal cord dysfunction. Am J Respir Crit Care Med 1995;152(4 Pt 1):1382–6.
38. Lee JW, Tay TR, Paddle P, et al. Diagnosis of concomitant inducible laryngeal obstruction and asthma. Clin Exp Allergy 2018;48(12):1622–30.
39. Christensen PM, Heimdal JH, Christopher KL, et al. ERS/ELS/ACCP 2013 International Consensus Conference nomenclature on inducible laryngeal obstructions. Eur Respir Rev 2015;24(137):445–50.
40. Olin JT, Clary MS, Deardorff EH, et al. Inducible laryngeal obstruction during exercise: moving beyond vocal cords with new insights. Phys Sportsmed 2015;43(1):13–21.
41. Cummings KJ, Fink JN, Vasudev M, et al. Vocal cord dysfunction related to water-damaged buildings. J Allergy Clin Immunol Pract 2013;1(1):46–50.
42. Denton E, Hoy R. Occupational aspects of irritable larynx syndrome. Curr Opin Allergy Clin Immunol 2020;20(2):90–5.
43. Vertigan AE, Bone SL, Gibson PG. Development and validation of the Newcastle laryngeal hypersensitivity questionnaire. Cough 2014;10(1):1.
44. Hoy RF, Ribeiro M, Anderson J, et al. Work-associated irritable larynx syndrome. Occup Med (Lond) 2010;60(7):546–51.
45. de la Hoz RE, Shohet MR, Bienenfeld LA, et al. Vocal cord dysfunction in former World Trade Center (WTC) rescue and recovery workers and volunteers. Am J Ind Med 2008;51(3):161–5.
46. Lyberg-Ahlander V, Rydell R, Fredlund P, et al. Prevalence of voice disorders in the general population, based on the Stockholm Public Health Cohort. J Voice 2019;33(6):900–5.
47. Ebersole B, Soni RS, Moran K, et al. The influence of occupation on self-perceived vocal problems in patients with voice complaints. J Voice 2018;32(6):673–80.
48. Mori MC, Francis DO, Song PC. Identifying occupations at risk for laryngeal disorders requiring specialty voice care. Otolaryngol Head Neck Surg 2017;157(4):670–5.
49. Morris MJ, Oleszewski RT, Sterner JB, et al. Vocal cord dysfunction related to combat deployment. Mil Med 2013;178(11):1208–12.
50. Rundell KW, Spiering BA. Inspiratory stridor in elite athletes. Chest 2003;123(2):468–74.
51. Irwin RS, French CT, Lewis SZ, et al. Overview of the management of cough: CHEST guideline and expert panel report. Chest 2014;146(4):885–9.
52. Irwin RS, French CL, Chang AB, et al. Classification of cough as a symptom in adults and management algorithms: CHEST guideline and expert panel report. Chest 2018;153(1):196–209.
53. Tarlo SM, Altman KW, Oppenheimer J, et al. Occupational and environmental contributions to chronic cough in adults: chest expert panel report. Chest 2016;150(4):894–907.
54. Tarlo SM, Altman KW, French CT, et al. Evaluation of occupational and environmental factors in the assessment of chronic cough in adults: a systematic review. Chest 2016;149(1):143–60.
55. Song WJ, Chang YS, Morice AH. Changing the paradigm for cough: does 'cough hypersensitivity' aid our understanding? Asia Pac Allergy 2014;4(1):3–13.
56. Vertigan AE, Bone SL, Gibson PG. Laryngeal sensory dysfunction in laryngeal hypersensitivity syndrome. Respirology 2013;18(6):948–56.
57. Vertigan AE, Kapela SM, Kearney EK, et al. Laryngeal dysfunction in cough hypersensitivity syndrome: a cross-sectional observational study. J Allergy Clin Immunol Pract 2018;6(6):2087–95.
58. Morice AH, Millqvist E, Belvisi MG, et al. Expert opinion on the cough hypersensitivity syndrome in respiratory medicine. Eur Respir J 2014;44(5):1132–48.
59. Gibson PG. Management of cough. J Allergy Clin Immunol Pract 2019;7(6):1724–9.
60. Morice AH, Jakes AD, Faruqi S, et al. A worldwide survey of chronic cough: a manifestation of enhanced somatosensory response. Eur Respir J 2014;44(5):1149–55.
61. Morice AH, Millqvist E, Bieksiene K, et al. ERS guidelines on the diagnosis and treatment of chronic cough in adults and children. Eur Respir J 2019;55(1):1901136.
62. Morice AH, Kitt MM, Ford AP, et al. The effect of gefapixant, a P2X3 antagonist, on cough reflex sensitivity: a randomised placebo-controlled study. Eur Respir J 2019;54(1):1900439.
63. Gibson P, Wang G, McGarvey L, et al. Treatment of unexplained chronic cough: CHEST guideline and expert panel report. Chest 2016;149(1):27–44.

Occupational Bronchiolitis
An Update

Randall J. Nett, MD, MPH[a,*], R. Reid Harvey, DVM, MPH[a], Kristin J. Cummings, MD, MPH[b]

KEYWORDS

- Constrictive bronchiolitis • Military deployment • Obliterative bronchiolitis • Flavoring • Diacetyl
- 2,3-Pentanedione • Styrene

KEY POINTS

- Workers in industries producing or using flavoring containing diacetyl or 2,3-pentanedione continue to be at risk for flavoring-related lung disease, although the disease is preventable.
- Cases of constrictive bronchiolitis have been associated with military deployments to Iraq and Afghanistan, but the causative exposure(s) have not been identified.
- Multiple reports in recent years have drawn attention to previously unrecognized risk factors for occupational bronchiolitis following exposures in several settings, such as fiberglass-reinforced plastic boatbuilding.

INTRODUCTION

Bronchiolitis is characterized by inflammation of the small airways (<2 mm).[1,2] The most common clinical presentation includes insidious onset of exertional dyspnea and cough. The complexities surrounding occupational bronchiolitis are many. At the forefront of those complexities is the terminology used to describe the wide range of pathologies and causative exposures that fall under the umbrella term occupational bronchiolitis (eg, bronchiolitis obliterans, constrictive bronchiolitis, obliterative bronchiolitis, proliferative bronchiolitis, popcorn lung disease). Consequently, small airways diseases resulting from occupational exposures are often defined by pathologic description[3]; however, most workers suspected of having occupational bronchiolitis do not undergo biopsy.[4] Thus, the most commonly used naming scheme is left open to interpretation because relatively few pathologic specimens are often the foundation for selected terminology. Noninvasive diagnostic tests including lung function testing and imaging are frequently nonspecific, particularly for the small airways. Further, when deciding whether to recommend surgical or thoracoscopic lung biopsy, health care providers are charged with performing risk-benefit analyses in which potential surgical and anesthetic risks might not justify anticipated results. Moreover, occupational bronchiolitis is relatively rare and workplace exposures might not be considered early during the diagnostic evaluation, which can result in the misdiagnoses of more common airways diseases, such as asthma or chronic obstructive pulmonary disease (COPD).[5]

In this report, we provide an update on some known causes of occupational bronchiolitis based on the published literature from 2009 to 2018. We cover flavoring-related lung disease caused by exposure to diacetyl and 2,3-pentanedione, constrictive bronchiolitis associated with military deployment, and emerging issues such as occupational bronchiolitis associated with the fiberglass-reinforced plastic industry and industrial machine manufacturing. For these

[a] Respiratory Health Division, National Institute for Occupational Safety and Health, Centers for Disease Control and Prevention, 1000 Frederick Lane, Morgantown, WV 26508, USA; [b] Occupational Health Branch, California Department of Public Health, 850 Marina Bay Parkway P-3, Richmond, CA 94804, USA
* Corresponding author.
E-mail address: gge5@cdc.gov

Clin Chest Med 41 (2020) 661–686
https://doi.org/10.1016/j.ccm.2020.08.011
0272-5231/20/Published by Elsevier Inc.

occupational exposures that can potentially result in small airways disease, our knowledge continues to expand as additional studies are published. Much of the literature to date consists of case reports, case series, and other observational epidemiologic studies, but research methods are beginning to include more systematic or standardized approaches to describe and understand these diseases. Inevitably, we will learn of novel occupational exposures that can cause small airways diseases in the future, and we will continue to rely on astute health care providers to suspect workplace exposures and public health agencies to conduct follow-up investigations.

FLAVORINGS

Flavoring-related lung disease (FRLD) was first described in 2002 among former workers at a sentinel microwave popcorn production facility.[6,7] Clinical progression was insidious and marked by exertional dyspnea and cough. The patients had fixed obstruction on spirometry testing, and lung pathology findings for those who underwent biopsy were consistent with bronchiolitis obliterans based on inflammation and fibrotic changes leading to narrowing of the bronchioles.[6,7] Diacetyl (2,3-butanedione), a butter flavoring chemical, was the predominant compound detected on air sampling, and a strong relationship between cumulative diacetyl exposure and airways obstruction was observed among current workers.[6] Experimental animal studies subsequently revealed inhalation exposure to diacetyl caused severe injury to the respiratory epithelium, implicating diacetyl as the cause of FRLD.[8–11] Alpha-diketones structurally similar to diacetyl that differ in the number of carbon groups, including 2,3-pentanedione, 2,3-hexanedione, and most recently methylglyoxol, have demonstrated similar toxicity in animal studies.[12–15] Additional epidemiologic investigations supported the association between occupational exposure to diacetyl and bronchiolitis in microwave popcorn production and flavoring manufacturing.[16–18]

Findings from select case reports, case studies, and epidemiologic studies related to FRLD from 2009 to 2018 are summarized in **Table 1**. Since the initial investigation of the sentinel microwave popcorn facility, additional cases of FRLD have been diagnosed among workers in other microwave popcorn facilities and other industries, including flavoring manufacturing, snack food production, pet food production, and coffee roasting and packaging facilities.[16,19–24] Most FRLD cases have been associated with occupational exposure, although in 2012 Egilman and Schilling[25] reported 3 cases of FRLD that they attributed to microwave popcorn consumption.

Understanding of the clinical characteristics has improved since the identification and description of the sentinel cluster. The most commonly reported symptoms are exertional dyspnea and dry cough; however, chest tightness and upper respiratory symptoms also can occur.[6,26,27] Fixed obstruction on spirometry is the most common pattern on lung function testing, although 28% (30 of 106) of flavoring manufacturing workers in one study had restrictive patterns on spirometry.[20,21,28–30] Mixed and normal spirometry patterns also have occurred.[5,25] High-resolution computed tomography (HRCT) commonly demonstrates mosaic attenuation consistent with air trapping, but results are not specific to FRLD.[20,28] The diagnosis of most FRLD cases is based on work and exposure history, signs and symptoms, and noninvasive diagnostic testing results.

Lung biopsy of workers with FRLD can lead to false negative results because of patchy distribution of bronchiolar inflammation.[31,32] Compared with transbronchial biopsy, surgical biopsy is the more sensitive method if pursuing a pathologic diagnosis. Several workers from the sentinel microwave popcorn plant who underwent lung biopsy and histopathology demonstrated narrowing and fibrosis of the bronchioles that led to the pathologic diagnosis of bronchiolitis obliterans.[7] However, as additional cases of FRLD have been diagnosed, the observed histopathology results have varied and included granulomatous inflammation, pleural proliferation of mesothelial cells or eosinophils, emphysema, and interstitial fibrosis.[17,20,21,33] A study analyzing a series of pathologic specimens from flavoring-exposed workers would be a useful contribution to our understanding of the potential disease spectrum.

FRLD is often misdiagnosed because more common obstructive lung diseases, including asthma or COPD, are typically considered.[5] The misdiagnoses are likely attributable to the relatively rare occurrence of FRLD, the absence of a thorough occupational exposure history, and the attribution of the condition to cigarette smoking.[34] Consequently, FRLD should be considered as a possible diagnosis in any worker who presents with breathing difficulty and is exposed at work to diacetyl or other flavoring-related compounds. There is no specific treatment for FRLD other than removing the individual from the exposure and supportive treatment.[35] There have been mixed results following treatment with steroids or other anti-inflammatory agents.[36] Lung transplantation is an option for end-stage disease, although lung function might stabilize after cessation of exposure.[37]

Table 1
Flavoring-related lung disease case reports, case series, or epidemiologic studies, 2009–2019

Authors	No. Cases (% Male)	Diagnosis/ Terminology	Symptoms	Pulmonary Function Testing	HRCT	Histology	Exposures/ Tobacco Exposures	No. Workers/ Other
Lockey et al.[38] 2019	–	–	–	Workers with historically higher exposure from first cohort (mixers) had a significant decline in % FEV1 during 7-y study period; study participants had increased restrictive lung patterns compared with general US population	–	–	3 exposure cohorts that represented dates of diacetyl substitution and introduction of engineering and administrative controls, and respiratory protection to reduce exposure	1105 workers evaluated; 7-y study at 4 microwave popcorn facilities with 3 cohorts

(continued on next page)

Table 1
(continued)

Authors	No. Cases (% Male)	Diagnosis/ Terminology	Symptoms	Pulmonary Function Testing	HRCT	Histology	Exposures/ Tobacco Exposures	No. Workers/ Other
Fechter-Leggett et al. [4] 2018	4 (pathologist-reported) (75%); 48 (probable) (50%)	Constrictive bronchiolitis or bronchiolitis obliterans	3 of 4 exertional dyspnea; 4 of 4 usual cough (pathology-reported); 92% exertional dyspnea, 65% usual cough (probable)	2 (50%) obstruction, 2 (50%) mixed (pathology reported); 21% obstruction; 79% mixed (probable)	—	Constrictive bronchiolitis or bronchiolitis obliterans (also granulomas, respiratory bronchiolitis, and emphysema in 4 pathology-reported cases)	Microwave popcorn or flavoring manufacturing facilities;3 of 4 never smoker (pathology-reported)35% never smoker (probable)	1407 workers evaluated from 8 microwave popcorn or flavoring manufacturing facilities; 7 of 11 workers with biopsy did not meet pathology-reported case definition (granulomas, respiratory bronchiolitis, chronic fibrous pleuritis, interstitial fibrosis, peribronchial inflammation, emphysema)
Harvey et al.[40] 2018	1 (100%)	Flavoring-related lung disease	Chest tightness, mucous membrane irritation, dyspnea, cough	Moderate mixed pattern	Mosaic attenuation consistent with diffuse bilateral air trapping	Focal mild cellular bronchiolitis and pleuritic, and focal peribronchial giant cells/ granulomas	Flavoring coffee: 521–2173 ppb diacetyl and 345–1445 ppb 2,3-PD; TWA 41–421 ppb diacetyl and 22–276 ppb 2,3-PD	

Warrior et al.[41] 2018	1 (100%)	Flavoring-induced bronchiolitis obliterans syndrome	Chronic cough	Severe obstruction with air trapping and mild gas transfer defect	Biapical scarring and bilateral bronchiectasis	—	Flavoring pet food	
Morales-Camino [24] 2016	-	—	—	5.6% of workers with excessive decline in FEV1 or FVC	—	—	—	479 workers evaluated at potato chips factory
Bailey et al.[39] 2015	5 former workers (NR)	Obliterative bronchiolitis	More dyspnea compared with general population	More obstruction compared with general population	—	2 former workers with biopsy-confirmed obliterative bronchiolitis	Maximum TWA 283 ppb combined diacetyl and 2,3-PD; maximum STEL 14,300 ppb diacetyl and 18,400 ppb 2,3-PD	75 current workers and 13 formers workers evaluated at coffee facility
Kreiss[29] 2014	-	—	—	More spirometric restrictive pattern than expected; excessive decline in FEV1 in 19% of workers	—	—	Maximum TWA 10.17 ppm diacetyl	106 flavoring manufacturing workers evaluated

(continued on next page)

Table 1
(*continued*)

Authors	No. Cases (% Male)	Diagnosis/ Terminology	Symptoms	Pulmonary Function Testing	HRCT	Histology	Exposures/ Tobacco Exposures	No. Workers/ Other
Cummings et al.[27] 2014	–	Subclinical obliterative bronchiolitis	Dyspnea associated with tenure $\geq$7 y, other chest symptoms associated with time in production	Mean spirometric parameters lower in workers with tenure $\geq$7 y or $\geq$1 h daily in production; mean diffusing capacity lower in workers with tenure $\geq$7 y	—	—	Flavoring manufacturing	367 current workers evaluated at flavoring manufacturer
CDC [20] 2013	2 (50%)	Obliterative bronchiolitis	Cough, exertional dyspnea	Obstruction	Bronchial wall thickening, prominent mosaic pattern, mild cylindrical bronchiectasis, fibrotic scarring	Constrictive bronchiolitis with narrowed and obliterated airways with surrounding fibrous tissue and variable mixed chronic inflammatory cell infiltrate; chronic and subacute small airways injury	Mixers in the flavoring room of a coffee processing facility	Both misdiagnosed before obliterative bronchiolitis diagnoses

Halldin et al.[5] 2013	4 (NR)	"Other COPD"-associated deaths	3 usual cough, 2 shortness of breath	1 obstruction, 2 mixed patterns	—	—	Microwave popcorn; diacetyl 1.99 ppm average exposure (range: 0.004–9.74 ppm); 2 never smokers	Respiratory-associated mortality study of 15 deaths identified among 511 workers at sentinel microwave popcorn facility; no ICD code for bronchiolitis obliterans
Huff et al.[23] 2013	5 (NR)	Bronchiolitis obliterans	Cough, wheeze, exertional dyspnea	Severe fixed obstruction	Upper lobe reticular nodular abnormalities with bronchial wall thickening, mild cylindrical bronchiectasis	2 of 5 with biopsy; chronic and subacute small airways injury suggestive of proliferative and obliterative constrictive bronchiolitis	Coffee flavoring	
Kreiss et al.[30] 2012	–	—	—	Excessive decline in lung function associated with companies using more diacetyl during production	—	—	Flavoring manufacturing	Evaluation of spirometry data from 724 flavoring manufacturing workers in California

(continued on next page)

Table 1
(continued)

Authors	No. Cases (% Male)	Diagnosis/ Terminology	Symptoms	Pulmonary Function Testing	HRCT	Histology	Exposures/ Tobacco Exposures	No. Workers/ Other
Cavalcanti et al.[21] 2012	4 (100%)	Brochiolitis obliterans	Cough, shortness of breath, wheeze	Moderate to severe obstruction	Hyperinflation, air trapping, bronchial thickening, mosaic perfusion	1 of 4 with biopsy; slight distortion of small airways with airway wall smooth muscle hypertrophy, mild mononuclear cell infiltrate, and area of air trapping and hyperinflation; single non-necrotic epithelioid granulation with multinucleated giant cells in subpleural space	Brazilian cookie factory with artificial butter flavoring	
Egilman and Schilling [25] 2012	3 (33%)	Bronchiolitis obliterans	Exertional dyspnea, cough, wheeze	1 normal spirometry; 1 decreased FEV1; 1 restriction pattern	1 ground glass opacity; 1 bibasilar atelectasis and lingular infiltrate; 1 mosaic pattern	Mild constrictive bronchiolitis with granulomas	Butter flavored microwave popcorn consumers	Nonoccupational exposure

Kanwal et al.[41] 2011	–	—	Workers with past high exposure had stable respiratory symptoms and new workers had fewer respiratory symptoms	New workers had higher lung function than worker with past high exposures	—	—	Engineering controls reduced diacetyl exposures by 1 to 3 orders of magnitude	373 current workers evaluated in follow-up study from sentinel microwave popcorn facility
Kim et al.[28] 2010	8 (NR)	Bronchiolitis obliterans or fixed obstructive related to flavorings	Dyspnea, cough, wheeze most common	Moderate to severe fixed obstruction	4 of 7 with HRCT consistent with bronchiolitis obliterans	2 biopsies: 1 consistent with bronchiolitis obliterans, 1 interpreted as hypersensitivity pneumonitis	Flavor manufacturing workers in California	467 workers evaluated from 16 flavoring manufacturing facilities using medical surveillance data
Van Rooy et al.[22] 2009	4 (NR)	Bronchiolitis obliterans syndrome	Trouble breathing, cough, wheeze, asthma attack	Excessive decline in FEV1 (cohort)	—	—	Dutch food flavoring production; 1.8–351 mg/m^3 historic exposure, 3–396 mg/m^3 for specific tasks	175 workers evaluated from plant producing diacetyl in historic cohort study

(continued on next page)

Table 1
(continued)

Authors	No. Cases (% Male)	Diagnosis/ Terminology	Symptoms	Pulmonary Function Testing	HRCT	Histology	Exposures/ Tobacco Exposures	No. Workers/ Other
Lockey et al.[18] 2009	–	Bronchiolitis obliterans	—	Lower % predicted FEV1 and 8-fold increased risk of airway obstruction associated with diacetyl exposure	—	—	High cumulative diacetyl exposure (≥8 ppm-y) prior to respiratory use associated with lower % predicted FEV1 and eight-fold increased risk of airway obstruction	765 workers evaluated from 4 microwave popcorn production plants

Abbreviations: '—', not performed/evaluated; 2, 3-PD, 2, 3-Petanedione; FEV1, forced expiratory volume in 1 second; FVC, forced vital capacity; HRCT, high-resolution computed tomography; NR, not reported; PFT, pulmonary function tests; ppb, parts per billion; ppm, parts per million; STEL, short term exposure; TWA, time-weighted average.

The risk of FRLD is established among microwave popcorn production workers. In response, strategies to reduce diacetyl exposure in the industry have included substitution, engineering controls, administrative controls, and respiratory protection. A recent study evaluated change in lung function over time in more than 1000 microwave popcorn workers and demonstrated the historically high-exposure group had a significant decrease in percent predicted FEV_1 during the 7-year study period.[38] Although the risk of FRLD has been recognized in microwave popcorn production for nearly 2 decades, FRLD cases continue to be identified in new industry settings in which flavorings are added during production.[39–41] Management in industrial settings where flavorings are used but where cases have not been identified might not be aware of the risk for occupational lung disease. In addition, the hazards might not be communicated appropriately in Safety Data Sheets of flavoring formulations, including those for diacetyl and 2,3-pentanedione.[42]

FRLD is preventable. Engineering controls such as enclosing the flavoring room in industries that use flavorings during production, or adding local exhaust ventilation can substantially reduce exposures.[43] These controls have also proven effective in stabilizing workers' lung function in some settings.[44] Personal protective equipment (PPE), such as a half mask respirator with organic vapor cartridge is required in some settings, although PPE should not be relied on as the primary source of protection. Substituting other alpha-diketones such as 2,3-petanedione or 2,3-hexanedione for diacetyl is not considered a safe alternative based on animal studies demonstrating similar pathologic findings following exposure. The National Institute for Occupational Safety and Health (NIOSH) recommends medical surveillance, including respiratory symptom screening and spirometry every 6 months for workers who regularly work in or enter areas where alpha-diketones are used.[45] Early detection of abnormal spirometry or excessive decline in lung function over time and subsequent removal from further exposure to diacetyl or other alpha-diketones is important to prevent the progression of FRLD.[28] In 2006, the California Department of Industrial Relations, Division of Occupational Safety and Health (Cal/OSHA), and California Department of Public Health initiated an industrywide surveillance program for flavoring manufacturing that included diacetyl exposure assessments, engineering controls, spirometry for workers, and PPE requirements.[28,30]

The US Department of Labor's Occupational Safety and Health Administration (OSHA) has no permissible exposure limits for alpha-diketones. NIOSH published recommended exposure limits of 5.0 parts per billion (ppb) for diacetyl and 9.3 ppb for 2,3-pentanedione for time-weighted averages (TWAs) for a 40-hour workweek in 2016. The NIOSH short-term exposure limits (STELs) are 25 ppb for diacetyl and 31 ppb for 2,3-pentanedione.[46] The American Conference of Governmental Industrial Hygienists published a threshold limit value (TLV) TWA of 10 ppb and an STEL of 20 ppb for diacetyl, and has placed 2,3-pentanedione on the 2017 list of Chemical Substances and Other Issues under study.[47,48]

Diacetyl has been detected during processes and tasks in industries not associated with FRLD. For instance, diacetyl is naturally produced during some production processes including coffee roasting and marijuana processing, although we are not aware of FRLD cases attributed to natural sources of diacetyl.[49–51] E-cigarette and vaping products commonly contain diacetyl and other flavorings[52]; case reports in e-cigarette and vaping product consumers include severe lung disease that is the subject of ongoing inquiry.[53–55]

SOUTHWESTERN ASIA DEPLOYMENT

Cases of constrictive bronchiolitis have been attributed to inhalation exposures that occurred during military deployments to Iraq and Afghanistan as part of Operation Iraqi Freedom (OIF) and Operation Enduring Freedom (OEF).[56–60] Military personnel who served in Southwestern Asia as part of OIF/OEF often experienced inhalation exposures to sandstorms, dust, diesel exhaust, open air burn pits, and cigarette smoke, and some experienced combat-related exposures, including weapons firing and exposures to blasts from improvised explosive devices.[61–64] These inhalation exposures prompted concerns for the development of long-term respiratory symptoms related to deployments during OIF/OEF and led to the Department of Veterans Affairs establishing the Airborne Hazards and Open Burn Pit registry to identify health effects associated with inhalation exposures during Southwestern Asia military deployments.[65] As of July 31, 2015, of 42,558 registry respondents who had deployed to Southwestern Asia since October 7, 2001, 433 (1%) self-reported a health care provider diagnosis of constrictive bronchiolitis; these respondents more often reported burn pit exposure compared with those without a diagnosis of constrictive bronchiolitis.[66]

From 2004 to 2009, King and colleagues[57] evaluated 80 soldiers from a single US Army base who were referred for evaluation of respiratory symptoms and exercise intolerance following deployments during OIF/OEF. Thirty-eight of the 49 soldiers who underwent video-assisted thoracoscopic lung biopsies were determined to have constrictive bronchiolitis following nonblinded specimen review by 2 pathologists (**Table 2**). More than 80% were never smokers or former smokers. Twenty-eight were exposed to a sulfur-mine fire near Mosul in 2003. Occupational histories varied and included exposure to burn pits, incinerated human waste, dust storms, and combat smoke. More than 33% had normal spirometry, lung volumes, and diffusing capacity of the lung for carbon monoxide (DLCO). One-half had normal spirometry and isolated low DLCO. Only 4 had abnormal spirometry, including 3 with a restrictive pattern and 1 with an obstructive pattern. Among the 37 soldiers who underwent HRCT, 25 (68%) had normal HRCTs and 6 (16%) had mild air trapping. Lacy black pigment was noted in the visceral pleural surface following lung biopsy for 37 of the 38 soldiers. Prominent pathologic features included pigment deposition (n = 37), polarizable material within pigment (36), peribronchiolar inflammation (34), hypertensive-type arterial change (28), and prominent bronchial-associated lymphoid tissue (19). Luminal constriction was observed in 64% of sampled terminal and respiratory bronchioles. The alveolar structures and larger airways were typically normal. This case series demonstrated the possibility for inhalation exposures that occurred during military deployments to Iraq to be the source of constrictive bronchiolitis, a rare lung disease, among this previously healthy cohort.

Since publication of the series of King and colleagues[57] in 2011, 50 other cases of bronchiolitis associated with military deployments during OIF/OEF have been described (see **Table 2**).[56,58,60,67–69] Forty-one of these patients were described as having bronchiolitis, 6 constrictive bronchiolitis, 2 respiratory bronchiolitis, and 1 as nonspecific interstitial pneumonitis and bronchiolitis. Krefft and colleagues[68] used a case definition to identify 87 cases of distal deployment-related lung disease (DDLD) among 127 military or civilian workers who presented consecutively to a specialty clinic with new-onset respiratory symptoms that began during or following military-related deployments. Thirty-one (60%) of 52 of these patients who underwent lung biopsies were identified as having bronchiolitis; each of the 52 patients who underwent lung biopsy had at least 1 histologic abnormality. No additional data were provided by Krefft and colleagues[68] specifically for the 31 biopsy-confirmed cases of bronchiolitis or by Madar and colleagues[69] for the 2 cases of respiratory bronchiolitis. For the remaining 17 patients from the 7 other studies that reported additional data, 16 (94%) patients presented with exertional dyspnea.[56,58–60] Seven of these patients had additional clinical information, of whom 2 had normal spirometry. Only 1 of the 6 patients who had HRCT findings reported a normal HRCT compared with 68% of the patients described by King and colleagues.[56–60] Each of the 5 patients who had an available smoking history was a never smoker.[56,58,60] Deployment histories included Iraq (n = 4), Afghanistan (n = 2), Middle East (n = 1), and not reported (n = 2). Since the identification of cases of constrictive bronchiolitis associated with OIF/OEF, 2 cases of constrictive bronchiolitis among veterans of Gulf War I also have been described (see **Table 2**).[70,71]

Following a systematic review, Banks and colleagues[72] analyzed 41 cases of military deployment–related constrictive bronchiolitis compared with a cohort of cases of constrictive bronchiolitis related to other causes including occupational exposure to artificial flavorings and exposure to sulfur mustard gas. Compared with constrictive bronchiolitis from other causes, the cohort of military deployment–related cases had the following statistically significant differences ($P<.05$) in prevalences of clinical findings: (1) lower prevalences of spirometric obstruction, abnormal chest radiography, and CT/HRCT not consistent with constrictive bronchiolitis; and (2) higher prevalences of abnormal diffusing capacity.[72] A small case series demonstrated that of 6 patients with deployment-related biopsy-proven bronchiolitis, each had abnormalities on noncontrast chest CT, including centrilobular nodularity (n = 6), bronchial wall thickening (2), air trapping (2), and ground glass opacities (1).[67] Further, investigators used field-emission scanning electron microscopy and laser ablation inductively coupled plasma mass spectrometry to analyze lung tissue specimens from 11 military personnel who had deployed to Southwestern Asia and undergone subsequent lung biopsy because of respiratory symptoms, several of whom were confirmed to have had constrictive bronchiolitis.[73,74] Compared with negative controls (n = 11) and positive controls (n = 11) who had autoimmune constrictive bronchiolitis, the lung tissue specimens from the symptomatic military personnel had higher abundances of silicon, cadmium, aluminum, and vanadium.[73] The findings from this small case series exhibit the possibility that these metals could play a role in the development of constrictive bronchiolitis related to military deployment.

Table 2
Southwestern Asia military deployment-related bronchiolitis cases

Authors	No. Cases (% Male)	Diagnosis	Symptoms	PFTs	HRCT	Histology	Deployment Exposures/ Tobacco Exposures	Other
Gulf War I								
Robinson and Barney[70] 2018	1 (100%)	Constrictive bronchiolitis	Progressive exertional dyspnea; episodic coughing and wheezing	Restriction; FVC = 45% predicted; TLC = 57% predicted; DLCO = 64% predicted Required 4 L oxygen on 6MWT to maintain normal oxygen saturation	Bilateral lower lobe atelectasis and bilateral air trapping on expiratory views	Constrictive bronchiolitis; airway-centered antraco-silicotic dust; SEM/EDX = aluminum and magnesium silicates; titanium dioxide; rare earth elements (cerium and lanthanum); antimony; chromium	Veteran of Gulf War (Saudi Arabia, Kuwait, Iraq during 1990–1991) Sandstorms, Kuwait oil fires Nonsmoker	

(continued on next page)

Table 2
(*continued*)

Authors	No. Cases (% Male)	Diagnosis	Symptoms	PFTs	HRCT	Histology	Deployment Exposures/ Tobacco Exposures	Other
Weiler et al.[71] 2018	1 (100%)	Constrictive bronchiolitis	Progressive exertional dyspnea	1992 — FEV1 = 5.41 L (123% predicted); FVC = 7.36 L (132%); FEV1/FVC = 0.73 1994 — FEV1 = 4.75 L (109%); FVC = 6.51 L (118%); FEV1/FVC = 0.73 2016 — FEV1 = 2.83 L (78%); FVC = 4.32 L (88%); FEV1/FVC = 0.65; TLC = 6.96 L (92%); RV = 2.26 L (86%); DLCO = 20.3 mL/min/mm Hg (70%)	Inspiratory = mild bibasilar atelectasis and old granulomatous disease Expiratory = diffuse air trapping	Small airways abnormalities (muscular hypertrophy, luminal narrowing, diminution of size compared with paired pulmonary artery) Middle lobe had focal organizing pneumonia and a few isolated granulomas No evidence of foreign material in sample No birefringent particulates	Two Persian Gulf deployments during 1991 and 1992 (burning oil wells; petrochemical cracking facilities; burned tanks that had been hit by depleted uranium penetrating rounds; downwind several hundred miles from plume from detonation of Khamisiyah Ammunition Storage Facility; dust storms; pesticide impregnated uniforms; weapons firing; CS tear gas) Never smoker	

Operation Iraqi Freedom/Operation Enduring Freedom							
King et al.[57] 2011	38 (92%)	Constrictive bronchiolitis	Exertional dyspnea	Normal = 13 (34%) Normal with low DLCO = 19 (50%) Obstructive = 2 (5%) Restrictive = 3 (8%) Mixed obstructive/ restrictive = 1 (3%)	Normal = 25 (68%)[a] Mild air trapping = 6 (16%) >1 nodules (<1 cm) = 2 (5%) Solitary nodule (<1 cm) = 1 (3%) Pleural thickening = 1 (3%) Bibasilar scarring = 1 (3%) Apical bullae = 1 (3%)	Bronchiolar luminal constriction = 38 (100%) Predominant c onstrictive stroma = 38 (100%; smooth muscle [7], fibrous tissue [3], mixed [28]) Pigment deposition = 37 (97%) Polarizable material within pigment = 36 (95%) Peribronchiolar inflammation = 34 (89%) Hypertensive-type arterial change = 28 (74%) Respiratory bronchiolitis = 27 (71%) Prominent bronchial-associated lymphoid tissue = 19 (50%) Mucus plugging = 13 (34%) Eosinophils in bronchiolar wall = 7 (18%) Luminal granulation = 2 (5%)	Dust storms = 33 (87%) Sulfur-mine fire in 2003 = 28 (74%) Incinerated solid waste = 24 (63%) Incinerated human waste = 18 (47%) Combat smoke = 17 (45%) Current smoker = 7 (18%) Former smoker = 6 (16%)

(*continued on next page*)

Table 2
(*continued*)

Authors	No. Cases (% Male)	Diagnosis	Symptoms	PFTs	HRCT	Histology	Deployment Exposures/ Tobacco Exposures	Other
						Obliteration of bronchioles = 0 (0%)		
Szema et al.[79] 2012	1 (100%)	Nonspecific interstitial pneumonitis and bronchiolitis	Cough, wheeze	NR	NR	Nonspecific interstitial pneumonitis with peribronchiolar inflammation; lung section had evidence of iron, copper, titanium	Deployed to Iraq and Kuwait; airborne dust in laundry facility; improvised explosive device; sandstorms; burn pits; occasional cigar	
Dhoma et al.[67] 2014	10 (NR)	Bronchiolitis	Exertional dyspnea	NR	NR	NR	NR	
Osman et al.[59] 2014	1 (100%)	Constrictive bronchiolitis	Progressive dyspnea on exertion	No obstruction; TLC = 74% predicted	Focal bronch-iectasis within right lower and middle lobes	Constrictive bronchiolitis	Deployed to Iraq in 2008; burn pits	Evaluated 6 y after deployment

Lentz et al.[58] 2016	3 (100%)	Constrictive bronchiolitis	Exertional dyspnea	Patient 1 PFT pattern = normal; FEV1 (% predicted) = 94%; FVC = 89%; TLC = 100%; DLCO = 108% Patient 2 PFT pattern = normal; FEV1 (% predicted) = 81%; FVC = 78%; TLC = 80%; DLCO = 92% Patient 3 PFT pattern = mixed obstruction/ restriction; FEV1 (% predicted) = 66%; FVC = 78%; TLC = 64%; DLCO = 97%	Patient 1 3 mm nodule Patient 2 Right middle lobe bronchial thickening Patient 3 Mild air trapping	Cryobiopsy diagnostic of constrictive bronchiolitis (n = 3) Peribronchial pigment deposition (n = 3)	Patient 1 Iraq Burn pits Combat smoke Never smoker Patient 2 Afghanistan Burn pits Never smoker Patient 3 Iraq Afghanistan Burn pits Never smoker	Diagnosis made following cryobiopsy
Madar et al.[69] 2017	2 (NR)	Respiratory bronchiolitis	NR	NR	NR	NR	NR	2 cases occurred among 137 deployed military personnel with lung biopsies (1%) compared with 4 cases among 254 non-deployed personnel (2%), p = NS
Papieniak et al.[60] 2018	1 (100%)	Constrictive bronchiolitis	Progressive exertional dyspnea	Pulmonary function testing lower limits of normal for age 6MWT reduced at 298 m; required 3 L oxygen with exertion	Normal	Constrictive bronchiolitis	Middle East deployment, multiple exposures, burn pits Never smoker	Former triathlete; 6MWT increased to 426m after beginning thrice weekly azithromycin

(*continued on next page*)

Table 2
(continued)

Authors	No. Cases (% Male)	Diagnosis	Symptoms	PFTs	HRCT	Histology	Deployment Exposures/ Tobacco Exposures	Other
Butzko et al.[56] 2019	1 (0%)	Constrictive bronchiolitis	Progressive dyspnea	Pre-BD spirometry (% predicted)[b] FEV1 = 2.35 L (81%); FVC = 2.86 L (81%); FEV1/FVC = 0.82; TLC = 3.68 L (80%); RV = 0.71 L (50%); DLCO = 19.10 mL/min/mm Hg (84%) Pre-BD FOT (%predicted) Rrs 4 = 8.06 hPa/L/s (148%); Rrs 4-Rrs 20 = 2.56; Xrs 4 = −2.42 (117%); Ax4 = 40.79 Hz•hPa/L/s (342%); Fres = 31.56 (183%) Post-BD FOT (% change)< Rrs 4 = 2.88 hPa/L/s (−64%); Rrs 4-Rrs 20 = −1.18 (−146%); Xrs 4 = −0.81 (−71%); Ax4 = 5.68 Hz•hPa/L/s (−86%); Fres = 5.68 (−51%)	Widespread large and small airway thickening, mild distortion most prominent in lung bases, subtle mosaic attenuation	Constrictive bronchiolitis with secondary airspace enlargement	12-mo deployment to Iraq in 2005; burn pits; dust; sand storms Never smoker	Respiratory symptoms began within 2 mo of arriving in Iraq and episode of pneumonia; frequent bronchitis and dyspnea on exertion; symptoms persisted post-deployment and refractory to therapy; diagnosis made 9.5 y post-deployment;

Krefft et al.[68] 2020	31 (NR)	Bronchiolitis	Cough, shortness of breath, chest tightness/ wheezing	Normal = 52/80 (65%); obstruction = 4/80 (5%); restriction = 20/80 (25%); air trapping (RV>120% predicted) = 36/77 (47%); abnormal DLCO = 18/77 (23%); any abnormality = 55/80 (69%)	34/118 (29%) met case definition for probable DDLD[c]	31/52 (60%) patients who underwent lung biopsies had bronchiolitis	For all DDLD cases: Iraq, Afghanistan, Iraq/Afghanistan, other conflict areas; mean deployment duration = 20.3 mo; mean number of deployments = 2.1 For all DDLD cases: Never smoker = 53%; ex-smoker = 43%; current smoker = 3%	All 52 patients who underwent lung biopsy had at least one histologic abnormality; hyperinflation/ emphysema = 69%; granulomatous pneumonitis accompanied by lymphocytic interstitial inflammation = 50% 18/77 (23%) of DDLD patients had abnormal DLCO compared with 0/20 (0%) with proximal respiratory disease, $P = .02$

Abbreviations: 6MWT, 6 minute walk test; Ax4, reactance curve area calculated either between 4 hertz and resonant frequency; BD, bronchodilator; cm, centimeter; DDLD, deployment-related distal lung disease; DLCO, diffusing capacity of the lungs for carbon monoxide; EDX, energy dispersive X-ray spectroscopy; FEV1, forced expiratory volume in 1 second; FOT, forced oscillation technique; Fres, resonant frequency; FVC, forced vital capacity; hPa, hectopascal; HRCT, high-resolution computed tomography; Hz, hertz; L, liter; min, minute; ml, milliliter; mm, millimeter; NR, not reported; NS, not significant; PFT, pulmonary function tests; Rrs, resistance; RV, residual volume; s, second; SEM, scanning electron microscopy; TLC, total lung capacity; Xrs, reactance.

[a] 37 of 38 soldiers underwent high-resolution computed tomography testing.

[b] No significant change post-bronchodilator.

[c] Deployment-related distal lung disease defined as military or civilian patients who had respiratory symptoms (ie, cough, shortness of breath, or chest tightness/wheezing) that began during or after deployment and (a) Definite = 1 or more of the following surgical lung biopsy findings: hyperinflation or emphysema; bronchiolitis, small airways inflammation, peribronchiolar fibrosis; or granulomatous pneumonitis, or (b) Probable = 2 or more of the following chest computed tomography findings: centrilobular nodularity, air trapping or mosaicism, or bronchial wall thickening.

Despite concerns over the potential for inhalation exposures experienced during OIF/OEF to be the source of constrictive bronchiolitis and other respiratory diseases, conclusive evidence remains elusive.[61,64,75] The Millennium Cohort study that evaluated deployment and burn pit exposure during 2004 to 2008 determined that no increased likelihood existed for newly reported asthma, newly reported chronic bronchitis or emphysema, or self-reported respiratory symptoms among military personnel exposed to burn pits compared with other deployed military personnel.[64] In addition, the Institute of Medicine's Committee on the Long-Term Health Consequences of Exposure to Burn Pits in Iraq and Afghanistan was unable to render a conclusion whether long-term health effects are caused by exposure to the burn pit at Joint Base Balad in Iraq, but did note that long-term health effects might result from air pollution in Iraq and Afghanistan that originates from sources other than burn pits.[61] More recently, investigators evaluated a cohort of 50 military personnel who had developed respiratory symptoms within 6 months of returning from deployment in 2010.[76] Initial health assessments failed to yield a clinical diagnosis for 21 patients. A total of 37 patients had normal HRCTs, but unlike the case series described by King and colleagues,[57] none of the patients underwent lung biopsy.[76]

The likelihood of identifying a specific causal agent as the source of deployment-related bronchiolitis is low considering that (1) to date, fewer than 50 of the more than 2.7 million service members deployed to OIF/OEF have been described in the published literature as having deployment-related bronchiolitis[56–60,67,69,77]; (2) establishing a standardized case definition for the histologic diagnosis of constrictive bronchiolitis has proven challenging[78]; (3) some patients were deployed multiple times to different locations[58,79]; (4) patients had multiple, varying, and not well-characterized exposures[56–60,67,69,79,80]; and (5) the challenge in characterizing the timing of specific known exposures with respect to disease onset.[81] Additional well-designed epidemiologic studies are needed to further describe the association between military deployments to Southwestern Asia and constrictive bronchiolitis with particular attention given to possible individual host susceptibility factors.

EMERGING ISSUES

Multiple reports in recent years have drawn attention to novel or previously unrecognized risk factors for occupational bronchiolitis. A case series published in 2013 described 6 cases of obliterative bronchiolitis in fiberglass-reinforced plastics workers: 5 boat builders and 1 water cooling tower fabricator from 5 different worksites.[82] The cases were remarkable for their severity with outcomes that included 2 lung transplants and 1 death. The industrial process associated with each case involved fabrication of fiberglass-reinforced plastics using a resin mixed with styrene and an accelerating agent. High concentrations of styrene and dimethyl phthalate were found in the workplace air of 1 patient, and for other cases chemical exposures were thought to include acetone, butyl acetate, butanone, N,N-diethylaniline, diethylene glycol, and isophorone diisocyanate. This series prompted the reporting of 2 additional cases in a yacht builder and water storage tank repairer, who shared exposures to chemicals used in lamination, including polyester resin, methyl ethyl ketone peroxide, and styrene.[83]

Epidemiologic studies of the fiberglass-reinforced plastics industry also indicate respiratory disease consistent with bronchiolitis. One clue originated from cancer mortality studies demonstrating unanticipated excess mortality from nonmalignant respiratory diseases such as COPD.[84] In particular, the occurrence of COPD deaths among short-tenure workers who had high styrene exposures raises the possibility of misdiagnosed bronchiolitis among workers who left employment early in their tenure after being disabled by occupational exposure.[85] In one example, longitudinal analysis of a cohort of 5204 workers from 2 fiberglass-reinforced plastic boatbuilding facilities found short-tenure, high-exposure workers had elevated standardized mortality ratios for nonmalignant respiratory disease (1.99; 95% confidence interval [CI] 1.38–2.79) and COPD (2.60; 95% CI, 1.70–3.81).[86] When we examined death certificates and available medical records for decedents from this cohort who died of nonmalignant respiratory disease, we found 1 case of bronchiolitis and 9 cases of early-onset COPD that could represent misdiagnosed bronchiolitis.[87] Planned follow-up of this cohort to characterize the respiratory health of survivors might further elucidate the risk of bronchiolitis among workers in this industry.

The fiberglass-reinforced plastics industry is notable for its chemical complexity and determining the exposure(s) responsible for occupational bronchiolitis among these workers is challenging. At a manufacturing facility that made fiberglass-reinforced windblades for the green energy sector, styrene was the predominant exposure, with high peak concentrations associated with certain tasks.[88] Evaluation of the workforce demonstrated associations between chest symptoms, spirometric obstruction, other functional deficits, and estimated styrene exposure using urinary metabolites.[89] Styrene is a readily absorbed volatile organic compound (VOC) and a plausible respiratory toxin given its observed effects on respiratory epithelium in some animal models.[84] Nevertheless, the toxicologic literature on styrene is not uniform,[90,91] and it is possible that associations between adverse respiratory outcomes and

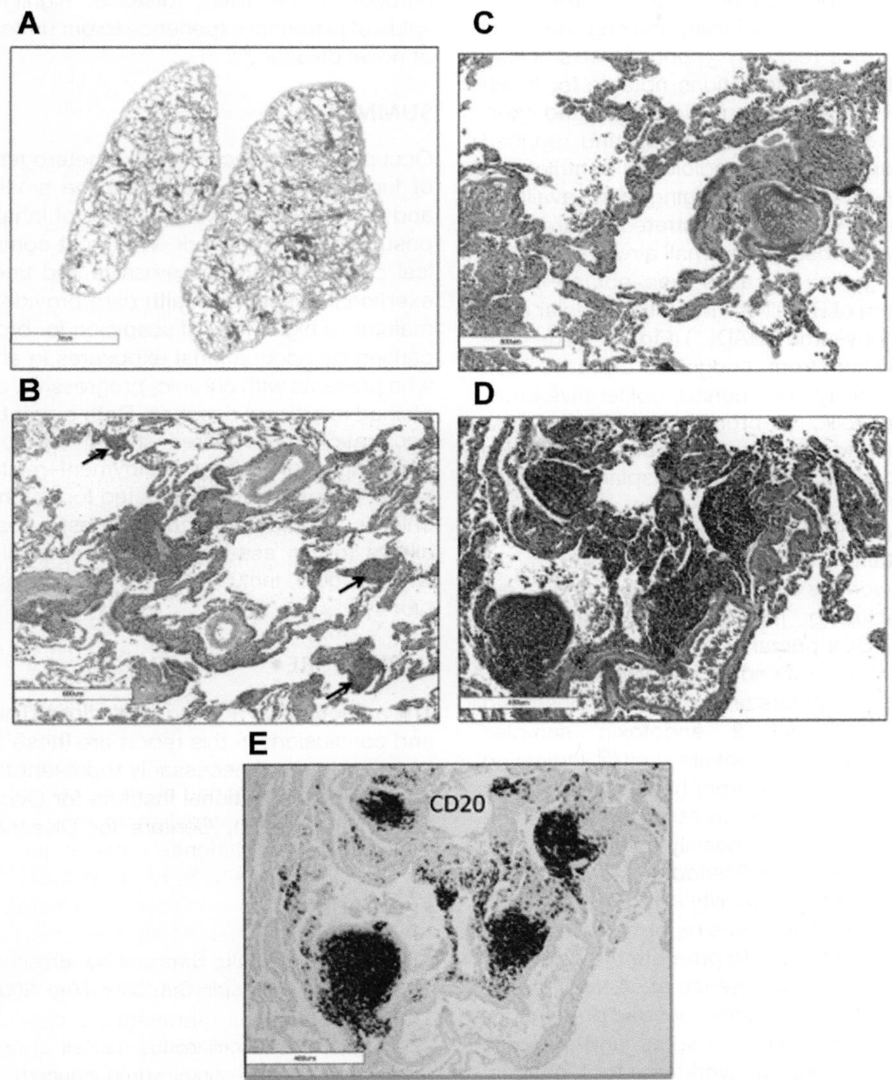

Fig. 1. Representative hematoxylin and eosin stains of explanted lung tissue and surgical lung biopsies from patients with lymphocytic bronchiolitis, alveolar ductitis, and emphysema (BADE). These specimens highlight the primary histologic features of lymphoplasmacytic infiltrates with primary lymphoid follicles around the distal airways and notable involvement of respiratory bronchioles and alveolar ducts, in addition to diffuse emphysema. (*A*) Low-power view, highlighting peribronchiolar lymphoid aggregates with widespread emphysema. (*B*) Medium-power view, showing nonreactive lymphoid follicles with nodular extensions into the alveolar ducts (*arrows*); emphysema also appreciated. (*C, D*) High-power views of nodular lymphoid aggregates around a respiratory bronchiole and chronic inflammatory infiltrates expanding the walls of the alveolar ducts. (*E*) Immunochemical staining for CD20, a B-cell marker, demonstrating B cells make up most of the primary follicles. (*From* Cummings KJ, Stanton ML, Nett RJ, et al. Severe lung disease characterized by lymphocytic bronchiolitis, alveolar ductitis, and emphysema (BADE) in industrial machine-manufacturing workers. Am J Ind Med. 2019;1-11. https://doi.org/10.1002/ajim.23038; with permission.)

styrene exposure in epidemiologic studies reflect the effects of another toxin that shares styrene's exposure profile. Planned studies using a novel humanized mouse model that accounts for differential styrene metabolism in mice and humans should better inform our understanding of bronchiolitis in this industry.

We recently reported a novel form of bronchiolitis among workers at a facility making industrial machines.[92] Five relatively young never-smoking men had clinical presentations notable for insidious post-hire onset of cough, wheeze, and exertional dyspnea; airflow obstruction and reduced diffusing capacity; and radiologic centrilobular emphysema. Expiratory imaging was available for 2 patients, which demonstrated air trapping consistent with obstructive small airways disease. Histopathology in all cases was notable for a unique pattern of B-cell bronchiolitis, alveolar ductitis, and emphysema ("BADE") (**Fig. 1**).[92] The findings were distinct from recognized diseases such as hypersensitivity pneumonitis, obliterative bronchiolitis, and follicular bronchiolitis. Clinical outcomes included chronic dyspnea, progressive functional decline, and lung transplantation in 1 patient to date.

The cause of this novel occupational bronchiolitis is uncertain.[92] The 5 BADE cases occurred in production workers who had multiple potential exposures including metals (mainly steel and aluminum), VOCs primarily associated with painting, and aerosols related to metalworking fluids. Air sampling for metals and VOCs demonstrated low exposures, but 2 endotoxin samples exceeded the Dutch exposure limit,[93] indicating potential to impair respiratory health. The evident source of endotoxin was aerosolization of metalworking fluid, which was heavily colonized by the gram-negative bacteria *Pseudomonas pseudoalcaligenes*; indeed, the facility's most commonly used metalworking fluid was reportedly designed, through its constituents, to promote the growth of this organism.[94] In the absence of certainty about the cause of BADE, we recommended precautionary measures to limit exposures and periodic spirometry to monitor the workforce for functional declines that would merit further evaluation. Multidisciplinary investigation of additional BADE cases or clusters could help to illuminate the cause and guide preventive strategies.

Other notable recent reports of occupational bronchiolitis include a small airways-centered granulomatous reaction in 4 workers chronically exposed to polytetrafluoroethylene (PTFE or Teflon) and acute fibrosing bronchiolitis in a construction worker 1 week after substantial dust and mold exposure.[95–97] In one of the PTFE cases, an extensive workplace exposure assessment concluded the disease was caused by aerosolization of PTFE during spray coating of frying pans.[97] The construction worker's histopathologic findings and robust response to steroids were reminiscent of the classic descriptions from the mid-20th century of proliferative bronchiolitis from oxides of nitrogen in silo-fillers' disease, highlighting the value of historical experience to our understanding of novel disease.[98]

SUMMARY

Occupational bronchiolitis is a heterogeneous set of lung conditions that affect the small airways and can occur following a range of inhalation exposures related to work. The most common clinical presentation is progressive and unexplained exertional dyspnea. Health care providers should maintain a high index of suspicion for bronchiolitis caused by occupational exposures in any patient who presents with chronic, progressive, and unexplained exertional dyspnea. Both current and past occupational exposures should be considered, including prior military deployment–related exposures. Patients being evaluated for potential bronchiolitis should undergo diagnostic testing that allows for an assessment of the small airways, which could include HRCT and possibly lung biopsy.

DISCLOSURE

The authors have nothing to disclose. The findings and conclusions in this report are those of the authors and do not necessarily represent the official position of the National Institute for Occupational Safety and Health, Centers for Disease Control and Prevention.

REFERENCES

1. Ryu JH, Myers JL, Swensen SJ. Bronchiolar disorders. Am J Respir Crit Care Med 2003;168(11):1277–92.
2. King TE Jr. Miscellaneous causes of bronchiolitis: inhalational, infectious, drug-induced, and idiopathic. Semin Respir Crit Care Med 2003;24(5):567–76.
3. Cummings KJ, Kreiss K. Occupational and environmental bronchiolar disorders. Semin Respir Crit Care Med 2015;36(3):366–78.
4. Fechter-Leggett ED, White SK, Fedan KB, et al. Burden of respiratory abnormalities in microwave popcorn and flavouring manufacturing workers. Occup Environ Med 2018;75(10):709–15.
5. Halldin CN, Suarthana E, Fedan KB, et al. Increased respiratory disease mortality at a microwave

popcorn production facility with worker risk of bronchiolitis obliterans. PloS one 2013;8(2):e57935.
6. Kreiss K, Gomaa A, Kullman G, et al. Clinical bronchiolitis obliterans in workers at a microwave-popcorn plant. N Engl J Med 2002;347(5):330–8.
7. Akpinar-Elci M, Travis WD, Lynch DA, et al. Bronchiolitis obliterans syndrome in popcorn production plant workers. Eur Respir J 2004;24(2):298–302.
8. Hubbs AF, Battelli LA, Goldsmith WT, et al. Necrosis of nasal and airway epithelium in rats inhaling vapors of artificial butter flavoring. Toxicol Appl Pharmacol 2002;185(2):128–35.
9. Hubbs AF, Goldsmith WT, Kashon ML, et al. Respiratory toxicologic pathology of inhaled diacetyl in Sprague-Dawley rats. Toxicol Pathol 2008;36(2): 330–44.
10. Morgan DL, Flake GP, Kirby PJ, et al. Respiratory toxicity of diacetyl in C57BL/6 mice. Toxicol Sci 2008;103(1):169–80.
11. Palmer SM, Flake GP, Kelly FL, et al. Severe airway epithelial injury, aberrant repair and bronchiolitis obliterans develops after diacetyl instillation in rats. PloS one 2011;6(3):e17644.
12. Flake GP, Morgan DL. Pathology of diacetyl and 2,3-pentanedione airway lesions in a rat model of obliterative bronchiolitis. Toxicology 2016;388:40–7.
13. Morgan DL, Jokinen MP, Price HC, et al. Bronchial and bronchiolar fibrosis in rats exposed to 2,3-pentanedione vapors: implications for bronchiolitis obliterans in humans. Toxicol Pathol 2012;40(3):448–65.
14. Morgan DL, Jokinen MP, Johnson CL, et al. Chemical reactivity and respiratory toxicity of the alpha-diketone flavoring agents: 2,3-Butanedione, 2,3-Pentanedione, and 2,3-Hexanedione. Toxicol Pathol 2016;44(5):763–83.
15. Hubbs AF, Kreis K, Cummings KJ, et al. Flavorings-related lung disease: a brief review and new mechanistic data. Toxicol Pathol 2019;47(8):1012–26.
16. Kanwal R, Kullman G, Piacitelli C, et al. Evaluation of flavorings-related lung disease risk at six microwave popcorn plants. J Occup Environ Med 2006;48(2): 149–57.
17. van Rooy FG, Rooyackers JM, Prokop M, et al. Bronchiolitis obliterans syndrome in chemical workers producing diacetyl for food flavorings. Am J Respir Crit Care Med 2007;176(5):498–504.
18. Lockey JE, Hilbert TJ, Levin LP, et al. Airway obstruction related to diacetyl exposure at microwave popcorn production facilities. Eur Respir J 2009;34(1):63–71.
19. Kreiss K. Occupational causes of constrictive bronchiolitis. Curr Opin Allergy Clin Immunol 2013;13(2): 167–72.
20. Centers for Disease Control and Prevention. Obliterative bronchiolitis in workers in a coffee-processing facility - Texas, 2008-2012. MMWR Morb Mortal Wkly Rep 2013;62(16):305–7.
21. Cavalcanti ZRAA, Pereira CA, Coletta EN. Bronchiolitis associated with exposure to artificial butter flavoring in workers at a cookie factory in Brazil. J Bras Pneumol 2012;38:395–9.
22. van Rooy FG, Smit LA, Houba R, et al. A cross-sectional study of lung function and respiratory symptoms among chemical workers producing diacetyl for food flavourings. Occup Environ Med 2009;66(2):105–10.
23. Huff SD, Levin JL, Azzi EJ, et al. Bronchiolitis obliterans from coffee flavoring. Am J Respir Crit Care Med 2013;187:A2081.
24. Morales-Camino JA. Pulmonary effects by diacetyl exposure. Toxicol Lett 2016;259:S53.
25. Egilman DS, Schilling JH. Bronchiolitis obliterans and consumer exposure to butter-flavored microwave popcorn: a case series. Int J Occup Environ Health 2012;18(1):29–42.
26. Hendrick DJ. "Popcorn worker's lung" in Britain in a man making potato crisp flavouring. Thorax 2008; 63(3):267–8.
27. Cummings KJ, Boylstein RJ, Stanton ML, et al. Respiratory symptoms and lung function abnormalities related to work at a flavouring manufacturing facility. Occup Environ Med 2014; 71(8):549–54.
28. Kim TJ, Materna BL, Prudhomme JC, et al. Industry-wide medical surveillance of California flavor manufacturing workers: cross-sectional results. Am J Ind Med 2010;53(9):857–65.
29. Kreiss K. Work-related spirometric restriction in flavoring manufacturing workers. Am J Ind Med 2014;57(2):129–37.
30. Kreiss K, Fedan KB, Nasrullah M, et al. Longitudinal lung function declines among California flavoring manufacturing workers. Am J Ind Med 2012;55(8): 657–68.
31. Ryu JH. Classification and approach to bronchiolar diseases. Curr Opin Pulm Med 2006;12(2):145–51.
32. Devakonda A, Raoof S, Sung A, et al. Bronchiolar disorders: a clinical-radiological diagnostic algorithm. Chest 2010;137(4):938–51.
33. Centers for Disease Control and Prevention. Fixed obstructive lung disease among workers in the flavor-manufacturing industry–California, 2004-2007. MMWR Morb Mortal Wkly Rep 2007;56(16): 389–93.
34. Pierce JS, Abelmann A, Spicer LJ, et al. Diacetyl and 2,3-pentanedione exposures associated with cigarette smoking: implications for risk assessment of food and flavoring workers. Crit Rev Toxicol 2014;44(5):420–35.
35. Rose CS. Early detection, clinical diagnosis, and management of lung disease from exposure to diacetyl. Toxicology 2017;388:9–14.
36. Parmet AJ, Von Essen S. Rapidly progressive, fixed airway obstructive disease in popcorn workers: a

new occupational pulmonary illness? J Occup Environ Med 2002;44(3):216–8.
37. Kreiss K. Flavoring-related bronchiolitis obliterans. Curr Opin Allergy Clin Immunol 2007;7(2):162–7.
38. Lockey JE, Hilbert TJ, LeMasters G, et al. Respiratory follow-up pre- and post-engineering controls or cessation of added diacetyl at four microwave popcorn facilities. ERJ Open Res 2019;5(3):00042.
39. Bailey RL, Cox-Ganser JM, Duling MG, et al. Respiratory morbidity in a coffee processing workplace with sentinel obliterative bronchiolitis cases. Am J Respir Crit Care Med 2015;58(12):1235–45.
40. Harvey RHB, Korbach E, Rawal A, et al. Flavoring-related lung disease in a worker at a coffee roasting and packaging facility. Am J Respir Crit Care Med 2018;197:A6075.
41. Warrior K, Gamino AJ. Every dog has its day: FIBOS caused by diacetyl exposure from an unusual source. Am J Respir Crit Care Med 2018;197:A6588.
42. LeBouf RF, Hawley B, Cummings KJ. Potential hazards not communicated in safety data sheets of flavoring formulations, including diacetyl and 2,3-Pentanedione. Ann Work Expo Health 2019;63(1): 124–30.
43. Hirst DV, Dunn KH, Shulman SA, et al. Evaluation of engineering controls for the mixing of flavorings containing diacetyl and other volatile ingredients. J Occup Environ Hyg 2014;11(10):680–7.
44. Kanwal R, Kullman G, Fedan KB, et al. Occupational lung disease risk and exposure to butter-flavoring chemicals after implementation of controls at a microwave popcorn plant. Public Health Rep 2011; 126(4):480–94.
45. Weissman DN. Medical surveillance for the emerging occupational and environmental respiratory diseases. Curr Opin Allergy Clin Immunol 2014;14(2):119–25.
46. National Institute for Occupational Safety and Health. Criteria for a recommended standard: occupational exposure to diacetyl and 2,3-pentanedione. U.S. Department of Health and Human Services, Centers for Disease Control and Prevention, National Institute for Occupational Safety and Health, DHHS (NIOSH) publication No. 2016-111. Available at: https://nam03.safelinks.protection.outlook.com/?url=https%3A%2F%2Fwww.cdc.gov%2Fniosh%2Fdocs%2F2016-Q12&data=02%7C01%7Cr.mayakrishnan%40elsevier.com%7Cb327dd696d2b4feaec0b08d863bc1226%7C9274ee3f94254109a27f9fb15c10675d%7C0%7C0%7C637369007460113610&sdata=3GPWKsTBGeAAWWhnx8kuGSSnp60Sty6U8Tx%2B9M%2BD904%3D&reserved=0 111/.
47. American Conference of Governmental Industrial Hygienists. TLVs® and BEIs®: threshold limit values for chemical substances and physical agents and biological exposure indices. Cincinnati (OH): American Conference of Governmental Industrial Hygienists; 2018.
48. American Conference of Governmental Industrial Hygienists. Chemicals substances and other issues under study (TLV®-CS). Available at: http://www.acgih.org/tlv-bei-guidelines/documentation-publications-and-data/under-study-list/chemical-substances-and-other-issues-under-study-tlv. Accessed September 28, 2020.
49. National Institute for Occupational Safety and Health. NIOSH. Evaluation of a medicinal cannabis manufacturing facility with an indoor and outdoor grow operation. In: Couch J, Wiegand D, Grimes GR, et al, editors. Health hazard evaluation report 2016- 0090-3317. Cincinnati, OH: US Department of Health and Human Services, Centers for Disease Control and Prevention, National Institute for Occupational Safety and Health; 2018. Available at: https://www.cdc.gov/niosh/hhe/reports/pdfs/2016-0090-3317.pdf.
50. Duling MG, LeBouf RF, Cox-Ganser JM, et al. Environmental characterization of a coffee processing workplace with obliterative bronchiolitis in former workers. J Occup Environ Hyg 2016;13(10):770–81.
51. Daglia M, Papetti A, Aceti C, et al. Isolation and determination of alpha-dicarbonyl compounds by RP-HPLC-DAD in green and roasted coffee. J Agric Food Chem 2007;55(22):8877–82.
52. Farsalinos KE, Kistler KA, Gillman G, et al. Evaluation of electronic cigarette liquids and aerosol for the presence of selected inhalation toxins. Nicotine Tob Res 2015;17(2):168–74.
53. Atkins G, Drescher F. Acutte inhalational lung injury related to the use of electronic nicotine delivery system (ENDS). Chest 2015;148(4):83A.
54. Hua M, Talbot P. Potential health effects of electronic cigarettes: a systematic review of case reports. Prev Med Rep 2016;4:169–78.
55. Ghinai I, Pray IW, Navon L, et al. E-cigarette product use, or vaping, among persons with associated lung injury - Illinois and Wisconsin, April-September 2019. MMWR Morb Mortal Wkly Rep 2019;68(39): 865–9.
56. Butzko RB, Sotolongo AM, Frnaks TJ, et al. Forced oscillation technique in the evaluation of constrictive bronchiolitis in a southwest Asia deployed veteran. Am J Respir Cell Mol Biol 2019;199:A1819.
57. King MS, Eisenberg R, Newman JH, et al. Constrictive bronchiolitis in soldiers returning from Iraq and Afghanistan. N Engl J Med 2011;365(3):222–30.
58. Lentz RJ, Fessel JP, Johnson JE, et al. Transbronchial cryobiopsy can diagnose constrictive bronchiolitis in veterans of recent conflicts in the middle east. Am J Respir Crit Care Med 2016;193(7):806–8.
59. Osman U, Bascom R. A case of constrictive bronchiolitis in a soldier with unexplained dyspnea. Chest 2014;146:78A, 4_MeetingAbstracts.

60. Papierniak K, Samra Y. Successful treatment of deployment-related constrictive bronchiolitis with azithromycin. Am J Respir Crit Care Med 2018; 197:A6081.
61. Institute of Medicine. Long-Term Health Consequences of Exposure to Burn Pits in Iraq and Afghanistan. Washington, DC: The National Academies Press; 2011.
62. Krefft SD, Meehan R, Rose CS. Emerging spectrum of deployment-related respiratory diseases. Curr Opin Pulm Med 2015;21(2):185–92.
63. Rose CS. Military service and lung disease. Clin Chest Med 2012;33(4):705–14.
64. The Armed Forces Health Surveillance Center, The Naval Health Research Center, Command TUSAPH. Epidemiological studies of health outcomes among troops deployed to burn pit sites. Silver Spring (MD): Armed Forces Health Surveillance Center; 2010.
65. Szema A, Mirsaidi N, Patel B, et al. Proposed Iraq/Afghanistan war-lung injury (IAW-LI) clinical practice recommendations: National Academy Of Sciences' Institute of Medicine burn pits workshop. Am J Mens Health 2017;11(6):1653–63.
66. Jani N, Falvo M, Sotolongo A, et al. Self-reports of constrictive bronchiolitis among service members participating in the veterans administration and department of defense airborne hazards and open burn pit registry. Chest 2017;152:A822.
67. Dhoma S, Cox C, Chung JH, et al. Chest tomography may predict histopathologic abnormalities in symptomatic deployers returning from Iraq and Afghanistan. Am J Respir Crit Care Med 2014;189: A5102.
68. Krefft SD, Wolff J, Zell-Baran L, et al. Respiratory diseases in post-9/11 military personnel following southwest Asia deployment. J Occup Environ Med 2020;62(5):337–43. [Epub ahead of print].
69. Madar CS, Lewin-Smith MR, Franks TJ, et al. Histological diagnoses of military personnel undergoing lung biopsy after deployment to southwest Asia. Lung 2017;195(4):507–15.
70. Robinson SW, Barney JB. When the smoke clears: constrictive bronchiolitis from Gulf War exposures. Am J Respir Crit Care Med 2018;197:A3538.
71. Weiler BA, Colby TV, Floreth TJ, et al. Small airways disease in an operation desert storm deployer: case report and review of the literature on respiratory health and inhalational exposures from Gulf War I. Am J Ind Med 2018;61(10):793–801.
72. Banks DE, Bolduc CA, Ali S, et al. Constrictive bronchiolitis attributable to inhalation of toxic agents: considerations for a case definition. J Occup Environ Med 2018;60(1):90–6.
73. Lowers HA, Todorov T, Strand MJ, et al. Lung biopsies from symptomatic military deployers have variable mineral particle types and higher abundances of silicon, aluminum, cadmium and vanadium compared to controls. Am J Respir Crit Care Med 2015;191:A2575.
74. Lowers HA, Breit GN, Strand M, et al. Method to characterize inorganic particulates in lung tissue biopsies using field emission scanning electron microscopy. Toxicol Mech Methods 2018;28(7):475–87.
75. Morris MJ, Rawlins FA, Forbes DA, et al. Deployment-related respiratory issues. US Army Med Dep J 2016;(2–16):173–8.
76. Morris MJ, Dodson DW, Lucero PF, et al. Study of active duty military for pulmonary disease related to environmental deployment exposures (STAMPEDE). Am J Respir Crit Care Med 2014;190(1): 77–84.
77. Wenger JW, O'Connell C, Cottrell L. Examination of recent deployment experience across the services and components. Santa Monica (CA): RAND Corporation; 2018.
78. Garshick E, Abraham JH, Baird CP, et al. Respiratory health after military service in southwest Asia and Afghanistan. an official American Thoracic Society workshop report. Ann Am Thorac Soc 2019; 16(8):e1–16.
79. Szema AM, Schmidt MP, Lanzirotti A, et al. Titanium and iron in lung of a soldier with nonspecific interstitial pneumonitis and bronchiolitis after returning from Iraq. J Occup Environ Med 2012;54(1):1–2.
80. Zell-Baran LM, Meehan R, Wolff J, et al. Military occupational specialty codes: utility in predicting inhalation exposures in post-9/11 Deployers. J Occup Environ Med 2019;61(12):1036–40.
81. Falvo MJ, Bradley M, Brooks SM. Is deployment an "exposure" in military personnel? J Occup Environ Med 2014;56(11):e139–40.
82. Cullinan P, McGavin CR, Kreiss K, et al. Obliterative bronchiolitis in fibreglass workers: a new occupational disease? Occup Environ Med 2013;70(5): 357–9.
83. Chen CH, Tsai PJ, Wang WC, et al. Obliterative bronchiolitis in workers laying up fiberglass-reinforced plastics with polyester resin and methylethyl ketone peroxide catalyst. Occup Environ Med 2013;70(9): 675–6.
84. Nett RJ, Cox-Ganser JM, Hubbs AF, et al. Non-malignant respiratory disease among workers in industries using styrene-A review of the evidence. Am J Ind Med 2017;60(2):163–80.
85. Cummings KJ, McCague AB, Kreiss K. Nonmalignant respiratory disease mortality in styrene-exposed workers. Epidemiology 2014;25(1):160–1.
86. Ruder AM, Meyers AR, Bertke SJ. Mortality among styrene-exposed workers in the reinforced plastic boatbuilding industry. Occup Environ Med 2016; 73(2):97–102.
87. Nett RJ, Edwards NT, Ruder AM, et al. Deaths from nonmalignant respiratory disease in styrene-

exposed workers: does obliterative bronchiolitis contribute to mortality? Ann Am Thorac Soc 2017; 14(5):810–1.
88. Hammond D, Garcia A, Feng HA. Occupational exposures to styrene vapor in a manufacturing plant for fiber-reinforced composite wind turbine blades. Ann Occup Hyg 2011;55(6):591–600.
89. McCague AB, Cox-Ganser JM, Harney JM, et al. Styrene-associated health outcomes at a windblade manufacturing plant. Am J Ind Med 2015;58(11): 1150–9.
90. Cruzan G, Bus J, Hotchkiss J, et al. CYP2F2-generated metabolites, not styrene oxide, are a key event mediating the mode of action of styrene-induced mouse lung tumors. Regul Toxicol Pharmacol 2012; 62(1):214–20.
91. Cruzan G, Bus JS, Andersen ME, et al. Based on an analysis of mode of action, styrene-induced mouse lung tumors are not a human cancer concern. Regul Toxicol Pharmacol 2018;95:17–28.
92. Cummings KJ, Stanton ML, Nett RJ, et al. Severe lung disease characterized by lymphocytic bronchiolitis, alveolar ductitis, and emphysema (BADE) in industrial machine-manufacturing workers. Am J Ind Med 2019;62(11):927–37.
93. Dutch Expert Committee on Occupational Standards (DECOS). Endotoxins: health-based recommended occupational exposure limit. The Hague (Netherlands): Health Council of the Netherlands; 2010.
94. Kuenzi P, Rufenact A, Di Maiuta N, et al. Microbiology in bioconcept metalworking. Proceedings of the Society of Tribologists and Lubrication Engineers. Annual Meeting and Exhibition, May 2014, Lake Buena Vista, Florida, USA. Available at: https://nam03.safelinks.protection.outlook.com/?url=https%3A%2F%2Fwww.stle.org%2FShared_Content%2FExtended_Abstracts%2FEA_AM2014%2FMetalworking_Fluids%2FMicrobiology%2520in%2520Bio-Concept%2520Metalworking%2520Fluids.aspx&data=02%7C01%7Cr.mayakrishnan%40elsevier.com%7Cb327dd696d2b4feaec0b08d863bc1226%7C9274ee3f94254109a27f9fb15c10675d%7C0%7C0%7C637369007460113610&sdata=nnzl9ra43%2FK%2BJnW9NN%2Bu8nlyNZiBT7Lqw9p1hwMVAVQ%3D&reserved=0. Accessed September 24, 2020.
95. Choi WI, Jung HR, Shehu E, et al. Small airway-centered granulomatosis caused by long-term exposure to polytetrafluoroethylene. Chest 2014; 145(6):1397–402.
96. Ryerson CJ, Olsen SR, Carlsten C, et al. Fibrosing bronchiolitis evolving from infectious or inhalational acute bronchiolitis. a reversible lesion. Ann Am Thorac Soc 2015;12(9):1323–7.
97. Lee N, Baek K, Park S, et al. Pneumoconiosis in a polytetrafluoroethylene (PTFE) spray worker: a case report with an occupational hygiene study. Ann Occup Environ Med 2018;30:37.
98. Cummings KJ, Kreiss K, Roggli VL. Bronchiolitis by any other name: describing bronchiolar disorders from inhalational exposures. Ann Am Thorac Soc 2016;13(1):143–4.

Coal Workers' Pneumoconiosis and Other Mining-Related Lung Disease

New Manifestations of Illness in an Age-Old Occupation

Leonard H.T. Go, MD[a,b,*], Robert A. Cohen, MD[a,b]

KEYWORDS

- Coal workers' pneumoconiosis • Coal mine dust lung disease
- Chronic obstructive pulmonary disease • Silicosis • Mixed-dust pneumoconiosis
- Dust-related diffuse fibrosis • Lung cancer • Coal mine dust

KEY POINTS

- Mine workers may develop diseases other than classic pneumoconiosis from their occupational exposures, including obstructive lung disease, pulmonary fibrosis, and lung cancer.
- A detailed occupational history incorporating details of the job tasks performed by the miner and dust control measures used is critical to the understanding of disease risk.
- Chest imaging and physiologic evaluation are the cornerstones of medical surveillance for mining-related lung disease.
- Diagnosis is made by compatible history, imaging, and physiologic findings. In selected cases, pathologic evaluation of lung tissue may be necessary.
- Mining-related lung diseases are untreatable. Therefore, primary prevention should be the primary public health concern.

INTRODUCTION

Mining-related lung diseases are a group of preventable chronic lung diseases associated with extractive activities performed at or below the surface of the earth. These diseases arise not only from the mineral dust generated from disrupting rock strata, but also from other exposures generated from the equipment and processes needed to perform mining. Of the diseases associated with mining, those associated with coal are the best known and understood, and are the primary focus of this article.

Although there is growing interest in renewable energy sources, such as solar and wind power, internationally, thermal coal remains a primary source of fuel for the generation of electricity and metallurgical coal is essential for steel manufacture. Despite the known contribution of coal mine dust to respiratory disease, coal mine dust lung disease (CMDLD; a spectrum of lung disease that includes not only coal workers' pneumoconiosis [CWP] and silicosis, but also obstructive lung disease and dust-related diffuse fibrosis [DDF]) remains a significant health concern in many parts of the world.

[a] Division of Environmental and Occupational Health Sciences, University of Illinois Chicago School of Public Health, 1603 West Taylor Street, Chicago, IL 60612, USA; [b] Department of Medicine, Northwestern University Feinberg School of Medicine, Chicago, IL, USA
* Corresponding author. Division of Environmental and Occupational Health Sciences, University of Illinois Chicago School of Public Health, 1603 West Taylor Street, Chicago, IL 60612.
E-mail address: lgo2@uic.edu

Clin Chest Med 41 (2020) 687–696
https://doi.org/10.1016/j.ccm.2020.08.002
0272-5231/20/

COMPOSITION OF THE MINE ATMOSPHERE

Because of its abundance in the earth's crust, exposure to respirable crystalline silica (RCS) is a potential hazard common to all mining. In addition to coal, this includes the mining of metals, salts, stone, sand, and oil shale. Most commonly the exposures are caused by dust generated from the drilling, blasting, earth moving, crushing, and processing of the desired commodity. Significant exposures occur whether the mining process is performed primarily at the surface, or by means of underground access.

Coal is a fossil fuel composed primarily of carbonized plant matter, and inorganic substances including silica and silicates; volatile compounds including hydrocarbons; and metals. Disruption of coal seams and neighboring rock layers during mining processes are the primary source of coal mine dust. Other coal mine atmosphere constituents include diesel exhaust from machinery and carbonates, such as crushed limestone, applied to mine surfaces to mitigate the risk of float coal dust explosions.

An individual mine worker's job duties and the mining methods used are the primary determinants of the exposures a worker experiences (**Fig. 1**). Workers in underground mines generally encounter greater dust exposures than those who work at surface mines, although some surface jobs, such as drilling, may be associated with heavy exposures. Mine dust exposure is generally greater for miners working near the point of production, usually the face, where the commodity, such as metal ore or coal, is extracted. Other areas where cutting or drilling occur, such as in mine development areas or securing the rock strata in the mine roof with bolts, have also been associated with excessive exposures.

Modern highly powerful and mechanized mining technology has increased output, allowing fewer miners to produce large quantities of material. However, these improvements may also have resulted in the generation of more dust, and smaller particles with greater toxicity.

Engineering controls used to mitigate dust exposures including local exhaust or dilution ventilation and water sprays are also major determinants of an individual mine worker's dust exposure.

Significant exposures may also occur in preparation or processing plants that take raw mine material and create finished products. Modern coal preparation plant technology permits the efficient separation of coal from large quantities of waste rock, permitting the cutting of large quantities of noncoal material and increasing the risk of exposing miners to greater quantities of RCS.

EPIDEMIOLOGY

Chest radiographs are the cornerstone of surveillance for pneumoconiosis in the workplace given wide international availability, portability, and low cost. The International Labor Office International Classification of Radiographs of Pneumoconioses[1] provides a widely accepted framework for evaluation of posteroanterior chest radiographs taken for medical surveillance of occupational lung disease. The system requires users to compare the images of the subject with standard calibration radiographs to classify the shape, size, and profusion (abundance) of pneumoconiotic opacities. This system improves the consistency in the reading of pulmonary parenchymal and pleural disease and placing an individual case in the context of available epidemiologic information.[1,2]

After the enactment of permissible respirable dust exposure limits in US coal mines in the 1970s, there was a marked decline in radiographic pneumoconiosis into the 1990s, as measured by the National Institute for Occupational Safety and Health Coal Workers' Health Surveillance Program, a voluntary chest radiographic screening program for active US coal miners. However, since the late 1990s, the rates of radiographic

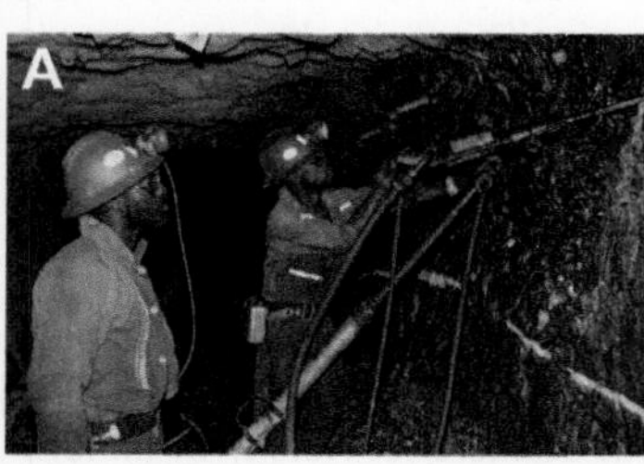

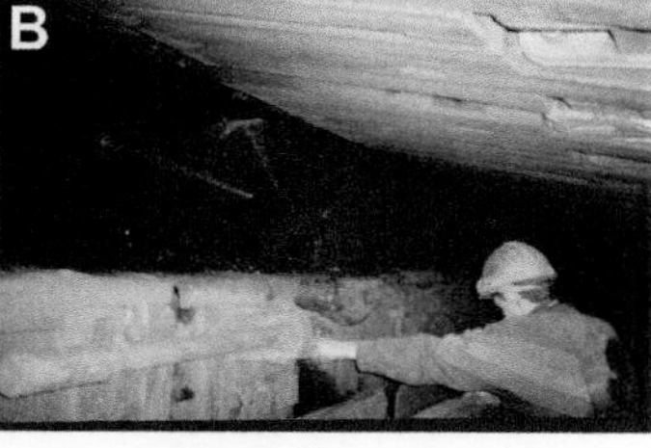

Fig. 1. Mine workers at risk of respiratory disease. (*A*) Gold miners in South Africa drilling holes into the mining face to allow blasting and extraction of gold ore. Drilling and blasting result in generation of dusts, including respirable crystalline silica. (*B*) Underground coal miner in Ukraine. The miner in the figure works underneath protective shields while a longwall shear moves across the mine face to cut coal. Water sprays are among the engineering controls used to reduce respirable dust levels. (*Courtesy of* R. Cohen MD, Chicago, Illinois.)

pneumoconiosis in the United States have risen to 10% of screened miners who have 25 years or more of coal mining tenure.[3] In central Appalachia, 20% of miners with 25 years or more of coal mining tenure have radiographic pneumoconiosis,[3] and progressive massive fibrosis (PMF) has returned to the high levels seen before the enactment of modern dust control regulations.[4]

The alarming trend of increasing pneumoconiosis prevalence and severity in US coal miners despite modern permissible exposure limits has been observed in workers' compensation data. An examination of the US Black Lung Benefits Program shows a rise in the claims awarded for PMF as a percentage of overall claims.[5]

The resurgence of pneumoconiosis is not limited to the United States. After approximately 30 years without reported cases of pneumoconiosis among coal miners in the state of Queensland in Australia, more than 100 cases have been reported since 2015.[6] Data are less complete for other countries. A systematic evaluation of pooled published data from 2001 to 2011 estimated a prevalence of 6.02% for CWP in China.[7] For the states of Madhya Pradesh and Orissa in India, Parihar and colleagues[8] reported a prevalence of CWP of 3.03%.

PATHOGENESIS

Although there is a substantial body of literature describing the cellular biology of lung disease caused by silica exposure, less is known about the pathogenesis of other mining-related lung diseases at the molecular and cellular level. Numerous case-control studies, mostly from China, have suggested multiple candidate genes that may confer differential risk of CWP and potentially provide insight into the mechanisms for the development of CWP.[9–12]

In addition to differences in host susceptibility, it is likely that the heterogeneity of exposures among mine workers contributes to the diversity of presentations. Dust composition, especially the overall quantity of RCS; total cumulative dust exposure; and particle size all likely contribute to the toxicity of dust retained within the lungs of individual mine workers.

DISEASE MANIFESTATIONS

Classic CWP and silicosis have historically been the diseases most associated with exposure to mining-related dust. Unlike a "pure" exposure, such as asbestos, coal mine dust inherently exhibits significant heterogeneity. This heterogeneity likely contributes to the wide spectrum of disease that has been described in coal miners, known as CMDLD. CMDLD includes not only CWP and silicosis, but also emphysema, chronic bronchitis, and pulmonary fibrosis, known as DDF.

Classic Coal Workers' Pneumoconiosis

CWP refers to the predominantly nodular interstitial lung disease that is most often diagnosed in an individual coal mine dust exposure of at least 10 years, although shorter durations of more intense coal mine dust exposure may be associated with the disease. Typical radiologic findings of CWP include nodular or mass-like opacities; areas of lucency consistent with emphysema; and, in advanced disease, architectural distortion caused by loss of lung volume.

The most important risk factor in the development of CWP is cumulative coal mine dust exposure.[13,14] Increasing coal rank, reflecting greater carbon content within the coal, and exposure to mine dust containing a greater proportion of RCS are also believed to contribute to the risk of disease.[14,15]

CWP is divided into "simple" and "complicated" disease based on the size of radiographic or pathologic lesions ($\leq$1 cm vs >1 cm, respectively). The abnormalities of simple CWP are often rounded and upper-zone predominant, although, contrary to prior dogma, significant proportions of workers have irregular and lower-zone predominant lesions.[16] Increasing profusion of simple CWP opacities is associated with reductions in lung function.[17]

PMF, also known as complicated CWP, may develop with the growth or conglomeration of smaller CWP lesions. The risk of PMF increases with age and cumulative dust exposure,[18] and with a higher baseline profusion of small opacities.[18,19] PMF lesions often become bilateral with continued progression of disease. They are typically polygonal in shape and are found in the upper lung zones, although more rounded lesions and lower-zone disease has been reported.[20] Workers with PMF also have a background of small opacities, although their profusion may be reduced as the nodules are subsumed into these larger scars. There may also be associated emphysema, volume loss, and architectural distortion with advanced disease.

Rapidly Progressive Pneumoconiosis

In the United States, rapidly progressive pneumoconiosis (RPP), defined as radiographic progression of more than one International Labor Office profusion subcategory within 5 years or the development of PMF after 1985, has been observed with increasing frequency.[21] RPP seems to be concentrated in the central Appalachian states of Kentucky, Virginia, and West Virginia. Histopathologic examination of lung tissue from workers with RPP demonstrates lesions of silicosis and mixed-dust pneumoconiosis, and pulmonary fibrosis (**Fig. 2**).[22] These findings implicate significant silica and silicate exposures as an important driving factor in this disease.

Mixed-Dust Pneumoconiosis

Coal miners are exposed to mixed dusts as part of many job tasks in modern mining. Silica is an important component of coal mine dust, and is prominent in dust created during mine construction; roof bolting; cutting through rock to build ventilation pathways (overcasts); and narrow-seam mining where miners cut through siliceous layers above, below, and within the coal seams. Mixed-dust pneumoconiosis can only be diagnosed pathologically by mineralogic analysis of lung tissue.[22] It cannot be differentiated from CWP or silicosis without this analysis because the patterns seen radiologically and physiologically are not readily distinguished.

Silicosis

Because of the abundance of silica in neighboring rock layers, inhalation of RCS represents a significant potential respiratory hazard for all miners, regardless of commodity mined. Thus, all miners are at risk for silicosis, much like nonminers exposed to silica. Silicosis and CWP cannot be readily distinguished radiologically or physiologically, although it has been suggested that silicosis is more likely to be associated with r-type (rounded, 3–10 mm diameter) radiologic opacities.[23] Silicosis is reviewed in further detail by Krefft and colleagues in this issue.

Obstructive Lung Disease and Lung Function Impairment

Chronic cough and sputum production are commonly encountered among active and former coal miners.[24,25] The prevalence of chronic bronchitis increases with increased coal mine employment history and greater cumulative dust exposure.[24] Chronic bronchitis symptoms are also associated with declines in forced expiratory volume in 1 second.[26]

Coal mine dust is an important cause of emphysema (**Fig. 3**).[23,27,28] The effect of coal mine dust on emphysema is independent of smoking status,[29] and is additive to the effect of cigarette smoking.[28] The pathologic severity of emphysema is associated with increased dust content.[29,30] All pathologic types of emphysema, including centriacinar, panacinar, and bullous emphysema, are observed with coal mine dust exposure.[31]

Coal mine dust exposure is also associated with lung function impairment as measured by spirometry, even in the absence of radiographic evidence of classic CWP[32] or silicosis.[33] After adjusting for age and smoking status, the magnitude of lung function decline is proportional to estimated cumulative coal mine dust exposure, and the effect is of the same order of magnitude as that caused by tobacco smoke exposure.[34–37]

Mineral dust airways disease refers to disease of the small airways, including fibrosis and pigmentation of respiratory bronchioles. This is seen in

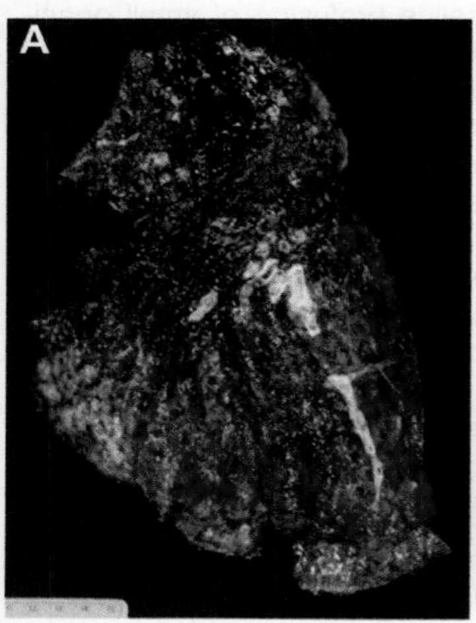

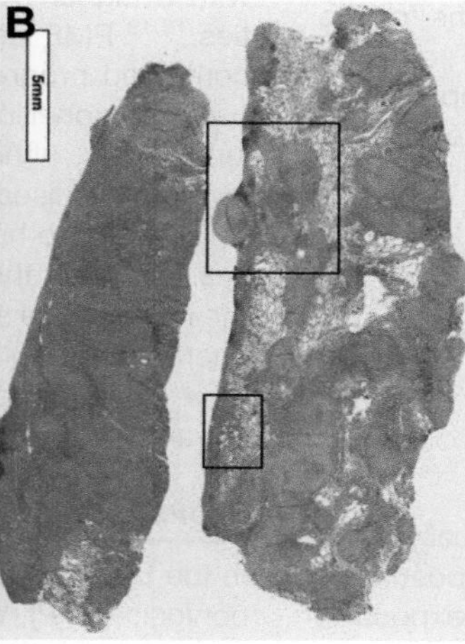

Fig. 2. Rapidly progressive pneumoconiosis. (*A*) Explanted left lung from a coal miner with 35 years of coal mining experience and no history of smoking. The upper lobe and apical portion of the lower lobe are completely replaced by PMF. Pale areas within the PMF are indicative of silicosis. (*B*) Low-magnification view from region of PMF seen in *A*. The parenchyma is largely replaced by silicotic nodules. In the *upper boxed area,* silicotic nodules and lymphoid pleural reaction are seen. Interstitial fibrosis is seen in areas without silicotic nodules, including in the *lower boxed area*. (*Adapted from* Cohen RA, Petsonk EL, Rose C, et al. Lung pathology in US coal workers with rapidly progressive pneumoconiosis implicates silica and silicates. Am J Respir Crit Care Med. 2015; 673-680; with permission.)

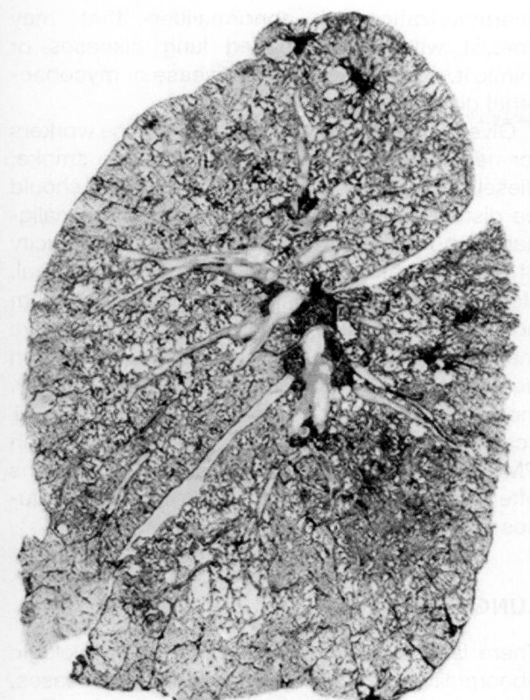

Fig. 3. Emphysema related to mineral dust exposure. Whole lung section from a never-smoker with 28 years of coal mining experience, showing coal workers' pneumoconiosis amid a background of severe emphysema. (*Adapted* with permission of the American Thoracic Society. Copyright © 2020 American Thoracic Society. All rights reserved. Cite: Kuempel ED, Wheeler MW, Smith RJ, et al. Contributions of dust exposure and cigarette smoking to emphysema severity in coal miners in the United States. Am J Respir Crit Care Med 2009;180(3): 257–64. The American Journal of Respiratory and Critical Care Medicine is an official journal of the American Thoracic Society. Readers are encouraged to read the entire article for the correct context at https://www.atsjournals.org/doi/full/10.1164/rccm.200806-840OC. The authors, editors, and The American Thoracic Society are not responsible for errors or omissions in adaptations.)

association with exposures to a variety of mineral dusts, including silica.[38] Tobacco smoke exposure may potentiate the effect of silica dust on airflow obstruction.[39] The magnitude of forced expiratory volume in 1 second decline is also associated with increased risk of death from cardiovascular and nonmalignant respiratory disease.[40]

Dust-Related Diffuse Fibrosis

Coal mine dust exposure is also associated with a pulmonary fibrosis phenotype, known as DDF. It may have features of usual interstitial pneumonia and is sometimes mistaken for idiopathic pulmonary fibrosis (IPF). It is, however, imperative to keep in mind that IPF is a diagnosis of exclusion, and that potential occupational and environmental exposures, among many other possibilities, should be excluded before arriving at a diagnosis of IPF. McConnochie and colleagues[41] showed that pulmonary fibrosis was common among autopsied coal miners, underscoring the importance of obtaining a careful occupational history in the evaluation of pulmonary fibrosis. This is particularly important in an era of efficacious, but costly, treatments for IPF that have not yet been demonstrated to be effective in treating DDF.

Workers with exposure to coal mine, silica, and mixed mineral dusts are at risk for DDF. The pulmonary fibrosis found in DDF may be pigmented or unpigmented,[22,41] and there may be a background of nodular interstitial disease. Analysis of these tissues using polarizing light microscopy or scanning electron microscopy with energy-dispersive x-ray spectroscopy may reveal the mineral particulate associated with this disease.[22,42] Desquamative interstitial pneumonia has been suggested as a possible precursor lesion to DDF.[43] DDF is believed to be generally less aggressive than IPF.

Rheumatoid Pneumoconiosis

Known eponymously as Caplan syndrome, rheumatoid pneumoconiosis is the association of rheumatoid arthritis with CWP. Rheumatoid pneumoconiosis is uncommon, observed in less than 1% of autopsied cases. Chest imaging typically demonstrates large well-defined nodules or masses, typically without a background of smaller opacities. These opacities represent rheumatoid nodules that may regress, in contrast to the lesions of classic CWP.[44] Pulmonary tuberculosis and fungal infections should be considered in some cases, particularly when nodules cavitate.

Lung Cancer

Historically, coal mine dust was not believed to contribute to the development of bronchogenic lung cancer. However, several recent studies with longer follow-up have demonstrated an increased association between coal mining and lung cancer.[45–47] The risk seems to be elevated even with a short coal mining career median of 7 years.[48] Mine dust may contain multiple constituents that contribute to lung cancer risk, including silica[49] and diesel exhaust.[50] Additionally, nonmalignant respiratory diseases, such as chronic obstructive pulmonary disease[51] and pulmonary fibrosis,[52] may be linked to subsequent development of lung cancer.

Other Lung Diseases

Other exposures within mines raise the possibility of other diseases. Bronchial asthma has been described in miners. It may be unrelated to work, exacerbated by work, or caused by occupational exposures. Occupational asthma has been reported in association with *Rhizopus* found in coal mine aerosols.[53] In one study of gold miners in Ghana, 37.5% of subjects reported having asthma.[54] Mines may contain several exposures that may cause or exacerbate asthma, including diesel particulates and isocyanates, ureaformol, and formophenolic compounds.[55] Exposure to isocyanates may occur with use of polyurethane products, such as glues, fillers, and binders used in ground and strata control, such as roof bolting in underground mines to prevent collapse.

In addition to occupational asthma, isocyanate exposure can potentially cause hypersensitivity pneumonitis. Also, some miners may have been exposed to asbestos, whether caused by mining through naturally occurring deposits, or through the use of asbestos with mining equipment, such as insulation in coal preparation plants or in the brake pads of heavy machinery.

CLINICAL FEATURES

Individuals with CMDLD and other mining-related lung diseases may initially be asymptomatic, as often occurs when disease is identified through screening. When they occur, symptoms typically develop insidiously, and may start while the individual is still working as a miner or after they have left employment. Dyspnea, cough, sputum production, and wheezing are common symptoms. Symptom severity may worsen even after the worker is no longer exposed to mine dust. The severity of symptoms may not correlate with the degree of observed radiographic abnormality. Advanced stages of disease may be complicated by cor pulmonale or by hypoxemia necessitating home oxygen therapy.

IMAGING

Although the chest radiograph is insensitive in detecting early lesions of CWP,[56] it remains a useful tool in the assessment of the severity of CWP because the number of small opacities correlates well with the number of small lesions observed on pathologic examination.[57] High-resolution computed tomography scanning is a more sensitive imaging modality for certain manifestations of CMDLD, including early pulmonary fibrosis and emphysema.[58,59] High-resolution computed tomography scans also permit better characterization of abnormalities that may coexist with mining-related lung diseases or mimic it, such as neoplastic disease or mycobacterial disease.

Given common risk factors among mine workers for neoplastic disease, such as tobacco smoke, diesel particulates, and silica, malignancy should be distinguished from PMF. Suspicion for malignancy should be stronger when there is a paucity of small opacities or when disease is unilateral. However, PMF is challenging to distinguish from nonpneumoconiotic lesions by noninvasive means. Prior imaging, when available, is useful in determining the likelihood of malignancy. Increased 18-fluorodeoxyglucose uptake on PET scanning may not be a useful finding to distinguish PMF from malignant lesions, because PMF lesions often demonstrate increased 18-fluorodeoxyglucose uptake.[60]

LUNG FUNCTION

There is no characteristic pattern of physiologic abnormality in mining-related lung diseases, reflective of their heterogeneous disease manifestations.[29,61] Spirometry demonstrates obstructive, restrictive, or mixed impairments. Diffusion impairment is common[23,62] even in the absence of abnormalities of spirometry. Abnormalities of spirometry and diffusion testing are associated with increased emphysema[58] and profusion of small irregular opacities[63] observed on chest imaging. Cardiopulmonary exercise testing may be useful in assessing gas exchange abnormalities and determining the cause of dyspnea when pulmonary function tests do not explain symptom severity.[64,65]

PATHOLOGY

Simple CWP may initially manifest as a coal macule, a collection of dust-laden macrophages containing reticulin and collagen located within the wall of respiratory bronchioles. Coal macules may be surrounded by centrilobular, or focal, emphysema. In contrast to coal macules, coal nodules contain more collagen and are not localized to respiratory bronchioles. Scarring from simple CWP may also be irregular, with resemblance to lesions of usual interstitial pneumonia.[66] Nodules may grow or coalesce into lesions of PMF, which are greater than 1 cm in size. PMF lesions might cavitate reflecting superimposed mycobacterial or fungal infection.[67] Silicotic nodules are frequently identified when there has been significant RCS exposure.[22]

DIAGNOSIS

Diagnosis of mining-related lung diseases is most commonly made based on exposure history and chest imaging findings. In addition to their job titles, mine workers should be asked about the specific tasks they performed, an assessment of the dustiness of the work environment, and the nature and degree of use of dust suppression technologies and personal protective equipment.

Surgical biopsy is appropriate in the setting of diagnostic uncertainty, such as concern for neoplastic disease, but should not be used routinely in the diagnosis of mining-related diseases in a sufficiently exposed individual with typical clinical findings. When evaluating a miner's pulmonary abnormalities, the broad spectrum of CMDLD and other mining-related lung diseases should be kept in mind, especially when considering the differential diagnosis of obstructive lung disease or pulmonary fibrosis.

MANAGEMENT

Medical surveillance often results in the identification of asymptomatic mine workers with early stage radiographic or physiologic abnormalities. Although it is generally accepted that workers with more advanced radiographic or physiologic abnormalities should not continue work in positions with additional significant mine dust exposures, workers with early milder disease present a challenge regarding removal from continued exposure. Clinicians should be mindful of the financial and psychosocial impacts of job loss when they prohibit a miner's return to work.

There is no specific treatment of mining-related lung diseases. Treatment is generally directed at specific disease manifestations, such as the use of bronchodilators for obstructive lung disease or supplemental oxygen for hypoxemia. In symptomatic individuals, avoidance of further exposure to respiratory hazards is advised, particularly tobacco smoke. Pulmonary rehabilitation should be considered in symptomatic patients. Lung transplantation is being performed with greater frequency in the United States.[68] Whole lung lavage has been evaluated as a possible treatment to remove mineral dust,[69] but insufficient evidence for its use exists to support its use outside of an investigational setting.

Mining-related lung diseases may progress or be initially diagnosed after a miner is no longer exposed to coal mine dust. CWP may initially appear or become more severe after an individual has stopped working as a miner.[70,71] Similarly, physiologic abnormalities may initially appear or worsen after cessation of mine dust exposure.[72] Therefore, former coal miners warrant ongoing follow-up to monitor for the development or progression of disease.

Clinicians may be asked to opine on whether mine dust exposure has contributed to a patient's respiratory disease and impairment. There is no uniform standard across workers' compensation programs with regard to causation or contribution of mine dust to respiratory disease. Therefore, the clinician should be aware of the standard for the compensation program of interest to provide a clear opinion for an individual worker's compensation claim.

PREVENTION

Primary prevention of mining-related lung diseases, in the form of reductions in worker exposure to mine dusts, is of paramount importance in preventing or reducing the severity of disease. Governmental regulation of permissible exposure levels of respirable mine dusts plays a central role in preventing or mitigating respiratory disease in mine workers.

Engineering controls to limit respirable mine dust exposure are the most effective means of reducing the risk of developing CMDLD and other mining-related lung diseases. Dilution ventilation and local exhaust ventilation measures and water sprays are the most commonly used engineering controls to reduce dust exposures in mine workers.

Respiratory personal protective equipment may be used and reduce individual exposure to mine dusts, but should be used only in conjunction with an effective dust control program within a mine. Several practical barriers reduce the effectiveness of respirators, including improper or inadequate training in their use, the impediment to communication in a noisy environment, difficulty coughing and expectorating, and the difficulty of breathing through high-efficiency loaded dust filters while performing heavy labor.

Secondary prevention of mining-related lung diseases through medical surveillance programs allows the detection of early lung disease, providing the worker the opportunity to modify their job tasks and environment to reduce their subsequent mine dust exposure. Surveillance data aggregated across a worker population also provide insight into the effectiveness of primary prevention measures, and can inform changes in individual mine practices. Medical surveillance data plays an important role in governmental regulation of respirable dust levels. For example, after the rise in CWP prevalence among US coal miners starting in the late 1990s, the national permissible exposure limit for respirable coal mine dust was reduced from 2.0 mg/m^3 to 1.5 mg/m^3.

SUMMARY

Providers must recognize that mine exposures may cause obstructive lung disease, pulmonary fibrosis, and lung cancer, in addition to the CWP and silicosis that receive greater attention. Given the potential impact a diagnosis of mining-related lung disease may have on a miner's ability to continue working, along with the financial and psychosocial aftereffects, the provider bears an important responsibility in the accurate detection and characterization of disease. Obtaining a thorough occupational and exposure history is a critical step in the provider's investigation, and provides important insights into clinical, physiologic, and radiologic findings. Because treatment options are limited and noncurative, prevention of disease or its progression through exposure controls and effective medical surveillance programs are of greatest importance in limiting the public health impacts of these diseases.

DISCLOSURE

The authors have nothing to disclose.

REFERENCES

1. International Labour Office. Guidelines for the use of the ILO international classification of radiographs of pneumoconioses. Revised edition. Geneva (Switzerland): International Labour Office; 2011.
2. Halldin CN, Blackley DJ, Petsonk EL, et al. Pneumoconioses radiographs in a large population of US coal workers: variability in A Reader and B Reader classifications by using the International Labour Office classification. Radiology 2017;284(3):870–6.
3. Blackley DJ, Halldin CN, Laney AS. Continued increase in prevalence of coal workers' pneumoconiosis in the United States, 1970–2017. Am J Public Health 2018;108(9):1220–2.
4. Blackley DJ, Halldin CN, Laney AS. Resurgence of a debilitating and entirely preventable respiratory disease among working coal miners. Am J Respir Crit Care Med 2014;190(6):708–9.
5. Almberg KS, Halldin CN, Blackley DJ, et al. Progressive massive fibrosis resurgence identified in U.S. coal miners filing for black lung benefits, 1970–2016. Ann Am Thorac Soc 2018;15(12):1420–6.
6. Queensland Department of Natural Resources Mines and Energy. Mine dust lung diseases. 2017. Available at: https://www.business.qld.gov.au/industries/mining-energy-water/resources/safety-health/mining/accidents-incidents-reports/mine-dust-lung-diseases. Accessed January 28, 2020.
7. Mo J, Wang L, Au W, et al. Prevalence of coal workers' pneumoconiosis in China: a systematic analysis of 2001-2011 studies. Int J Hyg Environ Health 2014;217(1):46–51.
8. Parihar YS, Patnaik JP, Nema BK, et al. Coal workers' pneumoconiosis: a study of prevalence in coal mines of eastern Madhya Pradesh and Orissa states of India. Ind Health 1997;35(4):467–73.
9. Ates I, Yucesoy B, Yucel A, et al. Possible effect of gene polymorphisms on the release of TNFα and IL1 cytokines in coal workers' pneumoconiosis. Exp Toxicol Pathol 2011;63(1–2):175–9.
10. Ji X, Wu B, Jin K, et al. MUC5B promoter polymorphisms and risk of coal workers' pneumoconiosis in a Chinese population. Mol Biol Rep 2014;41(7):4171–6.
11. Volobaev VP, Larionov AV, Kalyuzhnaya EE, et al. Associations of polymorphisms in the cytokine genes IL1β (rs16944), IL6 (rs1800795), IL12b (rs3212227) and growth factor VEGFA (rs2010963) with anthracosilicosis in coal miners in Russia and related genotoxic effects. Mutagenesis 2018;33(2):129–35.
12. Liu Y, Yang J, Wu Q, et al. LRBA gene polymorphisms and risk of coal workers' pneumoconiosis: a case–control study from China. Int J Environ Res Public Health 2017;14(10). https://doi.org/10.3390/ijerph14101138.
13. Hurley JF, Burns J, Copland L, et al. Coalworkers' simple pneumoconiosis and exposure to dust at 10 British coalmines. Br J Ind Med 1982;39(2):120.
14. Attfield MD, Seixas NS. Prevalence of pneumoconiosis and its relationship to dust exposure in a cohort of U.S. bituminous coal miners and ex-miners. Am J Ind Med 1995;27(1):137–51.
15. Bennett JG, Dick JA, Kaplan YS, et al. The relationship between coal rank and the prevalence of pneumoconiosis. Br J Ind Med 1979;36(3):206.
16. Laney AS, Petsonk EL. Small pneumoconiotic opacities on U.S. coal worker surveillance chest radiographs are not predominantly in the upper lung zones. Am J Ind Med 2012;55(9):793–8.
17. Blackley DJ, Laney AS, Halldin CN, et al. Profusion of opacities in simple coal worker's pneumoconiosis is associated with reduced lung function. Chest 2015;148(5):1293–9.
18. Hurley JF, Alexander WP, Hazledine DJ, et al. Exposure to respirable coalmine dust and incidence of progressive massive fibrosis. Br J Ind Med 1987;44(10):661.
19. Cochrane AL. The attack rate of progressive massive fibrosis. Br J Ind Med 1962;19(1):52–64.
20. Halldin CN, Blackley DJ, Markle T, et al. Patterns of progressive massive fibrosis on modern coal miner chest radiographs. Arch Environ Occup Health

2019;1–7. https://doi.org/10.1080/19338244.2019.1593099.
21. Antao VC, Petsonk EL, Sokolow LZ, et al. Rapidly progressive coal workers' pneumoconiosis in the United States: geographic clustering and other factors. Occup Environ Med 2005;62(10):670–4.
22. Cohen RA, Petsonk EL, Rose C, et al. Lung Pathology in U.S. coal workers with rapidly progressive pneumoconiosis implicates silica and silicates. Am J Respir Crit Care Med 2015;193(6):673–80.
23. Ruckley VA, Fernie JM, Chapman JS, et al. Comparison of radiographic appearances with associated pathology and lung dust content in a group of coalworkers. Br J Ind Med 1984;41(4):459.
24. Rae S, Walker DD, Attfield MD. Chronic bronchitis and dust exposure in British coalminers. Inhaled Part 1970;2:883–96.
25. Leigh J. 15 year longitudinal studies of FEV1 loss and mucus hypersecretion development in coal workers in New South Wales, Australia. In: Proceedings of the VIIth: International Pneumoconioses Conference Part II. Vol 2. U.S. Department of Health and Human Services, Public Health Service, Centers for Disease Control, National Institute for Occupational Safety and Health, DHHS (NIOSH); :112-121. Available at: http://www.cdc.gov/niosh/docs/90-108/. Accessed December 4, 2011.
26. Wang X, Yu IT, Wong TW, et al. Respiratory symptoms and pulmonary function in coal miners: looking into the effects of simple pneumoconiosis. Am J Ind Med 1999;35(2):124–31.
27. Ryder R, Lyons JP, Campbell H, et al. Emphysema in coal workers' pneumoconiosis. Br Med J 1970; 3(5721):481.
28. Kuempel ED, Wheeler MW, Smith RJ, et al. Contributions of dust exposure and cigarette smoking to emphysema severity in coal miners in the United States. Am J Respir Crit Care Med 2009;180(3): 257–64.
29. Leigh J, Driscoll TR, Cole BD, et al. Quantitative relation between emphysema and lung mineral content in coalworkers. Occup Environ Med 1994;51(6): 400–7.
30. Cockcroft A, Seal RM, Wagner JC, et al. Post-mortem study of emphysema in coalworkers and non-coalworkers. Lancet 1982;2(8298):600–3.
31. Green FHY, Brower PS, Vallyathan V, Attfield MD. Coal mine dust exposure and type of pulmonary emphysema in coal workers. In: Chiyotani K, Hosoda Y, eds Advances in the Prevention of Occupational Respiratory Diseases: Proceedings of the 9th International Conference on Occupational Respiratory Diseases, Kyoto, October 13–16, 1997. International congress series. New York; Amsterdam: Elsevier; 1998.
32. Morgan WK. Industrial bronchitis. Br J Ind Med 1978;35(4):285–91.
33. Cowie RL, Mabena SK. Silicosis, chronic airflow limitation, and chronic bronchitis in South African Gold Miners. Am Rev Respir Dis 1991;143(1):80–4.
34. Cowie HA, Miller BG, Rawbone RG, et al. Dust related risks of clinically relevant lung functional deficits. Occup Environ Med 2006;63(5):320–5.
35. Love RG, Miller BG. Longitudinal study of lung function in coal-miners. Thorax 1982;37(3):193–7.
36. Carta P, Aru G, Barbieri MT, et al. Dust exposure, respiratory symptoms, and longitudinal decline of lung function in young coal miners. Occup Environ Med 1996;53(5):312–9.
37. Soutar CA, Hurley JF. Relation between dust exposure and lung function in miners and ex-miners. Br J Ind Med 1986;43(5):307.
38. Churg A, Wright JL, Wiggs B, et al. Small airways disease and mineral dust exposure. Am Rev Respir Dis 1985;131(1):139–43.
39. Hnizdo E, Vallyathan V. Chronic obstructive pulmonary disease due to occupational exposure to silica dust: a review of epidemiological and pathological evidence. Occup Environ Med 2003; 60(4):237–43.
40. Beeckman LA, Wang ML, Petsonk EL, et al. Rapid declines in FEV1 and subsequent respiratory symptoms, illnesses, and mortality in coal miners in the United States. Am J Respir Crit Care Med 2001; 163(3 Pt 1):633–9.
41. McConnochie K, Green FHY, Vallyathan V, et al. Interstitial fibrosis in coal workers: experience in Wales and West Virginia. Ann Occup Hyg 1988; 32(inhaled particles VI):553–60.
42. Monso E, Tura JM, Marsal M, et al. Mineralogical microanalysis of idiopathic pulmonary fibrosis. Arch Environ Health 1990;45(3):185–8.
43. Jelic TM, Estalilla OC, Sawyer-Kaplan PR, et al. Coal mine dust desquamative chronic interstitial pneumonia: a precursor of dust-related diffuse fibrosis and of emphysema. Int J Occup Environ Med 2017;8(3):1066–153, 165.
44. Schreiber J, Koschel D, Kekow J, et al. Rheumatoid pneumoconiosis (Caplan's syndrome). Eur J Intern Med 2010;21(3):168–72.
45. Graber JM, Stayner LT, Cohen RA, et al. Respiratory disease mortality among US coal miners; results after 37 years of follow-up. Occup Environ Med 2014; 71(1):30–9.
46. Hosgood HD, Chapman RS, Wei H, et al. Coal mining is associated with lung cancer risk in Xuanwei, China. Am J Ind Med 2012;55(1):5–10.
47. Hoffmann B, Jöckel K-H. Diesel exhaust and coal mine dust. Ann N Y Acad Sci 2006;1076(1):253–65.
48. Taeger D, Pesch B, Kendzia B, et al. Lung cancer among coal miners, ore miners and quarrymen: smoking-adjusted risk estimates from the synergy pooled analysis of case-control studies. Scand J Work Environ Health 2015;41(5):467–77.

49. International Agency for Research on Cancer. Silica, Some Silicates, Coal Dust and para-Aramid Fibrils. Lyon, 1997.
50. International Association for Research on Cancer. Diesel and gasoline engine exhausts and some nitroarenes. IARC monographs on the evaluation of carcinogenic risks to humans. 2013;105.
51. Schroedl C, Kalhan R. Incidence, treatment options, and outcomes of lung cancer in patients with chronic obstructive pulmonary disease. Curr Opin Pulm Med 2012;18(2):131–7.
52. King C, Nathan SD. Identification and treatment of comorbidities in idiopathic pulmonary fibrosis and other fibrotic lung diseases. Curr Opin Pulm Med 2013;19(5):466–73.
53. Gamboa PM, Jáuregui I, Urrutia I, et al. Occupational asthma in a coal miner. Thorax 1996;51(8): 867–8.
54. Ayaaba E, Li Y, Yuan J, et al. Occupational respiratory diseases of miners from two gold mines in Ghana. Int J Environ Res Public Health 2017;14(3). https://doi.org/10.3390/ijerph14030337.
55. Tarlo SM, Lemiere C. Occupational asthma. N Engl J Med 2014;370(7):640–9.
56. Vallyathan V, Brower PS, Green FH, et al. Radiographic and pathologic correlation of coal workers' pneumoconiosis. Am J Respir Crit Care Med 1996; 154(3 Pt 1):741–8.
57. Fernie JM, Ruckley VA. Coalworkers' pneumoconiosis: correlation between opacity profusion and number and type of dust lesions with special reference to opacity type. Br J Ind Med 1987;44(4): 273–7.
58. Gevenois PA, Sergent G, De Maertelaer V, et al. Micronodules and emphysema in coal mine dust or silica exposure: relation with lung function. Eur Respir J 1998;12(5):1020–4.
59. Remy-Jardin M, Degreef JM, Beuscart R, et al. Coal worker's pneumoconiosis: CT assessment in exposed workers and correlation with radiographic findings. Radiology 1990;177(2):363–71.
60. Reichert M, Bensadoun ES. PET imaging in patients with coal workers pneumoconiosis and suspected malignancy. J Thorac Oncol 2009;4(5):649–51.
61. Miller BG, MacCalman L. Cause-specific mortality in British coal workers and exposure to respirable dust and quartz. Occup Environ Med 2010;67(4):270–6.
62. Wang XR, Christiani DC. Respiratory symptoms and functional status in workers exposed to silica, asbestos, and coal mine dusts. J Occup Environ Med 2000;42(11):1076.
63. Akkoca Yildiz O, Eris Gulbay B, Saryal S, et al. Evaluation of the relationship between radiological abnormalities and both pulmonary function and pulmonary hypertension in coal workers' pneumoconiosis. Respirology 2007;12(3):420–6.
64. Rasmussen DL. Patterns of physiological impairment in coal workers' pneumoconiosis. Ann N Y Acad Sci 1972;200(1 Coal Workers):455–62.
65. Petsonk EL, Stansbury RC, Beeckman-Wagner L-A, et al. Small airway dysfunction and abnormal exercise responses. A study in coal miners. Ann Am Thorac Soc 2016;13(7):1076–80.
66. Honma K, Chiyotani K. Diffuse interstitial fibrosis in nonasbestos pneumoconiosis: a pathological study. Respiration 1993;60(2):120–6.
67. Kleinerman J, Green F, Harley RA, et al. Pathology standards for coal workers' pneumoconiosis. Report of the pneumoconiosis Committee of the College of American Pathologists to the national Institute for occupational Safety and health. Arch Pathol Lab Med 1979;103(8):375–432.
68. Blackley DJ, Halldin CN, Cummings KJ, et al. Lung transplantation is increasingly common among patients with coal workers' pneumoconiosis. Am J Ind Med 2016;59(3):175–7.
69. Wilt JL, Banks DE, Weissman DN, et al. Reduction of lung dust burden in pneumoconiosis by whole-lung lavage. J Occup 1996;38(6):619–24.
70. Kimura K, Ohtsuka Y, Kaji H, et al. Progression of pneumoconiosis in coal miners after cessation of dust exposure: a longitudinal study based on periodic chest X-ray examinations in Hokkaido, Japan. Intern Med 2010;49(18):1949–56.
71. Francois P, Prevost JM, Courtois G, et al. Pneumoconiosis of delayed apparition: large scaled screening in a population of retired coal miners of the northern coal fields of France. In: Proceedings of the VIIth: International Pneumoconioses Conference Part II. Vol 2. U.S. Department of Health and Human Services, Public Health Service, Centers for Disease Control, National Institute for Occupational Safety and Health, DHHS (NIOSH); :979-984. Available at: http://www.cdc.gov/niosh/docs/90-108/. Accessed December 4, 2011.
72. Dimich-Ward H, Bates DV. Reanalysis of a longitudinal study of pulmonary function in coal miners in Lorraine, France. Am J Ind Med 1994;25(5):613–23.

Occupational Contributions to Interstitial Lung Disease

Carl Reynolds, MD*, Johanna Feary, MD, Paul Cullinan, MD

KEYWORDS

- Idiopathic pulmonary fibrosis • Asbestosis • Hypersensitivity pneumonitis • Occupational
- Epidemiology

KEY POINTS

- Globally, coal workers pneumoconiosis, silicosis, and asbestosis remain the most important pneumoconioses.
- Idiopathic pulmonary fibrosis (IPF) and asbestosis can be challenging to differentiate clinically, and there is clear evidence for an occupational contribution to IPF.
- Bacterial contamination of metal working fluid has recently emerged as an important cause of occupational hypersensitivity pneumonitis.

IMPORTANCE

The Global Burden of Disease Study provides a comprehensive assessment of mortality due to 264 causes in 195 locations from 1980 to 2016. Estimates for the burden of interstitial lung disease (ILD) are given under the heading of chronic respiratory diseases for "interstitial lung disease and pulmonary sarcoidosis" and, separately, for pneumoconiosis including "Silicosis," "Asbestosis," and "Coal workers." Global ILD and pulmonary sarcoidosis deaths increased from 48,000 in 1990 to 127,000 in 2016. A similar pattern was seen in the United States where deaths increased from 7000 in 1990 to 19,000 by 2016.[1]

In general, ILDs are difficult to manage and are frequently associated with serious comorbidities. Occupational and environmental exposures have a clear causal role in the pneumoconioses and hypersensitivity pneumonitis (HP) and early diagnosis and cessation of exposure is the gold standard of treatment. A high degree of suspicion is required for the early detection of disease even in the context of known exposure-disease relations, and long latency diseases can be a particular challenge. Detecting previously unknown exposure-disease relations in the context of latency, novel exposure, and polyexposure compounds the challenge. Missing the link is costly for patients, their coworkers, and future workers.[2]

The means available for estimating the contribution of occupational exposures to ILD are limited for 3 main reasons: occupational exposure data are not widely collected or readily available; exposure-disease relations and underlying pathologic processes are not well elucidated; and occupational ILDs are diverse and relatively uncommon. Case-control studies are invaluable for the study of less frequent entities and for investigating suspected exposure-disease relations. Toxicologic studies, including animal studies, are helpful for understanding underlying pathologic processes.[3]

OCCUPATIONAL IDIOPATHIC PULMONARY FIBROSIS

Idiopathic pulmonary fibrosis (IPF) is the most common ILD, and although by definition it is a

The authors declare that they have no conflicts of interest.
National Heart and Lung Institute, Imperial College London, 1b Manresa Road, London, UK
* Corresponding author.
E-mail address: carl.reynolds@imperial.ac.uk

Clin Chest Med 41 (2020) 697–707
https://doi.org/10.1016/j.ccm.2020.08.015

diagnosis made after the exclusion of known causes of lung fibrosis, including occupational exposures, the potential for misdiagnosis is well recognized. A recent meta-analysis published by the European Respiratory Society (ERS) and American Thoracic Society (ATS) of 12 case-control studies of occupational exposures in IPF estimated that 26% of cases were attributable to occupational exposures to vapors, gases, dusts, and fumes (VGDF).[4] There was considerable heterogeneity between studies, for example, $I^2 = 95\%$ for the 6 studies reporting on general (VGDF) occupational respiratory exposures[4] and to a lesser extent for wood, metal, and stone dust (**Figs. 1–4**).

This may be due to real clinical differences in the populations studied or due to chance, publication bias, or methodological issues. To investigate possible publication bias the authors looked for funnel plot asymmetry using data from the ERS/ATS meta-analysis.[4] They found evidence of publication bias for VGDF and metal dust (Egger test $P = .04$) but not for wood dust (Egger test $P = .1$) and not for agricultural dust (Egger test $P = .58$). However, caution must be exercised in the interpretation of these findings because tests of funnel plot asymmetry are underpowered to distinguish chance from real asymmetry when fewer than 10 studies are being considered.[5]

Considering the possibility of methodological issues the authors tabulated study case and control definitions and exposure measures and assessed the risk of bias using RoB-SPEO,[6] a tool for assessing risk of bias in studies estimating the prevalence of exposure to occupational risk factors (**Tables 1** and **2**). Case definitions and sources for cases varied between studies. For example, Scott (1990)[7] used a case definition that included a chest radiograph showing bilateral interstitial shadowing, whereas most other studies relied on high-resolution computed tomography. Four studies used mortality data[8–11] to identify cases, and one study[10] used a national register of patients receiving oxygen therapy. Differences in health care coverage and coding practices can result in selection bias in studies making use of mortality data.[12]

Seven[7,10,13–17] of the twelve case-control studies considered in the meta-analysis used population controls. One study[11] used a pension fund record to select cases and controls, one study used an orthopedic practice list,[18] and 3 studies used respiratory inpatients or a mix of respiratory inpatients and outpatients.[17,19,20] Only 2 studies

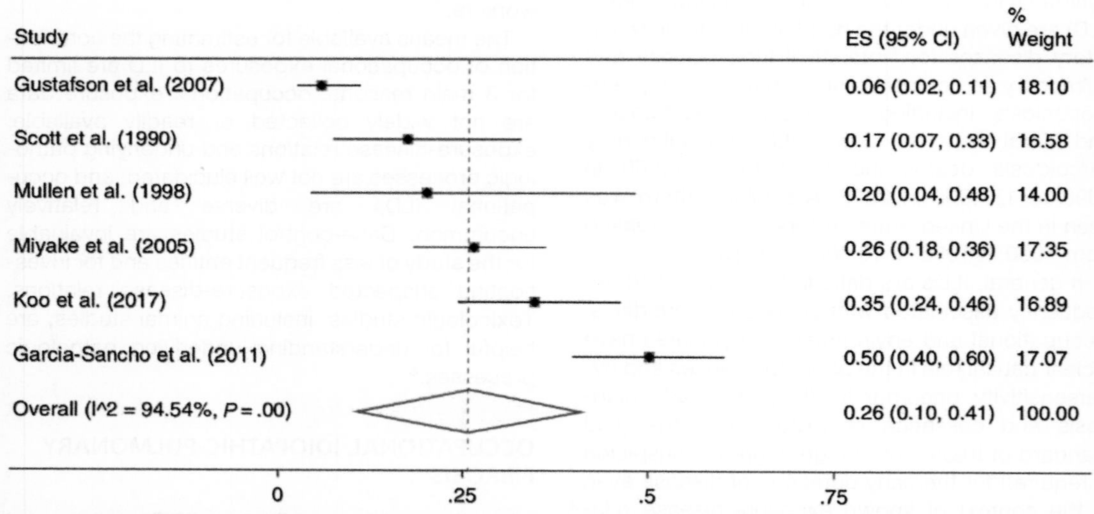

Fig. 1. Forest plot of pooled population attributable risk factors for occupational VGDF exposure and idiopathic pulmonary fibrosis. IPF: population attributable fraction (PAF) from VGDF. Forest plot of studies relevant to estimating the occupational contribution to IPF of VGDF (combined categories of exposure considered in the studies included). The estimated PAF, confidence interval (CI), and weighted contribution for each study are shown, as well as the calculated pooled estimate (red dashed line) and 95% CI. For IPF, the pooled PAF for VGDF is 26% (95% CI, 10%–41%). ES, effect size. (*From* Blanc PD, Annesi-Maesano I, Balmes JR, et al. The occupational burden of nonmalignant respiratory diseases. An official american thoracic society and european respiratory society statement. American journal of respiratory and critical care medicine. 2019;199(11):1312-1334. https://doi.org/10.1164/rccm.201904-0717ST. Reprinted with permission of the American Thoracic Society. Copyright © 2020 American Thoracic Society. All rights reserved.)

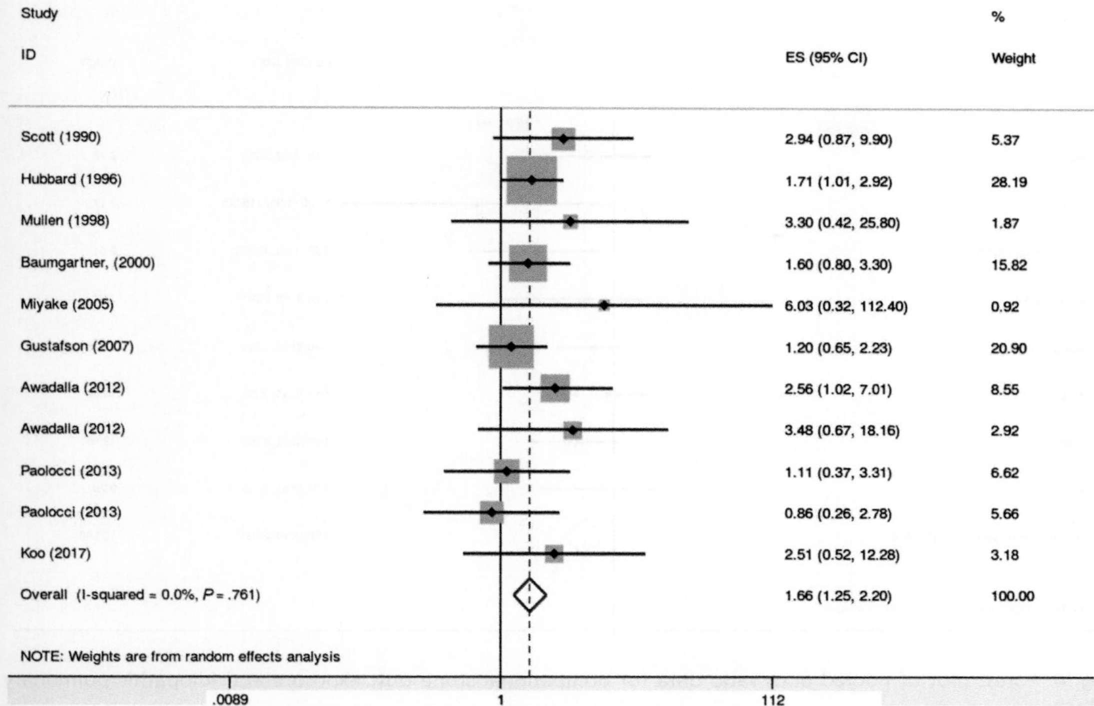

Fig. 2. Forest plot of pooled odds ratio data for occupational wood dust exposure and idiopathic pulmonary fibrosis.

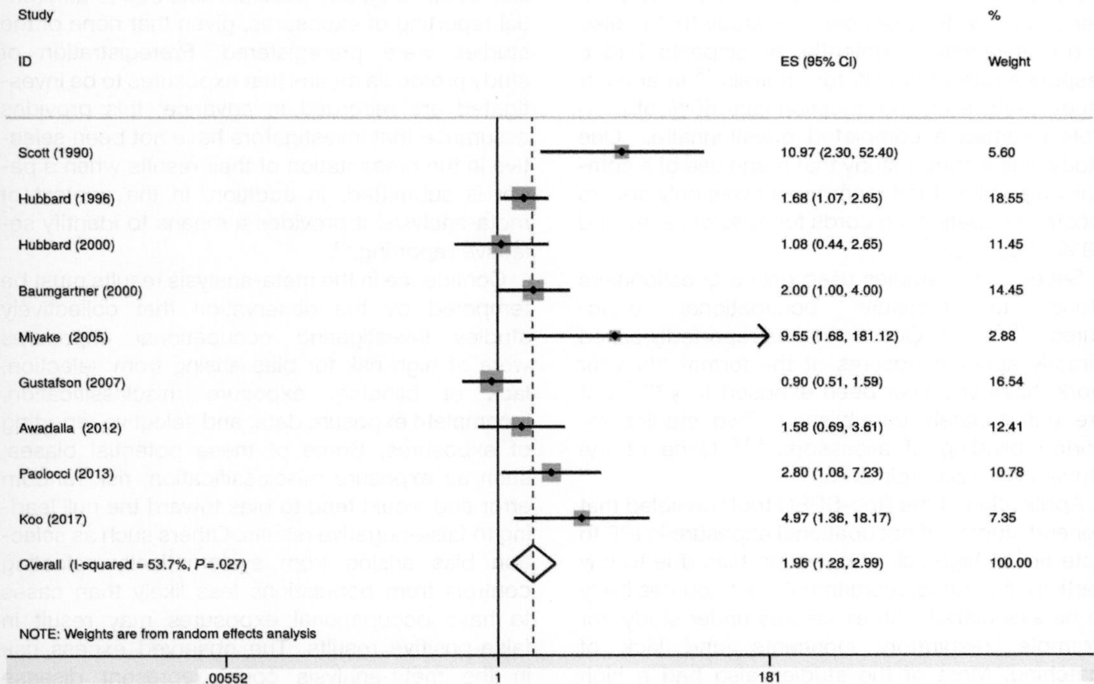

Fig. 3. Forest plot of pooled odds ratio data for occupational metal dust exposure and idiopathic pulmonary fibrosis.

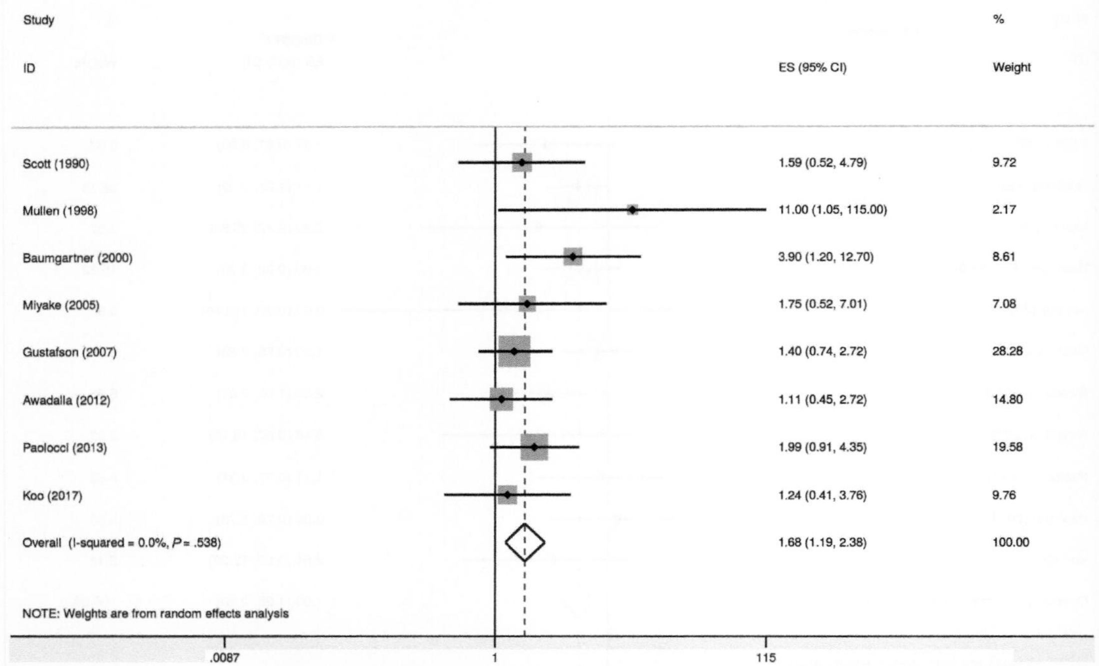

Fig. 4. Forest plot of pooled odds ratio data for occupational stone dust exposure and idiopathic pulmonary fibrosis.

did not match on age or sex[16,19] and one study matched on age only.[10] Where participation rates were reported for community controls they were generally low, for example, one study that mailed a questionnaire to potential participants had a response rate of 32.4% for controls.[18] In another study using a mailed questionnaire 60% of controls returned a completed questionnaire.[7] One study was a cohort study that made use of a company's pension fund records and was only able to locate occupational records for 40% of cases and 38% of controls.[11]

Seven of the studies used only a questionnaire alone to measure occupational exposures.[7,10,16,18–20] Questionnaires reportedly asked directly about exposures of the format "In your work, have you ever been exposed to y?"[10] but are unfortunately unpublished. Two studies reported blinding of assessors.[14,17] None of the studies were preregistered.

Application of the Rob-SPEO tool[6] revealed that general studies of occupational exposure in IPF to date are at high risk of selection bias due to low participation rates, recruitment from sources likely to be associated with exposures under study, for example, respiratory inpatients, and lack of matching. Most of the studies also had a high risk of bias from exposure misclassification and/or incomplete exposure data through reliance on questionnaires that used yes/no questions for a limited number of specific exposures, bias due to lack of blinding, and possible bias due to differential reporting of exposures, given that none of the studies were preregistered. Preregistration of study protocols means that exposures to be investigated are recorded in advance; this provides assurance that investigators have not been selective in the presentation of their results when a paper is submitted. In addition, in the context of meta-analysis, it provides a means to identify selective reporting.[21]

Confidence in the meta-analysis results must be tempered by the observation that collectively studies investigating occupational exposures were at high risk for bias arising from selection, lack of blinding, exposure misclassification, incomplete exposure data, and selective reporting of exposures. Some of these potential biases, such as exposure misclassification, risk random error and would tend to bias toward the null leading to false-negative results. Others such as selection bias arising from systematically selecting controls from populations less likely than cases to have occupational exposures may result in false-positive results. The observed excess risk in the meta-analysis could represent disease misclassification of pneumoconiosis or HP, but this is unlikely to fully explain the observed effects.

Table 1
Overview of occupational idiopathic pulmonary fibrosis studies

Author Year	N[a]	Case definition	Control Definition	Exposure Measure
Scott et al,[7] 1990	40	Clinical assessment, CXR, pulmonary function	Matched on age and sex of cases using general practice register, ratio 1:4	Questionnaire
Hubbard et al,[13] 1996	218	Clinical assessment, CXR, CT, pulmonary function	Matched on age and sex of cases using general practice register, ratio 1:4	Questionnaire and telephone interview
Mullen et al,[18] 1998	15	Clinical assessment, lung biopsy, CT	Matched on age and sex of cases using orthopedic practice list, ratio 1:6	Questionnaire
Baumgartner et al,[14] 2000	248	Clinical assessment, lung biopsy, BAL, CT	Matched on age, sex, and geographic region of cases using random digit dialling, ratio 1:2	Telephone interview
Hubbard et al,[11] 2000[b]	22	Death certificate diagnosis from pension fund records for Rolls Royce	Random sample of deceased Roll Royce employees, ratio 1:10	Company records and job group
Miyake et al,[19] 2005	102	Clinical assessment, lung biopsy, BAL, CT	Respiratory department inpatients at 21 participating hospitals, unmatched, 2:1 ratio	Questionnaire
Gustafson et al,[10] 2007	140	Pulmonary fibrosis of unknown cause, requiring LTOT, identified from LTOT register	Random age-matched population sample	Questionnaire
Garcia-Sancho et al,[15] 2011	100	Clinical assessment, CT, lung biopsy	Matched on age, sex, and geographic region of using neighborhood sampling ratio 1:1–3	Questionnaire
Awadalla et al,[20] 2012, men	95	Clinical assessment, CT, pulmonary function, inpatients	Matched on age, sex, respiratory inpatients 1:1	Questionnaire
Awadalla et al,[20] 2012, women	106	Clinical assessment, CT, pulmonary function	Matched on age, sex, respiratory inpatients 1:1	Questionnaire
Paolocci et al,[16] 2013, soft wood (abstract only)	65	Clinical assessment and CT	Matched on area but not age or sex	Questionnaire

(*continued on next page*)

Table 1
(continued)

Author Year	N[a]	Case definition	Control Definition	Exposure Measure
Paolocci et al,[16] 2013, hard wood (abstract only)	n/a	Cinical assessment and CT	Matched on area but not age or sex	Questionnaire
Koo et al,[17] 2017	78	Clinical assessment, CT, lung biopsy, recruited from inpatients and outpatients	Matched on age, sex, and area, ratio 1:1, recruited from respiratory inpatients and outpatients	Interview

Abbreviations: BAL, bronchoalveolar lavage; CT, computed tomography scan of the thorax; CXR, chest radiograph; LTOT, long-term oxygen therapy.
[a] Number of cases.
[b] This is a cohort study. All other studies are case-control studies.

The meta-analysis[4] supports an etiologic role for occupational exposures in IPF, potentially explaining up to 23% of the burden of disease and highlighting a role for workplace exposure reduction in disease prevention. Further studies are urgently needed to confirm and better characterize this risk; in addition to addressing study design issues outlined earlier, future studies should investigate host–environment interactions taking account of known genetic susceptibility factors.

An occupational asbestos–IPF association is notably absent; several investigators have argued that a proportion of IPF is likely due to asbestos exposure because asbestosis can present similarly to IPF, there are ecological correlations, and evidence of misclassification.[22,23] Seven of the case-control studies in the meta-analysis reported asking about occupational asbestos exposure and finding a nonsignificant association with IPF.[7,10,13,14,17–19] The possibility of asbestos

Table 2
Rob-SPEO risk of bias scores for occupational idiopathic pulmonary fibrosis studies

Author, Year	S	B	E	I	SR	C	D	O
Scott et al,[7] 1990	3	4	2	2	3	1	1	1
Hubbard et al,[13] 1996	3	3	2	2	3	1	1	1
Mullen et al,[18] 1998	3	3	2	2	3	1	1	4
Baumgartner et al,[14] 2000	3	2	2	2	3	1	1	1
Hubbard et al,[11] 2000	4	4	2	3	3	2	1	2
Miyake et al,[19] 2005	4	4	2	3	3	1	1	1
Gustafson et al,[10] 2007	4	4	2	3	3	1	1	1
Garcia-Sancho et al,[15] 2011	3	3	2	3	3	1	1	1
Awadalla et al,[20] 2012, men	4	3	2	3	3	1	1	1
Awadalla et al,[20] 2012, women	4	3	2	3	3	1	1	1
Paolocci et al,[16] 2013, soft wood (abstract only)	4	3	2	3	3	1	1	1
Paolocci et al,[16] 2013, hard wood (abstract only)	4	3	2	3	3	1	1	1
Koo et al,[17] 2017	4	1	2	2	3	1	1	1

Eight domains of bias were considered: S = selection, B = blinding, E = exposure misclassification, I = incomplete exposure data, SR = selective reporting of exposures, C = conflict of interests, D = differences in the numerator and denominator, O = other bias. Risk of bias was rated in each domain: 1 = low, 2 = prob low, 3 = prob high, 4 = high, 5 = no info.

coexposure confounding the observed association with metal and wood dust is intriguing; carpenters and metal plate workers, who have significant wood and metal dust exposure, are known to be high-risk groups for pleural mesothelioma, a disease almost entirely attributable to occupational asbestos exposure.[24,25] There is strong intuitive sense for occupational inhalation of silica or asbestos fibers being an underrecognized cause of IPF, because both are known to be fibrogenic and are frequently used in animal models of pulmonary fibrosis.[26] A common MUC5b-driven pulmonary fibrosis endotype has recently been suggested following the observation that the IPF genetic risk factor rs35705950 (whose main effect is to increase airway MUC5b) is also associated with asbestosis.[27,28] A potential mechanism for this is increased MUC5b expression secondary to interleukin-1β release resulting from activation of the asbestos-sensing NLRP3 inflammasome in alveolar macrophages,[29] and more research is needed.

ASBESTOSIS

Coal worker's pneumoconiosis and silicosis are discussed elsewhere, and this section is concerned with the third of the most important pneumoconiosis, asbestosis. Regional and national incidence rates of asbestosis have recently been examined through the Global Burden of Disease project.[30] Although unexpectedly high rates in North America, Australia, and South Africa were reported, the data must be interpreted with great care. In 2017, for example, a total of just 9397 new cases across the globe were recorded; this is surely a gross underestimate and a reminder that enumerating the disease requires not only access to sophisticated diagnostic services but also a common approach to attribution for a disease that can be clinically and radiologically indistinguishable from IPF. Moreover, with a latency of several decades, cases of asbestosis reflect working conditions long ago; taken together, these factors contribute to the apparent paradox that countries with currently the highest incidence rates tend to be those that have long abandoned the use of asbestos.

What is clearer is that a second wave of asbestosis is inevitable, as many parts of the world become increasingly industrialized and face the challenge of providing an infrastructure for a rapidly increasing urban population. Asbestos remains a very cheap means of reinforcing concrete and is widely used in manufacturing drainage and sewage systems and in roofing and cladding materials. Although worldwide rates of asbestos use peaked in the 1980s and declined, by around 50%, until the late 1990s they have since stabilized at about 2 million tons per year.[31] Virtually all this is in low- and middle-income countries—two-thirds of it in Asia[32]—supplied by chrysotile mining operations in Russia, China, Kazakhstan, and, until very recently, Brazil. In this global context it is important to recognize that asbestosis can arise not only from classical occupational exposures but also those acquired—from birth and equally in both sexes—by residence in the vicinity of poorly controlled industrial operations. Almost 10% of cases of asbestos-related disease in those living near, but not working in, the Fibronit plant in Broni, Italy were of asbestosis, with an average latency 10 years shorter than that of mesothelioma (82% of cases).[33] More than 50 cases of asbestosis have been reported in women and men living close to the asbestos mines in the Chung-Cheong province of South Korea.[34] The long history of asbestos use in Europe, North America, and Australia—and its ongoing, tragic legacy—suggests strongly that the risks cannot be adequately controlled by technology or by the regulation of work practices and that only the elimination of its use altogether is effective.

There is, currently, no effective medical treatment of asbestosis. The use of modern antifibrotic agents such as pirfenidone or nintedanib is generally restricted, although the finding, as mentioned earlier, that asbestosis and IPF share at least one genetic determinant[28] suggests that these treatments might be equally effective in both conditions. Lung transplant is rarely offered to patients with asbestosis, who tend to be older than those with other forms of pneumoconiosis, but the available evidence suggests that the outcome is no worse than it is for patients with nonoccupational causes of lung failure.[35]

OCCUPATIONAL HYPERSENSITIVITY PNEUMONITIS

HP is caused by an abnormal immune response to repeated exposure to an inhaled agent in a susceptible individual.[36] There are around 300 recognized causal agents in HP, most of which may be encountered in the workplace. They can be broadly grouped into microbial (fungi and bacteria) triggers, animal proteins, and a few chemical reagents.[36,37] Identification of the etiologic agent is associated with a better prognosis but is impossible in up to 50% of cases.[38] A meticulous occupational and environmental exposure history should be taken from all patients with suggestive symptoms to increase the likelihood of pinpointing putative causes. Historically, the most common causes of HP were bird fanciers' lung (due to avian antigens from occupational, recreational, or domestic exposure), with reported prevalence rates of up to 21%,[39] and farmer's lung (due to thermophilic actinomycetes), which showed significant geographic variation with higher rates in humid or damp climates.[40–42]

More recently, metalworking fluids (MWF) have become an increasingly important cause of occupational HP (OHP) and in the United Kingdom are now responsible for half of all cases of OHP and the most commonly reported cause of OHP in the last 10 years.[43] NIOSH estimates that 1.2 million workers in the United States are exposed to MWF, which is widely used in industry, and several workplace-related outbreaks have been reported both there and in Europe.[44–47] HP in this setting is thought to arise due to bacterial contamination of MWF (despite, or because of, the addition of biocides) and is more likely where MWF is repeatedly recycled and/or where machine use is prolonged. Even with the use of enclosed machines and use of exhaust ventilation, some MWF aerosol "mists" escape, becoming potentially respirable.[45,48,49] Nontuberculous mycobacterium including *Myobacterium immunogenum* and *Myobacterium avium* have been identified as the presumed etiologic agent in many cases of HP due to MWF.[50–52] Further sporadic newly reported causes of OHP and HP due to environmental agents are described in detail elsewhere.[2,53]

HP (regardless of the cause) is generally thought to be a rare disease. The reported prevalence of OHP depends on the diagnostic criteria used and is often based on cross-sectional surveys during outbreak investigation. A recent analysis estimated the occupational burden of HP to range from 0% to 81.3%, with a weighted meta-proportion of 19% (95% CI, 12%–28%), but this was based on 15 highly heterogeneous (I^2 of 97%) studies, almost all of which were case series.[4] NIOSH collected nationally comprehensive longitudinal data on OHP from 1980 to 2002 and reported 814 deaths and, over the same period, a significant increase in overall age-adjusted death rates from 0.09 to 0.29 per million.[54] Of these cases, farmer's lung accounted for 37.3%, bird fancier's lung for 4.4%, and no cause was specified in 55.5%. The highest death rate was reported in Wisconsin (1.04/million). Proportionate mortality ratios (PMR) by industry were significantly increased for agricultural production of livestock (PMR: 19.3; 95% confidence interval [CI]: 14.0 to 25.9) and crops (PMR: 4.3; 95% CI: 3.0–6.0). Similarly, a recent analysis of HP mortality data from the National Center for Health Statistics (2003–2017) identified the highest PMR (adjusted for age, sex, and race) for animal production (PMR, 9.9; 95% CI: 5.1–17.3) and crop production (PMR, 5.2; 95% CI: 2.9–8.7).[55]

The features of OHP do not differ from those of HP from other or unknown causes. The diagnosis of HP is challenging and should be based on clinical, immunologic, radiological, and pathologic findings following multidisciplinary team discussion although there is poor expert agreement about how to define a case of chronic disease.[56] The clinician should have a low index of suspicion for diagnosing HP in those exposed to a known etiologic agent. The relationship of symptoms to work is helpful in determining whether there is an occupational cause (**Box 1**).

HP causes diffuse, predominantly parenchymal inflammation but also importantly can involve the respiratory bronchioles (thus causing a "bronchioloalveolitis")[57] and so serial peak flow monitoring may show diurnal variability mimicking occupational asthma. Sampling of the putative antigen source at work to determine antigen-specific IgG antibodies can be valuable and is important when the commercial antigen is not available. Inhalation provocation tests with relevant specific antigen are not widely available, and the sensitivity and specificity of the investigations are not established.[53] Prediction tools may be of some value depending on the circumstances but rely heavily on exposure to a known cause (eg, Lacasse and colleagues[58] [diagnosis of HP] and Barber and colleagues[59] [MWF-HP for case definition in outbreaks]).

The key to management of HP is to remove the causative trigger if known; this is often more straightforward if the exposure is encountered at work than where a domestic or environmental

Box 1
Key questions which may be helpful in determining whether there is an occupational cause

The questions include whether

1. Symptoms developed after moving to a new job, moving to a different working environment, or starting work with different equipment.
2. Symptoms are better away from home (eg, on vacation) or away from work (vacations or at weekends)
3. There is a suggestion of a workplace outbreak with others affected (or where others recently left work due to ill health).

cause (such as mold within the home) is suspected. Temporary relocation with monitoring of symptoms, radiology, and lung physiology is often helpful but changes may not be apparent for several weeks. No decisions about work should be made before expert assessment of the patient to avoid any potentially life-changing relocation without a high chance of success. Where a case of occupational HP is identified, environmental controls of the exposure should be instituted for the benefit of the whole workforce. If removal of an affected individual from exposure is not possible, a reduction in exposure may be achieved by the use of appropriate respiratory protective equipment. For some patients this is not possible, and a change in employment may be necessary with significant socioeconomic consequences.

Workplace HP outbreaks usually occur sporadically, and it is common for only a few members of a workforce to be affected. Identification of one worker with OHP should trigger a prompt survey of the workplace, to identify potential environmental hazards, and of the workforce, to identify other cases who may have remained underdiagnosed without active case finding.[45,46,60,61] Surveillance programs, such as those recommended by NIOSH for MWF-exposed workers (**Box 2**), are useful in monitoring for and prompt identification of new cases, maintaining worker education on risks and symptoms of the condition, and helping to ensure that workplace hazards are controlled.[62] Employers generally have a duty to provide a safe working environment for their workers, and an employer who is deemed to be at fault may be vulnerable to legal action. In some countries, workers with HP may be entitled to compensation from the State (see **Box 2**).

Box 2
Key elements of an occupational hypersensitivity pneumonitis surveillance program[63]

1. Safety and health training,
2. Worksite analysis,
3. Hazard prevention and control, and
4. Medical monitoring of exposed workers:
   i. Initial examination (respiratory symptom questionnaire, baseline spirometry)
   ii. Periodic examination (respiratory symptom questionnaire, spirometry)
   iii. Detailed examination for selected workers
   iv. Physician's reports to the worker and employer
   v. Follow-up medical evaluations after transfer for workers transferred on medical grounds

UNCOMMON AND EMERGING OCCUPATIONAL INTERSTITIAL DISORDERS

Organizing pneumonia and other uncommon interstitial disorders have recently been covered in Parkes occupational lung disease.[64] Outbreaks of occupational ILD have occurred due to Ardystil,[65] nylon flock,[66] indium tin oxide,[67] and most recently artificial stone.[68]

REFERENCES

1. GBD 2016 Causes of Death Collaborators. Global, regional, and national age-sex specific mortality for 264 causes of death, 1980-2016: a systematic analysis for the global burden of disease study 2016. Lancet 2017;390(10100):1151–210.
2. Fishwick D. New occupational and environmental causes of asthma and extrinsic allergic alveolitis. Clin Chest Med 2012;33(4):605–16.
3. Sauler M, Gulati M. Newly recognized occupational and environmental causes of chronic terminal airways and parenchymal lung disease. Clin Chest Med 2012;33(4):667–80.
4. Blanc PD, Annesi-Maesano I, Balmes JR, et al. The occupational burden of nonmalignant respiratory diseases. An official american thoracic society and european respiratory society statement. Am J Respir Crit Care Med 2019;199(11):1312–34.
5. Deeks JJ, Higgins JP, Altman DG, et al. Analysing data and undertaking meta-analyses. Cochrane Handbook for Systematic Reviews of Interventions 2019;241–84.
6. Pega F, Norris SL, Backes C, et al. RoB-speo: a tool for assessing risk of bias in studies estimating the prevalence of exposure to occupational risk factors from the who/ilo joint estimates of the work-related burden of disease and injury. Environ Int 2020;135:105039.
7. Scott J, Johnston I, Britton J. What causes cryptogenic fibrosing alveolitis? A case-control study of environmental exposure to dust. BMJ 1990;301(6759):1015.
8. Iwai K, Mori T, Yamada N, et al. Idiopathic pulmonary fibrosis. Epidemiologic approaches to occupational exposure. Am J Respir Crit Care Med 1994;150(3):670–5.
9. Pinheiro GA, Antao VC, Wood JM, et al. Occupational risks for idiopathic pulmonary fibrosis mortality in the United States. Int J Occup Environ Health 2008;14(2):117–23.

10. Gustafson T, Dahlman-Höglund A, Nilsson K, et al. Occupational exposure and severe pulmonary fibrosis. Respir Med 2007;101(10):2207–12.
11. Hubbard R, Cooper M, Antoniak M, et al. Risk of cryptogenic fibrosing alveolitis in metal workers. Lancet 2000;355(9202):466–7.
12. Caminati A, Madotto F, Cesana G, et al. Epidemiological studies in idiopathic pulmonary fibrosis: Pitfalls in methodologies and data interpretation. Eur Respir Rev 2015;24(137):436–44.
13. Hubbard R, Johnston I, Coultas DB, et al. Mortality rates from cryptogenic fibrosing alveolitis in seven countries. Thorax 1996;51(7):711–6.
14. Baumgartner KB, Samet JM, Coultas DB, et al. Occupational and environmental risk factors for idiopathic pulmonary fibrosis: a multicenter case-control study. Collaborating centers. Am J Epidemiol 2000; 152(4):307–15.
15. García-Sancho C, Buendía-Roldán I, Fernández-Plata MR, et al. Familial pulmonary fibrosis is the strongest risk factor for idiopathic pulmonary fibrosis. Respir Med 2011;105(12):1902–7.
16. Paolocci G, Nicolic V, Folletti I, et al. Risk factors for idiopathic pulmonary fibrosis in Southern Europe: a case-control study [abstract]. Eur Respir J 2013; 42(Suppl 57):1912.
17. Koo J-W, Myong J-P, Yoon H-K, et al. Occupational exposure and idiopathic pulmonary fibrosis: a multicentre case-control study in korea. Int J Tuberc Lung Dis 2017;21(1):107–12.
18. Mullen J, Hodgson MJ, DeGraff CA, et al. Case-control study of idiopathic pulmonary fibrosis and environmental exposures. J Occup Environ Med 1998; 40(4):363–7.
19. Miyake Y, Sasaki S, Yokoyama T, et al. Occupational and environmental factors and idiopathic pulmonary fibrosis in Japan. Ann Occup Hyg 2005;49(3): 259–65.
20. Awadalla NJ, Hegazy A, Elmetwally RA, et al. Occupational and environmental risk factors for idiopathic pulmonary fibrosis in Egypt: a multicenter case-control study. Int J Occup Environ Med 2012;3(3):107–16.
21. Peat G, Riley RD, Croft P, et al. Improving the transparency of prognosis research: the role of reporting, data sharing, registration, and protocols. PLoS Med 2014;11(7):e1001671.
22. Barber C, Wiggans R, Young C, et al. UK asbestos imports and mortality due to idiopathic pulmonary fibrosis. Occup Med (Lond) 2015; 66(2):106–11.
23. Monsó E, Tura J, Pujadas J, et al. Lung dust content in idiopathic pulmonary fibrosis: a study with scanning electron microscopy and energy dispersive x ray analysis. Br J Ind Med 1991;48(5):327–31.
24. McElvenny DM, Darnton AJ, Price MJ, et al. Mesothelioma mortality in great britain from 1968 to 2001. Occup Med (Lond) 2005;55(2):79–87.
25. Rake C, Gilham C, Hatch J, et al. Occupational, domestic and environmental mesothelioma risks in the british population: a case-control study. Br J Cancer 2009;100(7):1175–83.
26. Moore B, Lawson WE, Oury TD, et al. Animal models of fibrotic lung disease. Am J Respir Cell Mol Biol 2013;49(2):167–79.
27. Seibold MA, Smith RW, Urbanek C, et al. The idiopathic pulmonary fibrosis honeycomb cyst contains a mucocilary pseudostratified epithelium. PLoS One 2013;8(3):e58658.
28. Platenburg MGJP, Wiertz IA, van der Vis JJ, et al. The muc5b promotor risk allele for idiopathic pulmonary fibrosis predisposes to asbestosis. Eur Respir J 2020. https://doi.org/10.1183/13993003.02361-2019.
29. Dostert C, Pétrilli V, Van Bruggen R, et al. Innate immune activation through nalp3 inflammasome sensing of asbestos and silica. Science 2008; 320(5876):674–7.
30. Shi P, Xing X, Xi S, et al. Trends in global, regional and national incidence of pneumoconiosis caused by different aetiologies: an analysis from the global burden of disease study 2017. Occup Environ Med 2020;77(6):407–14.
31. Stayner L, Welch LS, Lemen R. The worldwide pandemic of asbestos-related diseases. Annu Rev Public Health 2013;34:205–16.
32. Leong SL, Zainudin R, Kazan-Allen L, et al. Asbestos in a sia. Respirology 2015;20(4):548–55.
33. Visonà SD, Villani S, Manzoni F, et al. Impact of asbestos on public health: a retrospective study on a series of subjects with occupational and non-occupational exposure to asbestos during the activity of fibronit plant (Broni, Italy). J Public Health Res 2018;7(3):1519.
34. Kim HR. Overview of asbestos issues in korea. J Korean Med Sci 2009;24(3):363–7.
35. Joubert KD, Awori Hayanga J, Strollo DC, et al. Outcomes after lung transplantation for patients with occupational lung diseases. Clin Transplant 2019; 33(1):e13460.
36. Vasakova M, Selman M, Morell F, et al. Hypersensitivity pneumonitis: Current concepts of pathogenesis and potential targets for treatment. Am J Respir Crit Care Med 2019;200(3):301–8.
37. Costabel U, Bonella F, Guzman J. Chronic hypersensitivity pneumonitis. Clin Chest Med 2012;33(1): 151–63.
38. Fernandez Perez ER, Swigris JJ, Forssen AV, et al. Identifying an inciting antigen is associated with improved survival in patients with chronic hypersensitivity pneumonitis. Chest 2013;144(5): 1644–51.
39. Christensen LT, Schmidt CD, Robbins L. Pigeon breeders' disease–a prevalence study and review. Clin Allergy 1975;5(4):417–30.

40. Madsen D, Klock LE, Wenzel FJ, et al. The prevalence of farmer's lung in an agricultural population. Am Rev Respir Dis 1976;113(2):171–4.
41. Terho EO, Heinonen OP, Lammi S, et al. Incidence of clinically confirmed farmer's lung in Finland and its relation to meteorological factors. Eur J Respir Dis Suppl 1987;152:47–56.
42. Gruchow HW, Hoffmann RG, Marx JJJ, et al. Precipitating antibodies to farmer's lung antigens in a Wisconsin farming population. Am Rev Respir Dis 1981; 124(4):411–5.
43. Barber CM, Wiggans RE, Carder M, et al. Epidemiology of occupational hypersensitivity pneumonitis; reports from the sword scheme in the UK from 1996 to 2015. Occup Environ Med 2016. https://doi.org/10.1136/oemed-2016-103838.
44. Tillie-Leblond I, Grenouillet F, Reboux G, et al. Hypersensitivity pneumonitis and metalworking fluids contaminated by mycobacteria. Eur Respir J 2011; 37(3):640–7.
45. Cullinan P, D'Souza E, Tennant R, et al. Lesson of the month: extrinsic allergic (bronchiolo)alveolitis and metal working fluids. Thorax 2014;69(11):1059–60.
46. Robertson W, Robertson AS, Burge CB, et al. Clinical investigation of an outbreak of alveolitis and asthma in a car engine manufacturing plant. Thorax 2007;62(11):981–90.
47. Kreiss K, Cox-Ganser J. Metalworking fluid-associated hypersensitivity pneumonitis: a workshop summary. Am J Ind Med 1997;32(4):423–32.
48. Barber CM, Burton CM, Robinson E, et al. Hypersensitivity pneumonitis due to metalworking fluid exposures. Chest 2013;143(4):1189.
49. Lacasse Y, Girard M, Cormier Y. Recent advances in hypersensitivity pneumonitis. Chest 2012;142(1): 208–17.
50. Burton CM, Crook B, Scaife H, et al. Systematic review of respiratory outbreaks associated with exposure to water-based metalworking fluids. Ann Occup Hyg 2012;56(4):374–88.
51. Rosenman K. Occupational diseases in individuals exposed to metal working fluids. Curr Opin Allergy Clin Immunol 2015;15(2):131–6.
52. James PL, Cannon J, Barber CM, et al. Metal worker's lung: Spatial association with mycobacterium avium. Thorax 2018;73(2):151–6.
53. Quirce S, Vandenplas O, Campo P, et al. Occupational hypersensitivity pneumonitis: an eaaci position paper. Allergy 2016;71(6):765–79.
54. Bang KM, Weissman DN, Pinheiro GA, et al. Twenty-three years of hypersensitivity pneumonitis mortality surveillance in the United States. Am J Ind Med 2006;49(12):997–1004.
55. Hall NB, Wood JM, Laney AS, et al. Hypersensitivity pneumonitis mortality by industry and occupation. Am J Respir Crit Care Med 2019;200(4):518.
56. Walsh SL, Wells AU, Desai SR, et al. Multicentre evaluation of multidisciplinary team meeting agreement on diagnosis in diffuse parenchymal lung disease: a case-cohort study. Lancet Respir Med 2016;4(7):557–65.
57. Pickering CA, Newman Taylor AJ. Extrinsic allergic bronchioloalveolitis (hypersensitivity pneumonitis). Occupational Lung Disorders, 3rd ed. London: Butterworth Heinemann; 1994. p. 667-709.
58. Lacasse Y, Selman M, Costabel U, et al. Clinical diagnosis of hypersensitivity pneumonitis. Am J Respir Crit Care Med 2003;168(8):952–8.
59. Barber CM, Burton CM, Hendrick DJ, et al. Hypersensitivity pneumonitis in workers exposed to metalworking fluids. Am J Ind Med 2014;57(8):872–80.
60. Cormier Y, Israel-Assayag E, Bedard G, et al. Hypersensitivity pneumonitis in peat moss processing plant workers. Am J Respir Crit Care Med 1998; 158(2):412–7.
61. Veillette M, Cormier Y, Israel-Assayaq E, et al. Hypersensitivity pneumonitis in a hardwood processing plant related to heavy mold exposure. J Occup Environ Hyg 2006;3(6):301–7.
62. National Institute for Occupational Safety and Health (NIOSH). Criteria for a recommended standard. Occupational exposure to metalworking fluids 1998. Available at: http://www.cdc.gov/niosh/docs/98-102/pdfs/98-102.pdf. Accessed August 26, 2020.
63. NIOSH. What you need to know about occupational exposure to metalworking fluids. 1998. Available at: https://www.cdc.gov/niosh/docs/98-116/default.html.
64. Taylor AN, Cullinan P, Blanc P, et al, editors. Parkes' Occupational lung disorders. CRC Press; 2016.
65. Moya C, Antó JM, Taylor AJ. Outbreak of organising pneumonia in textile printing sprayers. Collaborative group for the study of toxicity in textile aerographic factories. Lancet 1994;344(8921):498–502.
66. Kern DG, Crausman RS, Durand KT, et al. Flock worker's lung: chronic interstitial lung disease in the nylon flocking industry. Ann Intern Med 1998; 129(4):261–72.
67. Cummings KJ, Donat WE, Ettensohn DB, et al. Pulmonary alveolar proteinosis in workers at an indium processing facility. Am J Respir Crit Care Med 2010; 181(5):458–64.
68. Hoy RF, Baird T, Hammerschlag G, et al. Artificial stone-associated silicosis: a rapidly emerging occupational lung disease. Occup Environ Med 2018; 75(1):3–5.

Silicosis: An Update and Guide for Clinicians

Silpa Krefft, MD, MPH[a,b,c,d,*], Jenna Wolff, BA[a], Cecile Rose, MD, MPH[a,c,d]

KEYWORDS

• Silicosis • Silicoproteinosis • Acute silicosis • Accelerated silicosis • OSHA Silica standard

KEY POINTS

- Outbreaks of silicosis and its associated diseases, most recently among younger workers in the engineered stone industry, pose growing international concern for severe progressive disease.
- Underrecognized clinical phenotypes include silicoproteinosis, diffuse fibrosis, and emphysema, often with associated lung infection, autoimmune diseases, and inflammatory kidney disease.
- In addition to diagnosis and treatment, clinicians should be knowledgeable about legal, regulatory, and public health issues linked to a diagnosis of silicosis.
- The 2017 Occupational Safety and Health Administration silica standard contain expanded medical surveillance recommendations and more stringent permissible exposure levels for primary prevention.

INTRODUCTION

There are 2 primary goals of this overview. The first is to provide an update on the already significant body of literature on silicosis, with emphasis on emerging exposure settings and clinical presentations of silicosis and associated diseases, along with an approach to diagnosis and management. The second goal is to provide clinicians with practical guidance to questions that may arise when evaluating silica-exposed patients and to the public health responses needed following a diagnosis of silica-related disease.

THE MINERALOGY OF CRYSTALLINE AND AMORPHOUS SILICA AND SILICATES

Silica, the most abundant mineral on earth, is structurally classified as crystalline or amorphous. Respirable crystalline silica (RCS) is associated with lung and other organ toxicity after inhalation. Crystalline forms of silica include quartz present in granite and sandstone as well as tridymite and cristobalite contained in volcanic rock.[1–3]

Free or pure crystalline silica consists of silicon and oxygen, often referred to as silicon dioxide. Silicates are silicon and oxygen-containing compounds combined with other minerals. Common silicates include kaolinite that is mined as kaolin for use in ceramics; and talc, a hydrous magnesium silicate used as an ingredient in cosmetics and pharmaceutical formulations.[4] The hydrated alumino-magnesium silicates of asbestos (eg, chrysotile, crocidolite, amosite, anthophyllite, actinolite, and tremolite) and the fibrous zeolites are associated with a different spectrum of health outcomes and are not included in this discussion.

Amorphous silica includes vitreous silica (glass) and biogenic forms from marine and aquatic microalgae called diatoms that extract silica for skeleton formation. A number of cosmetic products contain primarily synthetic amorphous silica with ingredients listed as fused or hydrated silica

[a] Division of Environmental and Occupational Health Sciences, National Jewish Health, 1400 Jackson Street, Denver, CO 80206, USA; [b] Division of Pulmonary and Critical Care Medicine, VA Eastern Colorado Health Care System, Aurora, CO, USA; [c] Division of Pulmonary and Critical Care Medicine, University of Colorado Anschutz Medical Campus, Aurora, CO, USA; [d] Department of Environmental and Occupational Health, Colorado School of Public Health, Aurora, CO, USA
* Corresponding author. Division of Environmental and Occupational Health Sciences, National Jewish Health, 1400 Jackson Street, Denver, CO 80206.
E-mail address: kreffts@njhealth.org

Clin Chest Med 41 (2020) 709–722
https://doi.org/10.1016/j.ccm.2020.08.012
0272-5231/20/Published by Elsevier Inc.

and conferring little known risk for lung toxicity. Although RCS is not used in cosmetic products, labels often are vague and may list "silica" as an ingredient. The Cosmetic Ingredient Review, funded by the cosmetics industry trade association with support from the US Food and Drug Administration and the Consumer Federation of America, concluded that silica and silicates (eg, alumina magnesium metasilicate, aluminum calcium sodium silicate, aluminum iron silicates, hydrated silica, sodium potassium aluminum silicate) used in cosmetics are safe when manufactured in larger nonrespirable particle sizes and developed to avoid eye or dermal irritation.[5]

SILICOSIS, AN ANCIENT DISEASE WITH EMERGING IMPORTANCE

Recognition of the devastating effects of exposure to dust from stone goes back to the earliest medical observers. Hippocrates described breathing disorders in metal diggers in 400 BC. In the 1500s, Agricola's observation that dusty working conditions led to lung disease was a particular reference to silica exposure.[6] In the 1600s, van Diemerbrock described injurious effects of granite dust. By the 1700s, more detailed descriptions of lung scarring in stone and coal workers were described by Ramazzini, who recommended methods for improving ventilation in these work settings.

With onset of the Industrial Revolution in the mid-eighteenth century, changes in production techniques and increasing mechanization placed workers at risk from exposure to high concentrations of silica dust. In 1832, for example, Thackrah showed that sandstone quarry workers had shorter life expectancies than brick and limestone workers, dying by age 40.[7] In 1930, silicosis risks in mining and quarrying workers were highlighted at the Johannesburg International Labor Office Conference where ground-breaking occupational lung disease research was emerging from the large South African gold mining industry. With research contributions from scientists in Australia, Belgium, Canada, Germany, Great Britain, the Netherlands, the United States, and Italy, this conference marked a major international focus on medical and pathologic findings in silicosis, prevention strategies, and compensation for affected workers.[8,9]

In the 1920s and 1930s, the United States was the site for one of the country's worst industrial disasters known as the Hawk's Nest Incident. A hydroelectric plant in West Virginia required construction of 2 power stations, 2 dams, and 2 tunnels. Workers drilled through rock to create the Hawk's Nest Tunnel near Gauley Bridge, generating high silica concentrations in confined spaces with no ventilation or respiratory protection. Many developed disabling respiratory symptoms from acute silicosis within a few months. Congressional hearings estimated the death toll between 1930 and 1935 at 476 people, although later estimates of silicosis deaths (including complications from tuberculosis) ranged from 700 to 2000 workers.[10] Throughout the twentieth century, recognition grew of other industries in which RCS exposure placed workers at risk for disease, including pottery and porcelain work and abrasive blasting. Similar to mining and tunneling, construction on underground subways, highways and dams exposed thousands of workers to silica.[9]

Despite centuries of knowledge about risks from exposure to silica dust, the twenty-first century has seen a surge in this preventable disease. Since 2000, there has been an increase in severe and rapidly progressive pneumoconiosis in Central Appalachian coal miners.[11–13] Rapidly progressive pneumoconiosis has been linked to silica exposure based on lung pathology showing features of accelerated silicosis along with classic silicotic nodules.[14] Mining coal from lower seam heights is associated with more rock cutting above and below the coal seam, likely leading to increased RCS exposure and more virulent disease.

An outbreak of silicosis was described in 2006 among Turkish workers using abrasive sandblasting to distress jean material for clothing. Sixteen workers, with an average age of 23, developed clinical findings of silicosis, with a mean latency of disease onset after only 3 years. Few exposure controls were present in these small, unregulated workplaces. All 16 workers had imaging findings of silicosis, including 2 with the most severe forms of disease who died of respiratory failure within less than a year of clinical presentation. Lung biopsies in 2 workers showed silicotic nodules and alveolar proteinosis; the other workers were diagnosed with acute or accelerated silicosis based on clinical findings.[15] A subsequent cross-sectional study of 157 former denim sandblasters in Turkey found that more than half (77/145) had radiographic evidence of silicosis associated with decreased lung function.[16] A follow-up study in 2011 reassessed 83 of the original 145 former denim sandblasters and found an alarmingly high rate of silicosis despite no further occupational silica exposure. Nine had died, and 66% of the remaining 74 had significant lung function declines. Mortality was associated with never smoking status, sleeping at the sandblasting work site, and job titles with higher exposures.[17] Although Turkey's Ministry of Health banned RCS use for abrasive sandblasting in 2009, and despite availability of other methods, silica exposure in denim sandblasting continues in other countries.[18,19]

Severe silicosis from exposure to high concentrations of RCS in engineered stone countertops is an emerging worldwide problem. Engineered stone (also known as artificial stone or quartz conglomerate) was first commercially available in the mid-1980s, and is made by mixing finely crushed rock with polymeric resins, then heat-curing the mixture in molds to make slabs. Workers are exposed to high concentrations of RCS from cutting, grinding, and polishing slabs, and performing housekeeping duties such as dry-sweeping in work areas around these processes. The first reported cases of engineered stone silicosis were published in 2010 in Italy, with later cases described in Israel, Spain, Australia, and the United States.[20–22] Engineered stone silicosis appears to affect younger workers, with shorter disease latencies (typically within 2 to 10 years), and with acute and accelerated clinical features leading to severe and rapidly progressive lung impairment and death.[23] This emerging epidemic has prompted pulmonologists to confront the need for a coordinated medical and public health response, both for exposure control and primary prevention and to reexplore treatment options for severe, progressive disease affecting younger workers.

Hydraulic fracturing operations for extracting oil and natural gas from underground sources, known as "fracking," in use since the 1940s, and greatly expanded in the twenty-first century, are another source of workplace RCS exposures. Fracking requires large volumes of water and a solid known as a proppant to increase recovery of hydrocarbons and overall yield of oil and gas. Silica sand, also referred to as "frac sand," is a less expensive proppant than other options such as ceramics, sintered bauxite, aluminum pellets or modified proppants (containing epoxy resin, furan, polyurethane, phenol aldehyde, or vinyl) that may be less crush-resistant than silica sand.[24,25] The National Institute for Occupational Safety and Health (NIOSH) conducted an exposure monitoring study with full-shift personal breathing zone samples collected from 11 hydraulic fracture sites in Arkansas, Colorado, North Dakota, Pennsylvania, and Texas.[24] More than 50% of samples exceeded the 2013 OSHA permissible exposure limit (PEL) for the 12-hour shift, with some RCS concentrations 10 to 20 times higher than the PEL, mainly in jobs with close proximity to sand-moving machinery. Based on these findings, NIOSH recommended substitution using nonsilica proppants, engineering controls to reduce dust levels, and administrative controls to decrease time spent near sand-moving machinery. NIOSH investigators also found that air-purifying half-face respirators often did not provide adequate respiratory protection.[24]

EPIDEMIOLOGY OF SILICOSIS IN THE TWENTY-FIRST CENTURY

Worldwide, there are an estimated 23 million workers in China, 11.5 million in India, 3.2 million in the European Union, and 2 million in Brazil at risk from exposure to RCS.[26–28] An estimated 5000 Turkish workers have silicosis, and silica sandblasting continues to thrive in other countries like Bangladesh.[29] While countries including Brazil, Chile, China, India, Peru, South Africa, Thailand, Turkey, and Vietnam have implemented the Outline for a National Programme for the Elimination of Silicosis, and Australia, Belgium, Canada, Finland, France, Germany, Switzerland, Sweden, United Kingdom, and the United States have longstanding regulatory and prevention programs, silicosis continues to afflict tens of millions of workers.[8]

An estimated 2.3 million workers in the United States are exposed to RCS.[30] State-based data from Michigan and New Jersey suggest that most US silicosis cases between 2003 and 2011 occurred in manufacturing and construction industries (63% and 19.5%, respectively).[31] Job duties with high silica exposure include cutting, sawing, grinding, drilling, and crushing stone, rock, concrete, brick, block and mortar, and abrasive blasting with sand.[32] Among young adults ages 15 to 44 in the United States who died of silicosis, 31% worked in manufacturing (crushing, grinding, polishing, mixing, and blending stone and silica-containing materials), 14% in minerals extraction and construction work, 9% as brick/block masons, and 37% worked in other jobs including health care (dentist offices, ambulatory care services, hospitals) and social assistance that are less commonly associated with silica exposure, and 3 in unknown occupations.[33]

NONOCCUPATIONAL SETTINGS WHERE RESPIRABLE CRYSTALLINE SILICA EXPOSURE CAN OCCUR

Most studies focus on occupational silica exposure and work-related silicosis. However, cottage industries and hobbies also contribute to the worldwide burden of silica-related lung disease. Examples include pottery and ceramics work where RCS levels may be substantial and where access to dust controls and respiratory protection may be variable or absent.[34,35]

Although there has been little research on community exposure to silica dust, such exposures have been linked to dusty environments worldwide. Concerns have arisen for geogenic (eg, silica-containing agricultural and desert dusts) and anthropogenic sources (eg, from a local agate industry) contributing to detectable ambient silica concentrations that may pose a long-term respiratory health risk.[36–38] A small case series of nonoccupational anthracosilicosis was described in 6 nonsmoking homemakers in Ladakh, a high-desert town in the Himalayan region of India. Three of the 6 women had lung histopathology notable for polarizing birefringent silicotic pigment. The other 3 cases (in whom polarizing light microscopy was not performed) had progressive massive fibrosis and nodules throughout both lung fields. In addition to exposure to biomass smoke from indoor cooking and heating, the authors noted commonly occurring dust storms as an additional source of silica exposure.[39] Another study sampled dust in living rooms of residences in the Himalayan village of Chuchot in the Ladakh region and identified particulate matter ranging in size from 0.5 to 5 μm, with a substantial portion comprising silica-containing mica and quartz. No industrial source of silica was identified, implicating exposure from dust storms and farming practices.[40]

Crystalline silica in concentrations that approach or exceed occupational permissible exposure levels have been detected in communities in close proximity to local industries in Madhya Pradesh, India. Residential area sampling of quartz concentrations averaged between 41.07 and 57.22 $\mu g/m^3$ in 2 communities surrounded by slate pencil manufacturing operations, substantially higher compared with an average quartz concentration of 3.51 $\mu g/m^3$ in a village 5 km away from the slate facilities.[41] A 1983 case of silicosis confirmed by lung tissue showing birefringent particles was diagnosed in a Pakistani farmer with decades of farming, followed over subsequent decades by increasing recognition of silica exposure from agricultural dusts.[42–44]

CLASSIFICATION AND CLINICAL PRESENTATION OF SILICOSIS AND ASSOCIATED DISEASES

Silicosis has been considered mainly a disease of long latency (>20 years), but as noted with denim sandblasters and engineered stone workers, disease can occur with much shorter latency, present with inflammatory and systemic features, and contribute to increased mortality among younger workers.[16,45] Classically, silicosis has been categorized as acute, accelerated, and chronic (both simple and complicated). Newer definitions from the Centers for Disease Control and Prevention (CDC) categorize silicosis as either acute (silicoproteinosis) or nodular (including both accelerated and chronic forms of silicosis).[46] Recent outbreaks of silicosis are notable for overlapping features of acute, accelerated, and chronic silicosis. For this overview, clinical presentations using conventional designations of acute, accelerated and chronic are discussed.

Acute Silicosis

Silicoproteinosis, a clinical presentation of acute silicosis that resembles primary pulmonary alveolar proteinosis, typically occurs within a few weeks to years following exposure to high concentrations of RCS. The alveolar proteinosis observed in acute silicosis may be a response to lung injury from inorganic particulate exposure.[47] Cases of acute silicosis have been reported in tombstone sandblasters, brick masons, quartz millers, workers who did both wet and dry grinding of cement containers, and more recently in denim sandblasters and artificial stone workers.[17,21,48–50]

Both respiratory and systemic symptoms are commonly reported and include shortness of breath, productive or nonproductive cough, chest tightness, pleuritic chest pain, fevers, headaches, and unintentional weight loss. Symptoms are nonspecific and may be confused with lung infections, especially in younger patients when occupational exposure to RCS is unrecognized.[50] These symptoms are often accompanied by hypoxemia.

There are no laboratory tests specific to a diagnosis of silicoproteinosis. The presence of Granulocyte macrophage–colony-stimulating factor (GM-CSF) antibodies are helpful in diagnosing primary autoimmune alveolar proteinosis (PAP). Evaluation for infections that mimic or may be linked with acute silicosis should be considered, and complete blood count, human immunodeficiency virus (HIV) serologic testing, sputum culture, and *Pneumocystis carinii* pneumonia (PCP) direct fluorescence antibody staining indicated. Lung function in the setting of acute silicosis shows spirometric reduction of forced vital capacity (FVC) and forced expiratory volume in 1 second (FEV1).[51] Although few studies report lung volume and diffusion capacity measurements, both typically are reduced.[21,52] Chest imaging in acute silicosis (**Fig. 1**) demonstrates bilateral patchy centrilobular nodularity, ground glass opacities,

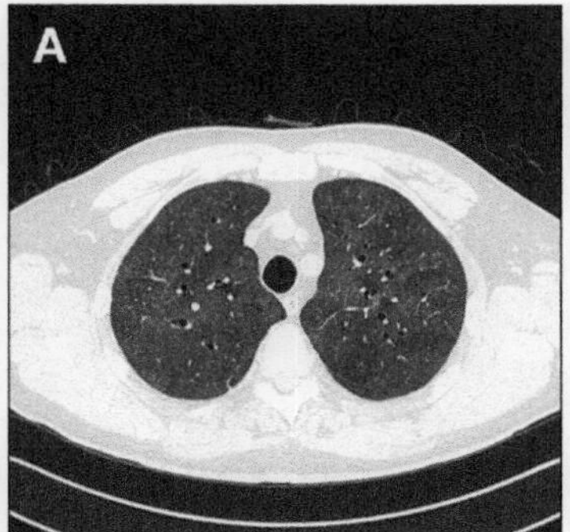

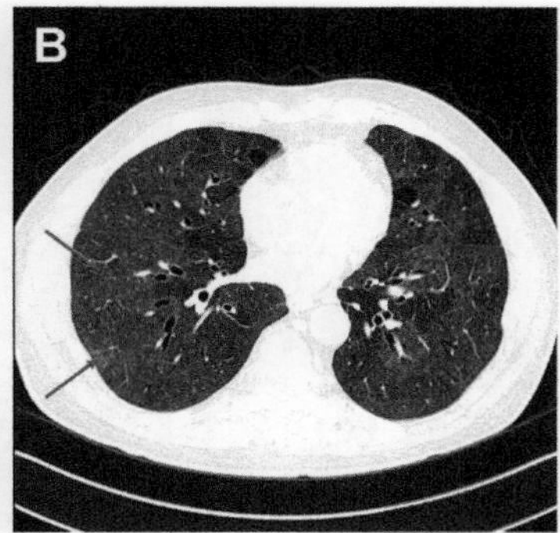

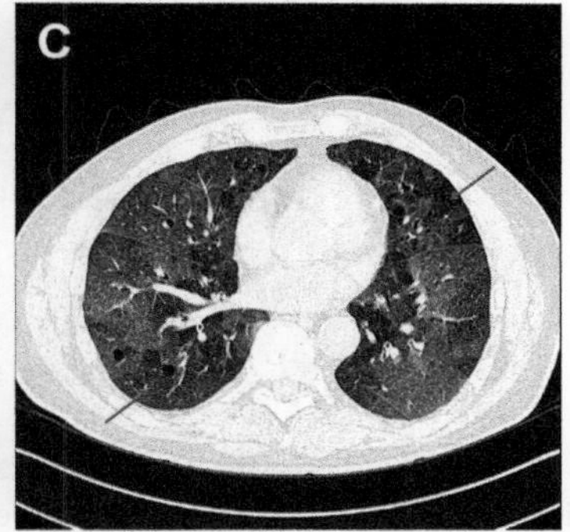

Fig. 1. (*A*) Diffuse faint centrilobular ground glass nodularity is visible at the lung apices in an engineered stone worker with silicosis. (*B*) Inspiratory image shows regional differences in lung attenuation due to mosaic perfusion and a background of ground glass abnormality with faint centrilobular nodularity (*arrows*). (*C*) Expiratory image demonstrates multilobular air trapping (*arrows*). Normal lung increases significantly in attenuation relative to (*B*).

interlobular septal thickening and consolidation in a perihilar distribution. A "crazy paving" appearance typical of other lung diseases (eg, PAP, PCP) can be present on chest imaging.[53] Pleural abnormalities may also manifest, including unilateral or bilateral pneumothorax.[54]

The prognosis of acute silicosis is poor, with patients often progressing to chronic respiratory failure, cor pulmonale, and death. Treatment with systemic steroids and whole lung lavage have been reported, but these interventions have not been systematically evaluated. They may be considered in severe cases despite the lack of evidence of in reducing morbidity or mortality.[55,56]

Chronic Silicosis

Symptoms of cough and dyspnea from chronic silicosis typically begin within 10 to 30 years after exposure onset.[57,58] Chronic silicosis is classified as either simple or complicated based on chest imaging. The chest imaging findings of simple silicosis include bilateral reticulonodular opacities that are typically upper lobe predominant, although lower lobe linear interstitial opacities also occur (**Fig. 2**).[59] Pleural thickening or, less commonly, pleural effusion may be present.[60,61] Complicated silicosis, also referred to as progressive massive fibrosis, is diagnosed by the presence of ILO (International Labour Organization) category large opacities on chest radiograph or with the chest HRCT finding of conglomerate opacities, typically with calcifications and fibrosis.[59] Lung function is variable and may be normal or abnormal, depending on disease stage. Mixed obstructive and restrictive ventilatory abnormalities have been described. Lung volumes show restrictive defects in advanced cases of chronic silicosis, especially in those with progressive massive fibrosis (PMF). Diffusion capacity of carbon monoxide (DLCO) may be normal in mild disease but typically worsens over time, especially in smokers.[62,63] Emphysema in silicosis patients may be correlated with reduced FVC, FEV1, lung volumes, and DLCO.[62,64] Lymph node and lung tissue biopsy and autopsy specimens show

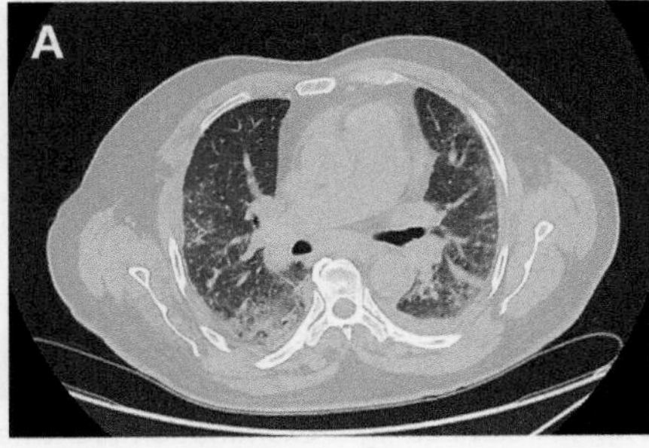

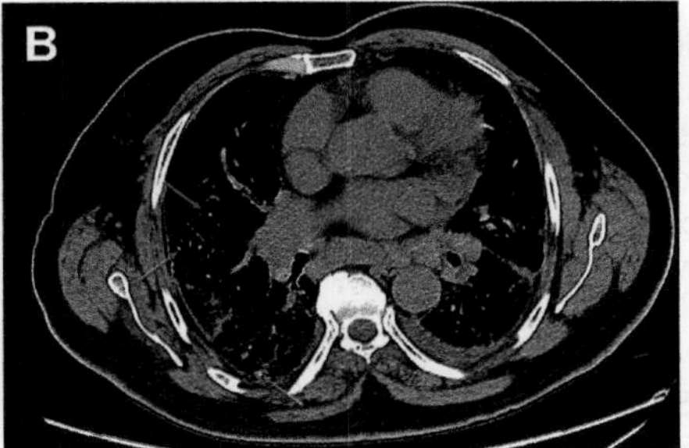

Fig. 2. (*A*) Engineered stone worker with multiple small calcified and noncalcified pulmonary nodules, ground glass opacities, and small pleural effusions. (*B*). Mediastinal window CT shows calcified lung nodules (*arrows*) and a small left pleural effusion.

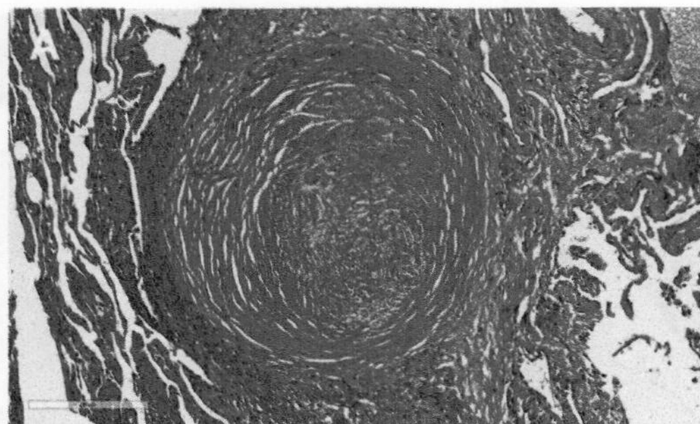

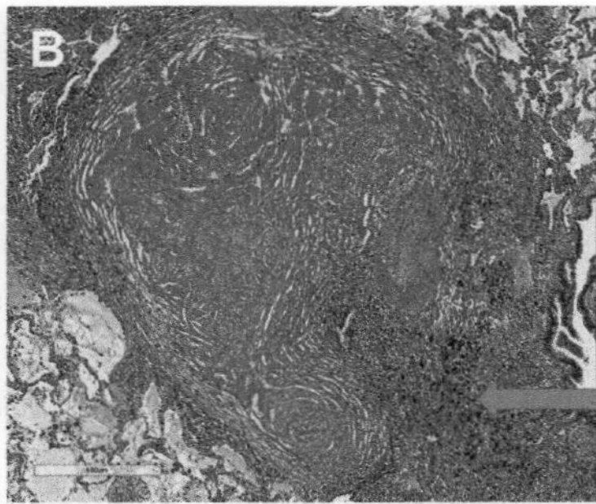

Fig. 3. (*A*) Classic silicotic nodule on hematoxylin-eosin stain that shows inner zone with concentric configuration of collagen fibrils surrounded by peripheral zone of inflammatory cells (eg, lymphocytes) and loose collagen. (*B*) Silicotic nodule with surrounding area of dusty macrophages/histiocytes and chronic inflammation.

silicotic nodules, birefringent silica particles, and interstitial fibrosis as shown in **Figs. 3** and **4**. Laboratory testing should be considered if there is concern for infection or autoimmunity.

Simple silicosis may progress to complicated silicosis as nodules coalesce. Prognosis is poor in complicated silicosis, as both progressively worsening lung function and infection with tuberculosis or nontuberculous mycobacteria are common. Although more indolent than acute silicosis, lung function decline in chronic silicosis may lead to significant ventilatory and gas exchange abnormalities and respiratory failure. Treatment is supportive, with use of supplemental oxygen in those with hypoxia, prompt treatment of infection, recommended vaccinations, and pulmonary rehabilitation.

Accelerated Silicosis

The major distinction between accelerated and acute or chronic silicosis is based on disease latency, with onset of accelerated disease within 5 to 10 years of exposure. Case descriptions based on lung histopathology and chest imaging are significant for overlapping features of silicoproteinosis (**Fig. 5**), a defining feature of acute silicosis, as well as silica nodules, birefringent silica particles, and interstitial fibrosis characteristic of chronic silicotic lung disease.[45,65] Disease progression is more rapid than in chronic silicosis. Recent outbreaks of accelerated (as well as acute and chronic) silicosis in denim sandblasters, Appalachian coal miners, and artificial stone workers have shown rapidly progressing and severe disease.[17,27]

OTHER DISEASES ASSOCIATED WITH SILICA EXPOSURE

Nonfibrotic lung diseases associated with RCS exposure include emphysema and related chronic obstructive pulmonary disease, lung infection, and lung cancer. There also are well-established links between silica exposure and autoimmune rheumatologic diseases as well as inflammatory kidney disease.

Emphysema

Although silicosis is widely recognized as an interstitial lung disease, emphysema is an underappreciated manifestation of silica-related pulmonary disease. The causal link between silica exposure and risk for emphysema is well-recognized. Although some earlier studies did not show statistically significant differences in chronic obstructive pulmonary disease (COPD) risk in miners versus nonminers or in degree of emphysema and lung function decline in nonsmoking miners,[66] there is mounting evidence demonstrating that emphysema and airflow obstruction may be present and significant even in the absence of smoking.[67,68] One study using chest computed

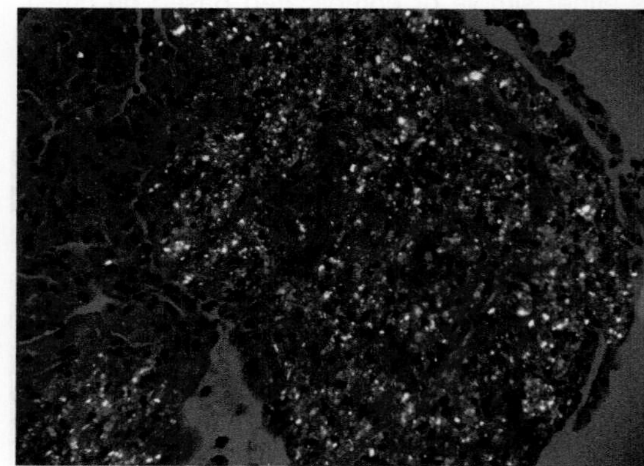

Fig. 4. Polarized light examination identifies multiple bright white silicate and dimmer silica particles in this fibrotic nodule. The collagen fibers appear pink under polarized light in this example.

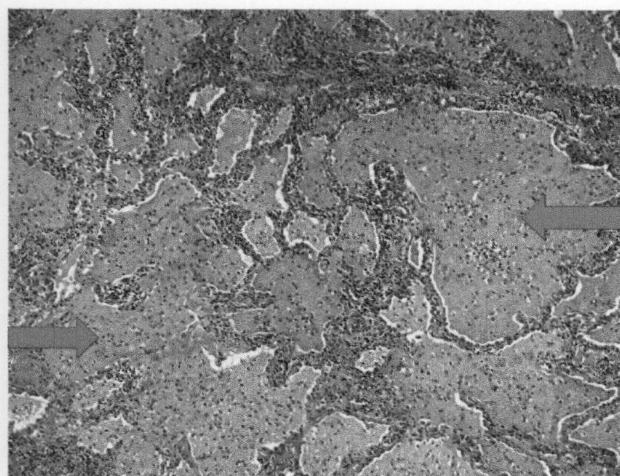

Fig. 5. Extensive alveolar proteinosis with arrows showing airspace filling with light pink proteinaceous material. (H&E stain and 200x magnification).

tomography (CT) found emphysema in silica-exposed workers who had smoked as well as in nonsmoking workers with radiographic evidence of silicosis based on ILO classification. A paracicatricial pattern of emphysema was noted in association with confluent silicotic opacities.[69] Studies in South African gold miners found evidence of a dose-response relationship between increasing cumulative silica exposure and airflow obstruction in both smokers and nonsmokers.[67,70] Not surprisingly, smoking appears to be a significant factor contributing to lung function decline and severity of emphysema in silica-exposed workers with and without radiologic evidence of silicosis.[69,70] A recent analysis of lung function and COPD adjusted for smoking status in Welsh slate miners found an association between slate mining and reduced FVC and FEV1 as well as a 1.38 higher odds of COPD risk.[71] Despite the compelling evidence of the link between RCS exposure and chronic bronchitis, COPD, and emphysema,[67,72,73] little is understood about pathogenic mechanisms. Intratracheal instillation of crystalline silica in rats resulted in increased amounts of desmosine (a marker of elastin breakdown) and hydroxyproline (associated with collagen breakdown), suggesting that silica-driven breakdown of lung connective tissue is linked to emphysema pathogenesis.[74]

Lung Infection

Mycobacterial infection, both tuberculous (TB) and nontuberculous (NTM), has long been recognized as a complication of silicosis and poses important challenges to global lung health.[75–78] Specific mechanisms and risk factors for mycobacterial lung infection in silica-exposed workers are not well understood, though underlying HIV infection, previous TB, and cumulative years and more intense RCS exposures increase risk.[78] Chemoprophylaxis for silica-exposed workers with latent TB infection (LTBI) is recommended by the CDC, and published guidelines should be followed based on country-specific TB epidemiologic profiles.[79] Notably, however, mass screening and treatment for LTBI among South African goal miners had no significant effect of tuberculosis control.[80] Treatment of mycobacterial lung infection in silicotic patients is challenging, with only 80% achieving sputum culture conversion to negative after 2 months in 1 randomized clinical trial.[79]

Lung Cancer

The International Agency for Research on Cancer recognized RCS as a human carcinogen as early as 1997, and reconfirmed its carcinogenicity in a 2009 report.[1] Case-control studies and meta-analyses in multiple industries and countries show higher risk of all histologic types of lung cancer based on cumulative duration of RCS exposure, mainly in workers with silicosis.[81] For example, a cohort study of over 34,000 silica-exposed Chinese workers, one-third of whom were never smokers, found that RCS exposure in the absence of smoking is associated with increased lung cancer risk. These investigators observed a 1.7-fold increased relative risk (RR) of lung cancer with high cumulative silica exposure and a 1.26-fold RR with low exposure workers compared to an unexposed group.[82] Proposed mechanisms for RCS-related carcinogenesis include impairment of lung epithelial expression of the G-protein-coupled receptor family C group 5 type A (GPRC5A), lung epithelial injury from reactive oxygen species generated by activated macrophages, and chronic inflammation through biopersistence of silica that may increase risk of DNA damage and tumorigenesis.[83]

The role of lung cancer screening in patients with silicosis is not straightforward, as the literature has focused primarily on lung cancer screening in smokers.[46,83] The US Preventive Services Task Force recommends an annual low-dose radiation chest CT for screening individuals between ages of 55 and 80 with a 30 pack-year or greater smoking history who are current smokers or who have stopped smoking for less than 15 years; additional lung cancer risk factors are not used to determine screening eligibility.[84] The 2012 National Comprehensive Cancer Network (NCCN) guidelines recommend similar lung cancer screening for smokers and former smokers between ages 55 to 74. Notably, NCCN criteria also include screening anyone age 50 or older who has a 20 pack-year or greater smoking history and occupational exposure to lung carcinogens such as silica.[85] Cui and colleagues[86] highlight some of the limitations of utilizing guidelines that focus only on smoking, since worldwide smoking accounts for only 80% of lung cancer in men and 50% in women, with many current guidelines overlooking other important causal factors (eg, silica, asbestos, radon). Early lung cancers may be missed due to a presumption of progressive silicosis on chest imaging studies; conversely parenchymal changes of silicosis may be confused for malignancy, making lung cancer screening interpretation challenging in cases of more advanced silicosis.[87] Screening for lung cancer in silica-exposed workers should be considered on a case-by-case basis after careful review of lung cancer guidelines in conjunction with a discussion of risks and benefits. Histopathologic confirmation should be considered in the context of a lung nodule that is increasing in size, as PET scanning can be positive in both cancer and silicotic nodules.

Autoimmune Disease

Exposure to RCS is associated with increased autoantibody production and risk for autoimmune diseases.[81] Early studies reported increased prevalence of antinuclear antibody (ANA) and topoisomerase autoantibodies in patients with silicosis, though these findings were not associated with risk for progression or severity of silicosis.[88] Although no specific autoantibody has been identified as unique or indicative of silica exposure, epidemiologic studies have established links between exposure and rheumatoid arthritis (RA), systemic sclerosis (SSc), systemic lupus erythematosus, and anti-neutrophil cytoplasmic antibody (ANCA)-related vasculitis.[89] Case reports of other autoimmune conditions such as Sjogren syndrome, dermatomyositis, Graves disease, autoimmune hemolytic anemia, and pemphigus vulgaris also have been reported in patients with occupational exposure to silica.[90–93] Treatment for silica-associated autoimmune conditions does not differ from treatment of idiopathic autoimmune disease.

The mechanisms of silica-related autoimmunity are not well understood, though abnormalities in T-cell function, humoral immunity, and immune complex deposition have been implicated in pathogenesis. Silica-related autoimmunity has been increasingly linked to chronic activation of responder and regulatory T cells that alter serum concentrations of soluble Fas, which is important in inhibiting lymphocyte apoptosis. Based on in vitro studies of T-cell activation, Lee and colleagues[94] proposed that, following silica-induced activation of T responder and regulatory cells, activated responder cells persist while regulatory T cells are lost due to Fas-mediated apoptosis. With reduced inhibition from loss of regulatory T cells, activated T responder cells may survive longer in peripheral CD4+25 fractions and result in autoreactive clones involved in progression to autoimmune disease.[94]

Kidney Disease

Reports of kidney disease in association with acute and chronic silicosis emerged in the 1970s, with accumulating evidence over the past decades. Early case reports described findings such as proteinuria and fatal renal failure in a young sandblaster with acute silicoproteinosis.[95] Using 1985 to 1995 data from the Michigan state-based silicosis surveillance system, Rosenman and colleagues found a higher prevalence of kidney disease in silica-exposed workers compared with healthy controls. Among 583 confirmed silicosis cases, kidney disease was mentioned in the medical records of 10%. An abnormal serum creatinine was present in 33% of 283 silicosis cases with available laboratory data. In contrast to earlier studies,[96–99] Rosenman and colleagues did not find evidence of a dose-response relationship between kidney disease and duration of silica exposure or profusion of scarring on chest radiograph. A follow-up cross-sectional study that included an additional 497 silicosis cases between 1987 and 2009 from the Michigan surveillance system found 69% with chronic kidney disease compared with 38.8% in an age-matched National Health and Nutrition Examination Study reference population. As with previous findings, they did not observe a dose-response relationship between kidney disease and silica exposure or silicosis severity.[100] A 2017 meta-analysis that reviewed 23 cohort and 4 case-control studies of silica-exposed workers found higher standardized mortality ratios for kidney disease. Aggregate data from multiple studies did not show a clear dose-response relationship between silica exposure and renal disease.[101]

There is evidence that 2 pathogenic mechanisms may be important in silica-related chronic kidney disease.[102,103] RCS may be directly nephrotoxic, resulting in glomerular and tubulointerstitial dysfunction. Alternatively, silica exposure may indirectly cause renal disease by triggering autoimmunity that manifests as ANCA-associated vasculitis, lupus, or other autoimmune/connective tissues disorders with kidney involvement.[102,104–106]

Silica and Sarcoidosis

Silicosis and sarcoidosis share a number of clinical features and, absent a careful history and comprehensive diagnostic evaluation, one may be mistaken for the other. Further complicating the diagnostic challenges for clinicians, epidemiologic studies assessing possible occupational and environmental exposure associations with sarcoidosis have suggested a link to RCS.[107] A 1998 case-control study described a significant association between occupational exposure to cristobalite and sarcoidosis (odds ratio of 13.2) at a diatomaceous earth processing facility in Iceland where amorphous silica was converted to crystalline silica containing up to 70% cristobalite and 1% to 2% quartz. Study investigators observed a higher annual sarcoidosis incidence of 9.3/100,000 in the health district surrounding the diatomaceous earth plant compared with the countrywide annual incidence of 0.5 to 2.7 per 100,000.[108] Higher rates of incident cases of sarcoidosis have been noted in World Trade Center–exposed workers compared with an unexposed and age-adjusted cohort, suggesting a link between inorganic dust exposure and sarcoidosis.[109] Animal studies describe granulomatous inflammation induced by exposure to low-dose aerosolized silica.[110] A case report of sarcoidosis diagnosed in a husband and wife residing in an urban area with nearby stone quarries raised concerns about a common environmental exposure to RCS.[111] A Swedish cohort study compared foundry workers with high and low RCS exposure to the unexposed Swedish population, and found an increased risk of sarcoidosis and seropositive RA linked to silica.[112] In contrast, a study of standard occupational classification codes and sarcoidosis-related deaths from US death certificates observed a mortality odds ratio less than 1 in standard occupational classification (SOC) codes with higher silica exposure.[113] Future investigation using occupational disease registries may provide additional insights into the possible connection between RCS exposure and sarcoidosis.

SILICOSIS PREVENTION AND SENTINEL CASE MANAGEMENT

As with most occupational lung diseases, primary prevention to control RCS dust levels remains the most important component to address this untreatable and often devastating fibrotic lung disease and its associated illnesses and complications. Unlike exposure control experts, clinicians focus mainly on early disease detection and secondary prevention to eliminate continued RCS dust exposures in their patients with silicosis and must implement approaches to both individual patient care as well as a public health response to this preventable disease.

The 2017 OSHA silica standard requires general industry and construction employers to provide baseline medical surveillance examinations as well as periodic examinations for those exposed to RCS above the permissible level for a defined number of days.[32,114] Surveillance includes a medical and work history, physical examination, chest x-ray, pulmonary function test, LTBI test, and any other tests deemed appropriate by the provider. The employer is responsible for providing a description of the employee's former, current, and anticipated job duties, information on workplace silica exposure concentrations, a description of personal protective equipment used, and information from employment-related medical examinations. After the initial examination, clinical follow-up must be offered at least every 3 years, unless more frequent evaluation is recommended by the physician or other licensed health care professional (PLHCP) during the initial visit. If the PLHCP suspects a case of silicosis, advanced COPD, or other respiratory conditions that may cause impairment, or if the chest x-ray is classified as 1/0 or higher profusion by an ILO-certified B-reader, the worker should be referred to a board-certified specialist in pulmonary or occupational medicine. The clinician must explain the results to the patient and provide them with a written medical report within 30 days, with recommendations for any limitations to exposure and information on risks of ongoing exposure and disease progression, personal risk factors, possible health outcomes, possible economic consequences, and referral to a specialist if necessary.

Under the 2017 OSHA silica standard, providers are also required to submit a medical opinion to the employer, guided by strict requirements to maintain patient confidentiality. These reports include the date of examination, a statement that guidelines for the examination have been met, any recommended limitations on the employee's use of respiratory protection or the employee's exposure to respirable silica, and recommendations for referral if needed. Evidence of active TB, acute or accelerated silicosis, or other silica-related diseases serve as a sentinel health event.

These events suggest that workers face ongoing risks from exposure to RCS that may require consultation with public health agencies such as local and state health departments, local and state OSHA, or NIOSH.[115] Reporting of a diagnosis of silicosis or other diseases associated with silica exposure to the appropriate agencies is essential and will enable investigation of similarly exposed coworkers who may also be at risk.

A diagnosis of silicosis has significant legal as well as medical implications for the patient.[116] Diagnosis of a work-related disease entitles the patient to apply for workers compensation to cover medical and other costs. In some states, there may be a statute of limitations within which timeframe the patient must file a workers compensation claim before losing the option to do so. It is important that the clinician who diagnoses a patient with work-related silicosis do so in writing, and should recommend that the patient obtain knowledgeable legal counsel to understand their rights and benefits.

Both national and international disease registries and silica surveillance programs are needed to track new cases of silicosis and other silica-related diseases so that public health programs can tailor education, outreach, and prevention strategies based on accurate incidence and prevalence data. Disease registries and national and international monitoring programs would also help identify new or emerging silica exposure settings, thereby providing an opportunity to prevent new and recurrent large-scale epidemics of silicosis.

CLINICS CARE POINTS

- Acute, chronic, and accelerated silicosis phenotypes may share overlapping lung histopathologic features of silicoproteinosis and interstitial fibrosis.
- Chest imaging abnormalities in accelerated and chronic silicosis are not limited to the upper lobes of the lungs and may involve lower lobe fibrosis and/or pleural disease.
- Chemoprophylaxis is indicated in silica-exposed workers with latent tuberculosis infection.
- Pharmacotherapeutic treatment for silica-associated autoimmune disease does not differ from that of idiopathic autoimmune disease.
- Although primary prevention is key, recent epidemics of acute and accelerated silicosis highlight the importance of the clinician's role in secondary and tertiary prevention strategies.

DISCLOSURE

S. Krefft provides medicolegal consulting in occupational lung disease. J. Wolff and C. Rose have nothing to disclose.

REFERENCES

1. World Health Organization IAfRoC. Silica, some silicates, coal dust and para-aramid fibrils. IARC Monogr Eval Carcinog Risks Hum 1997;68:86–149.
2. Lapp NL. Lung disease secondary to inhalation of nonfibrous minerals. Clin Chest Med 1981;2(2):219–33.
3. Merget R, Bauer T, Kupper HU, et al. Health hazards due to the inhalation of amorphous silica. Arch Toxicol 2002;75(11–12):625–34.
4. Fiume MM, Boyer I, Bergfeld WF, et al. Safety assessment of talc as used in cosmetics. Int J Toxicol 2015;34(1 Suppl):66S–129S.
5. Panel CIRE. Final report of the cosmetic ingredient review expert Panel. Safety assessment of silica and related cosmetic ingredients. 2009. Available at: https://pdfs.semanticscholar.org/b2aa/35e25a83f5b2e348a596f6bf08675f9a8a51.pdf?_ga=2.76527388.801858993.1580238050-760651985.1571255782. Accessed January 28, 2020.
6. Quaintance PA. Silicosis: a study of 106 pottery workers. Am J Public Health Nations Health 1934;24(12):1244–51.
7. Federation BPM. Lectures on the scientific basis of medicine. London: Athlone Press; 1954.
8. Office IL. Silicosis. Paper presented at: International Conference1930; Johannesburg, South Africa, August 13-27, 1930.
9. Sauve JF. Historical and emerging workplaces affected by silica exposure since the 1930 Johannesburg conference on Silicosis, with special reference to construction. Am J Ind Med 2015;58(Suppl 1):S67–71.
10. Cherniack M, Robbins A, Landigran PJ. The Hawk's nest incident: America's worst industrial disaster. New Haven (CT): Yale University Press; 1989.
11. Laney AS, Blackley DJ, Halldin CN. Radiographic disease progression in contemporary US coal miners with progressive massive fibrosis. Occup Environ Med 2017;74(7):517–20.
12. Almberg KS, Halldin CN, Blackley DJ, et al. Progressive massive fibrosis resurgence identified in U.S. coal miners filing for black lung benefits, 1970-2016. Ann Am Thorac Soc 2018;15(12):1420–6.
13. Blackley DJ, Reynolds LE, Short C, et al. Progressive massive fibrosis in coal miners from 3 clinics in Virginia. JAMA 2018;319(5):500–1.

14. Cohen ES, Elpern E, Silver MR. Pulmonary alveolar proteinosis causing severe hypoxemic respiratory failure treated with sequential whole-lung lavage utilizing venovenous extracorporeal membrane oxygenation: a case report and review. Chest 2001;120(3):1024–6.
15. Akgun M, Mirici A, Ucar EY, et al. Silicosis in Turkish denim sandblasters. Occup Med (Lond) 2006; 56(8):554–8.
16. Akgun M, Araz O, Akkurt I, et al. An epidemic of silicosis among former denim sandblasters. Eur Respir J 2008;32(5):1295–303.
17. Akgun M, Araz O, Ucar EY, et al. Silicosis appears inevitable among former denim sandblasters: a 4-year follow-up study. Chest 2015; 148(3):647–54.
18. Barmania S. Deadly denim: sandblasting-induced silicosis in the jeans industry. Lancet Respir Med 2016;4(7):543.
19. Weaver D. Levi's is replacing workers with lasers to give jeans that worn-down look. Englewood Cliffs (NJ): CNBC; 2018. Available at: https://www.cnbc.com/2018/03/02/levis-jeans-replacing-workers-with-lasers-distress.html. Accessed January 27, 2020.
20. Martinez C, Prieto A, Garcia L, et al. Silicosis: a disease with an active present. Arch Bronconeumol 2010;46(2):97–100.
21. Rose C, Heinzerling A, Patel K, et al. Severe silicosis in engineered stone fabrication workers — California, Colorado, Texas, and Washington, 2017–2019. MMWR Morb Mortal Wkly Rep 2019; 68(38):813–8.
22. Kirby T. Australia reports on audit of silicosis for stonecutters. Lancet 2019;393(10174):861.
23. Hoy RF, Baird T, Hammerschlag G, et al. Artificial stone-associated silicosis: a rapidly emerging occupational lung disease. Occup Environ Med 2018;75(1):3–5.
24. Esswein EJ, Breitenstein M, Snawder J, et al. Occupational exposures to respirable crystalline silica during hydraulic fracturing. J Occup Environ Hyg 2013;10(7):347–56.
25. Liang F, Sayed M, Al-Muntasheri GA, et al. A comprehensive review on proppant technologies. Petroleum 2016;2(1):26–39.
26. The Lancet Respiratory Medicine. The world is failing on silicosis. Lancet Respir Med 2019;7(4):283.
27. Leso V, Fontana L, Romano R, et al. Artificial stone associated silicosis: a systematic review. Int J Environ Res Public Health 2019;16(4):568.
28. Shih G. They built a Chinese boomtown. It left them dying of lung disease with nowhere to turn. The Washington Post. 2019. Available at: https://www.washingtonpost.com/world/asia_pacific/they-built-a-chinese-boomtown-it-left-them-dying-of-lung-disease-with-nowhere-to-turn/2019/12/15/4f070e54-0010-11ea-8341-cc3dce52e7de_story.html. Accessed January 29, 2020.
29. Hobson J. To die for? The health and safety of fast fashion. Occup Med (Lond) 2013;63(5):317–9.
30. Silica, crystalline. Occupational Safety and Health Administration. Safety and health Topics Web site. Available at: https://www.osha.gov/dsg/topics/silicacrystalline/. Accessed January 27, 2020.
31. Schleiff PL, Mazurek JM, Reilly MJ, et al. Surveillance for silicosis - Michigan and New Jersey, 2003-2011. MMWR Morb Mortal Wkly Rep 2016; 63(55):73–8.
32. Small Entity Compliance Guide for the Respirable Crystalline Silica Standard for Construction. In: Administration OSaH, ed2017.
33. Mazurek JMWJ, Schleiff PL, Weissman DN. Surveillance for silicosis deaths among persons aged 15-44 years - United States, 1999-2015. MMWR Morb Mortal Wkly Rep 2017;66(28):747–52.
34. Rose C. Silicosis. In: Post T, editor. UpToDate. Waltham (MA): UpToDate; 2020.
35. Forastiere F, Goldsmith DF, Sperati A, et al. Silicosis and lung function decrements among female ceramic workers in Italy. Am J Epidemiol 2002; 156(9):851–6.
36. Querol X, Tobias A, Perez N, et al. Monitoring the impact of desert dust outbreaks for air quality for health studies. Environ Int 2019;130:104867.
37. Bhagia LJ. Non-occupational exposure to silica dust. Indian J Occup Environ Med 2012;16(3): 95–100.
38. Saiyed HN, Sharma YK, Sadhu HG, et al. Non-occupational pneumoconiosis at high altitude villages in central Ladakh. Br J Ind Med 1991; 48(12):825–9.
39. Spalgais S, Gothi D, Jaiswal A, et al. Nonoccupational anthracofibrosis/anthracosilicosis from Ladakh in Jammu and Kashmir, India: a case series. Indian J Occup Environ Med 2015;19(3): 159–66.
40. Norboo T, Angchuk PT, Yahya M, et al. Silicosis in a Himalayan village population: role of environmental dust. Thorax 1991;46(5):341–3.
41. Bhagia LJ. Non-occupational exposure to silica dust in vicinity of slate pencil industry, India. Environ Monit Assess 2009;151(1–4):477–82.
42. Schenker M. Exposures and health effects from inorganic agricultural dusts. Environ Health Perspect 2000;108(Suppl 4):661–4.
43. Fennerty A, Hunter AM, Smith AP, et al. Silicosis in a Pakistani farmer. Br Med J (Clin Res Ed) 1983; 287(6393):648–9.
44. Swanepoel AJ, Rees D, Renton K, et al. Quartz exposure in agriculture: literature review and South African survey. Ann Occup Hyg 2010;54(3):281–92.
45. Levin K, McLean C, Hoy R. Artificial stone-associated silicosis: clinical-pathological-

radiological correlates of disease. Respirol Case Rep 2019;7(7):e00470.

46. Silicosis 2010 case definition. Centers for Disease Control and Prevention. Surveillance case definitions Web site. 2010. Available at: https://wwwn.cdc.gov/nndss/conditions/silicosis/case-definition/2010/. Accessed January 27, 2020.
47. Abraham JL, McEuen DD. Inorganic particulates associated with pulmonary alveolar proteinosis: SEM and X-ray microanalysis results. Appl Pathol 1986;4(3):138–46.
48. Buechner HA, Ansari A. Acute silico-proteinosis. A new pathologic variant of acute silicosis in sandblasters, characterized by histologic features resembling alveolar proteinosis. Dis Chest 1969;55(4):274–8.
49. Suratt PM, Winn WC Jr, Brody AR, et al. Acute silicosis in tombstone sandblasters. Am Rev Respir Dis 1977;115(3):521–9.
50. Palacio EJ, Champeaux A. Silicoproteinosis masquerading as community-acquired pneumonia. J Am Board Fam Pract 2000;13(5):376–8.
51. Xipell JM, Ham KN, Price CG, et al. Acute silicoproteinosis. Thorax 1977;32(1):104–11.
52. Duchange L, Brichet A, Lamblin C, et al. Acute silicosis. Clinical, radiologic, functional, and cytologic characteristics of the broncho-alveolar fluids. Observations of 6 cases. Rev Mal Respir 1998;15(4):527–34.
53. Satija B, Kumar S, Ojha UC, et al. Spectrum of high-resolution computed tomography imaging in occupational lung disease. Indian J Radiol Imaging 2013;23(4):287–96.
54. Srivastava GN, Prasad R, Meena M, et al. Acute silicosis with bilateral pneumothorax. BMJ Case Rep 2014;2014. bcr2013200089.
55. Goodman GB, Kaplan PD, Stachura I, et al. Acute silicosis responding to corticosteroid therapy. Chest 1992;101(2):366–70.
56. Stafford M, Cappa A, Weyant M, et al. Treatment of acute silicoproteinosis by whole-lung lavage. Semin Cardiothorac Vasc Anesth 2013;17(2):152–9.
57. Rosenman KD, Reilly MJ, Rice C, et al. Silicosis among foundry workers. Implication for the need to revise the OSHA standard. Am J Epidemiol 1996;144(9):890–900.
58. Verma DK, Ritchie AC, Muir DC. Dust content of lungs and its relationships to pathology, radiology and occupational exposure in Ontario hardrock miners. Am J Ind Med 2008;51(7):524–31.
59. Cox CW, Rose CS, Lynch DA. State of the art: imaging of occupational lung disease. Radiology 2014;270(3):681–96.
60. Arakawa H, Honma K, Saito Y, et al. Pleural disease in silicosis: pleural thickening, effusion, and invagination. Radiology 2005;236(2):685–93.
61. Salih M, Gashouta M, Pearson A, et al. Pacemaker induced post cardiac injury syndrome. Clin Med Case Rep 2015;2(4):88–9.
62. Gamble JF, Hessel PA, Nicolich M. Relationship between silicosis and lung function. Scand J Work Environ Health 2004;30(1):5–20.
63. Leung CC, Yu IT, Chen W. Silicosis. Lancet 2012;379(9830):2008–18.
64. Lopes AJ, Mogami R, Capone D, et al. High-resolution computed tomography in silicosis: correlation with chest radiography and pulmonary function tests. J Bras Pneumol 2008;34(5):264–72.
65. Marques da Costa F, Pierre de Oliveira E, Algranti E, et al. Accelerated silicosis: a report of three patients. Eur Respir J 2015;46(suppl 59):PA1163.
66. Hnizdo E, Sluis-Cremer GK, Baskind E, et al. Emphysema and airway obstruction in non-smoking South African gold miners with long exposure to silica dust. Occup Environ Med 1994;51(8):557–63.
67. Hnizdo E, Vallyathan V. Chronic obstructive pulmonary disease due to occupational exposure to silica dust: a review of epidemiological and pathological evidence. Occup Environ Med 2003;60(4):237–43.
68. Mohner M, Kersten N, Gellissen J. Chronic obstructive pulmonary disease and longitudinal changes in pulmonary function due to occupational exposure to respirable quartz. Occup Environ Med 2013;70(1):9–14.
69. Begin R, Filion R, Ostiguy G. Emphysema in silica- and asbestos-exposed workers seeking compensation. A CT scan study. Chest 1995;108(3):647–55.
70. Hnizdo E. Loss of lung function associated with exposure to silica dust and with smoking and its relation to disability and mortality in South African gold miners. Br J Ind Med 1992;49(7):472–9.
71. Reynolds CJ, MacNeill SJ, Williams J, et al. Chronic obstructive pulmonary disease in Welsh slate miners. Occup Med (Lond) 2017;67(1):20–5.
72. Humerfelt S, Eide GE, Gulsvik A. Association of years of occupational quartz exposure with spirometric airflow limitation in Norwegian men aged 30–46 years. Thorax 1998;53(8):649–55.
73. Hertzberg VS, Rosenman KD, Reilly MJ, et al. Effect of occupational silica exposure on pulmonary function. Chest 2002;122(2):721–8.
74. Li K, Keeling B, Churg A. Mineral dusts cause elastin and collagen breakdown in the rat lung: a potential mechanism of dust-induced emphysema. Am J Respir Crit Care Med 1996;153(2):644–9.
75. Ndlovu N, Richards G, Vorajee N, et al. Silicosis and pulmonary tuberculosis in deceased female South African miners. Occup Med (Lond) 2019;69(4):272–8.

76. Ndlovu N, Musenge E, Park SK, et al. Four decades of pulmonary tuberculosis in deceased South African miners: trends and determinants. Occup Environ Med 2018;75(11):767–75.
77. Ehrlich RI. Tuberculosis, mining and silica. Occup Environ Med 2018;75(11):763–4.
78. Corbett EL, Churchyard GJ, Clayton T, et al. Risk factors for pulmonary mycobacterial disease in South African gold miners. A case-control study. Am J Respir Crit Care Med 1999;159(1):94–9.
79. Yew WW, Leung CC, Chang KC, et al. Can treatment outcomes of latent TB infection and TB in silicosis be improved? J Thorac Dis 2019;11(1):E8–10.
80. Churchyard GJ, Fielding KL, Grant AD. A trial of mass isoniazid preventive therapy for tuberculosis control. N Engl J Med 2014;370(17):1662–3.
81. Manno M, Levy L, Johanson G, et al. Silica, silicosis and lung cancer: what level of exposure is acceptable? Med Lav 2018;109(6):478–80.
82. Liu Y, Steenland K, Rong Y, et al. Exposure-response analysis and risk assessment for lung cancer in relationship to silica exposure: a 44-year cohort study of 34,018 workers. Am J Epidemiol 2013;178(9):1424–33.
83. Sato T, Shimosato T, Klinman DM. Silicosis and lung cancer: current perspectives. Lung Cancer (Auckl) 2018;9:91–101.
84. USPSTF. Final recommendation statement: lung cancer: screening. U.S. Preventive Services Task Force. 2016. Available at: https://www.uspreventiveservicestaskforce.org/Page/Document/RecommendationStatementFinal/lung-cancer-screening. Accessed January 28, 2020.
85. Wood DE, Eapen GA, Ettinger DS, et al. Lung cancer screening. J Natl Compr Canc Netw 2012;10(2):240–65.
86. Cui JW, Li W, Han FJ, et al. Screening for lung cancer using low-dose computed tomography: concerns about the application in low-risk individuals. Transl Lung Cancer Res 2015;4(3):275–86.
87. Gungen AC, Aydemir Y, Coban H, et al. Lung cancer in patients diagnosed with silicosis should be investigated. Respir Med Case Rep 2016;18:93–5.
88. Doll R, Peto R. The causes of cancer: quantitative estimates of avoidable risks of cancer in the United States today. J Natl Cancer Inst 1981;66(6):1191–308.
89. Lee S, Hayashi H, Mastuzaki H, et al. Silicosis and autoimmunity. Curr Opin Allergy Clin Immunol 2017;17(2):78–84.
90. Koeger AC, Alcaix D, Gutmann L, et al. Silica, silicones and connectivitis. 20 cases. Rev Rhum Mal Osteoartic 1991;58(2):113–20.
91. Koeger AC, Nguyen JM, Fleurette F. Epidemiology of scleroderma among women: assessment of risk from exposure to silicone and silica. J Rheumatol 1997;24(9):1853–5.
92. Sanchez-Roman J, Wichmann I, Salaberri J, et al. Multiple clinical and biological autoimmune manifestations in 50 workers after occupational exposure to silica. Ann Rheum Dis 1993;52(7):534–8.
93. Haustein KO. Health consequences of passive smoking. Wien Med Wochenschr 2000;150(11):233–44.
94. Lee J, Taneja V, Vassallo R. Cigarette smoking and inflammation: cellular and molecular mechanisms. J Dent Res 2012;91(2):142–9.
95. Giles RD, Sturgill BC, Suratt PM, et al. Massive proteinuria and acute renal failure in a patient with acute silicoproteinosis. Am J Med 1978;64(2):336–42.
96. Calvert GM, Steenland K, Palu S. End-stage renal disease among silica-exposed gold miners. A new method for assessing incidence among epidemiologic cohorts. JAMA 1997;277(15):1219–23.
97. Ng TP, Ng YL, Lee HS, et al. A study of silica nephrotoxicity in exposed silicotic and non-silicotic workers. Br J Ind Med 1992;49(1):35–7.
98. Ng TP, Lee HS, Phoon WH. Further evidence of human silica nephrotoxicity in occupationally exposed workers. Br J Ind Med 1993;50(10):907–12.
99. Steenland NK, Thun MJ, Ferguson CW, et al. Occupational and other exposures associated with male end-stage renal disease: a case/control study. Am J Public Health 1990;80(2):153–7.
100. Millerick-May ML, Schrauben S, Reilly MJ, et al. Silicosis and chronic renal disease. Am J Ind Med 2015;58(7):730–6.
101. Mohner M, Pohrt A, Gellissen J. Occupational exposure to respirable crystalline silica and chronic non-malignant renal disease: systematic review and meta-analysis. Int Arch Occup Environ Health 2017;90(7):555–74.
102. Rosenman KD, Moore-Fuller M, Reilly MJ. Kidney disease and silicosis. Nephron 2000;85(1):14–9.
103. Mascarenhas S, Mutnuri S, Ganguly A. Silica - a trace geogenic element with emerging nephrotoxic potential. Sci Total Environ 2018;645:297–317.
104. Ghahramani N. Silica nephropathy. Int J Occup Environ Med 2010;1(3):108–15.
105. Mayeux JM, Escalante GM, Christy JM, et al. Silicosis and silica-induced autoimmunity in the diversity outbred mouse. Front Immunol 2018;9:874.
106. Gomez-Puerta JA, Gedmintas L, Costenbader KH. The association between silica exposure and development of ANCA-associated vasculitis: systematic review and meta-analysis. Autoimmun Rev 2013;12(12):1129–35.
107. Newman KL, Newman LS. Occupational causes of sarcoidosis. Curr Opin Allergy Clin Immunol 2012;12(2):145–50.
108. Rafnsson V, Ingimarsson O, Hjalmarsson I, et al. Association between exposure to crystalline silica and risk of sarcoidosis. Occup Environ Med 1998;55(10):657–60.

109. Webber MP, Yip J, Zeig-Owens R, et al. Post-9/11 sarcoidosis in WTC-exposed firefighters and emergency medical service workers. Respir Med 2017; 132:232–7.
110. Langley RJ, Mishra NC, Pena-Philippides JC, et al. Fibrogenic and redox-related but not proinflammatory genes are upregulated in Lewis rat model of chronic silicosis. J Toxicol Environ Health A 2011; 74(19):1261–79.
111. Leli I, Salimbene I, Varone F, et al. Husband and wife with sarcoidosis: possible environmental factors involved. Multidiscip Respir Med 2013;8(1):5.
112. Vihlborg P, Bryngelsson IL, Andersson L, et al. Risk of sarcoidosis and seropositive rheumatoid arthritis from occupational silica exposure in Swedish iron foundries: a retrospective cohort study. BMJ Open 2017;7(7):e016839.
113. Liu H, Patel D, Welch AM, et al. Association between occupational exposures and sarcoidosis: an analysis from death certificates in the United States, 1988-1999. Chest 2016;150(2):289–98.
114. Small Entity Compliance Guide for the Respirable Crystalline Silica Standard for General Industry and Maritime. In: Administration OSaH, ed2017.
115. Medical surveillance guidelines 1910.1053 App B. Occupational safety and health administration. Toxic and Hazardous Substances Web site. Available at: https://www.osha.gov/laws-regs/regulations/standardnumber/1910/1910.1053AppB. Accessed January 30, 2020.
116. Bukovitz B, Meiman J, Anderson H, et al. Silicosis: diagnosis and medicolegal implications. J Forensic Sci 2019;64(5):1389–98.

Screening for Occupational Lung Cancer

An Unprecedented Opportunity

Steven B. Markowitz, MD, DrPH*, Brittany Dickens, BA

KEYWORDS

• Lung cancer • Occupation • Screening • Carcinogens

KEY POINTS

- Occupational exposures play an important role in causing lung cancer.
- Occupation and smoking interact in multiple ways to increase lung cancer risk.
- Low-dose chest computed tomography scan–based screening is effective in identifying early lung cancers in occupational populations.
- Pulmonary physicians are critical in identifying patients with exposure to occupational lung carcinogens and ensuring that they participate in lung cancer screening.

INTRODUCTION

The enormous advances in early lung cancer detection and cure in the past decade are a potential paradigm shift in efforts to reduce the high burden of lung cancer mortality, These efforts are especially important in occupational populations, in which multiple lung cancer risk factors frequently coincide, permitting priority setting to identify and to facilitate candidates for low-dose CT-based lung cancer screening. Pulmonary physicians have a key role in realizing this potential, because they are skilled and practiced in discussing the occupational history with patients, which is the most accessible and reliable means to identify significant exposure to occupational lung carcinogens.

Occupational lung cancer is the most common cause of occupational mortality. Oddly, it can also be considered an orphan disease because of the near-universal lack of its recognition in clinical medicine, public health surveillance, and worker compensation systems.

Occupational lung cancer is widely underrecognized. In research covering diverse populations and industries across 3 continents (Asia, Europe, and North America), the number of recognized cases of occupational lung cancer has consistently been a small fraction (<3%) of the total number of estimated cases. Of the 5442 occupational lung cancer cases estimated to occur each year in the United Kingdom,[1] only 392 cases, or approximately 22 cases per year, were reported, according to the national voluntary reporting system, Surveillance of Work-Related and Occupational Respiratory Disease (SWORD), between 1996 and 2014.[2] Similarly, of the 4150 occupational lung cancer cases estimated to occur annually in Canada,[3] approximately 120 occupational lung cancers were compensated annually between 2005 and 2009.[4] In Korea, approximately 630 to 1181 occupational lung cancers are estimated to occur annually, but only 179 work-related lung cancers, or 10 per year on average, were compensated by the Korean national worker compensation system between 1994 and 2011.[5,6]

Funding sources: US Department of Energy and the Sheet Metal Workers Occupational Health Institute Trust.
Barry Commoner Center for Health and the Environment, Queens College, City University of New York, 65-30 Kissena Boulevard, Remsen Hall, Queens, NY 11367, USA
* Corresponding author.
E-mail address: smarkowitz@qc.cuny.edu

Clin Chest Med 41 (2020) 723–737
https://doi.org/10.1016/j.ccm.2020.08.016

chestmed.theclinics.com

The widespread under-recognition of occupational causes of lung cancer is a significant barrier to lung cancer prevention. Primary prevention of occupational lung cancer through the control of exposure to lung carcinogens in the workplace is assigned little urgency unless the burden of preventable disease is recognized. Secondary prevention through the advent of recently developed low-dose chest CT scan–based lung cancer screening receives few resources and little attention from physicians and workers alike unless the existence of occupational lung cancer is acknowledged. In addition, compensation, a form of tertiary prevention, entirely depends on clinical, administrative, and legal confirmation of the workplace origin of lung cancer.

OCCUPATIONAL CAUSES OF LUNG CANCER

Over the past 5 decades (1971–2020), the International Agency for Research on Cancer (IARC) has identified 19 IARC group 1 occupational lung carcinogens (substances or mixtures) and an additional 8 occupations, industries, or work processes in which occupational epidemiology studies were instrumental in establishing lung carcinogenicity.[7] These agents, occupations, and industries are listed in **Table 1**, adapted from IARC sources.[7,8] Nearly one-half (44% or 19 out of 47) of all agent-specific IARC group 1 carcinogens cause lung cancer. In addition, two-thirds of occupations, industries, or processes that cause occupational cancer cause lung cancer (see **Table 1**).

Probable human lung carcinogens (IARC group 2A) are numerous, although less broadly recognized within the occupational health community. They include cobalt, diazinon, and high-temperature frying emissions, and total 8 agents or mixtures and 4 occupations, industries, or processes (see **Table 1**).[8]

The number of recognized occupational lung carcinogens has grown within the past decade (see **Table 1**). Since 2010, IARC has added the following agents or processes (with year added) to its group 1 list: diesel engine exhaust (2013); outdoor air pollution, including particulate matter (2016); welding fumes (2017); and Acheson process (exposure to silicon carbide fibers) (2017).[7,8] Group 2A carcinogens that have been specifically designated by IARC to be linked to lung cancer within the past decade include biomass fuel (consisting of primarily wood and indoor emissions from household combustion) (2010), bitumens from roofing (2013), diazinon (2017), and hydrazine (2018).

It is important to recognize that only a small fraction of the estimated 86,000 chemicals on the Environmental Protection Agency's Toxic Substances Control Act Inventory have ever been tested for carcinogenicity.[9] In 5 decades, IARC has evaluated more than 1000 agents, occupations, and industries but found that available scientific studies are inadequate or lacking for approximately one-half of the exposure assessments.[7,10] Given the frequency of exposure of the respiratory system to inhaled toxicants and the demonstrated carcinogenicity of many chemical agents, it is likely that only a fraction of occupational lung carcinogens has been identified and the total burden of occupational lung cancer remains undefined.

HOW IMPORTANT IS OCCUPATIONAL LUNG CANCER?

Lung cancer is the most common cause of death from cancer in the world, causing nearly 1 in 5 (18.4%) cancer deaths. It is the most common cause of cancer death for men in most countries, including low-income, middle-income, and high-income nations, and the most frequent cause of cancer death among women in the United States, China, Australia, Scandinavia, and Canada. Tobacco is the dominant cause of lung cancer, and the maturity of the cigarette smoking epidemic and the adoption of smoking cessation determines much of the geographic and gender variation in lung cancer incidence and mortality.[11]

Lung cancer is by far the most common cancer caused by occupational exposures, accounting for 50% or more of occupational cancer. Excellent reviews of occupational cancer, including the relative prominence of lung cancer, are readily available.[3,7,12]

Occupational exposures cause or contribute to 10% to 15% of lung cancers.[1,13,14] This attributable fraction, obtained by combining estimates of the prevalence of exposure to recognized occupational lung carcinogens with relative risk estimates for each agent, has been remarkably consistent across studies over the past 2 decades, despite variation in agents, study populations, available exposure data, and modeling assumptions. A recent analysis by the British Occupational Cancer Burden study group applied estimates of working populations exposed to 21 occupational lung carcinogens (IARC groups 1 and 2A) to estimates of summary lung cancer relative risks for each agent and concluded that approximately 15% of all lung cancers in the United Kingdom have an occupational contribution (21.2% in men and 5.3% in women).[1] Dominant occupational causes identified in this analysis include asbestos, silica, and diesel engine exhaust. This estimate

Table 1
International Agency for Research on Cancer group 1 and 2A occupational human lung carcinogens

	IARC Group 1	IARC Group 2A
Agent	Arsenic and inorganic arsenic compounds Asbestos (all forms) Beryllium and beryllium compounds Bis(chloromethy)ether; chloromethyl methyl ether (technical grade) Cadmium and cadmium compounds Chromium (VI) compounds Coal, indoor emissions from household combustion Coal-tar pitch Engine exhaust, diesel[a] Nickel compounds Outdoor air pollution[a] Particulate matter in outdoor air pollution[a] Plutonium Radon-222 and its decay products Silica dust, crystalline Soot Tobacco smoke, secondhand Welding fumes[a] X-radiation, gamma radiation	Indoor emissions from household combustion of biomass fuel (primarily wood)[a] Bitumens, occupational exposure to oxidized bitumens and their emissions during roofing,[a] Alpha-chlorinated toluenes, and benzoyl chloride (combined exposures) Cobalt metal with tungsten carbide Creosotes Diazinon[a] Hydrazine[a]
Occupation, industry, or process	Occupational exposures associated with Acheson process[a] Aluminum production Coal gasification Coke production Hematite mining (underground) Iron and steel founding Painting Rubber production industry	Art glass, glass containers, and pressed ware (manufacture of) Carbon electrode manufacture[a] Emissions from high-temperature frying[a] Insecticides, nonarsenical, occupational exposures in spraying and application

[a] IARC group 1 and group 2A carcinogens identified as causing lung cancer within the past 10 years.
Adapted from IARC. List of Classifications by cancer sites with sufficient or limited evidence in humans, Volumes 1 to 125. International Agency for Research on Cancer: World Health Organization. With permission. Available at: https://monographs.iarc.fr/wp-content/uploads/2019/07/Classifications_by_cancer_site_127.pdf; and *Data from* IARC. Monograph Vol. 53, 58, 71, 86, 92, 95, 100F, and 112. International Agency for Research on Cancer: World Health Organization.

may be low because of the limited number of lung cancers attributed to asbestos exposure.[15]

Although 10% to 15% of lung cancer caused by occupation is modest compared with the proportion caused by smoking (≥80%), the high incidence of lung cancer worldwide results in a large number of people affected by occupational lung cancer. According to the recently published Global Burden of Disease Study 2015, worldwide, an estimated 525,000 deaths were caused by lung cancer in association with 9 occupational lung carcinogens: asbestos, arsenic, beryllium, chromium, diesel engine exhaust, secondhand smoke, nickel, polycyclic aromatic hydrocarbons, and silica.[16] This estimate represented a 25% increase over a 10-year period caused by increased mortality from exposure to asbestos, diesel engine exhaust, and silica. In the United States, Steenland and colleagues[17] at the National Institute for Occupational Safety and Health (NIOSH) estimate that 9677 to 19,901 lung cancer deaths were caused by occupational exposures. Other more recent national estimates of occupational lung cancer mortality include 4745 lung cancer deaths in the United Kingdom,[1] 2838 deaths in France,[14] and 4151 incident lung cancers in Canada.[3]

Asbestos exposure has been the most common cause of occupational lung cancer over the past 2 decades. Asbestos exposure accounted for 30% of occupational lung cancer deaths globally in 2015,[16] 41% of occupational lung cancer deaths in the United Kingdom,[12] and 46% of occupational lung cancer cases in Canada.[3] This rate may change in coming decades, given the banning of asbestos in 67 countries[18] and the relative salience of exposure to other lung carcinogens, especially diesel exhaust, silica, and welding fumes.

The proportion of lung cancer attributed to occupational exposures overlaps with the proportion caused by cigarette smoking, because of the high frequency of cigarette smoking among blue collar workers and the interaction between smoking and occupational agents in causing lung cancer (discussed later). There may also be overlap between occupational causes and other documented causes of lung cancer (eg, environmental radon, outdoor air pollution), but this overlap has been little studied.

EXPOSURE TO OCCUPATIONAL LUNG CARCINOGENS

Understanding the prevalence and distribution of occupational exposures is important in order (1) to prioritize efforts to control current exposures and prevent future disease, and (2) to provide a rational approach to identifying high-risk working populations for targeted lung cancer screening programs.

National surveys of workplace exposures have been conducted for 4 decades, beginning with the National Occupational Hazard Survey that NIOSH conducted in 1972 to 1974, later augmented by the National Occupational Exposure Survey in 1981 to 1983. There has been no systematic exposure survey of workplaces in the United States since the early 1980s. Since then, exposure to occupational carcinogens has been characterized using the FINJEM (Finnish job-exposure matrix) system in Finland, most recently in 2013,[19] and by the CAREX (carcinogen exposure) project for 15 countries in the European Union in the 1990 to 1993 period.[20] The most recent published efforts have been undertaken in Canada and Finland, using a modified European CAREX and FINJEM, respectively, incorporating available Canadian and Finnish workplace exposure measurements data, to produce exposure estimates for 2006 and 2008.[19,21] The Finnish estimates also project anticipated population workplace exposures for 2020.[19] These estimates are shown in **Table 2**.

The most prevalent occupational lung carcinogens in high-income countries at present are diesel exhaust, welding fumes, and silica. Based on data from Canada and Finland, more than 2% of the employed population is exposed to each of these lung carcinogens (see **Table 2**). The proportion of working populations estimated to be exposed to these 3 carcinogens has not changed in recent decades. Exposure to the carcinogenic metals chromium (hexavalent) and nickel affect up to 1% of the working population. Exposure to other metals, including cadmium and arsenic, are limited in high-income countries (see **Table 2**). Comparable data for middle-income and low-income countries are not available. Asbestos exposure in the United States, Europe, and Japan has clearly declined in the workplace since the 1980s, although accurate estimates of the prevalence of current exposure are not available. The continued high use of asbestos in China, Russia, India, and selected other countries is likely associated with large populations of workers at increased risk of asbestos-related lung cancer.[22] **Table 2** also highlights relevant exposures in the European Union in the early 1990s, which, in view of the long latency of occupational cancer, provides useful information for targeting current lung cancer screening efforts.

Salient industries and examples of occupations with current exposure to occupational lung carcinogens are provided in **Table 3**. Many construction workers are exposed to the most common lung carcinogens: diesel exhaust, silica, and welding. Diesel engine exhaust is highly prevalent among workers who drive or maintain diesel vehicles, including buses, trucks, and heavy equipment. Workers in many manufacturing industries have exposure to carcinogenic metals and silica.

Table 2
Estimated percentage of working population exposed to selected lung carcinogens

	European Union[20]	Canada[21]	Finland[19]
	Time Period Exposure		
Agent	1990–1993	2006	2008
Silica	2.3	2.3	2.2
Diesel exhaust	2.2	4.6	2.3
Welding fumes	—	—	2.3
Chromium (VI)	0.58	0.61	1.1
Nickel	0.40	0.69	1.4
Asbestos	0.86	0.90	0.2
Ionizing radiation	1.1	0.2–0.5	—
Cadmium	0.15	0.18	<0.1
Arsenic	0.11	0.15	0.1
Environmental tobacco smoke	5.4	—	0.1

Data from Refs.[19–21]

Table 3
Common occupational lung carcinogens by industry and selected occupations

Industry	Lung Carcinogen	Examples of Occupation
Manufacturing	Silica, chromium, nickel, cadmium	Metal fabricators, assemblers Metal processors, shaping workers Clay, stone, glass processors Forging workers Boilermakers, platers
Construction	Silica, diesel exhaust, painting, welding, coal-tar pitch, outdoor air pollution	Excavators Welders Painters Plumbers Other construction
Transportation	Diesel exhaust, outdoor air pollution	Bus drivers Truck drivers Mechanical maintenance
Mining, oil, gas, extraction	Silica, diesel exhaust	Drillers, blasters Miners, quarry workers Mineral ore treaters

Occupations listed are examples of workers with exposure within designated industries and do not represent a complete list of such occupations.

CIGARETTE SMOKING, CHRONIC LUNG DISEASES, AND OCCUPATIONAL LUNG CANCER

The overlap in cigarette smoking and exposure to occupational lung carcinogens has numerous critical ramifications for the risk of lung cancer and its control (**Box 1**).

Prevalence of Smoking by Occupation

Occupation is closely associated with cigarette smoking, highlighting its importance as a window to facilitate interventions designed to reduce lung cancer. In the United States, workers in construction, manufacturing, mining, and transportation smoke at much higher rates than workers in professional or managerial positions (**Fig. 1**). Data from middle-income or low-income countries are more limited, but the Global Adult Tobacco Survey conducted in 2010 showed similar findings. In China, for example, the prevalence of smoking among male machine operators (67%) was nearly twice that of male medical/health personnel or teaching staff (36%–38%).[23]

Smoking–Occupational Carcinogen Nexus

The relationship between tobacco use and occupational exposures is widely recognized but its full complexity is underappreciated and understudied. **Fig. 2** shows some causal connections between these exposures and their resultant diseases. Not only do these 2 exposures cause lung cancer but they also cause or contribute to chronic obstructive pulmonary disease (COPD) and pulmonary fibrosis, which are independent risk factors for lung cancer.[24] Occupational exposures to vapors, gases, dusts, or fumes increase the risk of COPD,[25] and some workplace dusts also cause pulmonary fibrosis (ie, asbestosis and silicosis). Smoking causes COPD and is also a risk factor for pulmonary interstitial fibrosis.[26] Key aspects of these relationships have been well studied (eg, smoking and asbestos interaction in lung cancer risk and the contribution of asbestosis and silicosis to risk of lung cancer.) Other relationships, such as the interaction between work-

Box 1
Smoking and occupation in lung cancer

1. Blue collar workers have an increased prevalence of smoking and exposure to occupational lung carcinogens.
2. Cigarette use and occupational toxins increase the risk of chronic obstructive pulmonary disease and pulmonary fibrosis, both of which are independent risk factors for lung cancer.
3. Smoking and occupational lung carcinogens interact to increase the risk of lung cancer.
4. Smoking cessation efforts may be more successful if they also address control of occupational exposure to lung carcinogens.

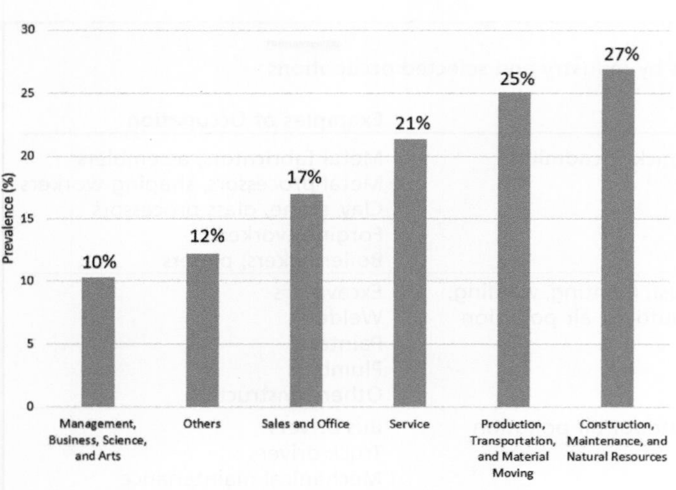

Fig. 1. Prevalence of cigarette smoking by occupation in the United States, 2012 to 2014. Standard Occupational Classification high-level aggregation codes are used. (*Data from* Syamlal G, Jamal A, Mazurek JM. Combustible tobacco and smokeless tobacco use among working adults—United States, 2012 to 2014. *J Occup Environ Med.* 2016;58:1185-1189.)

related COPD and lung cancer, have received less attention.

Interaction of Smoking and Occupational Lung Carcinogens

Asbestos

The interaction between smoking and asbestos exposure is well recognized, and seems principally supra-additive, although some studies show a multiplicative interaction.[27,28] The most recent studies from 2012 to 2020 support a supra-additive effect of the 2 combined exposures,[29–31] although a recent large pooled case-control study evaluating lower levels of asbestos exposure identified a multiplicative interaction.[32] Dr Selikoff's classic 1979 study of the asbestos-smoking interaction among insulators[33] has been updated, benefiting from long-term follow-up, an increased number of lung cancers among never smokers, and information about the presence or absence of radiographic asbestosis.[29] The main results of this study are shown in **Fig. 3**, showing an increased lung cancer mortality ratio for never-smoking insulators without asbestosis, an even higher mortality ratio for never-smoking insulators with asbestosis, and a supra-additive interaction between asbestos and smoking in causing lung cancer.[29]

Silica

Several large studies addressing the lung cancer risk among silica-exposed workers have been completed in the past decade.[34–38] Most studies support a supra-additive and possibly multiplicative interaction between silica exposure and cigarette smoking, although with some heterogeneity. Liu and colleagues[34] characterized the mortality of more than 34,000 Chinese metal mine and pottery factory workers over a 44-year period using Cox proportional hazards analysis. Compared with workers with no smoking or silica exposure, the hazard ratios for lung cancer mortality were 1.60 (95% confidence interval [CI], 1.01–2.55) in silica-exposed never smokers, 2.75 (95% CI, 1.74–4.35) in nonsilica-exposed smokers, and 5.07 (95% CI, 3.41–7.52) in silica-exposed smokers.[34] Consonni and colleagues[35] pooled data from 13 European case-control studies as part of the SYNERGY collaboration to evaluate 695 bricklayers with lung cancer and 468 controls.

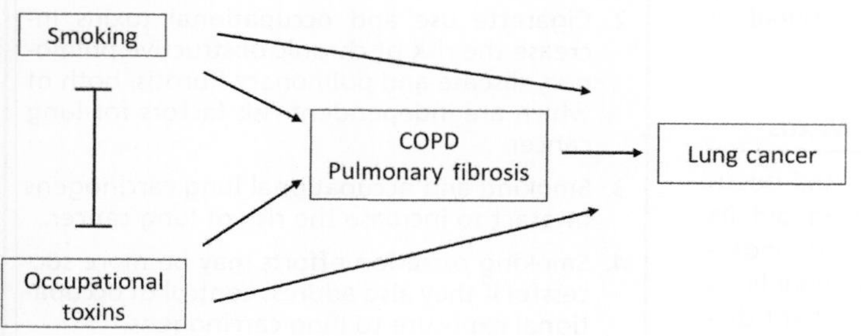

Fig. 2. Occupation and tobacco: nexus of disease. COPD, chronic obstructive pulmonary disease.

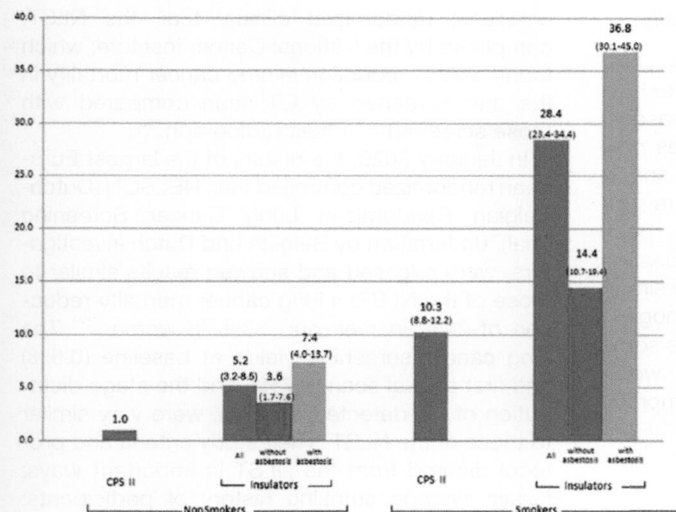

Fig. 3. Lung cancer mortality ratios (95% confidence intervals) by asbestos, asbestosis, and smoking status, North American Insulators versus Cancer Prevention Study (CPS) II, 1981 to 2008. (*From* Markowitz SB, Levin SM, Miller A, Morabia A. Asbestos, asbestosis, smoking, and lung cancer: new findings from the North American insulator cohort. *Am J Respir Crit Care Med.* 2013;188:90-96; with permission. Reprinted with permission of the American Thoracic Society. Copyright © 2020 American Thoracic Society. All rights reserved. Cite: Markowitz SB, Levin SM, Miller A, Morabia A. Asbestos, asbestosis, smoking, and lung cancer: new findings from the North American insulator cohort. *Am J Respir Crit Care Med.* 2013;188:90-96. The American Journal of Respiratory and Critical Care Medicine is an official journal of the American Thoracic Society.)

Compared with workers with no smoking or silica exposure, the odds ratios for lung cancer were 1.2 (95% CI, 0.66–2.08) in never smokers with silica exposure, 11.5 (95% CI, 10.4–12.7), in former smokers without silica exposure, and 18.5 (95% CI, 15.7–21.8) in former smokers with silica exposure.[35] In a large incident case-control study in northern Italy, De Matteis and colleagues[36] reported lung cancer odds ratios of 1.4 (95% CI, 0.5–3.9) in never smokers exposed to silica, 26.9 (95% CI, 17.3–41.6) in current smokers not exposed to silica, and 45.0 (95% CI, 27.2–74.5) in current smokers exposed to silica compared with workers with no exposure to smoking or silica. These results show clear amplification of the lung cancer risk in the presence of both silica and tobacco exposure, a result similar to that of asbestos.

Diesel exhaust

Silverman and colleagues[39] at the National Cancer Institute conducted a large case-control study of nonmetal miners with extensive assessment of diesel exhaust exposure, cigarette smoking, other occupational exposures, and history of lung disease. They found a dose-related increase in lung cancer risk with increasing level of diesel exhaust exposure, both among nonsmokers and mild to moderate smokers. Among heavy smokers, although lung cancer risk remained increased at all levels of diesel exhaust, it tended to be less increased with increasing diesel exhaust exposure. The odds ratio for lung cancer mortality among heavy smokers at the highest tertile of diesel exhaust exposure was 17.4 (95% CI, 3.5–86.7) versus 26.8 (95% CI, 6.2–116.6) at the lowest tertile of diesel exhaust exposure. These results may represent an example of negative interaction.

Pintos and colleagues[40] studied 1593 lung cancer cases and 1427 controls in Montreal in a population-based study between 1979 and 2001, semiquantitatively estimating diesel exhaust exposure based on occupational history and expert industrial hygiene opinion. They found a multiplicative or supra-additive interaction between smoking and diesel exhaust.[40]

Other occupational or environmental exposures

Studies of the joint effect of other occupational or environmental exposures and cigarette smoking on lung cancer are more limited. Multiple studies of uranium miners exposed to radon in the United States and Europe have found a supra-additive but submultiplicative interaction between smoking and radon exposure.[41–43] Ferreccio and colleagues[44] performed a large case-control study in northern Chile with endemic arsenic water contamination and found that water arsenic consumption and smoking synergistically increased lung cancer risk. They also found that exposure to other known lung carcinogens in the study population (eg, asbestos, silica, welding fumes) also interacted with arsenic exposure synergistically to increase lung cancer risk, controlling for tobacco consumption.[44] The interaction effects and risk of lung cancer from mixtures and other complex exposures remains an area of ongoing research.

Smoking Cessation Among Occupationally Exposed Workers

Smoking cessation is especially beneficial for blue collar workers for the aforementioned reasons. Ironically, workers in so-called dusty trades may be less likely than other workers to receive smoking cessation advice from their primary care providers.[45] In general, little research has been completed specifically on smoking cessation among blue collar workers, especially while simultaneously addressing workplace lung carcinogens or other workplace exposures.[46,47] There is some evidence that simultaneously addressing workplace health issues and smoking can improve smoking cessation efforts.[48]

SCREENING FOR LUNG CANCER

Current lung cancer screening guidelines in the United States reflect the recommendation of the United States Preventive Services Task Force (USPSTF) to implement annual low-dose chest CT scans for people aged 55 to 74 years who smoked at least 30 pack-years of cigarettes and currently smoke or quit less than 15 years prior.[49] This recommendation, first made in 2013, was based principally on the results of the National Lung Screening Trial (NLST). The USPSTF issued a draft modified recommendation in July 2020 after updating its literature review and decision analysis and proposed modified screening eligibility criteria to include people aged 50 to 80 years who smoked at least 20 pack-years of cigarettes and currently smoke or quit less than 15 years prior.[50] Occupational risk of lung cancer was not addressed in the current or the newly proposed USPSTF screening recommendation. A further revised recommendation is expected in 2020. USPSTF recommendations are important for screening practice, because public[51] and private insurers are required to offer health screening that is endorsed by the USPSTF under the Affordable Care Act.

CT-based lung cancer screening began in the United States in 1999, when Henschke and colleagues[52] showed that low-dose chest CT scanning successfully identified early-stage lung cancers: 23 of 27 (85%) low-dose CT–detected lung cancers among 1000 people screened were stage 1 lung cancers. In 2006, they further showed that, treated early, CT-detected lung cancers had excellent survival: a group of 412 stage 1 lung cancers detected by CT screening had an estimated 88% 10-year survival.[53] Further proof of the effectiveness of low-dose CT screening for lung cancer was provided in 2010 by a large (>53,000 enrollees) randomized clinical trial, the NLST, completed by the National Cancer Institute, which found a 20% reduction in lung cancer mortality in the arm screened by CT scan compared with those screened by chest radiograph.[54]

In January 2020, the results of the largest European randomized controlled trial, NELSON (Dutch-Belgian Randomized Lung Cancer Screening Trial), undertaken by Belgian and Dutch investigators, were released and showed results similar to those of the NLST: a lung cancer mortality reduction of 24% in men and 33% in women.[55] The lung cancer screening yields at baseline (0.9%) and first annual scan (0.7%), and the stage distribution of CT-detected cancers, were very similar to those of the NLST. Their study criteria and protocol differed from the NLST in important ways: lesser average smoking history of participants; use of CT-based volume measurements; screening intervals of 1, 2, and 2.5 years; a control group that received no imaging study; and a longer follow-up period (10 years).[55] One-half of the study participants did not meet the NLST screening criteria for age and smoking, but the results for that group were reported separately.

The NLST, NELSON, and USPSTF guidelines do not address occupational risks for lung cancer as a determinant of eligibility for lung cancer screening. However, the National Comprehensive Cancer Network (NCCN) and the American Society of Thoracic Surgeons have developed guidelines for including additional risk factors (ie, family history, history of chronic lung disease, and occupational exposures) to determine who should be screened. Specifically, NCCN group 2 eligibility criteria recommend screening people aged 50 years and older with a 20-pack-year smoking history if they have an additional risk factor for lung cancer, such as exposure to occupational lung carcinogens, chronic lung disease, or a family history of lung cancer, and had an aggregate 6-year risk of lung cancer greater than or equal to 1.3%.[56] NCCN group 2 criteria are similar to the proposed age and smoking criteria of USPSTF with the important exception that there is no limit to the number of years since quitting smoking under the NCCN group 2 criteria. NCCN group 1 eligibility criteria are similar to those of the USPSTF recommendation as formulated in 2013.

This broader risk-based approach embodied by the NCCN group 2 criteria that includes lung cancer risk factors other than age and smoking to determining eligibility for lung cancer screening has gained support over the past few years. National Cancer Institute (NCI) investigators compared the lung cancer mortality benefits of a risk-based model versus a USPSTF guidelines–

based model (restricted to age and smoking) and concluded that the former approach, which used family history, self-reported emphysema, body mass index, age, and a broader range of smoking history as eligibility criteria, prevented a greater number of lung cancer deaths than a model based on USPSTF screening guidelines.[57] Numerous risk prediction models and associated lung cancer risk calculators that include a broad set of risk factors beyond age and smoking history have been developed to identify optimal populations for screening and to allow patients and their providers to use individual values of risk factors to determine an overall risk for lung cancer and advisability of participating in low-dose CT screening.[57,58] Most of these calculators include no or little information about occupation in determining risk.

Empirical Studies of Lung Cancer Screening in Occupational Populations

In 2014, an international consensus of asbestos experts in Helsinki recommended that low-dose CT scanning be used for lung cancer screening in organized programs for asbestos-exposed workers if their aggregate risk of lung cancer met or exceeded the risk of the NLST population in which CT-based screening achieved reduction in lung cancer mortality.[59] Studies published since 2014 shed light on these guidelines.

From 2000 to 2013, Markowitz and colleagues[60] used low-dose CT scanning to screen 7189 US nuclear weapons workers in 9 nonmetropolitan US communities who were variably exposed to ionizing radiation, asbestos, beryllium, and other occupational toxins. Eligibility criteria included age ($\geq$50 years), smoking, occupation (production, maintenance, or laboratory worker), and, if present, radiographic evidence of asbestos-related fibrosis and/or a positive beryllium lymphocyte proliferation test. Among 7189 participants, all of whom had a smoking history, the proportions with screen-detected lung cancer were 0.83% at baseline and 0.51% on annual scan. Of 80 detected lung cancers, 59% (n = 47) were stage 1%, and 10% (n = 8) were stage 2, a result very similar to that of NLST. Study strengths include a large novel study population, high study compliance, excellent credibility with the study population through labor union cosponsorship, implementation in community settings, excellent follow-up, and use of a standardized protocol with demonstrated quality. A limitation included a lack of specific knowledge about occupational exposures.

To address the question about contribution of occupational risk to aggregate risk, the study results were analyzed for 3 separate study subgroups by screening eligibility criteria: (1) met NLST criteria for age ($\geq$55 years) and smoking history ($\geq$30 pack-years), (2) did not meet NLST criteria in (1) but did meet NCCN group 2 criteria (age $\geq$50 years, $\geq$20 pack-year smoking history, and occupational risk), and (3) did not meet the criteria in (1) or (2).[60] Results with comparison with NLST study results are shown in **Fig. 4**. The screening yield of the NCCN group 2 population (1.36% at baseline and 0.55% at first annual scan) was similar to that of the NLST study population. Study results show that participants who met neither the NLST criteria nor the NCCN group 2 criteria, despite a history of work in the nuclear weapons complex, have a lung cancer screening yield that is approximately one-third of that of the NLST study (see **Fig. 4**). There is no evidence at present that shows a reduction in lung cancer mortality with low-dose CT screening for the subpopulation with the lower level of lung cancer risk identified in group (3).

Although this study did not include mortality follow-up, the shift to diagnosis of earlier-stage lung cancers with CT screening is consistent with the NLST and NELSON trials that showed favorable mortality reductions.[60]

Welch, and colleagues[61] performed low-dose CT screening on 1260 construction workers, also from the US nuclear weapons complex. Only 43.5% of study participants met the eligibility criteria of the NLST, and the remainder met NCCN group 2 eligibility criteria. In addition to age ($\geq$50 years) and smoking ($\geq$20 pack-years), screening participants had a history of one of the following: (1) 5 years of work in the construction industry or exposure to asbestos, silica, beryllium, chromium, radiation, or welding; (2) chest radiographic findings consistent with asbestosis (even without smoking $\geq$20 pack-years of cigarettes) or pleural plaques (even without 5 years of construction); or (3) COPD by spirometry (even without 5 years of construction). They found a favorable stage distribution among CT-detected cancers: 20 of 30 (67%) detected lung cancers were stage 1 (57%) or stage 2 (10%) disease. As in the Markowitz and colleagues[60] study, the lung cancer screening yield at baseline scan was 1.7% (21 of 1260 participants), a result that was similar to the NLST results, despite less than one-half of participants meeting the NLST eligibility criteria.[61]

Dement and colleagues[62] recently extended their analysis of this construction worker cohort[61] by comparing different sets of screening eligibility criteria using a larger dataset of 17,060 nuclear weapons complex

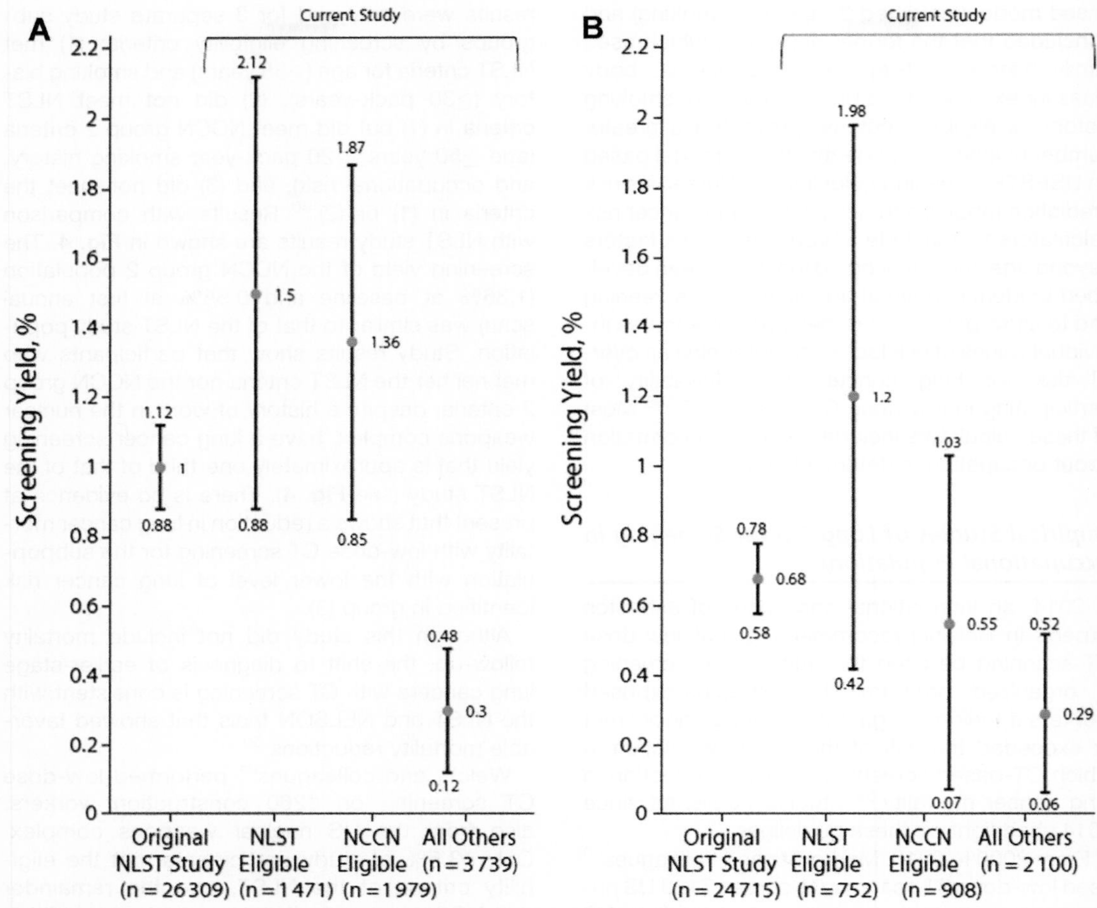

Fig. 4. Screening yields among nuclear weapons workers according to the eligibility criteria of the NLST and the NCCN at (*A*) baseline scan and (*B*) first annual scan, United States, 2000 to 2013. (*From* Markowitz SB, Manowitz A, Miller JA, et al. Yield of low-dose computerized tomography screening for lung cancer in high-risk workers: the case of 7,189 US nuclear weapons workers. *Am J Public Health.* 2018;108:1296-1302; with permission.)

construction workers, of whom 352 had died of lung cancer between 1998 and 2016. They developed a lung cancer risk prediction model (BTMed model) that includes age, gender, race, smoking history, spirometry, chest radiograph finding of parenchymal fibrosis and/or pleural plaques, occupational history of greater than or equal to 5 years of work in construction, body mass index, and personal history of cancer. Applying the lung cancer screening criteria described earlier in the Welch and colleagues[61] study yielded an 85.6% sensitivity, a 56.8% specificity, and a 4.2% positive predictive value. By contrast, application of the USPSTF-recommended screening criteria (age 50–80 years, ≥30 pack-years of smoking, and quitting <15 years in past) had a 50.9% sensitivity, an 81.2% specificity, and a 5.7% positive predictive value. Thus, the BTMed model substantially increased sensitivity with a concomitant decrease in specificity.[62]

Screening Asbestos-Exposed Populations

From 2002 to 2019, multiple studies have been published with a minimum of 150 participants that report results of the use of low-dose CT scan to screen asbestos-exposed populations for lung cancer.[63–73] The studies are heterogeneous in risk factors (age, smoking history, and extent of asbestos exposure), methods of assessing asbestos exposure, and details of the published reports. Summary results include:

1. Combining the 9 studies that had at least 150 participants, there were 86 lung cancers detected by screening CT scan among 5548 ever smokers (1.55%) and 6 lung cancers detected among 1787 never smokers (0.33%). Identifying the screening detection yields

according to the NLST study criteria or the NCCN group 2 criteria is not possible, because the published reports do not provide sufficient details on smoking history and age.

2. Although one-half of published studies screened people with a history greater than or equal to 15 years of asbestos exposure, one-half used a history of 1 or 5 years of significant asbestos exposure as a screening criterion. The studies with the highest screening yields tended to be the studies with a high prevalence (43% to 89%) of pleural plaques on low-dose CT scan.[65,69,72] However, importantly, these results do not signify that only asbestos-exposed workers with pleural plaques should be screened. Notably, the presence of pleural plaques was only identified after a low-dose CT scan was performed.

In a population environmentally or occupationally exposed to Libby amphibole asbestos, Loewen and colleagues[74] offered low-dose CT screening to people aged 50 to 84 years with a greater than or equal to 20 pack-year history of tobacco use and a history of asbestos-related pleural or pulmonary fibrosis on high-resolution CT scan. Most of the 567 screened participants had environmental (333, or 59%) or household exposure (145, or 25%) to Libby amphibole. Seventeen lung cancers were detected, mostly at a favorable stage distribution: 71% were stage 1 (59%) or stage 2 (11%).[74]

Should Asbestos-Exposed Populations Who Never Smoked Be Screened?

The 2 largest studies to address this issue, although still modestly sized (<500 never-smoking participants), have been published recently.[71,72] Kato and colleagues[72] performed a cross-sectional low-dose CT–based screening of 2132 asbestos-exposed workers between 2010 and 2012, mostly from shipbuilding, construction, and manufacturing sectors (asbestos products and nonasbestos products). Eligibility criteria included (1) work in asbestos manufacturing for greater than or equal to 1 year; (2) work in other asbestos-exposed industries for greater than 10 years; or (3) evidence of pleural plaques on chest radiograph or CT scan. Eighty-nine percent of participants had pleural plaques on CT scan. Three lung cancers (0.7%) were detected among 444 never smokers and 42 lung cancers among 1651 (2.5%) smokers. Details on the history of extent of smoking were not provided, precluding analysis by the NCCN eligibility categories.

Brims and colleagues[71] in Australia screened 960 individuals with a history of exposure to asbestos, defined as having at least 3 months of occupational exposure to asbestos or radiographic evidence of pleural plaques. Of the 325 never smokers, 2 lung cancers were found, a screening yield of 0.62%. The screening yield among 569 smokers was 0.88%. The overall screening yield was 0.77%, which is in the range of the screening yield among high-risk smokers in published studies, despite the fact that the mean cigarette consumption in the study population was modest (17 pack-years) and that only 4% of the cohort would have been eligible for screening under the USPSTF eligibility guidelines and 30% under the NCCN guidelines.

RECOMMENDATIONS: LUNG CANCER SCREENING OF OCCUPATIONAL POPULATIONS

Studies completed to date offer considerable evidence that a substantial history of occupational exposure (≥5 years of regular occupational exposure) to IARC group 1 or 2A lung carcinogens in combination with age (≥50 years old) and a limited smoking history (≥20 pack-years) constitute a reasonable indication for low-dose CT scan–based lung cancer screening. Completed studies among asbestos-exposed workers and workers with diverse exposures (nuclear weapons workers, construction workers) support this view and can probably be extended to workers with exposure to other occupational lung carcinogens, given the challenges in completing such studies. Workers with a shorter but more intense duration of exposure to occupational lung carcinogens should also be considered for screening with low-dose chest CT scan. Most studies to date have included only workers exposed to asbestos or to multiple carcinogens (ie, nuclear weapons workers), so the exposure eligibility parameters may need to be adjusted for the other documented occupational lung carcinogens. Among never smokers, there is inadequate evidence that exposure to occupational lung carcinogens increases the risk of lung cancer sufficiently close to the risk level identified in NLST as likely to be associated with a mortality benefit from low-dose CT scan screening. Whether the presence of lung cancer risk factors in addition to occupational exposures (eg, COPD or a family history of lung cancer) can sufficiently increase the lung cancer risk in the absence of smoking is an unanswered question. More fundamentally, whether screening people with an average lung cancer risk less than that of the CT arm in the NLST is associated with a benefit in life expectancy is uncertain. Additional reporting on results of the NELSON trial may shed light on this important question. Smoking cessation advice is a critical part of the lung cancer screening process, although most lung cancers that occur in the United States occur among former smokers.

If the USPSTF modifies its existing screening eligibility recommendation to reduce the age and smoking limits to 50 years of age and 20 cigarette pack-years, then a history of occupational exposures (or other lung cancer risk factors, such as chronic lung disease or family history) might justify further reducing the pack-year consumption for entry into occupational lung cancer screening programs. Modeling these risk-based scenarios may provide some helpful guidance.

IMPORTANT QUESTIONS THAT MAY ARISE IN CLINICAL PULMONARY PRACTICE

How Can Those at Increased Risk of Occupational Lung Cancer Be Identified?

A targeted occupational history can identify many, although not all, workers with exposure to the most common occupational lung carcinogens:

1. Have you worked with or near any of the following on a regular basis for at least 5 years?
   - Asbestos
   - Diesel exhaust
   - Silica
   - Welding
   - Metals: chromium, nickel, arsenic, and cadmium
2. Have you worked in the following occupation or industry on a regular basis for at least 5 years?
   - Painting
   - Construction
   - Metal or glass manufacture or processing
   - Transportation (eg, truck driver) or heavy machinery use

Such exposure identification is important to educating the patient about the need for lung cancer screening and justifying referral for a low-dose chest CT scan.

Which Occupational Populations Should Be Screened for Lung Cancer?

At present, workers aged greater than or equal to 50 years with a cigarette smoking history of greater than or equal to 20 pack-years and a history of 5 years of regular exposure to an occupational lung carcinogen (see **Table 1**) should be offered annual low-dose CT scan for lung cancer screening, assuming they are sufficiently healthy to undergo treatment of lung cancer. Workers with a shorter but especially intense exposure should also be offered screening. Workers with occupational exposure to lung carcinogens and who meet the age and smoking criteria cited earlier and who have COPD, pneumoconiosis, or a family history of lung cancer should be advised of the heightened importance of lung cancer screening.

The USPSTF may modify its existing screening eligibility recommendation to reduce the age and smoking limits to 50 years of age and 20 cigarette pack-years. If so, then adding occupational exposures (or other lung cancer risk factors such as chronic lung disease or family history) might justify further reducing the pack-year consumption for entry into occupational lung cancer screening programs.

How Can I Assist in Primary Prevention of Work-Related Lung Cancer?

Reduction or elimination of exposure to occupational lung carcinogens can prevent occupational lung cancer. A careful occupational history that includes exposure to lung carcinogens in the workplace (discussed earlier) is the principal means to identify workers at risk. Most occupational lung carcinogens are not associated with biomarkers, and exposure is best identified through an occupational history. For silica and asbestos, which may cause nonmalignant fibrosis of the lungs and/or pleura, workers are at increased risk of lung cancer even when they do not show evidence of nonmalignant disease of the chest. Workers who are exposed to occupational carcinogens should be made aware of such exposures and advised to reduce exposure through change in work practices, working with coworkers and employers to reduce or eliminate exposures, and to use of personal protective equipment. Smoking cessation is also important, although addressing this issue in combination with a discussion about reducing occupational exposures is likely to be the most effective way to address the topic.

Are Workers with Occupational Lung Cancer Entitled to Workers' Compensation or a Tort Judgment?

Such workers may be so entitled, depending on the jurisdiction. Workers with lung cancer and a history of exposure to any of the agents in **Table 1** should be advised to seek expert advice in a timely manner if they wish to pursue workers' compensation or a tort action. Physicians play a key role in providing a medical rationale for such compensation.

CLINICS CARE POINTS

- Probe the patient's occupational history by asking about major jobs held.

- Ask specifically about exposure to asbestos, silica, diesel exhaust, and welding fumes.
- Factor in occupational risk when considering patient's age and smoking history to decide if a low dose CT scan should be advised.

DISCLOSURE

Dr S. Markowitz has served as an expert witness in asbestos tort litigation. He has funding to conduct lung cancer screening from the US Department of Energy and the Sheet Metal Workers Occupational Health Institute Trust. Ms B. Dickens has nothing to declare.

REFERENCES

1. Brown T, Darnton A, Fortunato L, et al, British Occupational Cancer Burden Study Group. Occupational cancer in Britain: respiratory cancer sites: larynx, lung and mesothelioma. Br J Cancer 2012;107: S56–70.
2. Carder M, Darnton A, Gittins M, et al. Chest physician-reported, work-related, long-latency respiratory disease in Great Britain. Eur Respir J 2017;50:1700961.
3. Labrèche F, Kim J, Song C, et al. The current burden of cancer attributable to occupational exposures in Canada. Prev Med 2019;122:128–39.
4. Del Bianco A, Demers PA. Trends in compensation for deaths from occupational cancer in Canada: a descriptive study. CMAJ Open 2013;1:e91–6.
5. Ahn YS, Jeong KS. Epidemiologic characteristics of compensated occupational lung cancers among Korean workers. J Korean Med Sci 2014;29: 1473–81.
6. Kim EA, Lee HE, Kang SK. Occupational burden of cancer in Korea. Saf Health Work 2010;1:61–8.
7. Loomis D, Guha N, Hall AL, et al. Identifying occupational carcinogens: an update from the IARC monographs. Occup Environ Med 2018;75: 593–603.
8. IARC. List of classifications by cancer sites with sufficient or limited evidence in humans, volumes 1 to 127. Lyons (France): International Agency for Research on Cancer: World Health Organization Website; 2020. Available at: https://monographs.iarc.fr/wp-content/uploads/2019/07/Classifications_by_cancer_site_127.pdf. Accessed August 22, 2020.
9. Environmental Protection Agency. 2019. Available at: https://www.epa.gov/newsreleases/epa-releases-first-major-update-chemicals-list-40-years. Accessed February 2, 2020.
10. Cogliano VJ, Baan R, Straif K, et al. Preventable exposures associated with human cancers. J Natl Cancer Inst 2011;103:1827–39.
11. Bray F, Ferlay J, Soerjomataram I, et al. Global cancer statistics 2018: GLOBOCAN estimates of incidence and mortality worldwide for 36 cancers in 185 countries. CA Cancer J Clin 2018;68:394–424.
12. Rushton L, Bagga S, Bevan R, et al. Occupation and cancer in Britain. Br J Cancer 2010;102:1428–37.
13. Driscoll T, Nelson DI, Steenland K, et al. The global burden of disease due to occupational carcinogens. Am J Ind Med 2005;48:419–31.
14. Boffetta P, Autier P, Boniol M, et al. An estimate of cancers attributable to occupational exposures in France. J Occup Environ Med 2010;52: 399–406.
15. McCormack V, Peto J, Byrnes G, et al. Estimating the asbestos-related lung cancer burden from mesothelioma mortality. Br J Cancer 2012;106:575–84.
16. GBD 2015 Risk Factors Collaborators. Global, regional, and national comparative risk assessment of 79 behavioural, environmental and occupational, and metabolic risks or clusters of risks, 1990-2015: a systematic analysis for the Global Burden of Disease Study 2015. Lancet 2016;388:1659–724.
17. Steenland K, Burnett C, Lalich N, et al. Dying for work: the magnitude of US mortality from selected causes of death associated with occupation. Am J Ind Med 2003;43:461–82.
18. International Ban Asbestos Secretariat 2020. Available at: http://ibasecretariat.org/alpha_ban_list.php. Accessed February 5, 2020.
19. Kauppinen T, Uuksulainen S, Saalo A, et al. Trends of occupational exposure to chemical agents in Finland in 1950-2020. Ann Occup Hyg 2013;57: 593–609.
20. Kauppinen T, Toikkanen J, Pedersen D, et al. Occupational exposure to carcinogens in the European Union. Occup Environ Med 2000;57:10–8.
21. Peters CE, Ge CB, Hall AL, et al. CAREX Canada: an enhanced model for assessing occupational carcinogen exposure. Occup Environ Med 2015;72:64–71.
22. Flanagan D. USGS 2016 Minerals Yearbook May 2018. p. 10. Available at: https://s3-us-west-2.amazonaws.com/prd-wret/assets/palladium/production/mineral-pubs/asbestos/myb1-2016-asbes.pdf. Accessed January 20, 2020.
23. Gonghuan Y, Hsia J, Yan Y, editors. Global Adult Tobacco Survey (GATS) China 2010 Country report. Beijing (China): Chinese Center for Disease Control and Prevention. 2010. Available at: https://www.who.int/tobacco/surveillance/survey/gats/en_gats_china_report.pdf?ua=1. Accessed January 31, 2020.
24. Takiguchi Y, Sekine I, Iwasawa S, et al. Chronic obstructive pulmonary disease as a risk factor for lung cancer. World J Clin Oncol 2014;5:660–6.
25. Blanc PD, Annesi-Maesano I, Balmes JR, et al. The occupational burden of nonmalignant respiratory diseases. An official American Thoracic Society

and European Respiratory Society Statement. Am J Respir Crit Care Med 2019;199:1312–34.
26. Naccache JM, Gibiot Q, Monnet I, et al. Lung cancer and interstitial lung disease: a literature review. J Thorac Dis 2018;10:3829–44.
27. Nielsen LS, Baelum J, Rasmussen J, et al. Occupational asbestos exposure and lung cancer–a systematic review of the literature. Arch Environ Occup Health 2014;69:191–206.
28. Markowitz S. Cancer of the respiratory tract due to asbestos and zeolites. In: Taylor AN, Cullinan P, Blanc P, et al, editors. Parkes' occupational lung disorders. 4th edition. Beverly Farms (MA): OEM Press; 2016. p. 259–76.
29. Markowitz SB, Levin SM, Miller A, et al. Asbestos, asbestosis, smoking, and lung cancer: new findings from the North American insulator cohort. Am J Respir Crit Care Med 2013;188:90–6.
30. Wang X, Yano E, Qiu H, et al. A 37-year observation of mortality in Chinese chrysotile asbestos workers. Thorax 2012;67:106–10.
31. Offermans NS, Vermeulen R, Burdorf A, et al. Occupational asbestos exposure and risk of pleural mesothelioma, lung cancer, and laryngeal cancer in the prospective Netherlands cohort study. J Occup Environ Med 2014;56:6–19.
32. Olsson AC, Vermeulen R, Schüz J, et al. Exposure-response analyses of asbestos and lung cancer subtypes in a pooled analysis of case-control studies. Epidemiology 2017;28(2):288–99.
33. Hammond EC, Selikoff IJ, Seidman H. Asbestos exposure, cigarette smoking and death rates. Ann N Y Acad Sci 1979;330:473–90.
34. Liu Y, Steenland K, Rong Y, et al. Exposure-response analysis and risk assessment for lung cancer in relationship to silica exposure: a 44-year cohort study of 34,018 workers. Am J Epidemiol 2013;178:1424–33.
35. Consonni D, De Matteis S, Pesatori AC, et al. Lung cancer risk among bricklayers in a pooled analysis of case-control studies. Int J Cancer 2015;136: 360–71.
36. De Matteis S, Consonni D, Lubin JH, et al. Impact of occupational carcinogens on lung cancer risk in a general population. Int J Epidemiol 2012;41:711–21.
37. Kachuri L, Villeneuve PJ, Parent ME, Johnson KC, the Canadian Cancer Registries Epidemiology Group, Harris SA. Occupational exposure to crystalline silica and the risk of lung cancer in Canadian men. Int J Cancer 2014;135:138–48.
38. Lacourt A, Pintos J, Lavoué J, et al. Lung cancer risk among workers in the construction industry: results from two case-control studies in Montreal. BMC Public Health 2015;15:941.
39. Silverman DT, Samanic CM, Lubin JH, et al. The diesel exhaust in miners study: a nested case-control study of lung cancer and diesel exhaust. J Natl Cancer Inst 2012;104:855–68.
40. Pintos J, Parent ME, Richardson L, et al. Occupational exposure to diesel engine emissions and risk of lung cancer: evidence from two case-control studies in Montreal, Canada. Occup Environ Med 2012;69:787–92.
41. Schubauer-Berigan MK, Daniels RD, Pinkerton LE. Radon exposure and mortality among white and American Indian uranium miners: an update of the Colorado Plateau cohort. Am J Epidemiol 2009; 169:718–30.
42. Leuraud K, Schnelzer M, Tomasek L, et al. Radon, smoking and lung cancer risk: results of a joint analysis of three European case-control studies among uranium miners. Radiat Res 2011;176:375–87.
43. Kreuzer M, Sobotzki C, Schnelzer M, et al. Factors modifying the radon-related lung cancer risk at low exposures and exposure rates among German Uranium Miners. Radiat Res 2018;189:165–76.
44. Ferreccio C, Yuan Y, Calle J, et al. Arsenic, tobacco smoke, and occupation: associations of multiple agents with lung and bladder cancer. Epidemiology 2013;24:898–905.
45. Lee DJ, Fleming LE, McCollister KE, et al. Healthcare provider smoking cessation advice among US worker groups. Tob Control 2007;16:325–8.
46. Osinubi OY, Moline J, Rovner E, et al. A pilot study of telephone-based smoking cessation intervention in asbestos workers. J Occup Environ Med 2003;45: 569–74.
47. Sorensen G, Stoddard A, Quintiliani L, et al. Tobacco use cessation and weight management among motor freight workers: results of the gear up for health study. Cancer Causes Control 2010; 21(12):2113–22.
48. Sorensen G, Stoddard AM, LaMontagne AD, et al. A comprehensive worksite cancer prevention intervention: behavior change results from a randomized controlled trial (United States). J Public Health Policy 2003;24:5–25.
49. USPSTF 2020. Available at: https://www.uspreventiveservicestaskforce.org/BrowseRec/Index. Accessed February 3, 2020.
50. USPSTF 2020. Available at: https://uspreventiveservicestaskforce.org/uspstf/sites/default/files/file/supporting_documents/lung-cancer-screening-draft-rec-bulletin.pdf. Accessed July 23, 2020.
51. Centers for Medicare and Medicaid Services CMS. Decision memo for screening for lung cancer with low dose computed tomography. 2015. Available at: https://www.cms.gov/medicare-coverage-database/details/nca-decision-memo.aspx?NCAId=274. Accessed January 15, 2020.
52. Henschke CI, McCauley DI, Yankelevitz DF, et al. Early lung cancer action project: overall design and findings from baseline screening. Lancet 1999;354:99–105.

53. Henschke CI, Yankelevitz DF, Libby DM, et al. Survival of patients with stage I lung cancer detected on CT screening. N Engl J Med 2006;355:1763–71.
54. National Lung Screening Trial Research Team, Aberle DR, Adams AM, et al. Reduced lung-cancer mortality with low-dose computed tomographic screening. N Engl J Med 2011;365: 395–409.
55. de Koning HJ, van der Aalst CM, de Jong PA, et al. Reduced lung-cancer mortality with volume CT screening in a randomized trial. N Engl J Med 2020;382(6):503–13.
56. Wood DE, Kazerooni EA, Baum SL, et al. Lung cancer screening, version 3.2018: clinical practice guidelines in oncology. J Natl Compr Cancer Netw 2018;16:412–41.
57. Katki HA, Kovalchik SA, Berg CD, et al. Development and validation of risk models to select ever-smokers for CT lung cancer screening. JAMA 2016;315:2300–11.
58. Tammemägi MC. Application of risk prediction models to lung cancer screening: a review. J Thorac Imaging 2015;30:88–100.
59. Wolff H, Vehmas T, Oksa P, et al. Asbestos, asbestosis, and cancer, the Helsinki criteria for diagnosis and attribution 2014: recommendations. Scand J Work Environ Health 2015;41(1):5–15.
60. Markowitz SB, Manowitz A, Miller JA, et al. Yield of low-dose computerized tomography screening for lung cancer in high-risk workers: the case of 7,189 US nuclear weapons workers. Am J Public Health 2018;108:1296–302.
61. Welch LS, Dement JM, Cranford K, et al. Early detection of lung cancer in a population at high risk due to occupation and smoking. Occup Environ Med 2019;76(3):137–42.
62. Dement JM, Ringen K, Hines S, et al. Lung cancer mortality among construction workers: implications for early detection. Occup Environ Med 2020. https://doi.org/10.1136/oemed-2019-106196.
63. Tiitola M, Kivisaari L, Huuskonen MS, et al. Computed tomography screening for lung cancer in asbestos-exposed workers. Lung Cancer 2002; 35:17–22.
64. Minniti S, Valentini M, Pozzi Mucelli R. Low-dose helical chest CT in asbestos-exposed workers in the Veneto Region: preliminary results. Radiol Med 2005;110:317–24.
65. Das M, Mühlenbruch G, Mahnken AH, et al. Asbestos Surveillance Program Aachen (ASPA): initial results from baseline screening for lung cancer in asbestos-exposed high-risk individuals using low-dose multidetector-row CT. Eur Radiol 2007;17: 1193–9.
66. Fasola G, Belvedere O, Aita M, et al. Low-dose computed tomography screening for lung cancer and pleural mesothelioma in an asbestos-exposed population: baseline results of a prospective, non-randomized feasibility trial- an Alpe-Adria Thoracic Oncology Multidisciplinary Group study (ATOM 002). Oncologist 2007;12:1215–24.
67. Vierikko T, Järvenpää R, Autti T, et al. Chest CT screening of asbestos-exposed workers: lung lesions and incidental findings. Eur Respir J 2007; 29:78–84.
68. Mastrangelo G, Ballarin MN, Bellini E, et al. Feasibility of a screening programme for lung cancer in former asbestos workers. Occup Med 2008;58: 175–80.
69. Roberts HC, Patsios DA, Paul NS, et al. Screening for malignant pleural mesothelioma and lung cancer in individuals with a history of asbestos exposure. J Thorac Oncol 2009;4:620–8.
70. Clin B, Morlais F, Guittet L, et al. Performance of chest radiograph and CT scan for lung cancer screening in asbestos-exposed workers. Occup Environ Med 2009;66:529–34.
71. Brims FJH, Murray CP, de Klerk N, et al. Ultra-low-dose chest computer tomography screening of an asbestos-exposed population in Western Australia. Am J Respir Crit Care Med 2015;191:113–6.
72. Kato K, Gemba K, Ashizawa K, et al. Low-dose chest computed tomography screening of subjects exposed to asbestos. Eur J Radiol 2018;101:124–8.
73. Maisonneuve P, Rampinelli C, Bertolotti R, et al. Low-dose computed tomography screening for lung cancer in people with workplace exposure to asbestos. Lung Cancer 2019;131:23–30.
74. Loewen G, Black B, McNew T, et al. Lung cancer screening in patients with Libby amphibole disease: high yield despite predominantly environmental and household exposure. Am J Ind Med 2019;62: 1112–6.

Occupational Respiratory Infections

Marie A. de Perio, MD[a,*], Miwako Kobayashi, MD[b], Jonathan M. Wortham, MD[c]

KEYWORDS

• Tuberculosis • Psittacosis • Influenza • Coccidioidomycosis • Valley fever • Pneumonia
• Occupational • Respiratory infection

KEY POINTS

- Workers in specific settings are at increased risk for occupational respiratory infections, including tuberculosis, influenza, coccidioidomycosis, psittacosis, and other bacterial pneumonia.
- Clinicians should recognize that respiratory infections can be occupationally acquired.
- Considering occupational risk factors for infection, such as workplace factors and worker factors can help in implementing prevention and control strategies.
- Controlling exposures among workers according to the hierarchy of controls will help prevent disease transmission in the workplace.

INTRODUCTION

Occupational lung diseases caused by exposures to gases, chemicals, and dusts at work have been long recognized. However, recent experiences with occupationally acquired respiratory infections, including Middle East respiratory syndrome coronavirus, influenza, measles, and coronavirus disease 2019 (COVID-19) have highlighted the importance of understanding transmission of respiratory infections in the workplace.[1–3] Workplace exposures have been demonstrated to contribute substantially to the burden of community-acquired pneumonia, with an occupational population attributable fraction as high as 10% in 1 recent review.[4] Any infectious agent that is transmitted by airborne particles or by droplets can be acquired in the workplace.[5] Occupational respiratory infections can be caused by bacterial, viral, and fungal pathogens. Transmission in occupational settings can occur from other humans (such as co-workers or patients), animals, or the environment and occur in various occupations and industries. Factors that can facilitate transmission of infectious pathogens in the workplace include disease factors (such as mode of transmission), workplace factors (such as workplace conditions or work practices), and worker factors (such as impaired immunity).[6]

Occupational health and safety specialists have long used the hierarchy of controls (**Fig. 1**) as an approach to determine how to implement feasible and effective control solutions, and this can be applied to infectious agents.[6,7] Elimination (removing the hazard) and substitution (replacing the hazard) are the most effective ways to reduce occupational hazards but can be difficult to implement for infectious agents. Engineering controls are physical changes to work processes to remove the hazard or place a barrier between workers and hazards. They can effectively protect workers without placing the primary responsibility of

Disclaimer: The findings and conclusions in this report are those of the authors and do not necessarily represent the official position of the Centers for Disease Control and Prevention.

[a] Division of Field Studies and Engineering, National Institute for Occupational Safety and Health, Centers for Disease Control and Prevention, 1090 Tusculum Avenue, R-9, Cincinnati, OH 45226, USA; [b] Division of Bacterial Diseases, National Center for Immunization and Respiratory Diseases, Centers for Disease Control and Prevention, 1600 Clifton Road Northeast, MS H24-6, Atlanta, GA 30333, USA; [c] Division of Tuberculosis Elimination, National Center for HIV/AIDS, Viral Hepatitis, STD, and TB Prevention, Centers for Disease Control and Prevention, 1600 Clifton Road Northeast, MS US12-4, Atlanta, GA 30333, USA
* Corresponding author.
E-mail address: mdeperio@cdc.gov

Clin Chest Med 41 (2020) 739–751
https://doi.org/10.1016/j.ccm.2020.08.003
0272-5231/20/Published by Elsevier Inc.

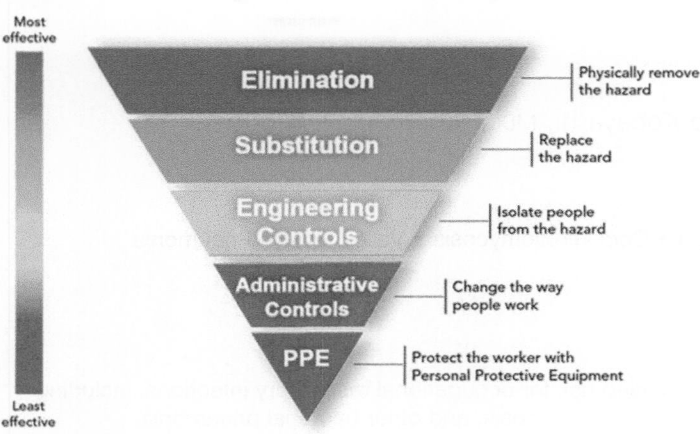

Fig. 1. Hierarchy of controls. (*From* The National Institute for Occupational Safety and Health (NIOSH). Hierarchy of Controls. Center for Disease Control. Available at: https://www.cdc.gov/niosh/topics/hierarchy/default.html With permission).

implementation on the worker. Ventilation is the most common engineering control, especially for airborne pathogens. Administrative controls are methods that change the way the work is performed, such as triaging and isolating ill patients or influenza vaccination of workers. Their effectiveness depends on the availability of the control and worker acceptance and commitment. Finally, use of personal protective equipment (PPE) provides a physical barrier between the worker and the hazard. PPE is considered the least effective control measure because it requires a comprehensive program and a high level of worker involvement and commitment for proper use.[7]

The National Institute for Occupational Safety and Health (NIOSH) Health Hazard Evaluation (HHE) program responds to requests from workers, employers, and public health agencies and conducts investigations of hazards, including infectious diseases, that occur in workplaces.[8] In this article, we describe 4 occupationally acquired respiratory infections at the focus of NIOSH investigations over the last decade: tuberculosis (TB), influenza, coccidioidomycosis, and psittacosis.[9–14] We describe their epidemiology, clinical manifestations, occupational risk factors, and prevention measures according to the hierarchy of controls. These examples demonstrate the breadth of infectious pathogens (bacterial, viral, and fungal) and transmission (from human, animals, and the environment) in the workplace.

TUBERCULOSIS

Tuberculosis (TB) is caused by *Mycobacterium tuberculosis*, an acid-fast bacillus that is most often transmitted from person to person through the air in contaminated respiratory droplets. These droplets can dry into tiny particles called droplet nuclei that remain suspended in air for long periods of time. Pulmonary TB often presents with a prolonged cough of 2 or more weeks' duration. While pulmonary TB is the most common form of disease, TB can affect other organs, such as the larynx, abdomen, meninges, and spine. Patients with TB involving any organ system often have nonspecific symptoms, such as fatigue, weight loss, loss of appetite, chills, and night sweats. Whereas some people become ill with TB soon after inhaling droplets contaminated with *M tuberculosis*, most do not. Approximately 20% to 30% of contacts develop latent TB infection (LTBI) with *M tuberculosis*.[15,16] Persons with LTBI are not infectious, and most persons with LTBI will have positive tests for TB infection (ie, the tuberculin skin test [TST] or an interferon-gamma release assay [IGRA]). Treating LTBI is an effective way of preventing symptomatic, potentially contagious TB.[17,18] Overall, among untreated persons with LTBI approximately 5% to 10% will develop symptomatic TB during their lifetimes; approximately half of those who develop TB will do so within 2 years of initially becoming infected with *M tuberculosis*.[15,16] The risk for progression from LTBI to TB is markedly higher among those living with HIV, young children less than 5 years, and persons with certain immune-suppressing medical conditions or those taking certain immune-suppressing medications.[15]

TB is extremely common worldwide; approximately one-fourth of the world's population is thought to have LTBI and approximately 10 million became ill with TB during 2018.[19] In the United States, TB incidence is very low; overall LTBI prevalence has been estimated at approximately 5%, and 9025 TB cases were reported during 2018, a 73% decline compared with 1991.[16,17] Just as is the case globally, TB is unevenly distributed in the United States; since 2001, most cases have occurred in persons born outside of the United States in countries with comparatively higher TB incidence.[20] Many cases among non-US-born persons likely represent infection acquired outside the United States in the remote past.[16] TB in the United States also disproportionately affects people experiencing homelessness, incarcerated persons, and persons with weakened immune systems.[16,20]

To maximize the predictive value of tests for TB infection and focus resources on evaluating and treating persons at risk for LTBI and TB given the relatively low LTBI prevalence and TB incidence in the United States, the Centers for Disease Control and Prevention (CDC) recommends testing only for persons with TB symptoms, epidemiologic risk factors for LTBI (eg, birth in a country with higher TB incidence), or medical risk factors for progression to TB.[17,21] To evaluate for TB, medical providers should perform a thorough diagnostic evaluation on all persons with positive tests for TB infection; this diagnostic evaluation should include a medical history and physical examination, chest radiography, and, in certain circumstances, acid-fast bacilli smear microscopy, culture, and nucleic acid amplification tests.[22]

M tuberculosis transmission is possible in any workplace with contagious persons; workplace-associated transmission has been described in health care settings, such as hospitals, long-term care facilities, and laboratories,[8,23] correctional facilities,[24] homeless shelters,[25] and even a refuge and zoo that housed elephants.[11,26] When pulmonologists, occupational medicine practitioners, or other health care providers identify workers with TB symptoms, they should collaborate with local and state public health programs to facilitate prompt TB diagnoses among workers. These collaborations should also facilitate worksite-based contact investigations, and focused efforts to identify persons exposed to infectious TB, so that they can be tested and treated for LTBI and TB.[15] Public health programs can use clinical, epidemiologic, and molecular data to determine whether LTBI and TB diagnoses among workers represent a cadre of workers with a high prevalence of risk factors for LTBI and TB or a workplace with *M tuberculosis* transmission.

M tuberculosis transmission in health care settings deserves special attention. Health care-associated transmission used to be common, and LTBI prevalence among health care personnel was higher than the overall population.[5] Recognizing the importance of preventing health care-associated transmission, CDC has published guidelines for preventing *M tuberculosis* transmission in health care settings since the 1980s.[27] The most recent version of these guidelines, published in 2005, promotes 3 categories of infection control measures: administrative, engineering (or environmental), and respiratory protection. The occupational health and safety hierarchy of controls typically prioritizes engineering controls over administrative controls. However, for TB, administrative controls, which are designed to reduce the risk of exposures to infectious TB, are prioritized over engineering controls and are the foundation of TB infection control and prevention strategies.[27] Examples of TB prevention measures according to the hierarchy of controls are shown in **Table 1**.

In the context of declining overall TB incidence in the United States, limited specificity of TSTs and IGRAs, and no TB cases identified in large cohorts of health care personnel despite widespread routine testing, CDC amended guidance for TB screening, testing, and treatment of health care personnel in 2019.[28] **Table 2** depicts the amended guidance for testing of health care personnel alongside the 2005 guidance. In the absence of ongoing transmission or exposure to infectious TB, CDC no longer recommends serial testing of health care personnel for LTBI or TB.[28] Current guidance recommends baseline screening for all health care personnel; screening includes assessing for TB symptoms, assessing for LTBI and TB risk factors, and performing a test for TB infection.[28] Those with positive tests should have a thorough diagnostic evaluation for TB; health care personnel with LTBI should be encouraged to take LTBI treatment to prevent TB unless medically contraindicated. Using the same test for TB infection (ie, a TST or IGRA) helps facilitate results interpretation for individuals and making inferences about whether transmission is occurring among cohorts of workers.[28] Recommendations regarding other aspects of infection control and prevention in health care settings remain unchanged from the 2005 guidelines.[27]

INFLUENZA

Influenza infections are thought to spread mainly through droplet transmission, although evidence for airborne transmission and transmission by direct contact also exists. Seasonal and pandemic influenza are important causes of morbidity and mortality in humans. Transmission occurs mostly from human to human. However, swine and poultry are 2 key reservoirs of influenza viruses

Table 1
Occupations at risk and examples of prevention measures according to the hierarchy of controls

	Tuberculosis[a]	Influenza	Coccidioidomycosis	Psittacosis
Example occupations at risk	Health care personnel Laboratory workers Correctional workers Homeless shelter workers	Health care personnel Swine and poultry farmers Veterinary personnel Meat processing workers	Agricultural workers Construction workers Archeological workers Military personnel Laboratory workers	Veterinary personnel Bird breeders Poultry processing workers Pet shop workers
Control type				
Elimination/substitution	Exclusion of infectious workers	Exclusion of ill workers from work Biosecurity/biosafety measures at farms, plants, live markets	Reduction in grading or need for trenching of land	Quarantine of newly acquired birds or birds exposed to ill birds Isolation of ill birds
Engineering controls	General ventilation to reduce concentrations in air Airborne infection isolation rooms (AIIRs) High efficiency particulate air filtration Ultraviolet germicidal irradiation	Partitions in triage areas Maintenance of air-handling systems Closed suctioning systems for airway suction Use of AIIRs for aerosol-generating procedures	Frequent, effective soil wetting Use of enclosed cabs Planting of vegetation, ground cover	Exhaust ventilation Cleaning/disinfection of cages Repair of malfunctioning tools
Administrative controls	Written TB control plan Prompt identification, isolation of persons with TB Treatment of TB and latent TB infection TB screening of exposed or at-risk workers Thorough and efficient contact investigations	Influenza vaccination Non-punitive sick leave policies Infection prevention training Triage, isolation of infectious patients Hand hygiene Cull infected animals	Suspension of work during excessive dust/wind Training workers about risks, symptoms Have onsite monitoring personnel to implement additional control measures	Maintain accurate records of bird-related transactions Good animal husbandry practices Educating workers about risks Hand hygiene Appropriate cleaning, disinfection protocols for cages

Personal protective equipment	Airborne precautions Use of NIOSH-approved filtering facepiece respirators[b]	Droplet precautions: surgical masks Standard precautions: gowns, gloves as needed Use of NIOSH-approved filtering facepiece respirators[b] for aerosol-generating procedures and for novel strains	Use of NIOSH-approved filtering facepiece respirators[b] for workers at high risk of exposure	Use of NIOSH-approved filtering facepiece respirators[b] for workers at high risk of exposure (ie, handling ill birds or cleaning cages) Gloves, eye protection as needed based on job duties

[a] For the hierarchy of controls for tuberculosis, administrative controls take priority over engineering controls.
[b] Respirators for employees must be used within an Occupational Safety and Health Administration (OSHA)-compliant respiratory protection program that includes medical clearance, fit testing, training, and procedures for disposing, cleaning, and maintaining respirators.

Table 2
CDC recommendations for tuberculosis screening, testing, and treatment of US health care personnel[a]

Category	2005 Recommendations[27]	2019 Recommendations[28]

Baseline (preplacement) screening and testing	• Symptom evaluation
	• Test for TB infection (eg, TST or IGRA) for those without documented history of TB or LTBI[b]
		• Symptom evaluation
		• Test for TB infection (eg, TST or IGRA) for those without documented history of TB or LTBI[b]
		• Individual risk assessment[c]
		  ○ Previous residency ≥1 mo in country with high TB rates[d]
		  ○ Current or planned immune suppression[e]
		  ○ Close contact with someone with infectious TB

Serial screening and testing for health care personnel without LTBI	Varies according to facility and setting risk assessment
	• Potential for ongoing transmission:
	  ○ Test for TB infection every 8–10 wk until effective infection controls implemented and no additional evidence for ongoing transmission
	• Medium risk:
	  ○ Annual symptom evaluation
	  ○ Annual test for TB infection
	• Low risk:
	  ○ None in the absence of exposure to *M tuberculosis*
		Not routinely recommended except for:
		• Selected groups who might be at increased occupational risk of exposure (eg, pulmonologists or respiratory therapists)
		• Certain settings if transmission has occurred in the past (eg, selected emergency departments)
		• Contact investigations[f]
		• Exposure to infectious TB outside of workplace
		• Evidence for ongoing TB transmission[f]

Annual TB education for health care personnel	Recommended	Recommended, with emphasis on: • Risk factors • Signs and symptoms of TB • Discussing occupational and nonoccupational TB exposures with primary care and occupational health providers as soon as practical after exposure
Evaluation and treatment of positive test results	Referral to determine whether LTBI treatment is indicated	Encouraged for all with untreated LTBI unless medically contraindicated

Abbreviations: IGRA, interferon-gamma release assay; LTBI, latent tuberculosis infection; TB, tuberculosis; TST, tuberculin skin test.

[a] Recommendations outside of the scope of health care personnel screening, testing, treatment, and education, including facility risk assessments for guiding infection control policies and procedures, remain unchanged from the 2005 guidelines.[27,28]

[b] Asymptomatic health care personnel who have positive tests are unlikely to be infected with *M tuberculosis*, and are at low risk for progression based on their risk assessment, should have a second test (either an IGRA or a TST) as recommended in the TB diagnostic guidelines of the American Thoracic Society, Infectious Diseases Society of America, and CDC.[22] These health care personnel should be considered infected with *M. tuberculosis* only if both the first and second tests are positive.

[c] CDC's Health care personnel baseline individual TB risk assessment found at: https://www.cdc.gov/tb/topic/infectioncontrol/pdf/healthCareSettings-assessment.pdf.

[d] This includes any country other than Australia, Canada, New Zealand, the United States, and those in western or northern Europe.

[e] Includes human immunodeficiency virus (HIV) infection, receipt of an organ transplant, treatment with a TNF-alpha antagonist, chronic steroids (equivalent of prednisone ≥15 mg/d for ≥1 mo), or other immunosuppressive medication.

[f] Consultation with the local or state health department is encouraged in making these determination.

Data from Refs.[22,27,28]

and cause zoonotic infection. Influenza A viruses cause the most morbidity in both humans and animals among influenza viruses.[29] CDC has estimated that the number influenza-related illnesses that have occurred during influenza season in the United States has ranged from 9.2 to 35.6 million, including 140,000 to 710,000 influenza-related hospitalizations.[30] The seasonal incidence of symptomatic influenza has been estimated at 8.9% for adults aged 18 to 64 years.[31]

Symptoms of influenza infection include fever, cough, sore throat, runny or stuffy nose, body aches, headache, chills, and fatigue. Some patients have vomiting and diarrhea, whereas others have respiratory symptoms without a fever. Influenza illness can range from mild to severe. Health conditions known to increase the risk of serious complications from influenza include pregnancy, asthma, and other chronic lung disease; diabetes mellitus; heart, neurologic, and kidney disease; and immunocompromising conditions.[32]

Health care personnel are considered to be at risk for influenza infections from both seasonal and pandemic influenza through exposure to patients with influenza and may also transmit influenza to patients and other health care personnel.[32] A meta-analysis of 15 studies demonstrated a significantly increased odds for influenza A (H1N1) for health care personnel (odds ratio = 2.08, 95% CI, 1.73, 2.51) during the 2009 H1N1 influenza epidemic.[33] Influenza has caused outbreaks of severe respiratory illness in hospitals and long-term care facilities.[34] For pandemic influenza, the Occupational Safety and Health Administration (OSHA) considers health care personnel performing aerosol-generating procedures on known or suspected influenza patients and laboratory personnel handling specimens from these patients to be at very high exposure risk. Other health care personnel involved in health care delivery and support or transport are considered at high exposure risk. Workers with high-frequency contact with the general population, such as those in schools, high population density work environments, and some high volume retail settings are considered at medium exposure risk.[35]

Studies have shown that occupational risk factors have been associated with infection among health care personnel including job type (ie, physicians and nurses), number of patient contacts, vaccination history, inadequate hand hygiene, and inadequate PPE use.[33] These occupational risk factors highlight the need for comprehensive infection prevention strategies in health care settings. Institutional strategies, primarily engineering and administrative controls, to prevent transmission of influenza among health care personnel and patients are shown in **Table 1**.[36,37]

Employer influenza vaccination requirements are associated with higher coverage rates, and, although controversial, mandatory influenza vaccination is supported by many health care personnel and multiple health care professional societies.[38–40] Mandatory influenza vaccination is increasingly common in health care settings, and multiple states have established influenza vaccination requirements for hospital health care personnel.[41] However, concerns have been raised related to the variable effectiveness of the vaccine and the ethical and legal impact of these policies.[41–43] The duty of health care personnel to protect the health of individual patients and the public competes with their right to personal autonomy. Mandates also invoke legal issues, including the applicability of state and federal constitutional laws and statutes.[41–43]

Provision of appropriate PPE with adequate training and an expectation of consistent use may also prevent transmission of influenza to health care personnel (see **Table 1**).[37] N95 filtering facepiece respirators have been demonstrated to have a protective advantage over surgical masks in laboratory settings.[44] However, 2 meta-analyses and multiple newer studies have concluded mixed results about the difference between surgical masks and N95 respirators in the incidence of laboratory-confirmed influenza, influenza-like illness, and acute respiratory infection.[44–47]

Animal workers have also been shown to be at higher risk for zoonotic transmission of influenza viruses. Influenza transmission from pigs was first recognized during the Spanish influenza pandemic of 1918 to 1919.[48] Swine farmers, swine production workers, veterinarians, and meat processing workers have been shown to have higher risk of infection from swine influenza virus.[49,50] In addition, there is significant evidence of zoonotic transmission of avian influenza viruses from birds to humans with the 1997 outbreak of human H5N1 infections in Hong Kong and the 2013 outbreak of human H7N9 infections primarily in China.[2] H7 and H5 strains are the avian influenza viruses that have most commonly infected humans and often cause severe disease after exposures to infected or dead birds.[29] Poultry farmers and cullers, veterinarians, commercial poultry workers, and poultry vendors at live animal markets are considered at higher risk of infection with avian influenza viruses.[3,5,29] Poultry contact involving mass culling during outbreaks, slaughtering and preparing of ill or deceased birds, and burial of carcasses have been implicated as modes of transmission.[3] More recently, transmission of influenza A (H7N2) infection has been documented from felines to humans in a city animal shelter.[51,52]

Measures to prevent animal-to-human transmission of influenza involves a OneHealth approach that includes comprehensive biosecurity and biosafety measures and training at the farms, processing plants, and live markets, surveillance for influenza viruses, culling infected animals, and vaccination of poultry and swine.[28,30] Strategies to minimize risk among individual workers include training on their risk and preventive measures, annual influenza vaccination, and appropriate hand hygiene (see **Table 1**).[2,50]

COCCIDIOIDOMYCOSIS

Coccidioidomycosis, also known as Valley fever, is caused by inhalation of spores of the fungus *Coccidioides* spp, which grows in soil in semiarid areas. The infection is an example of transmission from the environment, and it is not generally spread from to person to person, or from animals to people. Coccidioidomycosis is endemic in the southwestern United States, particularly parts of Arizona and California, Mexico, and parts of Central and South America.[53] During 2011 to 2017, a total of 95,371 cases of coccidioidomycosis were reported to CDC from 26 states and the District of Columbia, with greater than 95% of cases reported from Arizona and California.[54] An estimated 150,000 new infections occur annually in the United States,[55] although only approximately 10,000 cases are reported annually, suggesting that the disease is greatly underdetected and underreported.[56]

About 60% of coccidioidomycosis infections are asymptomatic.[53] People who develop symptoms, typically after a 1 to 3 week incubation period, may experience a flu-like illness. The infection can be clinically indistinguishable from community-acquired pneumonia caused by other pathogens, which can lead to inappropriate treatment.[54] A small percentage of infected persons (<1%) may develop widespread disseminated infection.[53] People at greater risk for developing disseminated infection include people of African American and Asian (particularly Filipino) descent, pregnant women during their third trimester, and immunocompromised persons.[53] Coccidioidomycosis has been shown to be costly and debilitating, with nearly 75% of patients in whom the disease has been recognized missing work or school because of their illness and more than 40% requiring hospitalization.[57]

This disease has important occupational risk factors. First, laboratory-acquired coccidioidomycosis has been documented, mostly arising from accidental laboratory exposure to *Coccidioides* spp.[58,59] Second, environmental exposures exist through disruption of soil or strong dust-raising winds, which can aerosolize spores. Therefore, in *Coccidioides*-endemic areas, persons who work outdoors are at particular risk for coccidioidomycosis when their duties include soil-disruptive work or when working in dusty or windy conditions. Workers in endemic areas involved in soil disturbance, including but not limited to agricultural, construction, and archeological workers, military personnel, and workers in mining, quarrying, and oil and gas extraction industries have been shown to be at higher risk for coccidioidomycosis.[6,60,61] A review of 47 coccidioidomycosis outbreaks during 1940 to 2015 revealed that 25 (53%) were associated with occupational exposures, including the military, construction, archaeology or other field studies, and laboratory activities.[62] Clusters of infections have also been found among employees and inmates at state prisons located in endemic areas.[11,63] Another paper reviewed 4 occupational coccidioidomycosis outbreaks from 2007 to 2014 in California, involving construction workers in several excavation projects and an outdoor filming event involving cast and crew.[64] It is important that health care providers consider a diagnosis of coccidioidomycosis in patients who live or work in or have traveled to areas with known geographic risk for *Coccidioides*.

The 4 occupational outbreaks in California illustrated multiple factors that facilitated transmission, including operating heavy equipment without enclosed cabs or closed windows, inconsistent soil-wetting practices, little or no risk communication to workers, and infrequent use of respiratory protection.[64] Reducing the risk of coccidioidomycosis among workers in endemic areas can be accomplished through the hierarchy of controls approach (see **Table 1**).[64] However, the efficacy of engineering and administrative methods in preventing infection can be difficult to measure.[62] In addition, prevention can be challenging because of the limited understanding of the distribution of *Coccidioides* spp in the environment, the effect of weather patterns, and the effectiveness of environmental mitigation efforts and respiratory protection.[54,62] In 2019, the state of California passed a bill requiring construction employers in highly endemic areas to provide awareness training on coccidioidomycosis for employees.[65]

PSITTACOSIS

Psittacosis refers to human infection by the bacteria *Chlamydia psittaci*. Psittacosis is most commonly associated with atypical pneumonia but can cause manifestations in multiple organ systems, including hepatic, central nervous system, cardiac, renal, and rheumatic disease.[66] Patients may develop mild illness with abrupt onset of fever, chills, headache, malaise, and myalgia after an incubation period of 5 to 14 days.[67] Dry cough is often present. Although rare, severe illness can occur.[68] *C psittaci* can infect birds, humans, and other mammals; most human infections occur from exposure to infected birds, such as psittacines, pigeons, or poultry.[69] Eighteen psittacosis outbreaks were investigated by the CDC's Epidemic Intelligence Service officers during 1946 to 2005. Of those, pet psittacine birds and turkeys were identified as frequent causes of outbreaks, affecting psittacine bird handlers and workers in turkey-processing plants.[70]

C psittaci is transmitted to humans through inhalation of aerosolized dried droppings or secretions of infected birds.[67] Transmission can also occur through direct contact with feathers, tissues, secretions of infected birds, or by mouth-to-beak contact.[67,69] Human-to-human transmission has been reported but is thought to be rare.[68] Workers in occupations that involve contact with live birds or bird carcasses, such as veterinarians,[71] bird breeders,[72] poultry handlers,[14,73,74] and pet shop workers[75] are at increased risk of infection. Prevention can be challenging, as infected birds may be asymptomatic or have few signs of illness.[69] Stress factors, such as transportation, relocation, crowding, injury, and illness may exacerbate shedding from infected birds.[67,76] In addition, workers who develop psittacosis may remain undiagnosed because symptoms are often mild and nonspecific and patients may not seek medical care. Moreover, the widely available serologic test for psittacosis diagnosis requires acute and convalescent serum samples collected a few weeks apart, and can cross-react with other *Chlamydia* species.[67] Currently in the United States, a real-time polymerase chain reaction assay for human specimens (more sensitive and specific than serology) is only available at CDC.[67] Psittacosis is a reportable condition in most jurisdictions in the United States, and cases are voluntarily reported to CDC. However, during 2008 to 2017, only 60 cases (6 cases per year on average) were reported,[77] which likely represents under detection.

Exposure to *C psittaci* in the workplace varies by occupation. The OSHA does not have a workplace standard for *C psittaci* exposure[78]; however, professional organizations provide recommendations to prevent transmission to humans.[67] Basic principles can be categorized following a hierarchy of controls to prevent occupational exposures to *C psittaci* (see **Table 1**). These include quarantine procedures of newly acquired birds or birds exposed to ill birds and other animal husbandry practices.

A REEMERGING OCCUPATIONAL RESPIRATORY INFECTION

Several studies have shown increased risk of pneumonia (defined as bacterial, lobar, and pneumococcal) and mortality among welders and other workers exposed to metal fumes and mineral dusts.[79–84] A recent review demonstrated that the median population attributable fraction was 10% for the occupational burden of pneumonia. The review also demonstrated that metal fumes/welding exposures had a median occupational attributable fraction of community-acquired pneumonia of 52% in cohort studies.[4] Several hypotheses have been posed that might explain this increased occupational risk. Theories have included that metal fumes (or iron) act as a growth nutrient for bacteria, enhance the binding of bacteria to lung tissues, or impair immune responses in the lung through oxidative stress.[79,83–85] Therefore, it is hypothesized that the occupational risk of this infection is not primarily from exposures to the pathogen at work but rather that the occupational exposure (metal fumes) is a risk factor for infection and subsequent disease. While further research is needed to establish this association and quantify the dose response relationship, a preventive approach using the hierarchy of controls has already been implemented at workplaces and corporations in some countries, including the United Kingdom. Engineering controls have consisted of methods to minimize fume inhalation through local exhaust ventilation. Administrative measures have included offering welders the 23-valent pneumococcal polysaccharide vaccination and cleaning workpieces to remove contaminants before welding.[86,87]

AN EMERGING OCCUPATIONAL RESPIRATORY INFECTION

In the United States, SARS-CoV-2, the novel coronavirus that causes COVID-19, was first detected during January 2020.[88] Since then, more than 2.1 million cases have been reported in the United States, including more than 116,000 associated deaths as of June 17, 2020.[89]

Data suggest that close-range aerosol transmission by droplet is the primary mode of transmission.[90] However, contact transmission is also possible following self-delivery to the eyes, nose, or mouth.[90] Transmission by asymptomatic and presymptomatic individuals has been described.[91–93]

In their occupational risk pyramid similar to the one for influenza, OSHA has divided jobs into 4 risk exposure levels for COVID-19: very high, high, medium, and lower risk. These categories are based on the industry type and the need for contact within 6 feet of people with suspected or confirmed COVID-19[94] and form the basis of recommendations for preventing transmission in the workplace. Health care personnel are considered to be at very high or high risk of exposure.[94] Characteristics of health care personnel with COVID-19 reported to CDC from February 12 to April 9 have been summarized.[95] As of June 17, more than 78,000 COVID-19 cases and 422 deaths have been reported among health care personnel.[89] In the first several months of the COVID-19 pandemic, COVID-19 outbreaks occurred in several types of medium-risk and high-risk workplaces, including long-term care facilities, meatpacking plants, correctional facilities, and homeless shelters.[93,96–99] Efforts to characterize the occupational burden of COVID-19 are ongoing, and prevention measures in workplaces have emphasized the use of engineering and administrative controls and PPE.

SUMMARY

Emerging and reemerging work-related infectious diseases will continue to threaten workers' health. It is important for clinicians to recognize that respiratory infections can be occupationally related. Communication and cooperation between clinicians and public health practitioners is important to identify work-related clusters of respiratory infections. Considering occupational risk factors and controlling exposures among workers according to the hierarchy of controls will help prevent disease transmission in the workplace.

DISCLOSURE

The authors have nothing to disclose.

REFERENCES

1. Brown CK. A call for improved occupational surveillance for measles in the United States. Am J Infect Control 2019;47(12):1519–20.
2. Suwantarat N, Apisarnthanarak A. Risks to health-care workers with emerging diseases: lessons from MERS-CoV, Ebola, SARS, and avian flu. Curr Opin Infect Dis 2015;28(4):349–61.
3. Ho PL, Becker CM, Chan-Yeung M. Emerging occupational lung infections. Int J Tuberc Lung Dis 2005; 11:710–21.
4. Blanc PD, Annesi-Maesano I, Balmes JR, et al. The occupational burden of nonmalignant respiratory diseases. an official American Thoracic Society and European Respiratory Society statement. Am J Respir Crit Care Med 2019;199(11): 1312–34.
5. Trajman A, Menzies D. Occupational respiratory infections. Curr Opin Pulm Med 2010;16(3):226–34.
6. Su CP, de Perio MA, Cummings KJ, et al. Case investigations of infectious diseases occurring in workplaces, United States, 2006–2015. Emerg Infect Dis 2019;25(3):397–405.
7. Raterman SM. Methods of control. In: Plog B, editor. Fundamentals of industrial hygiene. Itasca (IL): National Safety Council; 2000. p. 585–605.
8. National Institute for Occupational Safety and Health. Health hazard evaluations (HHEs) 2019. Available at: https://www.cdc.gov/niosh/hhe/default.html. Accessed: January 6, 2020.
9. Jackson DA, Mailer K, Porter KA, et al. Challenges in assessing transmission of *Mycobacterium tuberculosis* in long-term-care facilities. Am J Infect Control 2015;43(9):992–6.
10. de Perio MA, Niemeier RT. Evaluation of exposure to tuberculosis among employees at a medical center. J Occup Environ Hyg 2014;11(6):D63–8.
11. Murphree R, Warkentin JV, Dunn JR, et al. Elephant-to-human transmission of tuberculosis, 2009. Emerg Infect Dis 2011;17(3):366–71.
12. de Perio MA, Brueck SE, Mueller CA, et al. Evaluation of 2009 pandemic influenza A (H1N1) exposures and illness among physicians in training. Am J Infect Control 2012;40(7):617–21.
13. de Perio MA, Niemeier RT, Burr GA. *Coccidioides* exposure and coccidioidomycosis among prison employees, California, United States. Emerg Infect Dis 2015;21(6):1031–3.
14. Shaw KA, Szablewski CM, Kellner S, et al. Psittacosis outbreak among workers at chicken slaughter plants, Virginia and Georgia, USA, 2018. Emerg Infect Dis 2019;25:2143–5.
15. National Tuberculosis Controllers Association, Centers for Disease Control and Prevention (CDC). Guidelines for the investigation of contacts of persons with infectious tuberculosis. MMWR Recomm Rep 2005;54(RR-15):1–47.
16. Jereb J, Etkind SC, Joglar OT, et al. Tuberculosis contact investigations: outcomes in selected areas of the United States, 1999. Int J Tuberc Lung Dis 2003;7:S384–90.
17. Centers for Disease Control and Prevention. Targeted tuberculin testing and treatment of latent

tuberculosis infection. MMWR Recomm Rep 2000; 49(RR-6):1–51.
18. Borisov AS, Bamrah Morris S, Njie GJ, et al. Update of recommendations for use of once-weekly isoniazid-rifapentine regimen to treat latent *Mycobacterium tuberculosis* infection. MMWR Morb Mortal Wkly Rep 2018;67:723–6.
19. World Health Organization. Global tuberculosis report 2019. Geneva (IL): World Health Organization; 2019. Licence: CC BY-NC-SA 3.0 IGO.
20. Centers for Disease Control and Prevention. Reported tuberculosis in the United States, 2018. Atlanta (GA): U.S. Department of Health and Human Services, CDC; 2019.
21. US Preventive Services Task Force. Screening for latent tuberculosis infection in adults: US preventive services task force recommendation statement. JAMA 2016;316(9):962–9.
22. Lewinsohn DM, Leonard MK, LoBue PA, et al. Official American Thoracic Society/Infectious Diseases Society of America/Centers for Disease Control and Prevention clinical practice guidelines: diagnosis of tuberculosis in adults and children. Clin Infect Dis 2017;64(2):e1–33.
23. Sewell DL. Laboratory-associated infections and biosafety. Clin Microbiol Rev 1995;8(3):389–405.
24. Lambert LA, Armstrong LR, Lobato MN, et al. Tuberculosis in jails and prisons: United States, 2002-2013. Am J Public Health 2016;106(12):2231–7.
25. Centers for Disease Control and Prevention. Tuberculosis outbreak associated with a homeless shelter—Kane County, Illinois, 2007-2011. MMWR Morb Mortal Wkly Rep 2012;61(11):186–9.
26. Zlot A, Vines J, Nystrom L, et al. Diagnosis of tuberculosis in three zoo elephants and a human contact—Oregon, 2013. MMWR Morb Mortal Wkly Rep 2016;64(52):1398–402.
27. Jensen PA, Lambert LA, Iademarco MF, et al. Guidelines for preventing the transmission of *Mycobacterium tuberculosis* in health-care settings, 2005. MMWR Recomm Rep 2005;54(RR-17):1–141.
28. Sosa LE, Njie GJ, Lobato MN, et al. Tuberculosis screening, testing, and treatment of U.S. health care personnel: recommendations from the national tuberculosis controllers association and CDC, 2019. MMWR Morb Mortal Wkly Rep 2019;68(19):439–43.
29. Borkenhagen LK, Salman MD, Ma MJ, et al. Animal influenza virus infections in humans: a commentary. Int J Infect Dis 2019;88:113–9.
30. Rolfes MA, Foppa IM, Garg S, et al. Annual estimates of the burden of seasonal influenza in the United States: a tool for strengthening influenza surveillance and preparedness. Influenza Other Respir Viruses 2018;12(1):132–7.
31. Tokars JI, Olsen SJ, Reed C. Seasonal incidence of symptomatic influenza in the United States. Clin Infect Dis 2018;66(10):1511–8.
32. Grohskopf LA, Alyanak E, Broder KR, et al. Prevention and control of seasonal influenza with vaccines: recommendations of the advisory committee on immunization practices—United States, 2019–20 influenza season. MMWR Recomm Rep 2019;68(3): 1–21.
33. Lietz J, Westermann C, Nienhaus A, et al. The occupational risk of influenza A (H1N1) infection among healthcare personnel during the 2009 pandemic: a systematic review and meta-analysis of observational studies. PLoS One 2016;11(8):e0162061.
34. Centers for Disease Control and Prevention. Immunization of health-care personnel. Recommendations of the Advisory Committee on Immunization Practices (ACIP). MMWR Recomm Rep 2011;60(7):1–45.
35. Litchfield SM. A new occupational safety and health administration directive regarding H1N1 influenza in the workplace. AAOHN J 2010;58(1):3–4.
36. Black CL, Yue X, Ball SW, et al. Influenza vaccination coverage among health care personnel—United States, 2017–18 influenza season. MMWR Morb Mortal Wkly Rep 2018;67(38):1050–4.
37. Wise ME, De Perio M, Halpin J, et al. Transmission of pandemic (H1N1) 2009 influenza to healthcare personnel in the United States. Clin Infect Dis 2011;52(Suppl 1):S198–204.
38. de Perio MA, Yue X, Laney AS, et al. Agreement with employer influenza vaccination requirements among us healthcare personnel during the 2016–2017 season. Infect Control Hosp Epidemiol 2018;39(8):1019–20.
39. Pitts SI, Maruthur NM, Millar KR, et al. A systematic review of mandatory influenza vaccination in healthcare personnel. Am J Prev Med 2014;47(3):330–40.
40. Maurer J, Harris KM, Black CL, et al. Support for seasonal influenza vaccination requirements among US healthcare personnel. Infect Control Hosp Epidemiol 2012;33(3):213–21.
41. Stewart AM, Caplan A, Cox MA, et al. Mandatory vaccination of health-care personnel: good policy, law, and outcomes. Jurimetrics 2013;53(3):341–59.
42. Quan K, Tehrani DM, Dickey L, et al. Voluntary to mandatory: evolution of strategies and attitudes toward influenza vaccination of healthcare personnel. Infect Control Hosp Epidemiol 2012;33(1):63–70.
43. Randall LH, Curran EA, Omer SB. Legal considerations surrounding mandatory influenza vaccination for healthcare workers in the United States. Vaccine 2013;31(14):1771–6.
44. Smith JD, MacDougall CC, Johnstone J, et al. Effectiveness of N95 respirators versus surgical masks in protecting health care workers from acute respiratory infection: a systematic review and meta-analysis. CMAJ 2016;188(8):567–74.
45. Radonovich LJ Jr, Simberkoff MS, Bessesen MT, et al. N95 respirators vs medical masks for preventing influenza among health care personnel: a randomized clinical trial. JAMA 2019;322(9):824–33.

46. MacIntyre CR, Chughtai AA, Rahman B, et al. The efficacy of medical masks and respirators against respiratory infection in healthcare workers. Influenza Other Respir Viruses 2017;11(6):511–7.
47. Offeddu V, Yung CF, Low MSF, et al. Effectiveness of masks and respirators against respiratory infections in healthcare workers: a systematic review and meta-analysis. Clin Infect Dis 2017;65(11):1934–42.
48. Webster RG, Sharp GB, Claas EC. Interspecies transmission of influenza viruses. Am J Respir Crit Care Med 1995;152(4 Pt 2):S25–30.
49. Myers KP, Olsen CW, Gray GC. Cases of swine influenza in humans: a review of the literature. Clin Infect Dis 2007;44(8):1084–8.
50. Myers KP, Olsen CW, Setterquist SF, et al. Are swine workers in the United States at increased risk of infection with zoonotic influenza virus? Clin Infect Dis 2006;42(1):14–20.
51. Poirot E, Levine MZ, Russell K, et al. Detection of avian influenza A(H7N2) virus infection among animal shelter workers using a novel serological approach—New York City, 2016–2017. J Infect Dis 2019;219(11):1688–96.
52. Lee CT, Slavinski S, Schiff C, et al. Influenza A(H7N2) response team. Outbreak of influenza A(H7N2) among cats in an animal shelter with cat-to-human transmission—New York City, 2016. Clin Infect Dis 2017;65(11):1927–9.
53. Galgiani JN, Ampel NM, Blair JE, et al. 2016 Infectious Diseases Society of America (IDSA) clinical practice guideline for the treatment of coccidioidomycosis. Clin Infect Dis 2016;63(6):e112–46.
54. Benedict K, McCotter OZ, Brady S, et al. Surveillance for coccidioidomycosis—United States, 2011–2017. MMWR Surveill Summ 2019;68(7):1–15.
55. Galgiani JN, Ampel NM, Blair JE, et al. Coccidioidomycosis. Clin Infect Dis 2005;41(9):1217–23.
56. McCotter OZ, Benedict K, Engelthaler DM, et al. Update on the epidemiology of coccidioidomycosis in the United States. Med Mycol 2019;57:S30–40.
57. Tsang CA, Anderson SM, Imholte SB, et al. Enhanced surveillance of coccidioidomycosis, Arizona, USA, 2007–2008. Emerg Infect Dis 2010;16(11):1738–44.
58. Baron EJ, Miller JM. Bacterial and fungal infections among diagnostic laboratory workers: evaluating the risks. Diagn Microbiol Infect Dis 2008;60(3):241–6.
59. Stevens DA, Clemons KV, Levine HB, et al. Expert opinion: what to do when there is coccidioides exposure in a laboratory. Clin Infect Dis 2009;49(6):919–23.
60. Laniado-Laborin R. Expanding understanding of epidemiology of coccidioidomycosis in the western hemisphere. Ann N Y Acad Sci 2007;1111:19–34.
61. Das R, McNary J, Fitzsimmons K, et al. Occupational coccidioidomycosis in California: outbreak investigation, respirator recommendations, and surveillance findings. J Occup Environ Med 2012;54(5):564–71.
62. Freedman M, Jackson BR, McCotter O, et al. Coccidioidomycosis outbreaks, United States and worldwide, 1940–2015. Emerg Infect Dis 2018;24(3):417–23.
63. Pappagianis D, Coccidioidomycosis Serology Laboratory. Coccidioidomycosis in California state correctional institutions. Ann N Y Acad Sci 2007;1111:103–11.
64. de Perio MA, Materna BL, Sondermeyer Cooksey GL, et al. Occupational coccidioidomycosis surveillance and recent outbreaks in California. Med Mycol 2019;57(Supplement_1):S41–5.
65. State of California. Assembly Bill No. 203. Available at: https://leginfo.legislature.ca.gov/faces/billTextClient.xhtml?bill_id=201920200AB203. Accessed: June 15, 2020.
66. Basarab M, Macrae MB, Curtis CM. Atypical pneumonia. Curr Opin Pulm Med 2014;20:247–51.
67. Balsamo G, Maxted AM, Midla JW, et al. Compendium of measures to control *Chlamydia psittaci* infection among humans (psittacosis) and pet birds (avian chlamydiosis), 2017. J Avian Med Surg 2017;31:262–82.
68. Wallensten A, Fredlund H, Runehagen A. Multiple human-to-human transmission from a severe case of psittacosis, Sweden, January–February 2013. Euro Surveill 2014;19:20937.
69. Geens T, Dewitte A, Boon N, et al. Development of a *Chlamydophila psittaci* species-specific and genotype-specific real-time PCR. Vet Res 2005;36:787–97.
70. Hadler SC, Castro KG, Dowdle W, et al. Epidemic intelligence service investigations of respiratory illness, 1946–2005. Am J Epidemiol 2011;174:S36–46.
71. Heddema ER, van Hannen EJ, Duim B, et al. An outbreak of psittacosis due to *Chlamydophila psittaci* genotype A in a veterinary teaching hospital. J Med Microbiol 2006;55:1571–5.
72. Vanrompay D, Harkinezhad T, van de Walle M, et al. *Chlamydophila psittaci* transmission from pet birds to humans. Emerg Infect Dis 2007;13:1108–10.
73. Vorimore F, Thebault A, Poisson S, et al. *Chlamydia psittaci* in ducks: a hidden health risk for poultry workers. Pathog Dis 2015;73:1–9.
74. Centers for Disease Control and Prevention. Psittacosis at a turkey processing plant—North Carolina, 1989. MMWR Morb Mortal Wkly Rep 1990;39:460–1.
75. Maegawa N, Emoto T, Mori H, et al. Two cases of *Chlamydia psittaci* infection occurring in employees of the same pet shop. Nihon Kokyuki Gakkai Zasshi 2001;39:753–7.

76. Longbottom D, Coulter LJ. Animal chlamydioses and zoonotic implications. J Comp Pathol 2003; 128:217–44.
77. Centers for Disease Control and Prevention. MMWR: summary of notifiable infectious diseases. Available at: https://www.cdc.gov/mmwr/mmwr_nd/index.html. Accessed September 8, 2020.
78. Occupational Safety and Health Administration. OSHA hazard information bulletins contracting occupationally related psittacosis. United States Department of Labor; 1994. Available at: https://www.osha.gov/dts/hib/hib_data/hib19940808.html. Accessed September 8, 2020.
79. Torén K, Blanc PD, Naidoo RN, et al. Occupational exposure to dust and to fumes, work as a welder and invasive pneumococcal disease risk. Occup Environ Med 2020;77(2):57–63.
80. Koh DH, Moon KT, Kim JY, et al. The risk of hospitalisation for infectious pneumonia in mineral dust exposed industries. Occup Environ Med 2011; 68(2):116–9.
81. Torén K, Qvarfordt I, Bergdahl IA, et al. Increased mortality from infectious pneumonia after occupational exposure to inorganic dust, metal fumes and chemicals. Thorax 2011;66(11):992–6.
82. Wong A, Marrie TJ, Garg S, et al, SPAT Group. Welders are at increased risk for invasive pneumococcal disease. Int J Infect Dis 2010;14(9):e796–9.
83. Palmer KT, Cullinan P, Rice S, et al. Mortality from infectious pneumonia in metal workers: a comparison with deaths from asthma in occupations exposed to respiratory sensitisers. Thorax 2009;64(11):983–6.
84. Marongiu A, Hasan O, Ali, et al. Are welders more at risk of respiratory infections? Findings from a cross-sectional survey and analysis of medical records in shipyard workers: the WELSHIP project. Thorax 2016;71(7):601–6.
85. Coggon D, Harris EC, Cox V, et al. Pneumococcal vaccination for welders. Thorax 2015;70(2):198–9.
86. Donoghue AM, Wesdock JC. Pneumococcal vaccination for welders: global deployment within a multi-national corporation. Am J Ind Med 2019; 62(1):69–73.
87. Palmer KT, Cosgrove M. Vaccinating welders against pneumonia. Occup Environ Med 2012; 69(12):932.
88. Holshue ML, DeBolt C, Lindquist S, et al. First case of 2019 novel coronavirus in the United States. N Engl J Med 2020;382(10):929–36.
89. Centers for Disease Control and Prevention. Coronavirus disease 2019 (COVID-19): cases in the U.S. Available at: https://www.cdc.gov/coronavirus/2019-ncov/cases-updates/cases-in-us.html. Accessed June 16, 2020.
90. Jayaweera M, Perera H, Gunawardana B, et al. Transmission of COVID-19 virus by droplets and aerosols: a critical review on the unresolved dichotomy. Environ Res 2020;188:109819.
91. Huff HV, Singh A. Asymptomatic transmission during the COVID-19 pandemic and implications for public health strategies. Clin Infect Dis 2020. https://doi.org/10.1093/cid/ciaa654.
92. Wei WE, Li Z, Chiew CJ, et al. Presymptomatic transmission of SARS-CoV-2—Singapore, January 23–March 16, 2020. MMWR Morb Mortal Wkly Rep 2020;69(14):411–5.
93. Kimball A, Hatfield KM, Arons M, et al. Asymptomatic and presymptomatic SARS-CoV-2 infections in residents of a long-term care skilled nursing facility—King County, Washington, March 2020. MMWR Morb Mortal Wkly Rep 2020;69(13):377–81.
94. Occupational Safety and Health Administration. COVID-19: hazard recognition. Available at: https://www.osha.gov/SLTC/covid-19/hazardrecognition.html. Accessed: June 16, 2020.
95. CDC COVID-19 Response Team. Characteristics of health care personnel with COVID-19—United States, February 12–April 9, 2020. MMWR Morb Mortal Wkly Rep 2020;69(15):477–81.
96. Dyal JW, Grant MP, Broadwater K, et al. COVID-19 among workers in meat and poultry processing facilities—19 States, April 2020. MMWR Morb Mortal Wkly Rep 2020;69(18).
97. Wallace M, Hagan L, Curran KG, et al. COVID-19 in correctional and detention facilities—United States, February–April 2020. MMWR Morb Mortal Wkly Rep 2020;69(19):587–90.
98. Mosites E, Parker EM, Clarke KEN, et al. Assessment of SARS-CoV-2 infection prevalence in homeless shelters—four U.S. Cities, March 27–April 15, 2020. MMWR Morb Mortal Wkly Rep 2020;69(17): 521–2.
99. McMichael TM, Clark S, Pogosjans S, et al. COVID-19 in a long-term care facility—King County, Washington, February 27–March 9, 2020. MMWR Morb Mortal Wkly Rep 2020;69(12):339–42.

Update on Climate Change

Its Impact on Respiratory Health at Work, Home, and at Play

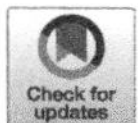

Hari M. Shankar, MD[a,*], Mary B. Rice, MD, MPH[b]

KEYWORDS

• Global warming • Climate change • Air pollution • PM2.5 • Extreme weather • Wildfires • Children

KEY POINTS

- Climate change affects respiratory health in several ways.
- Children, elderly patients, and those with lung disease are particularly vulnerable.
- At-risk individuals should stay indoors or use protective equipment during days with high air pollution.
- There is a grave need for a rapid transition to clean energy in order to protect lung health.

HOW IS CLIMATE CHANGE RELEVANT TO PULMONARY MEDICINE?

There is no dispute among climate scientists that the Earth's climate system is warming due to emissions of carbon dioxide (CO_2) and other greenhouse gases.[1] As early as 1896, it was known that atmospheric CO_2 increases ground temperatures by trapping infrared radiation from the planet's surface, a phenomenon now known as the greenhouse effect.[2] CO_2 levels have increased dramatically in concert with industrialization and continue to increase at alarming rates due to human activities, resulting in more frequent heat waves, droughts, storms, floods, wildfires, and worsening air quality, among other consequences. Climate change already affects the health of people of all ages, in every part of the world, and without rapid intervention, it will imperil the health of the next generation.[3]

Climate change is of particular concern to patients with chronic lung disease (CLD) because these patients are especially susceptible to extreme heat, pollen, wildfire smoke, and photochemical smog—each of which is intensified by climate change. A 2015 survey of American Thoracic Society members found that most had already observed symptoms among their patients that they attributed to climate change.[4] For example, 77% of respondents noted increases in the severity of chronic illness resulting from spikes in air pollution as a consequence of climate change; 58% noted increases in symptoms of allergic disease; and 48% observed heat-related health effects among patients.[4]

Heat waves are linked to increased hospitalizations among the elderly for a long list of respiratory, infectious, and metabolic conditions that are poorly tolerated in the setting of thermal stress.[5–8] Studies have found that elderly patients with CLD are particularly susceptible to heat-related death.[9] For instance, heat waves are associated with chronic obstructive pulmonary disease (COPD) hospitalization among the elderly[8] and possibly also increased hospitalizations for asthma among children and adults.[10,11] City-dwellers, particularly low-income families, are especially vulnerable to extreme heat because of an urban "heat island" effect.[12]

The intensification of the pollen season is particularly concerning for patients with allergic asthma. Warmer temperatures lengthen the pollen season due to earlier spring blooms and later first frosts

[a] Division of Pulmonary, Allergy and Critical Care, University of Pennsylvania, 3400 Spruce Street, 839 West Gates Building, Philadelphia, PA 19104, USA; [b] Department of Medicine, Beth Israel Deaconess Medical Center, Harvard Medical School, KS/BM23, 330 Brookline Avenue, Boston, MA 02215, USA
* Corresponding author.
E-mail address: hari.shankar@pennmedicine.upenn.edu

Clin Chest Med 41 (2020) 753–761
https://doi.org/10.1016/j.ccm.2020.08.004

in the fall; in fact, between 1995 and 2009, the ragweed season increased by 13 to 27 days above 44°N in the United States.[13] Moreover, higher atmospheric levels of CO_2 have been found to increase the pollen productivity of ragweed.[14,15] These changes in pollen production result in greater over-the-counter allergy medication use[16] as well as more emergency room and outpatient visits for allergic disease.[17,18]

Climate change worsens air quality in several ways. Hot, dry conditions lengthen the wildfire season and lead to more frequent wildfires in many parts of the world. Wildfires result in serious air pollution events that worsen respiratory disease, especially asthma and COPD, both near the fire and more distantly due to the spread of wildfire smoke.[19,20] Higher temperatures promote the formation of ground-level ozone, a respiratory irritant and component of smog, and may also promote higher levels of airborne particulate matter due to increased energy use for cooling.[21]

Climate change results in storms that can interrupt medical supply chains and access to treatment and medications. Warmer temperatures and coastal flooding each promote the formation of mold, which may trigger respiratory symptoms in sensitized patients with asthma. Although the United States ranks first among the world's nations in terms of the frequency of coastal hurricanes, there are many regions of the world that are much less equipped to cope with these natural disasters.[22]

Patients with CLD are especially vulnerable to the effects of climate change. It is therefore important for pulmonologists to recognize these health risks and help their patients anticipate and minimize them. Just as physicians advocated for smoking cessation programs and public smoking bans in eras past, there is a need for physicians to advocate for a rapid transition to clean energy for the sake of respiratory health.

MY PATIENT LIVES IN AN AREA WITH SIGNIFICANT POLLUTION. HOW DOES CLIMATE CHANGE AFFECT AIR QUALITY?

Climate change worsens air quality through multiple mechanisms. In suburban and urban areas, hot temperatures promote the formation of ground-level ozone, a major component of the photochemical smog that is formed through the interactions of nitrogen oxides and volatile organic compounds (VOCs)—both emitted by motor vehicles and fossil fuel burning—in the presence of sunlight. Both sunlight and higher temperatures favor the formation of ozone, and the frequency and intensity of ozone episodes during summer months are projected to increase as a result of increasing temperatures.[23,24] Recent heat waves have been associated with ozone levels that exceed air quality standards.[25] Forecasts in California have concluded that climate-related increases in ozone production could overwhelm and even negate emission reduction efforts, especially in the Los Angeles and the San Francisco areas.[26,27]

Ozone is a respiratory irritant that causes bronchial inflammation and hyperresponsiveness,[28,29] and people with preexisting obstructive lung disease are particularly susceptible to adverse health effects of ozone exposure. Even modest short-term increases in ozone increase the risk of acute care visits and hospitalization for asthma[30–33] and COPD.[34,35] Ozone exposure has also been associated with cough, dyspnea, and deterioration in asthma control, resulting in increased medication use and missed school and work days.[36,37] There is emerging evidence that obesity may increase susceptibility to pulmonary effects of ozone exposure, which is of particular importance, given the increasing prevalence of obesity in many parts of the world.[38,39]

Wildfire smoke poses a major air quality problem that affects populations around the world. Over the last decade, fires have occurred around the world with increasing frequency, duration, and destructive power, notably in Australia, South America, Russia, the United States, and Indonesia.[40] Wildfires are a growing health hazard not just because of longer wildfire seasons but also due to years of fire suppression (and biomass accumulation) and the expanding wildland-urban interface, which places more people at risk of wildfire exposure. Depending on fuel composition, fire temperature, and other factors, wildfire smoke may contain potentially toxic levels of thousands of compounds, including complex hydrocarbons, carbon monoxide (CO), nitrogen oxides, VOCs, particulate matter, and several carcinogens.[19,40] Wildfire smoke exposure increases the risk of respiratory admissions, particularly for exacerbations of asthma and COPD.[6,7] Of particular concern is recent evidence suggesting that, per unit mass, particulate matter from wildland fires may be more toxic to asthmatics than particulate matter from other sources.[41] The health effects of wildfires may vary based on distance from the fire's origin but are not limited to the geographic areas in which they arise: for example, smoke from the 2018 Camp Fire stretched more than 3000 miles, from California to New York.[42]

HOW DOES CLIMATE CHANGE AFFECT THE RESPIRATORY HEALTH OF PEOPLE AT WORK?

The respiratory effects of climate change extend into the workplace. Although workers of all kinds are vulnerable to the temperature and air quality effects of climate change, populations at elevated risk include wildland firefighters (WFs) and those who work outdoors.

WFs are primarily responsible for the suppression of fires driven by natural fuels, such as forests, grasslands, and brush, whereas structural firefighters work in built environments. WFs often must engage in longer firefighting campaigns measured in weeks to or months, compared with their structural counterparts, whose work is often completed in hours or days. Because of the intense physical demands of outdoor firefighting, most WFs do not wear any form of respiratory protective equipment other than a cotton bandana,[43,44] which offers scant protection from smoke inhalation. In addition, the physical exertion of firefighting increases pulmonary ventilation, resulting in substantial smoke inhalation.[44]

A large number of studies have found that both short- and long-term exposure to fine particulate matter from fossil fuel combustion sources is associated with premature cardiopulmonary mortality. Although the literature directly examining the health effects of organic fuel smoke on health is more limited, the evidence suggests that particulate matter originating from the combustion of biomass may be similarly damaging to human health.[45] Wildland firefighting entails intermittent but often prolonged exposures to respirable particles and gases, including CO, suspended particulate matter and respirable particulate matter,[43] as well as other toxins such as formaldehyde and acrolein.[46] Measurements of smoke and particulate exposure from the 1990s and 2000s show that exposure to respirable particulate matter among firefighters is often higher than occupational exposure standards.[44]

Surveys of WFs have shown an increase in respiratory symptoms such as cough, sputum production, and wheezing following smoke exposure.[45] Studies of spirometry after acute smoke exposure have also shown decrements in lung function associated with wildfire smoke exposure.[45] Analysis of sputum samples and bronchoalveolar lavage specimens following smoke exposure have shown an increase in sputum neutrophils, suggesting a state of lung inflammation that may lead to systemic inflammation mediated by alveolar macrophages, lung epithelial cells, neutrophils, and cytokines.[45] However, there is a paucity of studies examining the long-term impacts of vegetation smoke exposure on pulmonary function in WFs.

Although wildfires are a dramatic manifestation of climate change, increasing global temperatures affect health in other ways. In addition to WFs, a variety of workers including those in the construction, maintenance, and agricultural industries spend most of their working hours outdoors, making them vulnerable to wildfire smoke as well as extreme heat and other weather events.[47] Climate change is expected to increase employment in these industries as well as many others, where occupational hazards will be compounded by worsening heat, air pollution, and other safety hazards.[48] It is estimated that 5 to 10 million workers experience unsafe levels of outdoor heat exposure every year in the United States alone.[49] Heat affects health through air pollution and its attendant effects on cardiopulmonary dysfunction and also by causing heatstroke.[50] For instance, ozone concentrations increase in correlation with ambient temperatures, and outdoor workers may have increased exposure to it due to increased pulmonary ventilation rates resulting from physical exertion. One study examining the effects of daily short-term ozone exposure on outdoor farm workers showed lower lung function at the end of each workday,[51] and a study exploring the effects of daily outdoor air exposure showed possible DNA damage in urban outdoor workers in Mexico.[52] Outdoor workers may also be susceptible to other pulmonary effects of climate change, although many of these are not well studied: increased dust concentrations during arid conditions; elevated risk of pulmonary pathogens such as Legionella during warm and humid conditions; and exposure to chemicals and toxins.[49]

ARE CHILDREN VULNERABLE TO CLIMATE CHANGE?

It has been suggested that the life of every child born today will be affected by climate change.[3] Children are especially vulnerable because they are born with only 20% of the lung alveoli that they will eventually develop by adulthood. Compared with adults, children breathe in more air per unit of body weight and generally spend more time outdoors. Therefore, their lungs experience a higher dose of air pollution than adults exposed to the same air.

The high levels of $PM_{2.5}$, VOCs, and gaseous pollutants released by wildfires are very harmful to the respiratory health of children. Acute respiratory effects of wildfire smoke exposure among children include upper respiratory symptoms (including nose, eye, and throat irritation), lower respiratory symptoms (cough, bronchitis, wheeze), and an increased risk of asthma attacks.[53] Although the long-term consequences of repeated wildfire events on child respiratory health are poorly studied, they are likely similar to those of long-term exposure to $PM_{2.5}$ from other sources. Studies of urban pollution have found that $PM_{2.5}$ is associated with decreased lung function in healthy children,[54,55] slower childhood lung growth,[56,57] and aggravated asthma.[58] Long-term $PM_{2.5}$ exposure may increase the risk of developing asthma in childhood.[59,60] Children experience similar dangers from exposure to ground-level ozone, with elevated risks of developing asthma (among ozone-exposed children who exercise outdoors),[61] asthma attacks, and hospitalizations for pneumonia and other causes.[62–66] It has been estimated that climate-related increases in ozone may increase summer ozone-related asthma emergency department visits for children by 7.3% across the New York City metropolitan region by the 2020s compared with the 1990s.[67]

Impaired respiratory health during childhood can have long-term consequences for adult lung function,[68] and it is likely that some of the pulmonary effects of early life pollution exposure are irreversible. The need to protect children's respiratory health adds to the urgency of eliminating fossil fuel combustion.

HOW DO STORMS AND OTHER EXTREME WEATHER EVENTS AFFECT MY PATIENT WITH CHRONIC LUNG DISEASE?

One of the most dramatic manifestations of climate change is an increase in the number of extreme weather events (EWE), including longer and more intense heat waves,[69] stronger and slower-moving hurricanes,[70] intensified flooding, more damaging winter storms, as well as increased downpours and droughts.[71] Such events are particularly devastating for the poor, the elderly, children, and patients with CLD, as their physiologic vulnerability puts them at disproportionate risk for morbidity and mortality.[72] This vulnerability depends both on their physiologic status and on structural and geographic factors that influence access to health care.

Flooding, storms, and droughts can promote the growth and transmission of microorganisms and vectors in unpredictable ways, depending on the specific infectious organism, local ecology, and human factors. Several historical examples show the potential for increased respiratory illness after natural disasters. For example, the extensive flooding that occurred after Hurricanes Rita and Katrina in Louisiana in 2005 caused heavy indoor mold growth, with levels of fungal antigens commensurate with agricultural environments,[73] at concentrations concerning for adverse respiratory effects. Increased ambient temperatures and atmospheric CO_2 levels may likewise encourage the growth of mold like *Alternaria*, a species associated with allergies and asthma.[14] In addition to driving microbial growth, EWEs may also increase the transmission of infectious diseases because of overcrowded conditions, food shortages, and malnutrition, as well as reduced access to medical care and other infrastructure deficits.[74] Epidemiologic studies performed in Mozambique and India[74] found an increased rate of respiratory infections after flooding in those countries in the early 2000s, and a Bangladeshi study showed that respiratory infections were responsible for nearly 13% of mortality after a flood there.[75] Overcrowding has been associated with a variety of infectious diseases, including tuberculosis, measles, meningitis, influenza, and diarrheal illnesses, and patients with CLDs such as COPD are more likely to die as a result of severe infections.[76]

EWEs create surges in demand for health care while simultaneously straining the health care system's capacity to provide care. The modern health care system functions across a broad spectrum of inpatient and outpatient settings, which are highly reliant on critical services such as electricity, clean water, and waste disposal.[77] Patients with CLD and other conditions rely on frequent interactions with this system, but climate shocks place this reliance in jeopardy. Powerful storms and floods over the last few decades have laid bare the fragility of America's health care infrastructure in the face of climate shocks. Hurricane Katrina, for instance, resulted the closure of several of New Orleans' hospitals including Tulane Medical Center and its medical school,[78] a setback from which New Orleans took many years to recover. EWEs can disrupt the health care supply chain. For example, Hurricane Maria's devastation of Puerto Rico resulted in an acute shortage of intravenous saline throughout the United States due to a closure of one of the only factories that produced saline bags.[79] Depending on the severity of the weather event, the health system's level of preparedness, local geography, and other factors, EWEs can cause a variety of disruptions to health systems, including facility closures, patient evacuations, outages of electrical and water systems, and by preventing medical staff from reaching their places of work.[78]

Those with CLD are likely more vulnerable to extreme heat due to their limited physiologic reserve, age, or simply their decreased ability to access timely medical care in the setting of extreme heat. During the 2006 heat wave in Europe for example, COPD mortality increased by 5.4% for each 1°C increase in mean temperature.[80,81] Similarly, an analysis of in-hospital mortality in Italy showed that patients with CLD had a more than 2-fold increased odds of death with a 10°C increase in ambient outdoor temperature.[9] Heat stress may lower the threshold for bronchoconstriction, and inhalation of dust particles, such as during droughts or dust storms, may interfere with pulmonary endothelial cell signaling.[82] These effects may be accentuated and poorly tolerated in those with CLD and highlight the importance of bolstering communities and health systems against the future effects of climate change.

HOW SHOULD I COUNSEL MY PATIENTS TO BEST PREVENT OR ADAPT TO THE ANTICIPATED RESPIRATORY EFFECTS OF CLIMATE CHANGE?

Climate change has potentially serious consequences for all patients and particularly for those with CLD. Although none of these effects are entirely avoidable, there are measures that patients can take to adapt to the changing climate and protect themselves from some of its consequences.

Even low levels of fine particulate air pollution in the United States has been shown to carry significant health risks, particularly for those with chronic respiratory or cardiovascular disease.[81] Patients should be counseled to take pragmatic measures, by staying indoors during wildfires and other periods of poor air quality; avoiding smoking or other activities that generate indoor air pollution; and shutting off devices that circulate polluted outdoor air into the house, such as evaporative coolers or fresh-air ventilation systems.[40] Clinicians practicing in urban or suburban settings where summertime ozone levels often exceed US Environmental Protection Agency (EPA) standards can counsel their patients to minimize the health effects of ozone exposure. The EPA maintains an up-to-date Air Quality Index online (www.airnow.gov/), allowing patients to look up air quality in their region based on EPA monitoring data. If avoidance of polluted air is impossible, use of an N95 or N100 particulate respirator, available at many hardware stores and pharmacies, may also provide protection to the vulnerable patient.[40] Air filtration systems are also recommended to reduce exposure to particular matter and other harmful airborne biological contaminants. Indoor air filtration using high-efficiency particulate air (HEPA) filters can be provided by the house's heating, ventilation, and air conditioning system, by portable room air cleaners or both,[83] and deserve particular consideration.

A growing body of literature suggests that HEPA filters, which are effective at removing 99.97% of particles 0.3 μm or greater in diameter, can reduce indoor $PM_{2.5}$ with potential improvements in cardiovascular and respiratory health. A meta-analysis suggested that the use of HEPA filters is associated with fewer symptoms among patients with allergies and asthma.[84] Similarly, a trial of air purifier use demonstrated that air purification resulted in a 57% reduction in indoor $PM_{2.5}$, associated with a 17% decrease in the fractional exhaled nitric oxide, a marker of airway inflammation.[85] Studies have also shown cardiovascular benefits of air filtration and decreased $PM_{2.5}$ exposure, including decreased blood pressure[86] and reductions in serum inflammatory biomarkers.[85]

The interaction between air pollution and summer heat waves is especially concerning, as this combination causes excess hospital admissions as well as mortality in patients with CLDs such as COPD and asthma,[80,87] and this is particularly problematic in developed areas due to the urban heat island effect, putting increasing numbers of people at risk for heat-related complications.[88] Studies in the United States indicate that air conditioning serves an important protective role against heat-related mortality and that individuals both at home and in nursing homes are at risk for heat-related complications.[89] It may also be protective for patients with CLD; however, more research is needed to investigate the best ways to mitigate heat stress in other populations, given the cost barriers of air conditioning. Also important to consider is the fact that the long-term use of air conditioning will ultimately perpetuate the cycles that drive climate change.[90]

SUMMARY

Climate change poses a serious threat to the respiratory health of people all over the world, particularly those at extremes of age, workers with outdoor exposure, and patients with chronic respiratory disease. These health effects are mediated by extremes of weather and heat and worsening air quality due to smog formation and the increasing frequency of large wildfires that affect people thousands of miles away.

Although much is known about the interactions between climate change and pulmonary health, much remains to be understood. As global temperatures are projected to continue increasing in the next few decades, more research is needed in order to determine the most effective ways to mitigate the effects of air pollution on chronically ill and vulnerable populations. Above all, drastic action is needed to transition the economy away from its dependence on unhealthy fossil fuel combustion.

DISCLOSURE

The authors have no relevant disclosures.

REFERENCES

1. Stocker TF, Qin D, Plattner M, et al. IPCC, 2013: Climate Change 2013: The Physical Science Basis. Contribution of Working Group I to the Fifth Assessment Report of the Intergovernmental Panel on Climate Change. Cambridge University Press, Cambridge, United Kingdom and New York, NY, USA. p. 1535.
2. Arrhenius S. On the influence of carbonic acid in the air upon the temperature of the ground. Philos Mag J Sci 1896;41(251):237–76.
3. Watts N, Amann M, Arnell N, et al. The 2019 report of the Lancet Countdown on health and climate change: ensuring that the health of a child born today is not defined by a changing climate. Lancet 2019;394(10211):1836–78.
4. Sarfaty M, Bloodhart B, Ewart G, et al. American Thoracic Society member survey on climate change and health. Ann Am Thorac Soc 2015;12(2):274–8.
5. Bhaskaran K, Armstrong B, Hajat S, et al. Heat and risk of myocardial infarction: hourly level case-crossover analysis of MINAP database. BMJ 2012; 345:e8050.
6. Dematte JE, O'Mara K, Buescher J, et al. Near-fatal heat stroke during the 1995 heat wave in Chicago. Ann Intern Med 1998;129(3):173–81.
7. Bobb JF, Obermeyer Z, Wang Y, et al. Cause-specific risk of hospital admission related to extreme heat in older adults. JAMA 2014;312(24):2659.
8. Anderson GB, Dominici F, Wang Y, et al. Heat-related emergency hospitalizations for respiratory diseases in the Medicare population. Am J Respir Crit Care Med 2013;187(10):1098–103.
9. Stafoggia M, Forastiere F, Agostini D, et al. Factors affecting in-hospital heat-related mortality: a multi-city case-crossover analysis. J Epidemiol Community Health 2008;62(3):209–15.
10. Mireku N, Wang Y, Ager J, et al. Changes in weather and the effects on pediatric asthma exacerbations. Ann Allergy Asthma Immunol 2009;103(3):220–4.
11. Lim Y-H, Hong Y-C, Kim H. Effects of diurnal temperature range on cardiovascular and respiratory hospital admissions in Korea. Sci Total Environ 2012; 417-418:55–60.
12. Huang G, Zhou W, Cadenasso ML. Is everyone hot in the city? Spatial pattern of land surface temperatures, land cover and neighborhood socioeconomic characteristics in Baltimore, MD. J Environ Manage 2011;92(7):1753–9.
13. Ziska L, Knowlton K, Rogers C, et al. Recent warming by latitude associated with increased length of ragweed pollen season in central North America. Proc Natl Acad Sci U S A 2011; 108(10):4248–51.
14. Wolf J, O'Neill NR, Rogers CA, et al. Elevated atmospheric carbon dioxide concentrations amplify Alternaria alternata sporulation and total antigen production. Environ Health Perspect 2010;118(9): 1223–8.
15. Wayne P, Foster S, Connolly J, et al. Production of allergenic pollen by ragweed (Ambrosia artemisiifolia L.) is increased in CO2-enriched atmospheres. Ann Allergy Asthma Immunol 2002;88(3): 279–82.
16. Sheffield PE, Weinberger KR, Ito K, et al. The association of tree pollen concentration peaks and allergy medication sales in New York city: 2003-2008. ISRN Allergy 2011;2011:537194.
17. Cakmak S, Dales RE, Burnett RT, et al. Effect of airborne allergens on emergency visits by children for conjunctivitis and rhinitis. Lancet 2002; 359(9310):947–8.
18. Villeneuve PJ, Doiron M-S, Stieb D, et al. Is outdoor air pollution associated with physician visits for allergic rhinitis among the elderly in Toronto, Canada? Allergy 2006;61(6):750–8.
19. Reid CE, Brauer M, Johnston FH, et al. Critical review of health impacts of wildfire smoke exposure. Environ Health Perspect 2016;124(9):1334–43.
20. Delfino RJ, Brummel S, Wu J, et al. The relationship of respiratory and cardiovascular hospital admissions to the southern California wildfires of 2003. Occup Environ Med 2009;66(3):189–97.
21. Ebi Kristie L, McGregor G. Climate change, tropospheric ozone and particulate matter, and health impacts. Environ Health Perspect 2008;116(11): 1449–55.
22. Shultz JM, Russell J, Espinel Z. Epidemiology of tropical cyclones: the dynamics of disaster, disease, and development. Epidemiol Rev 2005;27:21–35.
23. Knowlton K, Rosenthal JE, Hogrefe C, et al. Assessing ozone-related health impacts under a changing climate. Environ Health Perspect 2004;112(15): 1557–63.
24. Murazaki K, Hess P. How does climate change contribute to surface ozone change over the United States? J Geophys Res 2006;111(D5):D05301.
25. Doherty RM, Heal MR, Wilkinson P, et al. Current and future climate- and air pollution-mediated impacts on human health. Environ Health Glob Access Sci Source 2009;8(Suppl 1):S8.

26. Millstein D, Harley R. Impact of climate change on photochemical air pollution in Southern California. Atmos Chem Phys Discuss 2009;9:1561–83.
27. Steiner AL, Tonse S, Cohen RC, et al. Influence of future climate and emissions on regional air quality in California. J Geophys Res 2006;111(D18): D18303.
28. Alexis NE, Lay JC, Hazucha M, et al. Low-level ozone exposure induces airways inflammation and modifies cell surface phenotypes in healthy humans. Inhal Toxicol 2010;22(7):593–600.
29. Song H, Tan W, Zhang X. Ozone induces inflammation in bronchial epithelial cells. J Asthma 2011; 48(1):79–83.
30. Moore K, Neugebauer R, Lurmann F, et al. Ambient ozone concentrations cause increased hospitalizations for asthma in children: an 18-year study in Southern California. Environ Health Perspect 2008; 116(8):1063–70.
31. Glad JA, Brink LL, Talbott EO, et al. The relationship of ambient ozone and PM(2.5) levels and asthma emergency department visits: possible influence of gender and ethnicity. Arch Environ Occup Health 2012;67(2):103–8.
32. Babin S, Burkom H, Holtry R, et al. Medicaid patient asthma-related acute care visits and their associations with ozone and particulates in Washington, DC, from 1994-2005. Int J Environ Health Res 2008;18(3):209–21.
33. Babin SM, Burkom HS, Holtry RS, et al. Pediatric patient asthma-related emergency department visits and admissions in Washington, DC, from 2001-2004, and associations with air quality, socio-economic status and age group. Environ Health Glob Access Sci Source 2007;6:9.
34. Ko FWS, Tam W, Wong TW, et al. Temporal relationship between air pollutants and hospital admissions for chronic obstructive pulmonary disease in Hong Kong. Thorax 2007;62(9):780–5.
35. Brunekreef B, Holgate ST. Air pollution and health. Lancet 2002;360(9341):1233–42.
36. Meng Y-Y, Wilhelm M, Rull RP, et al. Traffic and outdoor air pollution levels near residences and poorly controlled asthma in adults. Ann Allergy Asthma Immunol 2007;98(5):455–63.
37. Jacquemin B, Kauffmann F, Pin I, et al. Air pollution and asthma control in the epidemiological study on the genetics and environment of asthma. J Epidemiol Community Health 2012;66(9): 796–802.
38. Alexeeff SE, Litonjua AA, Suh H, et al. Ozone exposure and lung function: effect modified by obesity and airways hyperresponsiveness in the VA normative aging study. Chest 2007;132(6):1890–7.
39. Shore SA, Rivera-Sanchez YM, Schwartzman IN, et al. Responses to ozone are increased in obese mice. J Appl Physiol 2003;95(3):938–45.
40. Balmes JR. Where there's wildfire, there's smoke. N Engl J Med 2018;378(10):881–3.
41. Deflorio-Barker S, Crooks J, Reyes J, et al. Cardiopulmonary effects of fine particulate matter exposure among older adults, during wildfire and non-wildfire periods, in the United States 2008-2010. Environ Health Perspect 2019. https://doi.org/10.1289/EHP3860.
42. CNN AW. Smoke from the California wildfires is visible across the country in New York City. CNN. Available at: https://www.cnn.com/2018/11/20/us/california-wildfires-new-york-city-trnd/index.html. Accessed December 29, 2019.
43. DHS science and technology directorate: wildland firefighter respiratory protection. Available at: https://www.dhs.gov/sites/default/files/publications/931_R-Tech_Wildland-Firefighter-Respiration-Protection-FactSheet_180606-508.pdf. Accessed December 29, 2019.
44. Naeher LP, Brauer M, Lipsett M, et al. Woodsmoke health effects: a review. Inhal Toxicol 2007;19(1): 67–106.
45. Swiston JR, Davidson W, Attridge S, et al. Wood smoke exposure induces a pulmonary and systemic inflammatory response in firefighters. Eur Respir J 2008;32(1):129–38.
46. Youssouf H, Liousse C, Roblou L, et al. Non-accidental health impacts of wildfire smoke. Int J Environ Res Public Health 2014;11(11):11772–804.
47. Postma J. Protecting outdoor workers from hazards associated with wildfire smoke. Workplace Health Saf 2019. https://doi.org/10.1177/2165079919888516.
48. Roelofs C, Wegman D. Workers: the climate canaries. Am J Public Health 2014;104(10):1799–801.
49. Applebaum KM, Graham J, Gray GM, et al. An overview of occupational risks from climate change. Curr Environ Health Rep 2016;3(1):13–22.
50. Gordon CJ, Johnstone AFM, Aydin C. Thermal stress and toxicity. In: Terjung R, editor. Comprehensive physiology. Hoboken (NJ): John Wiley & Sons, Inc; 2014. p. 995–1016. https://doi.org/10.1002/cphy.c130046.
51. Brauer M, Blair J, Vedal S. Effect of ambient ozone exposure on lung function in farm workers. Am J Respir Crit Care Med 1996;154(4 Pt 1):981–7.
52. Tovalin H, Valverde M, Morandi MT, et al. DNA damage in outdoor workers occupationally exposed to environmental air pollutants. Occup Environ Med 2006;63(4):230–6.
53. Künzli N, Avol E, Wu J, et al. Health effects of the 2003 Southern California wildfires on children. Am J Respir Crit Care Med 2006;174(11):1221–8.
54. Rice MB, Rifas-Shiman SL, Litonjua AA, et al. Lifetime exposure to ambient pollution and lung function in children. Am J Respir Crit Care Med 2016;193(8):881–8.
55. Urman R, McConnell R, Islam T, et al. Associations of children's lung function with ambient air pollution:

joint effects of regional and near-roadway pollutants. Thorax 2014;69(6):540–7.
56. Gauderman WJ, Urman R, Avol E, et al. Association of improved air quality with lung development in children. N Engl J Med 2015;372(10):905–13.
57. Gauderman WJ, Avol E, Gilliland F, et al. The effect of air pollution on lung development from 10 to 18 years of age. N Engl J Med 2004;351(11):1057–67.
58. Slaughter JC, Lumley T, Sheppard L, et al. Effects of ambient air pollution on symptom severity and medication use in children with asthma. Ann Allergy Asthma Immunol 2003;91(4):346–53.
59. Gehring U, Wijga AH, Hoek G, et al. Exposure to air pollution and development of asthma and rhinoconjunctivitis throughout childhood and adolescence: a population-based birth cohort study. Lancet Respir Med 2015;3(12):933–42.
60. Garcia E, Berhane K, Islam T, et al. Association of changes in air quality with incident asthma in children in California, 1993-2014. JAMA 2019;321(19):1906–15.
61. McConnell R, Berhane K, Gilliland F, et al. Asthma in exercising children exposed to ozone: a cohort study. Lancet 2002;359(9304):386–91.
62. Strickland MJ, Klein M, Flanders WD, et al. Modification of the effect of ambient air pollution on pediatric asthma emergency visits: susceptible subpopulations. Epidemiology 2014;25(6):843–50.
63. Strickland MJ, Darrow LA, Klein M, et al. Short-term associations between ambient air pollutants and pediatric asthma emergency department visits. Am J Respir Crit Care Med 2010;182(3):307–16.
64. Gleason JA, Bielory L, Fagliano JA. Associations between ozone, PM2.5, and four pollen types on emergency department pediatric asthma events during the warm season in New Jersey: a case-crossover study. Environ Res 2014;132:421–9.
65. Silverman RA, Ito K. Age-related association of fine particles and ozone with severe acute asthma in New York City. J Allergy Clin Immunol 2010;125(2):367–73.e5.
66. Darrow LA, Klein M, Flanders WD, et al. Air pollution and acute respiratory infections among children 0-4 years of age: an 18-year time-series study. Am J Epidemiol 2014. https://doi.org/10.1093/aje/kwu234.
67. Sheffield PE, Knowlton K, Carr JL, et al. Modeling of regional climate change effects on ground-level ozone and childhood asthma. Am J Prev Med 2011;41(3):251–7 [quiz: A3].
68. McGeachie MJ, Yates KP, Zhou X, et al. Patterns of growth and decline in lung function in persistent childhood asthma. N Engl J Med 2016;374(19):1842–52.
69. Meehl GA, Tebaldi C. More intense, more frequent, and longer lasting heat waves in the 21st century. Science 2004;305(5686):994–7.
70. Shultz J, Sands D, Kossin J, et al. Double environmental injustice — climate change, hurricane dorian, and the Bahamas. N Engl J Med 2020;382(1):1–3.
71. Reidmiller DR, Avery DR, Easterling KE, et al. USGCRP, 2018: Impacts, Risks, and Adaptation in the United States: Fourth National Climate Assessment, Volume II. Washington, DC: U.S. Global Change Research Program; 2018. p. 1515.
72. WHO | Operational framework for building climate resilient health systems. WHO. Available at: http://www.who.int/globalchange/publications/building-climate-resilient-health-systems/en/. Accessed January 5, 2020.
73. Impact of weather and climate change with indoor and outdoor air quality in asthma: a work group report of the AAAAI environmental exposure and respiratory health committee - Journal of Allergy and Clinical Immunology. Available at: https://www.jacionline.org/article/S0091-6749(19)30281-7/fulltext. Accessed January 4, 2020.
74. Kondo H, Seo N, Yasuda T, et al. Post-flood–infectious diseases in Mozambique. Prehosp Disaster Med 2002;17(3):126–33.
75. Mirsaeidi M, Motahari H, Taghizadeh Khamesi M, et al. Climate change and respiratory infections. Ann Am Thorac Soc 2016;13(8):1223–30.
76. Ivers LC, Ryan ET. Infectious diseases of severe weather-related and flood-related natural disasters. Curr Opin Infect Dis 2006;19(5):408–14.
77. Paterson J, Berry P, Ebi K, et al. Health care facilities resilient to climate change impacts. Int J Environ Res Public Health 2014;11(12):13097–116.
78. Guenther R, Balbus J. Primary protection: enhancing health care resiliency for a changing climate. Washington, DC: U.S. Department of Health & Human Services; 2014.
79. Wong JC. Hospitals face critical shortage of IV bags due to Puerto Rico hurricane. The Guardian. 2018. Available at: https://www.theguardian.com/us-news/2018/jan/10/hurricane-maria-puerto-rico-iv-bag-shortage-hospitals. Accessed January 6, 2020.
80. Monteiro A, Carvalho V, Oliveira T, et al. Excess mortality and morbidity during the July 2006 heat wave in Porto, Portugal. Int J Biometeorol 2013;57(1):155–67.
81. Bernstein AS, Rice MB. Lungs in a warming world: climate change and respiratory health. Chest 2013;143(5):1455–9.
82. Ärzteblatt DÄG Redaktion Deutsches. The effects of climate change on patients with chronic lung disease. 2015. Deutsches Ärzteblatt. Available at: https://www.aerzteblatt.de/int/archive/article?id=173351. Accessed January 5, 2020.
83. Sublett JL. Effectiveness of air filters and air cleaners in allergic respiratory diseases: a review of the recent literature. Curr Allergy Asthma Rep 2011;11(5):395–402.

84. McDonald E, Cook D, Newman T, et al. Effect of air filtration systems on asthma: a systematic review of randomized trials. Chest 2002;122(5): 1535–42.
85. Chen R, Zhao A, Chen H, et al. Cardiopulmonary benefits of reducing indoor particles of outdoor origin: a randomized, double-blind crossover trial of air purifiers. J Am Coll Cardiol 2015;65(21): 2279–87.
86. Morishita M, Adar SD, D'Souza J, et al. Effect of portable Air filtration systems on personal exposure to fine particulate matter and blood pressure among residents in a low-income senior facility: a randomized clinical trial. JAMA Intern Med 2018;178(10): 1350–7.
87. Lin S, Luo M, Walker RJ, et al. Extreme high temperatures and hospital admissions for respiratory and cardiovascular diseases. Epidemiology 2009;20(5): 738–46.
88. Lundgren-Kownacki K, Hornyanszky ED, Chu TA, et al. Challenges of using air conditioning in an increasingly hot climate. Int J Biometeorol 2018; 62(3):401–12.
89. Kovats RS, Hajat S. Heat stress and public health: a critical review. Annu Rev Public Health 2008;29: 41–55.
90. McCormack MC, Belli AJ, Waugh D, et al. Respiratory effects of indoor heat and the interaction with air pollution in chronic obstructive pulmonary disease. Ann Am Thorac Soc 2016;13(12):2125–31.

Working in Smoke:
Wildfire Impacts on the Health of Firefighters and Outdoor Workers and Mitigation Strategies

Kathleen Navarro, PhD, MPH

KEYWORDS

• Wildfire • Smoke • Firefighters • Outdoor workers • Particulate matter

KEY POINTS

- Wildland firefighters do not wear respiratory protection while working long hours and can be exposed to elevated concentrations of smoke.
- There is very limited research on long-term health of wildland firefighters from smoke exposure across an entire career.
- New emergency regulations have been enacted in California to protect outdoor workers from wildfire smoke.

INTRODUCTION

During the peak of the 2018 wildfire season, approximately 30,000 personnel including wildland firefighters were mobilized across the United States to suppress wildland fires.[1] Wildland firefighters suppressing wildland fires or conducting prescribed burns work under arduous conditions often for long hours (commonly shifts are 16 hours) and can be exposed to smoke. Wildfire smoke can contain carbon monoxide, benzene, formaldehyde, particulate matter (PM), acrolein, and polycyclic aromatic hydrocarbons (PAHs).[2] Unlike structural firefighters, wildland firefighters do not wear any respiratory protection, as there is no respirator currently available that meets specifications recommended by the National Fire Protection Association.[2] In addition to air contaminants in smoke, wildland firefighters may also be exposed to crystalline silica from soil and ash.[3] As the total number of burned acres has increased, so has the number of lost homes and structures due to the expansion of the wildland-urban interface (WUI), where wildland vegetation and urban areas meet.[4,5] For wildland firefighters working in the WUI, not only are they exposed to wildfire smoke but they may also experience smoke exposure from urban fire sources without the personal protective equipment or decontamination procedures used by structural firefighters.

Wildland firefighters complete a variety of job tasks to suppress fires including operating a fire engine, constructing fireline, holding, mop-up, and firing operations. **Fig. 1** includes photos of some of these job tasks. Engine operators work as a part of an engine crew (3–7 firefighters) and operate the diesel pumps on an engine that provides water to crews working near the fire. Fireline construction involves clearing vegetation (first with chainsaws) and digging or scraping down to mineral soil with hand tools to create a break in burnable vegetation to stop the spread of a fire. Firefighters engaged in holding ensure that the active fire has not crossed the fireline or fuel break. After the fire has been controlled, crews will mop-up the area by extinguishing any burning or smoldering material by digging out the burning material or applying water to stop anything that may re-ignite a fire. Firing operations involve setting an intentional fire, typically with torches filled with a

National Institute for Occupational Safety and Health, Centers for Disease Control and Prevention, 1090 Tusculum Avenue MS 13, Cincinnati, OH, USA
E-mail address: knavarro@cdc.gov

Clin Chest Med 41 (2020) 763–769
https://doi.org/10.1016/j.ccm.2020.08.017
0272-5231/20/Published by Elsevier Inc.

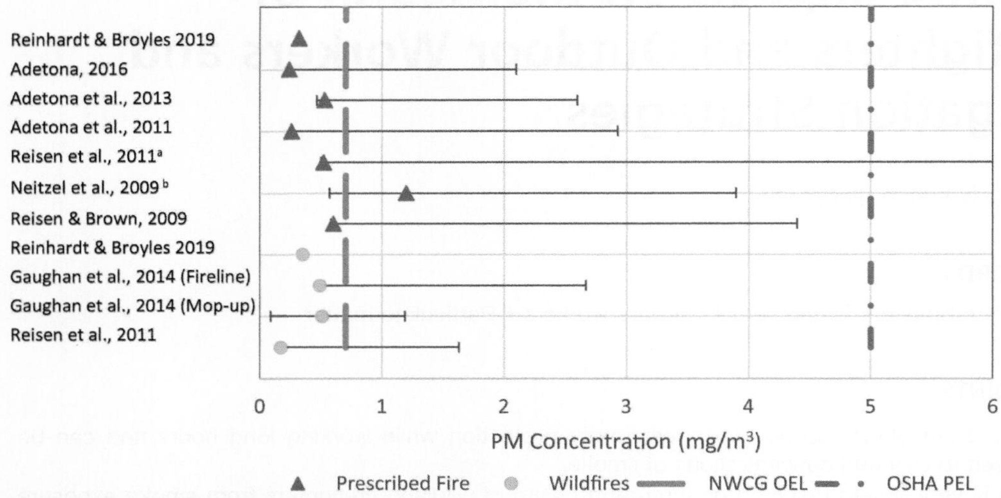

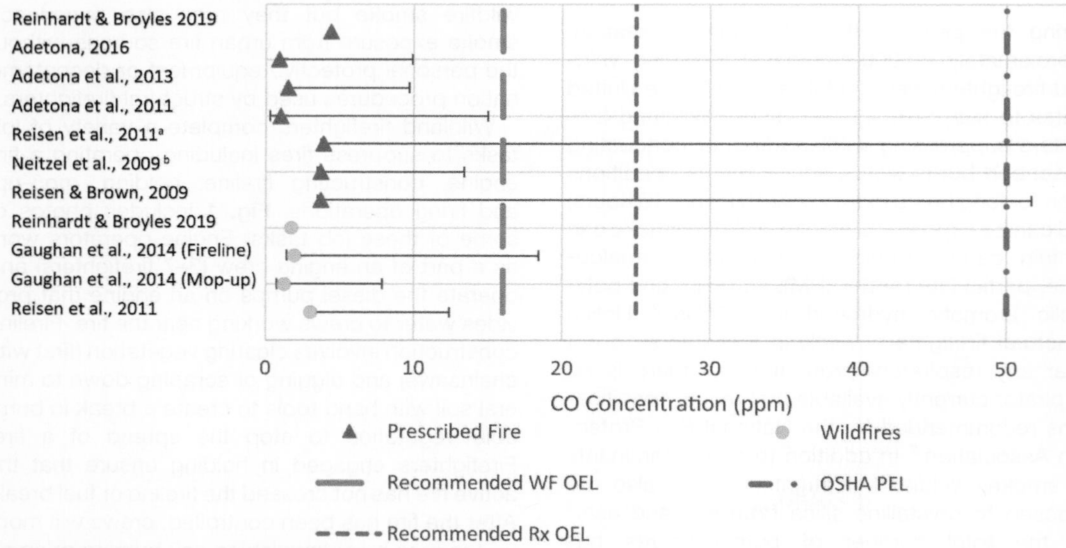

Fig. 1. Summary of PM and carbon monoxide concentrations measured on wildland firefighters in the past 10 years. (*Data from* Refs.[3,9–15])

3:2 diesel/unleaded gasoline mixture, to reduce the available flammable material for the wildfire to consume. Firing, holding and mop-up are common tasks that are performed on prescribed fires as well. In addition, when working on a large wildland fire, firefighters will sleep and eat at a base camp (incident command post) that can be close to the fire and experience exposure to smoke, emissions from vehicles and generators (diesel exhaust), and road dust.

EXPOSURES FACED BY WILDLAND FIREFIGHTERS

Measuring exposure to toxic compounds in smoke for wildland firefighters is difficult due to the extreme work conditions, remote locations, and the high variability of smoke conditions in the fire environment. Past assessments of wildland firefighter exposures to smoke have commonly measured and reported concentrations of CO and fine PM with an aerodynamic diameter of $\leq$2.5 μm ($PM_{2.5}$) and respirable particulate matter with an aerodynamic diameter of $\leq$4 μm (PM_4) (**Fig. 2**).[6] The permissible exposure limits set by the Occupational Health and Safety Administration (OSHA) for an 8-hour work day is 35 ppm for CO and 5 mg/m^3 for respirable fraction for particles not otherwise regulated ("inert" dust that can include some PM_4 as well as larger particles).[7] However, wildland firefighters do not often work only an 8-hour day and PM from wildfire smoke is more comparable to diesel PM than it is to the inert dust on which the OSHA regulation is based.[6] For these reasons, more conservative occupational exposure limits (OEL) of 16 ppm and 25 ppm for CO at wildfires and prescribed fires, respectively, and 0.7 mg/m^3 for PM_4 have been recommended by Domitrovich and colleagues[2] and the National Wildfire Coordinating Group.[3] Although field studies report different size fractions of PM ($PM_{2.5}$ or PM_4), it is likely that the particle size of combustion-generated particles is comparable across these wildfire smoke studies.[8]

Mean CO and PM concentrations measured across most prescribed fires and wildfires over the past 10 years did not exceed the OELs for CO or PM_4 (see **Fig. 2**). Mean CO and PM concentrations measured at prescribed fires were consistently higher than those measured at wildfires. Mean PM_4 and CO concentrations were highest for wildland firefighters performing mop-up (0.51 mg/m^3) and fireline construction (1.93 ppm). The highest mean concentration of $PM_{2.5}$ (1.2 mg/m^3) was reported by Neitzel and colleagues[9] for firefighters conducting a prescribed burn in the southeast United States. This mean concentration is above the OEL set for wildland firefighters. Reinhardt and Broyles[3] collected smoke field data across many prescribed fires and wildfires in the continental United States and reported the highest mean concentration for CO (4.4 ppm) at prescribed burns. Reisen and colleagues[10] reported the highest maximum concentrations for $PM_{2.5}$ (16 mg/m^3) and CO (120 ppm) during prescribed fires in Australia. On wildfires, the highest maximum concentration for PM was 2.2 mg/m^3 and CO was 19.8 ppm reported by Miranda and colleagues.[11] Wildland firefighters constructing fireline had higher maximum concentrations of PM_4 (2.18 mg/m^3) compared with firefighters performing mop-up (0.68 mg/m^3).[12]

In addition, Reinhardt and Broyles[3] examined factors in the wildfire environment that may

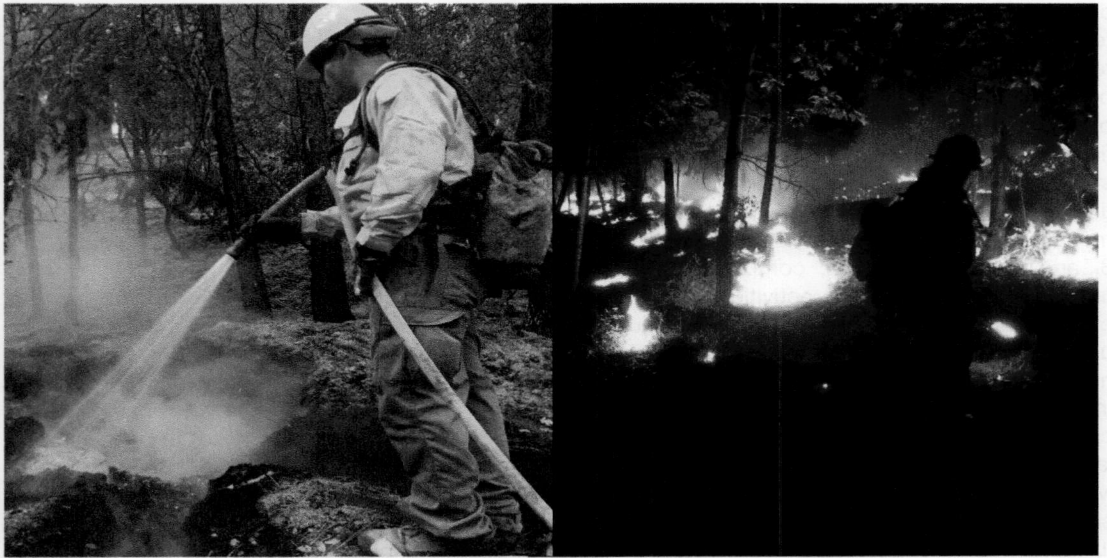

Fig. 2. Photo depicting mop-up and firing operations.

predict PM_4 exposures for wildland firefighters and reported that work task, time spent performing the work task, wind position, and type of wildfire crew were important factors predicting exposure at wildfires. Using the same data for CO, Henn and colleagues[13] also reported that fuel model, relative humidity, type of suppression strategy, and wind speed were significantly associated with elevated levels of CO exposure. Furthermore, Reinhardt and Broyles[3] reported that 22% and 20% of the measured PM_4 exceed OELs (derived specifically for wildland firefighters) at wildland fires and prescribed fires, respectively.[3]

HEALTH RISKS FOR WILDLAND FIREFIGHTERS

Previous health assessments for wildland firefighters generally measured acute health effects across work shifts or a whole fire season. Lung function has often been used to examine acute health effects from smoke exposure. Across one fire season, Liu and colleagues[14] found significant declines in lung function (forced vital capacity, forced expiratory volume at 1 second, and forced expiratory flow at 25% to 75%) and an increase in airway responsiveness as measured by methacholine dose-response slopes for more than 60 wildland firefighters in California. For one Interagency Hotshot Crew in Colorado, Gaughan and colleagues[12] measured a significant decline in lung function associated with high exposure to levoglucosan (a marker for wood smoke) across work shifts.

In addition, biomarkers of exposure and effects have been measured in wildland firefighters to understand exposures from smoke as well as systemic inflammatory and oxidative stress responses.[15–17] After conducting a prescribed burn, 9 hydroxylated metabolites of PAHs were reported to be elevated in the urine of 14 wildland firefighters.[18] Adetona and colleagues[19] demonstrated that firefighters engaged in lighting operations during a prescribed burn had elevated measurements for serum amyloid, interleukin (IL)-8, and C-reactive protein, compared with firefighters involved in holding activities. In addition, cross-work shift changes in creatinine-adjusted urinary mutagenicity, a urinary polycyclic aromatic hydrocarbon metabolite, malondialdehyde (marker of oxidative stress), and light-absorbing carbon were measured in the same group of wildland firefighters conducting prescribed burns.[20] Most recently, Main and colleagues[21] reported a significant increase after a 12-hour work shift for IL-6 and IL-8 among wildland firefighters working in Australia a week after a wildfire outbreak.

Long-term health risks for wildland firefighters have not been as well studied as acute health effects. Semmens and colleagues[22] surveyed wildland firefighters and found significant associations between the number of years worked as a wildland firefighter and history of ever being diagnosed with 2 cardiovascular health outcomes: hypertension and arrhythmias. To examine lung cancer and cardiovascular disease (CVD) risk for wildland firefighters, Navarro and colleagues[8] conducted a risk assessment to estimate mortality risk due to exposure to PM from smoke at wildfires. This study estimated that wildland firefighters were at an increased risk of lung cancer mortality (8%–43%) and CVD (16%–30%) across different exposure scenarios and career durations.

To examine health impacts across multiple seasons, the National Institute for Occupational Safety and Health (NIOSH) is partnering with the US Forest Service and National Park Service to measure exposure to smoke on fire lines and acute, sub-chronic and chronic health outcomes for 6 wildland fire crews across 3 fire seasons. This study will measure biomarkers of renal, cardiovascular, and respiratory function, in the blood and conduct tests of cardiovascular and lung function. In addition, exposure to smoke will be measured through air sampling and biomarkers of exposure, and audiometric tests will be performed to examine hearing loss.[23] More information can be found on the NIOSH study topic page (https://www.cdc.gov/niosh/topics/firefighting/wffhealthstudy.html) and in this video: https://www.youtube.com/watch?v=Ikb9LFvr-dY.

POTENTIAL SOLUTIONS FOR REDUCING SMOKE EXPOSURE FOR WILDLAND FIREFIGHTERS

For wildland firefighters, there is no easy way to reduce exposure to smoke; it is part of the wildland fire environment. Future research should examine how administrative controls on the fireline could reduce exposure to smoke. Fire managers and firefighters should take every precaution possible to reduce exposure to smoke. Small reductions in levels of smoke or the duration of exposure over a career may reduce health impacts.[8] Below are tasks that have been shown to be associated with higher exposures to PM and other chemicals in smoke.[3,9,12,23] Included are possible administrative controls that may be considered to limit exposure to particulate matter and other chemicals in smoke.

- *Mop-up:* Exposure to PM_4 can be significantly higher for firefighters completing mop-up compared with non-arduous ancillary tasks such as operational breaks or waiting for assignments.[3] Firefighters may reduce exposure to ash and smoldering material by limiting the amount of time spent in the burned area to reduce exposure to smoke. They should consider mopping-up to secure the line, and not go farther into the burned area (the black) than needed to extinguish the fire and secure the fire perimeter.
- *Holding:* Reinhardt and Broyles[3] specifically identified holding, as one in which firefighters could reduce cumulative exposure to PM_4. Firefighters performing holding can be instructed to stand along a fireline and watch for the fire escaping control lines, which can involve being in areas of high smoke and low visibility. Firefighters may use personnel as patrols, periodically walking a fireline and checking for spots, rather than standing directly in the smoke for long periods of time.
- *Fireline construction:* When constructing and digging fireline, firefighters may be close to the active fire's edge to stop forward progression of the fire. Firefighters are likely to be exposed to smoke when working close to this active fire edge. Gaughan and colleagues[12] reported that wildland firefighters constructing fireline had higher PM exposures compared with those performing mop-up. Using roads or natural features (rock bands or creeks) as an indirect fireline may reduce time near an active fireline and smoke.
- *Firing:* Adetona and colleagues[19] report that wildland firefighters who performed firing using torches filled with diesel and gasoline had elevated inflammatory markers compared with firefighters tasked with holding. The investigators hypothesized that the additional exposure to combustion of diesel and gasoline could have led to this increase in inflammatory markers. To reduce the concentration of smoke during firing operations, firefighters may consider starting firing operations when winds are favorable and will not send smoke toward the firefighters who are lighting the burn. How the burn is ignited (through firing patterns) may produce more heat and result in more complete combustion and reduce the amount of PM in the smoke.

Fire managers and firefighters should continue to discuss strategies to reduce exposure at all levels of the fire organization. In addition, researchers assessing exposure to smoke should also evaluate how mitigations may reduce exposure to smoke. The Interagency Standards for Fire and Fire Aviation Operations states that any respiratory protection used must be certified by NIOSH; however, respirators that are marketed to wildland firefighters are not NIOSH-approved.[24] Negative pressure half face air purifying respirators with organic vapor and formaldehyde filters were evaluated previously for wildland firefighters in Australia. This study found that the respirators were effective in reducing exposures and provided protection for firefighter's airway; however, these firefighters wore respiratory protection for only 2 hours, not representative of a full shift (over 24 hours), did not perform any firefighting tasks, and were not protected against carbon monoxide exposure.[25] No respirator can currently provide protection to gases and particles for wildland firefighters working in extreme environments performing physically demanding work (**Box 1**).

OUTDOOR WORKERS

In addition to wildland firefighters, workers in other outdoor occupations, such as agriculture, construction, landscape, utility, and facility maintenance workers, can be exposed to wildfire smoke. Depending on how much time these workers spend outdoors on days when wildfire smoke concentrations are high and how much exertion their jobs require, the effective smoke exposures can be substantially greater than for the general public. Unfortunately, little direct evidence of health impacts of these exposures is available. That said, based on the $PM_{2.5}$ health effects exposure-response literature, estimated health risks can be generated.[27,28] In general, outdoor workers with preexisting respiratory diseases and CVDs could experience increased risk of exacerbations of these diseases when air quality is poor due to wildfire smoke.

Current Policy Efforts to Reduce Exposures for Outdoor Workers

Recently, California adopted an emergency regulation, regulation 5141.1, *Protection from Wildfire Smoke under the California Code of Regulations*, Title 8, Division 1, Chapter 4, of the General Industry Safety Orders, to protect outdoor workers (excluding wildland firefighters) from wildfire smoke using $PM_{2.5}$ as an indicator for exposure to smoke.[29] The regulation requires employers to determine the Air Quality Index (AQI) for $PM_{2.5}$ throughout a work shift, communicate and train employees about the hazards of smoke, and reduce exposures that are above an AQI of 151 for $PM_{2.5}$ (0.055 mg/m^3). To reduce exposures to

Box 1
Federal interagency wildland firefighter medical standards arduous duty wildland firefighter

Minimum medical fitness for arduous duty wildland firefighters are established by the Federal Interagency Wildland Firefighter Medical Standards based on *5 CFR Part 339 Medical Qualifications Determinations*.[26] According to the standard, medical examinations are required for arduous duty wildland firefighters to determine an individual's ability to meet the medical standard by a designated physician. Standards included in the chest and respiratory system ensures that firefighters have a health respiratory system and can perform arduous exertion, carry heavy loads, and perform extensive movement across difficult terrain. Although not mandatory, a pulmonary function test should show a forced vital capacity (FVC) of at least 70% of the predicted value; a forced expiratory volume at 1 second (FEV1) of at least 70% of the predicted value; the ratio FEV1/FVC of at least 70%; and no evidence by physical examination and medical history of respiratory conditions likely to present a safety risk or to worsen as a result of carrying out the essential functions of the job. These standards are intended as a screen for further evaluation. Firefighters may be disqualified if they are diagnosed with an active pulmonary tuberculosis, history of bronchitis associated with decreased pulmonary function, lung access, spontaneous pneumothorax, emphysema, sarcoidosis, pulmonary embolism, pulmonary infraction, or pneumonectomy. Asthma is considered on a case-by-case basis and the use of an inhaler requires agency review. Any condition that may impair a firefighter's ability to perform their job tasks efficiently or safely should be evaluated on a case-by-case basis.

From NIFC. FEDERAL INTERAGENCY WILDLAND FIREFIGHTER MEDICAL STANDARDS. 2020; Available at: https://www.nifc.gov/medical_standards/documents/Federal_Interagency_Wildland_Firefighter_Medical_Standards.pdf Accessed 8/12/2020.

under an AQI of 151, employers can implement engineering or administrative controls such as providing enclosed spaces with filtered air or changing work schedules, reducing work intensity, or providing more rest breaks. At an AQI of 151 but below 500, the regulation requires that NIOSH-approved respirators are provided to employees for voluntary use, which does not require fit testing or medical evaluations. If the AQI is above 500, employers are required to provide respirators, and follow requirements under the respiratory protection regulation, which will reduce a worker's exposure to $PM_{2.5}$ to less than 0.055 mg/m^3.

SUMMARY

Whether on a prescribed fire or wildfire, occupational exposure of wildland firefighters to smoke can have both short-term and long-term negative health effects. Decreases in lung function, increases in systematic inflammation, and an estimated higher risk for lung cancer and cardiovascular disease mortality have been reported in wildland firefighter research studies.[8,12,20,21] For outdoor workers exposed to smoke, there is little research measuring smoke exposure and possible associated adverse health effects. Increased residential development in the WUI has correspondingly increased the risk of catastrophic fires spreading into urban neighborhoods where buildings and motor vehicles burn, which likely only increases the risk of adverse health impacts for the public and firefighters, as there is more than just vegetation burning. For wildland firefighters, there is no easy way to reduce exposure to smoke, it is part of the wildfire environment. It is important for all fire personnel to understand the hazards of smoke and develop ways to mitigate exposure.

CLINICS CARE POINTS

- Clinicians should recommend regular health screenings including lung function testing for workers regularly exposed to wildfire smoke.
- Healthcare providers should consider advising patients working in the wildland fire environment on how to minimize exposure to high levels of air pollution.

ACKNOWLEDGMENTS

The findings and conclusions in this report are those of the author(s) and do not necessarily represent the official position of the National Institute for Occupational Safety and Health (NIOSH) or Centers for Disease Control and Prevention (CDC). Mention of any company name or product does not constitute endorsement by NIOSH/CDC.

REFERENCES

1. NIFC. National Interagency Coordination Center incident management situation report Wednesday, August 8, 2018. Boise (ID): NIFC; 2018.
2. Domitrovich J, Broyles G, Ottmar R, et al. Final report: wildland fire smoke health effects on wildland firefighters and the public. Joint fire science program, Boise, ID 2017.

3. Reinhardt TE, Broyles G. Factors affecting smoke and crystalline silica exposure among wildland firefighters. J Occup Environ Hyg 2019;16(2):151–64.
4. NIFC. National Interagency Coordination Center - fire statistics. 2019. Available at: https://www.nifc.gov/fireInfo/fireInfo_statistics.html. Accessed January 31, 2020.
5. Ager AA, Palaiologou P, Evers CR, et al. Wildfire exposure to the wildland urban interface in the western US. Appl Geogr 2019;111:102059.
6. Adetona O, Reinhardt TE, Domitrovich J, et al. Review of the health effects of wildland fire smoke on wildland firefighters and the public. Inhal Toxicol 2016;28(3):95–139.
7. Occupational Safety and Health Administration. (2017). Occupational safety and health standards: TABLE Z-1 Limits for Air Contaminants. (Standard No. 1910.1000). Available at: https://www.osha.gov/laws-regs/regulations/standardnumber/1910/1910.1000TABLEZ1.
8. Navarro KM, Kleinman MT, Mackay CE, et al. Wildland firefighter smoke exposure and risk of lung cancer and cardiovascular disease mortality. Environ Res 2019;173:462–8.
9. Neitzel R, Naeher LP, Paulsen M, et al. Biological monitoring of smoke exposure among wildland firefighters: a pilot study comparing urinary methoxyphenols with personal exposures to carbon monoxide, particular matter, and levoglucosan. J Expo Sci Environ Epidemiol 2009;19(4):349–58.
10. Reisen F, Hansen D, Meyer CP. Exposure to bushfire smoke during prescribed burns and wildfires: firefighters' exposure risks and options. Environ Int 2011;37(2):314–21.
11. Miranda AI, Martins V, Cascão P, et al. Monitoring of firefighters exposure to smoke during fire experiments in Portugal. Environ Int 2010;36(7):736–45.
12. Gaughan DM, Piacitelli CA, Chen BT, et al. Exposures and cross-shift lung function declines in wildland firefighters. J Occup Environ Hyg 2014;11(9):591–603.
13. Henn SA, Butler C, Li J, et al. Carbon monoxide exposures among US wildland firefighters by work, fire, and environmental characteristics and conditions. J Occup Environ Hyg 2019;16(12):793–803.
14. Liu D, Tager IB, Balmes JR, et al. The effect of smoke inhalation on lung function and airway responsiveness in wildland fire fighters. Am Rev Respir Dis 1992;146(6):1469–73.
15. Adetona O, Hall DB, Naeher LP. Lung function changes in wildland firefighters working at prescribed burns. Inhal Toxicol 2011;23(13):835–41.
16. Hejl AM, Adetona O, Diaz-Sanchez D, et al. Inflammatory effects of woodsmoke exposure among wildland firefighters working at prescribed burns at the Savannah River Site, SC. J Occup Environ Hyg 2013;10(4):173–80.
17. Swiston JR, Davidson W, Attridge S, et al. Wood smoke exposure induces a pulmonary and systemic inflammatory response in firefighters. Eur Respir J 2008;32(1):129–38.
18. Adetona O, Simpson CD, Li Z, et al. Hydroxylated polycyclic aromatic hydrocarbons as biomarkers of exposure to wood smoke in wildland firefighters. J Expo Sci Environ Epidemiol 2017;27(1):78–83.
19. Adetona AM, Adetona O, Gogal RM, et al. Impact of work task-related acute occupational smoke exposures on select proinflammatory immune parameters in wildland firefighters. J Occup Environ Med 2017;59(7):679–90.
20. Adetona AM, Kyle Martin W, Warren SH, et al. Urinary mutagenicity and other biomarkers of occupational smoke exposure of wildland firefighters and oxidative stress. Inhal Toxicol 2019;31(2):73–87.
21. Main LC, Wolkow AP, Tait JL, et al. Firefighter's acute inflammatory response to wildfire suppression. J Occup Environ Med 2019;62(2):145–8.
22. Semmens EO, Domitrovich J, Conway K, et al. A cross-sectional survey of occupational history as a wildland firefighter and health. Am J Ind Med 2016;59(4):330–5.
23. Fent KW. Comprehensive Study of Wildland Firefigthers' Health Over Multiple Seasons: Overview and Update. 15th International Wildland Fire Safety Summit and 5th Human Dimensions of Wildland Fire Conference. Asheville, NC, December 18, 2018.
24. NIFC. Interagency standards for fire and fire aviation operations Boise, ID 2020.
25. De Vos AJ, Cook A, Devine B, et al. Effect of protective filters on fire fighter respiratory health: field validation during prescribed burns. Am J Ind Med 2009;52(1):76–87.
26. NIFC. Federal interagency wildland firefighter medical standards. 2020. Available at: https://www.nifc.gov/medical_standards/documents/Federal_Interagency_Wildland_Firefighter_Medical_Standards.pdf. Accessed August 12, 2020.
27. Orellano P, Quaranta N, Reynoso J, et al. Effect of outdoor air pollution on asthma exacerbations in children and adults: systematic review and multilevel meta-analysis. PLoS One 2017;12(3):e0174050.
28. Rajagopalan S, Al-Kindi SG, Brook RD. Air pollution and cardiovascular disease: JACC state-of-the-art review. J Am Coll Cardiol 2018;72(17):2054–70.
29. California Occupational Safety and Health Administration. Subchapter 7. General Industry Safety Orders. §5141.1 Protection from Wildfire Smoke. Available at: https://www.dir.ca.gov/title8/5141_1.html.

The Changing Nature of Wildfires

Impacts on the Health of the Public

John R. Balmes, MD[a,b,*]

KEYWORDS

• Wildfire • Smoke • Public health • Particulate matter

KEY POINTS

- The public are exposed to air contaminants from wildfire smoke that are associated with adverse respiratory and cardiovascular outcomes.
- There is very limited research on long-term health of the public from smoke exposure across multiple fire seasons.
- Patients with preexisting respiratory or cardiovascular disease should take particular care to protect themselves from exposure to wildfire smoke.

INTRODUCTION

Why Are More Catastrophic Wildfires Occurring Around the World?

The danger of catastrophic wildfires is increasing around the globe, with large fires occurring in Australia, Canada, Chile, Indonesia, Portugal, Russia, as well as in the United States over the past decade.[1] A major driver globally is climate change, which is expected to increase the frequency and severity of wildfires because of drier fire seasons, warmer temperatures, reduced precipitation, and snowpack.[2] Large forest fires in the western United States have been nearly 5 times as frequent on an annual basis as they were 50 years ago. These fires are burning more land area (**Fig. 1**) and requiring multiweek or month fire suppression campaigns.[3] The wildfire season has also become much longer, as exemplified by the severe fires in California during November and December 2018 to 2019. The wildfire season in California typically ended in October when autumn rains began, but there has not been sufficient rain to prevent wildfires in the fall months when high winds occurred for the last several years.

Wildfire Policy in the United States

A risk factor for large wildfires in the western United States that amplifies climate change and drought is a multidecade legacy of fire suppression that has allowed overgrowth of underbrush and small trees in forests where periodic lightning-sparked wildfires are part of the natural ecosystem. For more than a century, the primary objective of wildland fire policy in the United States was to suppress any wildland fires to protect communities and natural resources.[4] This policy was developed after the Great Fire of 1910, one of the largest fires in American history, where 86 people died, most of whom were firefighters.[5] Since the 1930s, with the introduction of the US Forest Service's "10 AM Policy" that instructed that every reported wildland fire be put out by 10 AM the next day, there have been fewer small fires allowed to burn on our landscape.[6] This policy has been very successful in reducing the number of wildland

[a] Department of Medicine, University of California, San Francisco, San Francisco, CA, USA; [b] School of Public Health, University of California, Berkeley, Berkeley, CA, USA
* UCSF, Box 0843, San Francisco, CA 94143-0843.
E-mail address: john.balmes@ucsf.edu

Clin Chest Med 41 (2020) 771–776
https://doi.org/10.1016/j.ccm.2020.08.006

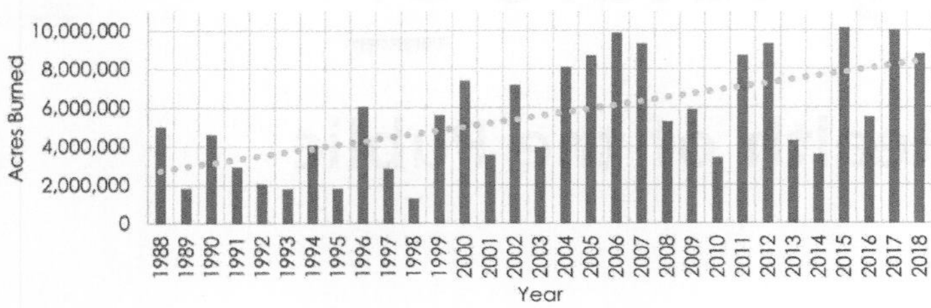

Fig. 1. Acres burned by wildfires per year. (*Data from* NIFC. National Interagency Coordination Center - Fire Statistics. 2019; Available at: https://www.nifc.gov/fireInfo/fireInfo_statistics.html. Accessed 1/31/2020.)

fires that burn every year, but has excluded fire from fire-dependent ecosystems.[7]

Fire exclusion can change ecosystem structure and reduce resilience to ecosystem disturbances. When fire is excluded from a forest, the forest can become denser with young trees that are fire-intolerant and can act as "ladder" fuels. These ladder fuels can aid in the spread of fire from the surface of a forest floor to the canopy resulting in a crown fire that can lead to a large catastrophic high-severity fire.[8] In addition, fire exclusion leads to an increase in tree density and forest fuels, and there is a decrease in forest heterogeneity and understory plant diversity.[8] The increased amount of fuel load and ladder fuels available increases the likelihood that high-severity crown fires will occur.[9]

If we want to reduce future catastrophic wildland fires, we need to work on restoring forest conditions that allowed small low to moderate fires to maintain open stand forests that were more resilient to fire. Forest thinning and burning could provide a method for restoring historical forest structure with increased heterogeneity that would allow wildland fires to burn at low or moderate severity. Prescribed fire, intentionally ignited low-intensity fires, and managed wildland fires, wildfires that are allowed to burn for land management benefit, could be used to treat the abundance of fuel in forests and restore fire-adapted landscapes across a larger area.[9] If our forests were more resilient to wildland fire, we could have fewer large catastrophic wildfires in the future.

Fires in the Wildland-Urban Interface

As urban populations grow around the world and the total number of burned acres has increased, so has the number of lost homes and structures because of the expansion of the wildland urban interface (WUI), where wildland vegetation and urban areas meet.[10] Between 1990 and 2010, areas classified as WUI grew by 33%, and new homes built increased by 41% in WUI areas.[11] Recent wildfires in both California and Australia have shown that catastrophic wildfires cannot be easily controlled, meaning that homes built in and adjacent to wooded areas cannot be defended and emergency evacuations become necessary. The social costs of protecting homes and lives at the WUI is becoming prohibitive in wildfire-prone areas of multiple jurisdictions in the United States and other countries.[12]

What Is in Wildfire Smoke?

Wildfire smoke contains carbon dioxide, water vapor, carbon monoxide (CO), particulate matter (PM), complex hydrocarbons (including polycyclic aromatic hydrocarbons), nitrogen oxides, trace minerals, and several thousand other compounds.[13] The actual composition of smoke depends on the fuel type (eg, deciduous vs coniferous), fire behavior, and environmental conditions. Wood smoke contains many of the same toxic and carcinogenic substances as cigarette smoke, including benzene, benzo(a)pyrene, and dibenz(a,h)anthracene.[14]

PM, typically a mixture of solid particles and liquid droplets, is the principal pollutant of health concern from wildfire smoke. Most PM in wood smoke is very small (0.4–0.7 μm) and falls in the fine particle ($PM_{2.5}$ or particles smaller than 2.5 μm in diameter) size range. CO is another pollutant that is always emitted when carbon-based fuels are burned, and CO levels are highest during the smoldering stages of a fire.

Like tobacco smoke, there are literally thousands of chemical compounds present in wood smoke. From a mass or number-based concentration standpoint, many of these other organics (acrolein, benzene, and formaldehyde), metals, shorter-lived radicals, and complex hydrocarbons are at lower concentrations than $PM_{2.5}$ or CO, but even low levels of these toxicologically potent materials raises some concern regarding potential adverse health effects.[14]

COMMUNITY EXPOSURES AND HEALTH EFFECTS FROM WILDFIRE SMOKE

Exposure to Wildfire Smoke for the Public

Fine PM ($PM_{2.5}$) is the pollutant in wildfire smoke that is of greatest public health concern and used to assess public exposure to smoke. The 24-hour air-quality standard set by the Environmental Protection Agency (EPA) for $PM_{2.5}$ to protect public health is 35 $\mu g/m^3$. For comparison, during the Camp Fire of November 2018, the air quality in terms of $PM_{2.5}$ was the worst that has ever been recorded in northern California, with the highest 24-hour concentration in Sacramento exceeding 250 $\mu g/m^3$, and in San Francisco exceeding 140 $\mu g/m^3$ despite the fact that the wildfire area was many miles away from both cities.[15] Similar 24-hour levels have occurred during the 2019 to 2020 summer wildfires in Australia. Hourly levels greater than 400 $\mu g/m^3$ were recorded in Sacramento during the Camp Fire and Sydney during the 2019 to 2020 summer bush fires.[16]

During catastrophic wildfires that devastate neighborhoods or whole towns at the WUI, many homes, other buildings, and motor vehicles burn. Fire emissions from these man-made structures and vehicles include more metal oxides and combustion products of synthetic materials, some of which are extremely toxic, such as hydrogen cyanide, phosgene, and dioxins.[17] By the time the plume of a large wildfire has traveled many miles, however, most of the smoke particles are from wood because that is the primary fuel source.

Respiratory Outcomes

The epidemiologic literature on the associations between short-term exposures to wildfire smoke and respiratory outcomes at the community level is fairly robust.[18,19] Major findings include increased symptoms of cough and wheeze, health care utilization for exacerbations of asthma and chronic obstructive pulmonary disease, and incidence of acute lower respiratory tract infections. Among adults, women and people with lower socioeconomic status may be at increased risk.[19] Published studies on the respiratory effects of wildfire smoke exposure in children are few, but the reported findings are consistent with the increased risk of exacerbations of asthma observed among adults.

Cardiovascular Outcomes

Reviews of epidemiologic studies of the associations between short-term community exposures to wildfire smoke and cardiovascular outcomes have found the published evidence less robust than for respiratory outcomes.[18,19] Since those reviews were published, however, several studies have documented increased health care utilization for cardiovascular outcomes in both the United States and Australia, including myocardial infarction, stroke, and out-of-hospital cardiac arrest.[20] In at least 1 study during the wildfire season in northern California in 2015, a not particularly intense fire season, the magnitude of the increased risk for cardiovascular outcomes was similar to that of the more well-established association between wildfire smoke and respiratory outcomes.[21]

Health Effects from Prescribed Fire

The published literature on the health effects of exposure to smoke from prescribed fire is almost exclusively limited to occupational exposures of wildland firefighters. A study of the effects of smoke from prescribed fire among the general public in the US state of Georgia reported an increase in emergency department visits for asthma in association with estimated $PM_{2.5}$ exposures from prescribed burns.[22]

Long-Term Health Effects from Reoccurring Smoke Exposure

Although multiple studies have evaluated the short-term health effects of exposure to wildfire smoke events, many communities have been exposed to prolonged (weeks to months) and/or repeated episodes of summertime wildfire smoke. The effects of these prolonged or repeated exposures on respiratory health have not been studied. Infants and children with developing lungs may be particularly vulnerable to such exposures. Research is also needed on long-term effects of short-term high-intensity exposures (eg, whether new-onset asthma can be triggered).

Adverse birth, neurologic, and metabolic outcomes have been associated with chronic exposure to $PM_{2.5}$.[23] Whether these outcomes might be associated with prolonged or repeated exposure to wildfire smoke PM is largely unknown, although there is limited evidence of increased risk of low birth weight and preterm birth.[24,25]

Recommendations for Reducing Exposures for Communities

Personal protections

The general public need clear and consistent messaging to understand that wildland fire smoke poses a health risk, especially to young children, the elderly, and those with preexisting respiratory or cardiovascular disease.[26,27] The public also need to know that relatively simple measures can effectively reduce the risk to health of exposure to wildfire smoke. These measures start with staying indoors if possible and, if it is necessary to go outdoors, taking steps to minimize exposure to smoke. Residents of wildfire-prone areas need to become informed and prepared for wildfire smoke events.[28] The communications tool for air quality health risk developed by the EPA, the Air Quality Index (AQI), is what most jurisdictions in the United States use to communicate the severity of health risk as a consequence of wildfire smoke events. The AQI was not developed for wildfire smoke messaging and can be misleading in that it is calculated based on the 24-hour concentration average. In hot summer months, the AQI during a wildfire smoke event might include non-fire-related increases in ozone levels as well as wildfire-related $PM_{2.5}$. In addition to media-based communication, the AQI is available to the public on AirNow.gov.

Home protections

In addition to staying indoors with closed windows during wildfire smoke events, one can improve home air quality by turning the ventilation system to recirculate if such a setting is available and, even better, to outfit the system with an MERV 13 filter if possible. MERV stands for Minimum Efficiency Reporting Value, and the values range from 1 to 16, with higher values representing greater filtration efficiency of fine particles. Another approach is to use portable HEPA filtration devices or "air cleaners."[29] These devices can substantially reduce $PM_{2.5}$ levels in a single room, although the quality of the devices varies. Fortunately, there are relatively good-quality devices available at reasonable prices.

Protecting children at schools

Whether to close schools when there is poor air quality due to wildfire smoke events is a difficult decision for school administrators. School-aged children might have lower exposures to wildfire smoke if they are inside a school building with good ventilation and filtration than if they are at home. To protect school-aged children from the detrimental effects of wildland fire smoke, the California Air Resources Board developed the *Air Quality Guidance Template for Schools* to standardize decision making among school districts across the state.[30] The guidelines advise school administrators to (1) monitor air quality using AirNow.gov and local tracking tools before making decisions about school closures or event cancellations, (2) assess and update classroom air conditioning systems, and (3) install portable HEPA filtration devices if central air filtration is poor. The guide also provides clear recommendations for safe and unsafe activities at all air quality levels and appropriate use of masks for adult learners. Unfortunately, no N95 masks have been certified for use by children.

How Should Physicians Advise Their Patients and the Public When There Is Poor Air Quality due to Wildfire Smoke?

Patients who are at greatest risk for symptoms owing to smoke, those with preexisting respiratory or cardiovascular disease, should be advised to stay indoors and, if they must go outdoors, to avoid prolonged activity.[31–33] Healthy young children and older adults should follow the same advice. Because even healthy adults can experience symptoms such as eye, nose, and throat irritation, they should take some basic precautions to reduce exposure to wildfire smoke, including minimizing or stopping outdoor activities, especially those involving vigorous exercise; staying indoors with windows and doors closed as much as possible; not running ventilation devices that bring smoky outdoor air inside (eg, swamp coolers, whole-house fans, fresh-air-ventilation systems, and some air-conditioning systems); using the "recirculate" or "recycle" setting on the ventilation-system control; and avoiding smoking, frying food, or other activities that will create indoor air pollution.

Patients with preexisting respiratory or cardiovascular disease should take particular care to stay indoors. If it is necessary to go outdoors, wearing an N95 or N100 particulate respirator provides some protection. These designations mean that the masks have been certified by NIOSH [National Institute for Occupational Safety and Health] to filter out least 95% or 100%, respectively, of very small (0.3 μm) test particles. Recommended use of N95 masks for patients with preexisting respiratory or cardiovascular disease has been criticized for 2 reasons. First, their use can give people a false sense of protection about going outside. Second, there is concern expressed about harm because of increased work of breathing and CO_2 retention. Wearing an N95 mask can be uncomfortable, but there is little evidence to support a substantial increase in work of breathing. CO_2 retention can be avoided by using N95 masks with an exhalation valve.

Patients with preexisting respiratory or cardiovascular disease who develop wheezing, chest tightness, excessive coughing, shortness of breath, chest pain, palpitations, or other acute symptoms during a wildfire smoke event should consider evacuating to an area with better air quality. If evacuation is not possible, staying indoors with windows closed should reduce exposure.

SUMMARY

The duration of the wildfire season and number of catastrophic wildfires are increasing because of climate change and the legacy of decades of fire suppression. Poor air quality because of wildfire smoke is becoming a major threat to public health in the United States and in multiple countries around the world. Increased residential development in the wildland-urban interface has correspondingly increased the risk of catastrophic fires spreading into urban neighborhoods where buildings and motor vehicles burn, which only increases the risk of adverse health impacts for the public and firefighters.

When considering community exposure to wildfire smoke, acute respiratory effects of exposure are well documented, but new studies suggest acute cardiovascular effects as well. Long-term effects of high and/or recurrent exposures need further study, for both wildland firefighters and the public. Adverse effects on birth outcomes, neurologic outcomes, and metabolic outcomes are not well studied, but are likely to be associated with exposure to wildfire smoke based on what is known from the robust outdoor $PM_{2.5}$ epidemiologic and toxicologic literature. An important area of future research is the relative toxicity of wildfire smoke $PM_{2.5}$ compared with that of $PM_{2.5}$ from transportation and coal-fired power generation.

Public messaging about the health risks of poor air quality because of wildfire smoke needs to be clear, consistent, and easily comprehensible. Physicians need to advise their patients, especially those with preexisting respiratory and cardiovascular disease who are most vulnerable, to reduce their exposure during wildfire smoke episodes. The best advice is to stay indoors with windows closed, ventilation systems both at home and in cars turned to recirculate, and to wear N95 masks if it is necessary to go outdoors. Preparation in advance of the wildfire season is key with a medication plan, outfitting the home ventilation system with a MERV 13 filter if possible, and purchase of one or more home HEPA air cleaners.

DISCLOSURE

Dr. Balmes is the Physician Member of the California Air Resources Board.

REFERENCES

1. Balmes JR. Where there's wildfire, there's smoke. N Engl J Med 2018;378(10):881–3.
2. Westerling AL. Increasing western US forest wildfire activity: sensitivity to changes in the timing of spring. Philos Trans R Soc Lond B Biol Sci 2016;371(1696): 20150178.
3. NIFC. National interagency coordination center - fire statistics 2019. Available at: https://www.nifc.gov/fireInfo/fireInfo_statistics.html. Accessed January 31, 2020.
4. Busenberg G. Wildfire management in the United States: the evolution of a policy failure. Rev Pol Res 2004;21(2):145–56.
5. United States Forest Service. The Great Fire of 1910. https://www.fs.usda.gov/Internet/FSE_DOCUMENTS/stelprdb5444731.pdf. Accessed January 31, 2020.
6. Dale L. Wildfire policy and fire use on public lands in the United States. Soc Nat Resour 2006;19(3): 275–84.
7. North MP, Stephens SL, Collins BM, et al. Reform forest fire management. Science 2015;349(6254): 1280–1.
8. Schoennagel T, Veblen TT, Romme WH. The interaction of fire, fuels, and climate across Rocky Mountain forests. BioScience 2004;54(7):661–76.
9. Ryan KC, Knapp EE, Varner JM. Prescribed fire in North American forests and woodlands: history, current practice, and challenges. Front Ecol Environ 2013;11(s1):e15–24.
10. Ager AA, Palaiologou P, Evers CR, et al. Wildfire exposure to the wildland urban interface in the western US. Appl Geogr 2019;111:102059.
11. Radeloff VC, Helmers DP, Kramer HA, et al. Rapid growth of the US wildland-urban interface raises wildfire risk. Proc Natl Acad Sci U S A 2018; 115(13):3314–9.
12. Baylis P, Boomhower J. Moral hazard, wildfires, and the economic incidence of natural disasters. Cambridge (MA): NBER Working Papers 26550, National Bureau of Economic Research, Inc; 2019.
13. Naeher LP, Brauer M, Lipsett M, et al. Woodsmoke health effects: a review. Inhal Toxicol 2007;19(1): 67–106.
14. Adetona O, Reinhardt TE, Domitrovich J, et al. Review of the health effects of wildland fire smoke on wildland firefighters and the public. Inhal Toxicol 2016;28(3):95–139.
15. United States Environmental Protection Agency. Pre-Generated data files. Available at: https://aqs.epa.gov/aqsweb/airdata/download_files.html. Accessed January 31, 2020.
16. Remeikis A. Canberra chokes on world's worst air quality as city all but shut down. The Guardian. 1/3/2020, 2020. Avaiable at: https://www.theguardian.com/australia-news/2020/jan/03/canberra-chokes-on-worlds-worst-air-quality-as-city-all-but-shut-down. Accessed Januray 31, 2020.
17. Stefanidou M, Athanaselis S, Spiliopoulou C. Health impacts of fire smoke inhalation. Inhal Toxicol 2008; 20(8):761–6.
18. Liu JC, Pereira G, Uhl SA, et al. A systematic review of the physical health impacts from non-occupational exposure to wildfire smoke. Environ Res 2015;136:120–32.

19. Reid CE, Brauer M, Johnston FH, et al. Critical review of health impacts of wildfire smoke exposure. Environ Health Perspect 2016;124(9):1334–43.
20. Haikerwal A, Akram M, Del Monaco A, et al. Impact of fine particulate matter (PM 2.5) exposure during wildfires on cardiovascular health outcomes. J Am Heart Assoc 2015;4(7):e001653.
21. Wettstein ZS, Hoshiko S, Fahimi J, et al. Cardiovascular and cerebrovascular emergency department visits associated with wildfire smoke exposure in California in 2015. J Am Heart Assoc 2018;7(8): e007492.
22. Huang R, Hu Y, Russell AG, et al. The impacts of prescribed fire on $PM_{2.5}$ air quality and human health: application to asthma-related emergency room visits in Georgia, USA. Int J Environ Res Public Health 2019;16(13):2312.
23. EPA U. Integrated science assessment (ISA) for particulate matter. Research Triangle Park (NC): Center for Public Health and Environmental Assessment, Office of Research and Development, U.S. Environmental Protection Agency; 2019. EPA/600/R-19/188.
24. Abdo M, Ward I, O'Dell K, et al. Impact of wildfire smoke on adverse pregnancy outcomes in Colorado, 2007–2015. Int J Environ Res Public Health 2019;16(19):3720.
25. Holstius DM, Reid CE, Jesdale BM, et al. Birth weight following pregnancy during the 2003 Southern California wildfires. Environ Health Perspect 2012;120(9):1340–5.
26. Fish JA, Peters MDJ, Ramsey I, et al. Effectiveness of public health messaging and communication channels during smoke events: a rapid systematic review. J Environ Manag 2017;193:247–56.
27. Mott JA, Meyer P, Mannino D, et al. Wildland forest fire smoke: health effects and intervention evaluation, Hoopa, California, 1999. West J Med 2002; 176(3):157.
28. EPA U. Air quality Index: a guide to air quality and your health. Research Triangle Park (NC): U.S. Environmental Protection Agency, Office of Air Quality Planning and Standards, Outreach and Information Division; 2014.
29. Barn PK, Elliott CT, Allen RW, et al. Portable air cleaners should be at the forefront of the public health response to landscape fire smoke. Environ Health 2016;15(1):116.
30. California Air Pollution Control Officers Association. Air Quality Guidance Template for Schools California Air Pollution Control Officers Associaton;2019. Available at: http://www.capcoa.org/wp-content/uploads/downloads/2019/06/Air-Quality-Guidance-Template-for-Schools-Updated-5.13.2019.pdf. Accessed January 31, 2020.
31. ATS. Disaster guidance: 10 tips for staying healthy during wildfires 2018. Available at: https://www.thoracic.org/about/newsroom/press-releases/10-tips-for-staying-healthy-during-wildfires-ats-recommendations.php. Accessed January 31, 2020.
32. EPA U. Wildfire smoke: a guide for public health officials. Research Triangle Park (NC): United States Environmental Protection Agency, Office of Air Quality Planning and Standards, Health and Environmental Impacts Division; 2019.
33. CDC. Wildfire smoke. 2013. Available at: https://www.cdc.gov/disasters/wildfires/smoke.html. Accessed January 31, 2020.

Indoor Microbial Exposures and Chronic Lung Disease

From Microbial Toxins to the Microbiome

Molly Wolf, MD[a], Peggy S. Lai, MD, MPH[a,b,*]

KEYWORDS

- Microbiome • Built environment • Bacteria • Endotoxin • Fungus • Asthma
- Chronic obstructive pulmonary disease

KEY POINTS

- Humans are exposed to a variety of microbial exposures on a daily basis in the home and work environments, which may impact chronic lung diseases, such as asthma and chronic obstructive pulmonary disease (COPD).
- Current studies have shown that both bacterial and fungal exposures can protect from or increase the risk of developing chronic obstructive lung diseases.
- Methods of quantification of microbial exposure have inherent limitations and likely explain contradictory results on lung health.
- The effects of bacterial and fungal exposure can be modified by other environmental factors, including tobacco smoke, vitamin levels, synthetic plastics, and by human genetic polymorphisms.
- Future studies need to determine which method of measuring environmental microbial exposure is most clinically relevant to human health and chronic lung diseases.

INTRODUCTION

Microbial exposures have been implicated in the development or exacerbation of many noncommunicable lung diseases, including asthma and chronic obstructive pulmonary disease (COPD). There has been significant debate over whether the effect of microbial exposures is harmful, neutral, or beneficial to lung health. For example, in the case of asthma, although a large number of studies have demonstrated that endotoxin exposure protects against asthma development or asthma symptoms,[1–8] an equal number have demonstrated evidence of harm associated with endotoxin exposure,[9–16] and several have shown no association between endotoxin exposure and asthma at all[17–20] (**Table 1**). Even more confusingly, a single publication based on 3 European birth cohorts have shown that early-life endotoxin exposure was associated with a protective effect against physician-diagnosed asthma by the age of 10 in the Spanish cohort, no effect in the German cohort, and a harmful effect in the Dutch cohort.[21] The purpose of this review is to try and reconcile these seeming paradoxes by rethinking how we measure microbial exposures and determine their association with chronic lung diseases.

SEARCH STRATEGY

For this review, our goal was to identify publications that focused on environmental bacterial

[a] Division of Pulmonary and Critical Care Medicine, Massachusetts General Hospital, Harvard Medical School, 55 Fruit Street, Bulfinch 148, Boston, MA 02114, USA; [b] Department of Environmental Health, Harvard T.H. Chan School of Public Health, Boston, MA, USA

* Corresponding author. Division of Pulmonary and Critical Care Medicine, Massachusetts General Hospital, Harvard Medical School, 55 Fruit Street, Bulfinch 148, Boston, MA 02114.

E-mail address: pslai@hsph.harvard.edu

Clin Chest Med 41 (2020) 777–796
https://doi.org/10.1016/j.ccm.2020.08.005

Table 1
The endotoxin paradox

Friend	Neutral	Foe
Braun-Fahrlander et al,[1] 2002	Bertelsen et al,[79] 2010	Bolte et al,[9] 2003
Campo et al,[2] 2006	Delfino et al,[77] 2015	Carlsten et al,[3] 2011
Carlsten et al,[3] 2011	Ege et al,[17] 2007	Celedon et al,[10] 2007
Douwes et al,[3] 2006	Gehring et al,[18] 2001	Gillespie et al,[11] 2006
El-Sharif et al,[5] 2006	Jacobs et al,[78] 2014	Lai et al,[12] 2015
Feng et al,[70] 2016	McSharry et al,[54] 2015	Lawson et al,[73] 2011
Gehring et al,[6] 2008	Moniruzzaman et al,[76] 2012	Oluwole et al,[75] 2018
Karvonen et al,[7] 2012	Norback et al,[80] 2016	Oluwole et al,[74] 2018
Lawson et al,[71] 2012	Rullo et al,[19] 2009	Perzanowski et al,[13] 2006
Morcos et al,[72] 2011	Tischer et al,[21] 2015	Smit et al,[14] 2010
Sordillo et al,[66] 2010	Wickens et al,[20] 2002	Tavernier et al,[15] 2005
Stein et al,[8] 2016		Thorne et al,[16] 2005
Tischer et al,[81] 2011		Tischer et al,[21] 2015
Tischer et al,[21] 2015		

Studies supporting the beneficial, neutral, or harmful effects of environmental endotoxin exposure on asthma development or asthma severity. Note that even in a single study,[21] protective, neutral, and harmful effects of environmental endotoxin exposure on asthma development have been described.

and/or fungal exposures and chronic lung diseases. Given the volume of literature on this topic, our literature search focused on original scientific articles based on human studies published in the last 10 years. The following search terms were used to identify relevant literature; "(environment*[tiab] OR environment*[Mesh] OR expos*[tiab] OR indoor[tiab] OR school[tiab] OR home [tiab])

AND ("Microbiota"[Mesh] OR "Bacteria"[Mesh] OR "Antigens, Bacterial"[Mesh] OR "Bacterial Toxins"[Mesh] OR "Enterotoxins"[Mesh] OR "Fungi"[Mesh] OR "Mycotoxins"[Mesh] OR bacteria [tiab] OR bacterial[tiab] OR endotoxin*[tiab] OR enterotoxin*[tiab] OR fungal[tiab] OR fungi[tiab] OR fungus[tiab] OR lipopolysaccharides[tiab] OR microbial [tiab] OR microbiome[tiab] OR microbiota*[tiab] OR mold[tiab] OR molds[tiab] OR mycotoxin*[tiab] OR peptidoglycan[tiab] OR staph[tiab] OR Staphylococcus[tiab] OR teichoic acid*[tiab]) AND (pulmonary[tiab] OR lung[tiab] OR asthma [tiab] OR copd[tiab] OR "ipf"[tiab]) AND ("2009/01/01"[PDat]: "2019/12/31"[PDat]) AND English [lang]

NOT (pneumonia[tiab] OR pneumonia[Mesh] OR tuberculos*[tiab] OR tuberculos*[Mesh] OR mycobact*[tiab] OR infection*[tiab] OR cancer[tiab]) NOT (Rodentia[Mesh] OR equine[tiab] OR murine [tiab] OR cell[tiab] OR cells[tiab] OR Cells[Mesh]) NOT "Review"[pt]". This yielded 1170 publications that we manually reviewed for relevance, and chose 149 pertaining to chronic lung disease (ie, asthma or COPD). An additional 25 citations were obtained from selected articles were also included in this review.

WAYS TO MEASURE MICROBES

Motivating Example: Why Does It Matter How Microbes Are Measured in the Environment?

There are several approaches to measure environmental microbial exposures as outlined in **Table 2**. It is important to consider the type of information each approach provides because it may explain seeming paradoxes in the literature. As noted above, one example of this paradox is the continued controversy over the role environmental endotoxin exposure plays in either preventing or promoting asthma development and/or asthma symptoms as outlined in **Table 1**. Historically, it has been difficult to reconcile the large number of well-designed studies that have supported both the protective and harmful effects of endotoxin exposure on asthma. Some authors suggest that perhaps gene-by-environment interactions of common genetic polymorphisms[22,23] with environmental endotoxin exposure are the explanation, although in the example of polymorphisms in the *CD14* gene, different investigative groups have shown conflicting evidence on which allele is protective.[24] An alternative explanation exists, which is that our method of measuring endotoxin in epidemiologic studies may not provide the type of information required to specify human health effects.

In almost all epidemiologic studies, environmental endotoxin exposure is measured using the Limulus amebocyte lysate (LAL) assay, an assay that to this day relies on the blood of *Limulus polyphemus*, the Atlantic horseshoe crab. In 1964, Dr. Bang, a marine biologist at Marine Biological

Table 2
Approach to measuring environmental microbial exposures

Technique	What Is Measured	What It Tells Us	Limitations
Microscopy	• Visible microbes • Spore count	• What we can see	• Labor-intensive and not easily reproducible • Morphology does not always predict taxonomy or function
Culture	• Colony-forming units	• Which organisms are culturable • Can isolate microbes for further study	• Labor-intensive, disruptive to the environment • Most environmental microbes are difficult to culture with conventional culture techniques; some are impossible to isolate in culture due to symbiotic relationships with other microbes
Microbial fragments • Gram-negative bacteria: endotoxin (lipopolysaccharide, or LPS) • Gram-positive bacteria: peptidoglycan, miramic acid, teichoic acid • Fungi: 1,3-beta-glucan, ergosterol	• Cell wall components of microbes	• Microbial load (specific to marker used)	• Only detects 1 subclass of microbe (depending on marker used)
Quantitative polymerase chain reaction[a]	• Gene fragments of microbes	• Microbial load	• Only detects 1 type of microbe (depending on the primer)
Amplicon sequencing • 16S (bacteria) • 18S (fungi or archaea) • ITS (fungi)	• Sequencing of marker gene	• Taxonomy of microbial community	• Only detects 1 class of microbe (depending on the primer) • Primer amplification bias described • Typically only provides relative not absolute abundance unless spike-in microbes added • Reliably detects taxonomy at the genus level

(*continued on next page*)

Table 2
(*continued*)

Technique	What Is Measured	What It Tells Us	Limitations
Metagenomics	• Sequencing of all genes in the sample (host and microbial)	• Taxonomy of microbial community • Predicted function of microbial community, including potential function, metabolites, antimicrobial resistance genes	• Costly • Typically only provides relative not absolute abundance unless spike-in microbes added • Sequences all DNA (including host-derived DNA) • Data generated more complex to analyze
Metatranscriptomics	• Actively transcribed genes of microbial community	• Actively expressed genes, and their relative levels	• Costly • Metatranscriptome may fluctuate rapidly

[a] Quantitative polymerase chain reaction (qPCR), is also known as real-time PCR. A refinement on qPCR is droplet digital PCR, which allows more precise quantification of nucleic acid amounts.

Labs made the observation that, when gram-negative bacteria came into contact with the blood of horseshoe crabs, a clotting cascade was activated,[25,26] which allowed the development of an assay to quantify endotoxin based on turbidity. This assay was later converted to a colorimetric assay[27] and the LAL assay remains today the primary approach by which endotoxin is measured in a wide range of applications, including the asthma studies described in **Table 1**. However, a number of investigators have demonstrated that a horseshoe crab-based assay for endotoxin does not approximate the biological response elicited in human-based assays, such as incubation with either human whole blood[28] or human immune cells.[29] Furthermore, endotoxin from different microbial species elicits differential responses in mammalian immune cells,[30] something not captured in the LAL assay.[28]

A recent microbiome study based on shotgun metagenomics sequencing has further provided evidence that not all endotoxin is the same, and that a different approach to measuring microbes may explain conflicting roles of endotoxin on health.[31] Karelia, a region that encompasses Russia, Estonia, and Finland, has long been known to have a gradient of allergic and autoimmune diseases, such as asthma and type I diabetes. Birth cohorts were established in each of these 3 countries and stool was collected from infants on a monthly basis for shotgun metagenomics sequencing and microbiome profiling. Differences in the infant gut microbiome were observed by country, with a higher relative abundance of *Bacteroides dorei* in the Finnish infants and simultaneously a higher proportion of type I diabetes-associated antibodies. On functional analysis of the sequencing data, differences in lipid A (the bioactive component of endotoxin) biosynthesis were noted between these cohorts leading the investigators to isolate a range of bacterial strains from the infants' stool and purify endotoxin from each strain. In an assay where endotoxin from each strain was incubated with human peripheral blood mononuclear cells (PBMCs) and a multiplex inflammatory cytokine assay was performed on the supernatant, endotoxin from *E coli* was associated with inflammatory cytokine production in a dose-dependent manner, whereas no amount of endotoxin from *B dorei* could elicit an inflammatory response. Interestingly, when endotoxin from *B dorei* was mixed with endotoxin from *E coli* and incubated with human PBMCs, no inflammatory response was elicited. In further work on a nonobese mouse model of diabetes, injection of *E coli* but not *B dorei* endotoxin led to a delay in the onset of diabetes. Development of immune tolerance requires a balance of proinflammatory and anti-inflammatory commensals in the gut; disruption of this balance leads to dysbiosis and development of autoimmune diseases, such as type I diabetes.[32] This study highlights the possibility that different types of endotoxin may have opposing effects on eliciting inflammation, therefore explaining the conflicting results from epidemiologic studies listed in **Table 1**. Different mixtures of endotoxin from different gram-negative bacteria may lead to protective, null, or harmful effects on asthma in mammalian systems. Whereas the use of the LAL assay to quantify microbial exposure is not able to differentiate between differences in the immunostimulatory effects of endotoxin from different bacteria, the use of microbial sequencing to quantify microbial taxonomy and function can offer the granularity needed to disentangle these effects. Thus, it is critical to consider how microbial exposures are measured in any given study to interpret the literature on microbial exposures and chronic lung disease.

Measuring What Is Alive and Easily Culturable

Before the availability of molecular methods, epidemiologic studies largely relied on direct microscopy or volumetric sampling onto culture media to characterize microbial exposures. Currently, microscopy is used infrequently as it is labor-intensive, although in various studies it remains a useful tool to quantify fungal spores[33] as this approach does not require an investigator to prespecify in advance which fungi to test for. Typically, these methods involve volumetric sampling with capture of the spores on a filter, slide, or spore trap followed by time-consuming manual identification and counting under light microscopy. Culture is sometimes used today, although techniques such as the use of an Andersen cascade impactor where air samples can be directly inoculated onto culture plates. However, this method is noisy and therefore disruptive to inhabitants of an indoor space.[34] An additional challenge with culture-based methods is that most microbes are metabolically active yet remain unculturable using conventional techniques.[35,36] We are often unable to easily replicate optimal growth conditions for environmental microbes in the laboratory setting, and typical clinical microbiology laboratories do not keep cultures for prolonged periods of time to detect slow-growing microbes. With the use of sequencing to identify members of microbial communities most relevant to health, there is renewed interest in "culturomics" to culture and characterize specific microbes identified using sequencing for further mechanistic studies, and in the future it is likely that approaches combining sequencing with culture will be more common.

Measuring Microbial Load

Approximating the burden of microbial exposure using microbial fragments (typically parts of microbial cell walls) has been one of the most common methods of evaluating microbial exposures. The popularity of this approach is in part due to available standardized assays (which in the case of endotoxin is the use of the LAL assay calibrated to endotoxin purified from *E coli*[37]) as well as the possibility of setting exposure limits based on an easy-to-interpret numeric threshold.[38] Other microbial fragments used to measure microbial load include peptidoglycan[39] and associated components, such as teichoic acid[40] or muramic acid[41] (which favors detection of gram-positive bacteria), or ergosterol[41] and 1,3-beta-D-glucan[41] for fungal exposures. More recently, quantitative polymerase chain reaction (qPCR) and related methods have been used to quantify microbial load. In this approach, nucleic acid is extracted from the sample of interest and specific primers are used to amplify the target gene of interest (for example, primers for the 16S rRNA gene for bacteria, or primers for the internal transcribed spacer [ITS] region to quantify fungi[42]), with fluorophores (that act as reporters) incorporated into the amplified product allowing quantification of the amount of PCR product produced with each cycle. All of these approaches to measure microbial load do require the investigator to prespecify in advance which microbial component (for example, bacteria versus fungi if using qPCR, or gram-positive versus gram-negative bacteria if measuring cell wall components) they are interested in studying.

Measuring Microbial Communities and Function Using Culture-Independent Methods

The ability to identify members of a microbial community through sequencing was made possible when Carl Woese,[43] an evolutionary microbiologist, discovered that the primary structure of the 16S ribosomal RNA gene was conserved, allowing it to serve as a "marker gene" for certain microbes where variations in this gene essentially could be used as a molecular fingerprint to differentiate between different microbes. This led to the discovery of archaea,[44] a prokaryotic kingdom closely related to bacteria but evolutionarily distinct, and enabled the ability of researchers to leverage sequencing to identify microbes in a culture-independent method in what we know as microbiome research today. There have been attempts to standardize terms in this field,[45] with "microbiota" referring to the taxonomic identity of the microbes in a sample, "metagenome" referring to the potential function of a microbial community based on its genetic composition, and "microbiome" referring to the microbiota, their metagenome, and the environmental conditions for that microbial community. In addition, "mycobiome" or the fungal microbiome refers to the fungal community in and on an organism.

What is probably more important is the distinction between amplicon sequencing and shotgun metagenomics sequencing in terms of the types of information provided. This topic has been extensively reviewed elsewhere,[46,47] but amplicon-based sequencing refers to marker gene-based methods where typically a single marker gene, such as the 16S ribosomal RNA gene is amplified, sequenced, and aligned to existing databases to determine the microbiota in a sample. Shotgun metagenomics sequencing is an approach where all DNA present in a sample is sequenced, and so in this way the investigator does not have to prespecify the microbial domain of interest (ie, bacteria, fungi, viruses, or archaea), and both the microbiota and their potential function (metagenome) can be identified. There are additional considerations for an investigator when choosing a sequencing approach. For example, amplicon sequencing is affected by primer amplification bias (thus distorting the relative abundance of the microbes detected) and may not reliably identify microbes beyond the genus level, whereas shotgun metagenomics sequencing is significantly more costly, can be technically difficult to perform in low-biomass samples, and also sequences human (or other host-derived) DNA, which needs to be removed as part of downstream bioinformatics pipelines. However, these culture-independent methods have allowed us to document the true diversity of microbial exposures present in our environment, demonstrated that in many cases microbial function rather than taxonomy is more relevant to human health,[48] and may identify characteristics of environmental microbial exposures that may be more relevant for human health effects.[31]

Considerations for Measuring Fungal Exposures

There are additional complexities for measuring environmental fungal exposures due to the lack of agreement on how best to quantify environmental fungal exposure and the diversity of phenotypes resulting from fungal exposures. This includes clinical entities due to a detrimental immune response (eg, allergic sensitization or hypersensitivity pneumonitis), effect of mycotoxins (many of which are volatile in nature[49]), or direct infection. Here, we will only provide a brief overview as this topic has previously been extensively reviewed.[50,51] Several studies use survey-based assessments focused on the presence of reported dampness, visible mold, or perceived moldy odor as a proxy for environmental fungal exposure. This is inherently subjective, subject to recall bias (particularly if it is participant self-report), and focuses on presence/absence, thereby precluding establishment of an exposure-response relationship with health effects. Some studies have relied on direct microscopy to quantify the total amount of exposure and the types of fungi present,[52] although this approach is labor-intensive and results are not easily reproducible. Other studies have relied on volumetric sampling onto culture media, which as noted may be insensitive although this approach is still widely used in studies evaluating fungal exposures. Measuring cell wall components or fungal metabolites is particularly challenging with fungal exposures given that this does not distinguish between fungi that may cause versus those that are not known to cause allergic sensitization. In addition, the LAL assay cross-reacts with 1,3-beta-D-glucan, thus requiring additional steps in the laboratory to measure 1,3-beta-D-glucan specifically. Before the widespread use of sequencing to identify the fungal mycobiome, a mold-specific qPCR assay focused on 36 common molds[53] has been used in several epidemiologic studies. These molds are subdivided into group 1 molds, which are molds commonly found in homes with water damage, and group 2 molds, which are commonly found in homes without water damage. Investigators have proposed an Environmental Relative Moldiness Index (ERMI) score that can then be calculated using this PCR approach based on the ratio of group 1 (defined as molds typically found in water-damaged homes) to group 2 molds (defined as molds not typically found in water-damaged homes, ie, many outdoor molds) to create a simple numerical score typically ranging from −10 to +20 to characterize the indoor mold environment. A high ERMI (ie, molds typically found in water-damaged homes) in the home environment has been associated with lower lung function in asthmatic adults[54] and with increased risk of asthma development in a birth cohort study, although in this study the authors found that the sum of 3 group 1 molds was a stronger predictor than the ERMI of asthma risk.[55] One challenge with the ERMI is that common allergenic molds, such as *Alternaria alternata* are classified as a group 2 molds (thus if there is a predominance *Alternaria* then the ERMI would be low). In addition, the ERMI approach inherently limits the diversity of fungi assessed by prespecifying the molds of interest, and both culture- and qPCR-based assessment of the ERMI molds have been shown to underestimate fungal diversity compared with sequencing-based approaches.[56] More recently, amplicon sequencing of either the 18S rRNA gene or the ITS region has been used to describe the environmental mycobiome and linked to health effects.[57] Deciding on which approach to measure fungal exposures will require studies that compare all of the above approaches and link them to health effects, and currently there are few studies that meet this criterion.

LUNG DISEASES

As mentioned in our introduction, there has been conflicting literature regarding the effect of microbial exposures on chronic lung disease. Here, we will discuss the existing literature on asthma and COPD, focusing primarily on bacterial and fungal studies.

It is important to mention that viral and archaeal exposures almost certainly impact the development or severity of chronic lung diseases. However, the literature is sparse in the case of archaea, and in the case of viruses focus almost exclusively on pathogenic viruses. For example, studies of high-risk atopic children with early-in-life acute respiratory illnesses, most commonly with rhinovirus or respiratory syncytial virus (RSV), were found to have increased risk of wheeze and physician-diagnosed asthma.[58] Other birth cohorts have noted that episodes of RSV infection early in life are associated with asthma development, and that RSV immunoprophylaxis administered to preterm infants reduced recurrent wheezing.[59] Little is known about exposure to archaea, but there are some case reports of gut microbiome alterations of archaea species, such as *Methanosphera stadtmanae*, which may reduce risk of asthma in children.[60] Given that there are more data on bacterial and fungal exposures, we will focus the rest of this review on the effect of these microbial exposures on common chronic lung diseases.

In this next section, we will outline the existing data published over the past 10 years with regard to effect of bacterial exposures on first asthma and then COPD. The mechanism of action of the bacterial microbiome is likely multifactorial. Current data suggest it likely encompasses exposure to environmental bacteria (measured by endotoxin levels, sequencing, and culture), but the degree to which each of these contribute is not clear. Some of these exposures likely lead to infection, but some may condition the immune system through colonization or exposure to microbial-derived metabolites, such as volatile organic compounds. We thus try to break down published studies into sections based on the method of quantification, followed by age groups.

EFFECTS OF BACTERIAL EXPOSURES ON ASTHMA

For many years, endotoxin has been used as the standard measure of overall bacterial exposure in epidemiologic studies. Endotoxin is thought to induce neutrophilic asthma and wheeze after binding to Toll-like receptor 4 to produce proinflammatory cytokines,[61] and is present inside gram-negative bacterial cell walls. There have been numerous studies examining endotoxin levels with relation to pediatric asthma. These are largely divided into early-exposure studies (ie, birth cohorts) versus late childhood exposure. Studying the effects of microbiome on infants is difficult, because almost 50% of children will have at least 1 episode of wheezing before age 6 years, but these are expressed in different phenotypes, and only a subset of these will develop asthma.[62] Furthermore, children cannot formally be diagnosed with asthma until age 3 years. Thus, most birth cohort studies focus on early childhood wheezing, with some extending into later childhood to determine if there is an eventual asthma diagnosis. A large birth cohort study examining an "environmental score" consisting of family size, number of children, sharing a bedroom, and number of pets at home (all of which are used as a proxy for microbial exposure) found that a higher environmental score early in life predisposes children to wheezing.[63] Other cross-sectional studies have found that mattress dust endotoxin levels can increase frequency of wheeze, but do not alter lung function and so the outcome cannot be classified as asthma.[64,65] Interestingly, a birth cohort study that followed these birth cohorts to school age found that early exposure to endotoxin may protect from progression to physician-diagnosed asthma.[66] Multiple cohort studies demonstrate a lower prevalence of asthma among children raised on farms,[67–69] with some association with greater environmental biodiversity.[67] A particularly large birth cohort study from Bacharier and colleagues[62] examined 442 children in the Urban Environment and Childhood Asthma cohort, from birth to age 7 years and performed cluster analysis on different wheezing phenotypes. They found 5 distinct phenotypes that differentiated participants based on patterns of wheezing and allergic sensitization, with the highest eventual diagnosis of asthma in children with high-wheeze and high-atopy phenotypes[62]; interestingly, this phenotype was associated with low household allergen microbial richness and diversity.[62] Thus, although it is difficult to draw conclusions from birth cohort data, there is a general trend toward the possibility that endotoxin increases infant wheezing but perhaps protects against eventual development of asthma.

On examination of endotoxin exposure effects on school-aged children, there have also been mixed results. Some have found home dust endotoxin protects against asthma,[70–72] whereas others have found a higher risk of asthma with endotoxin exposure,[3,73–75] some found no effect[54,76–80] and still others have found contradictory results in different populations[21,81] (see **Table 1**). A recent review article by Mendy and colleagues[82] concluded that endotoxin may positively correlate with wheeze in toddlers, but start to have a protective effect in school-aged children and protect against eventual development of asthma, but conceded that there are contradictory data. Once we move beyond school age, there is again conflicting data regarding effects of endotoxin. Adult studies have found that endotoxin levels in the bedroom can significantly increase wheezing,[83,84] whereas others have shown no effect.[85]

There are several hypotheses for these inconsistent results. First, measuring home dust endotoxin levels only measures one environment in a child's life. Recent cohort studies of asthmatic children have demonstrated that the school dust microbiome can differ significantly from the home dust microbiome.[12] In fact, after adjustment for home, school endotoxin levels alone have been shown to correlate with asthma diagnoses[86] and thus we may need more complete sampling. Second, endotoxin can be produced from different species of bacteria, and different strains of bacteria may have different effects. Third, there are likely effect modifiers, including environmental coexposures and genetics that can potentiate effects of endotoxin, as discussed below.

Given the difficulty with endotoxin data, there has been a recent shift in switching toward sequencing to evaluate the bacterial microbiome. Simultaneous measurement of endotoxin levels and microbial diversity (measured by sequencing) show that these 2 metrics do not correlate,[87] thus it cannot be assumed that high endotoxin environments also have high microbial diversity. For asthma prevention, as suggested from the farm studies, low household microbial richness early in life is associated with development of asthma.[62] Examination of microbial exposure by sequencing of mattress dust in school-aged children found that high microbial diversity decreased asthma frequency and severity.[88,89] Interestingly, after sequencing samples from both nasal passages and mattress dust samples, the association between asthma and mattress dust sample diversity was stronger than asthma and nasal passage diversity, suggesting involvement of the environmental microbiome beyond mere colonization of the nares.[88] It has been difficult to identify a single protective species, and cohort studies have rather suggested that some bacterial communities are more protective than others.[90,91] Some authors have performed sequencing of dust samples, and noted that specific species, including *Acinetobacter*, *Lactobacillus*, *Neisseria*, *Staph jeotgalicoccus*, and *Corynebacterium* exposures offered protective effects against asthma,[92] and others have found increasing levels of *Clostridium* to be protective.[93] Others have found that lower exposure to *Firmicutes* and *Bacteroidetes* is associated with atopy and atopic wheeze.[89] At present, no specific bacterial species has emerged as being independently protective or harmful. However, it must be noted that although high microbial diversity early in life may be protective against asthma, studies show that for children already diagnosed with asthma, high microbial diversity seems to promote asthma symptoms.[94,95] It is possible that a specific indoor microbial environment may be beneficial for asthma prevention yet harmful for asthma symptoms.

In other attempts to quantify human exposure to bacteria, some researchers have measured microbial volatile organic compounds (MVOCs), which are a variety of compounds formed during metabolic processes in fungi and bacteria. A case study of asthmatic children and health controls was performed where 28 MVOCs were measured and summed as a single exposure metric and was found to be associated with asthma risk in a dose-dependent manner, which was exacerbated by humidity in the home.[96] This method of quantification has the same risk of error as endotoxin, as it does not specify which types of bacteria or fungi the exposure includes and may simply represent a poorly ventilated home.

Beyond everyday exposures from inhalation, there are also data that colonization of the upper airway by pathogens may affect atopy and risk of asthma. A pediatric cohort study examining nasal carriage of *Staphylococcus aureus* found carriage was associated with severe asthma, as well as eczema and allergic rhinitis.[97] A case study of inner-city adolescents examining concentrations of *S aureus* in the home found some evidence that high-exposure days were associated with increased respiratory symptoms, but longitudinally *S aureus* concentrations did not correlate with a significant decline in lung function or FeNO.[98] A large case-control study by Sintobin and colleagues[99] of European adults, found that sensitization toward *S aureus* enterotoxins is associated with increased risk of severe asthma, and that this sensitization was associated with severe asthma assessed even 10 to 20 years later.

Another potential microbial exposure in the home environment is ingestion of raw milk. A cross-sectional study of children who consume raw milk found that it was protective against asthma; interestingly it was the raw milk itself rather than total bacterial count.[100]

Given that bacterial exposures clearly affect profiles for asthma, there is interest in identifying modifiable factors than can potentiate or alleviate their effects. Gene-by-environment interactions have long been postulated to explain the contradictory effect of environmental endotoxin on asthma. One case-control study examined 26 single-nucleotide polymorphisms (SNPs) among 824 children, and found that 2 variants were specifically associated with asthma-related hospital admissions.[101] These SNPs included CD14 SNP rs5744455 and LY96 SNP rs17226566, which are genetic variants in the endotoxin response pathway.[101] Another pediatric school-based study focused on polymorphism in the interleukin-4 receptor alpha chain gene (*IL4R*). Higher classroom endotoxin levels were associated with fewer asthma symptoms for children with the *Q/Q* genotype, an equivocal effect for the *Q/R* genotype and increased asthma symptoms for the *R/R* genotype.[23] The *R/R* genotype was much more prevalent in African American or mixed race children. These findings suggest that identified gene-by-environment interactions may explain health disparities, and may be used to target future therapies.

Other effect modifiers may be candidates for intervention, for example, second-hand smoke exposure.[102–104] A case-control pediatric study examining endotoxin levels in mattress dust found that high endotoxin levels were associated with decreased FEV_1, an association that was potentiated by concurrent tobacco smoke exposure.[102] Two separate cohort studies found that in smoke-free homes endotoxin was protective against asthma, whereas in homes with nicotine exposure through second-hand smoke, endotoxin was associated with asthma.[103,104] One of these was a large pediatric cohort study by Matsui and colleagues,[104] who found that the respiratory effects of household endotoxin are modified by coexposure to common indoor pollutants, including air nicotine and nitrogen dioxide. In a similar fashion, it has been shown that suspended particulate matter has been associated with worsening respiratory symptoms (ie, wheezing, cough, and breathlessness)[105] and may modify effects of endotoxin. Environmental particulate matter and endotoxin both vary by season, with peak levels in the autumn months.[106] An interesting large cohort study by Mendy and colleagues[107] examined the effects of ambient coexposure to levels of endotoxin and ambient particular matter, and found that these act synergistically. The combination of ambient particulate matter and endotoxin was associated with increased rate of emergency room visits for asthma, compared with either one alone.[107] Another cohort study noted that endotoxin effects may differ based on climate, and that in cold environments endotoxin exposure may more strongly predispose to wheezing.[108]

The role of vitamin D as an effect modifier has also been investigated. Given that endotoxin is thought to induce neutrophilic asthma through production of proinflammatory cytokines, and that vitamin D might inhibit lipopolysaccharide-induced cytokines, Mendy and colleagues[61] performed a large cohort analysis to look for interactions. They found that the combination of vitamin D deficiency and endotoxin was associated with current asthma (odds ratio = 1.56; 95% CI, 1.09–2.23).[61]

Phthalates, which are ingredients used to increase flexibility and durability of plastic products, are another coexposure that may potentiate the effects of endotoxin. A cross-sectional study of adults with asthma noted that, under medium or high endotoxin levels, exposure-response relationships were observed between specific phthalates and asthma.[109] This effect was not seen in low-endotoxin environments, suggesting that these exposures may modify each other.[109]

These studies raise the possibility that there are potential interventions to alter risk. A recent pilot randomized controlled trial examined classroom microbiome exposure in school-aged children, and found that the microbiome was modifiable with use of an integrated pest management intervention.[95] Another cohort study examining home endotoxin levels found that structured education on home cleaning can reduce endotoxin exposure and improve asthma symptoms.[110] These studies suggest that the microbial environment in an indoor space is modifiable.

Overall, the effects of environmental microbial exposure have conflicting results, in part due to a wide variety of exposure assessment techniques. The endotoxin data suggest some early-life protection, which is likely modified by other environmental exposures. Culture and sequencing data suggest that there are likely bacterial communities that increased risk of asthma. Future studies will need to establish which method of measuring bacterial exposure is most pertinent to human health. Studies that measure microbial exposure using a variety of methods are likely to be most helpful, although such studies may be costly to perform.

EFFECTS OF FUNGAL EXPOSURE ON ASTHMA

We next turn to the examination of data regarding fungal exposures and development of asthma. There are multiple methods of measuring environmental fungal exposures, although it has not been well established which of these markers is most accurate for identifying associations with lung diseases.

On review of clinical studies relating asthma to fungal exposures, there have been variable results (**Table 3**). There have been numerous cross-sectional studies suggesting that dampness, visible mold, and/or moldy odors are associated with increased severity of asthma symptoms.[111–124] The seasonal variations in visible mold have been associated with concurrent seasonal variations in asthma exacerbations.[125] There are some data that exposures to mold in pregnancy can increase risk of childhood asthma for the fetus.[126] In pediatric populations, there are multiple birth cohort studies suggesting early exposure to visible mold can increase risk of developing asthma[127–129] and interestingly this seems to be largely nonallergic asthma.[130] Some studies suggest that mold exposure can even lead to a decline in FEV_1 among nonasthmatic patients.[131] One potential advantage of using visible mold as a proxy, however, is that it is modifiable, that is, it can be easily identified by patients leading to cleanup efforts. Studies of workers with asthma symptoms found that remediation of damp buildings did seem to decrease rates of asthma.[132] Although these observational studies suggest that fungal exposure may increase risk and severity of asthma, they are subjective based largely on patient reporting of home conditions, and may be particularly vulnerable to recall bias.

Given the difficulty with visible mold reporting, various studies have attempted quantification of beta-glucan levels in the home as a surrogate for total mold levels. Examination of house dust samples for beta-glucan found that exposure to high levels of 1,3-beta-glucan is associated with reduced risk of wheezing during infancy,[75,133,134]

Table 3
Studies on fungal exposures (stratified by exposure assessment method) on asthma development or asthma severity

Friend	Neutral	Foe
Dampness, moldy odor, visible mold		
		Chen et al,[129] 2011
		Iossifova et al,[134] 2009
		Karvala et al,[132] 2011
		Karvonen et al,[128] 2015
		Thacher et al,[130] 2017
		Tischer et al,[127] 2011
Culture		
Behbod et al,[142] yeast protective	Huang et al[139]	Behbod et al,[142] 2013, outdoor fungi harmful
Behbod et al,[143] 2015, yeast protective		Behbod et al,[143] 2015, outdoor fungi harmful
		Bundy et al,[145] 2009
		Carreiro-Martins et al,[137] 2016
		Gunnbjornsdottir et al,[138] 2009
		Oluwole et al,[136] 2017
		Rosenbaum et al,[144] 2010
		Vicendese et al,[146] 2015
		Zubairi et al,[147] 2014
1,3-beta-D-Glucan (high)		
Oluwole et al,[75] 2018		Seo et al,[135] 2014
Iossifova et al,[134] 2009		
QPCR		
Karvonen et al,[149] 2014, high microbial diversity score	Rosenbaum et al,[159] 2015	Eiffert et al,[157] 2016, high ERMI
Mueller-Rompa et al,[151] 2017, specific taxa protective		McSharry et al,[54] 2015, high ERMI
Tischer et al,[148] 2016, high microbial diversity score		Reponen et al,[153] 2011, high ERMI
		Reponen et al,[55] 2012, high ERMI
		Segura-Medina et al,[150] 2019, specific molds
		Sinclair et al,[158] 2018, high ERMI
		Vesper et al,[154] 2013, high ERMI
		Vesper et al,[155] 2016, high ERMI
		Vesper et al,[156] 2017, high ERMI
Sequencing		
Dannemiller et al,[94] 2016, yeast genera *Kondoa* protective		Dannemiller et al,[94] 2016, total fungal concentration
		Dannemiller et al,[57] 2014, low fungal diversity

A score based on the ratio of group 1 molds (defined as molds typically found in water-damaged homes) compared with group 1 molds (defined as molds not typically found in water-damaged homes).
Abbreviation: ERMI, Environmental Relative Moldiness Index.

whereas others have shown that high 1,3-beta-D-glucan levels are a risk factor for wheezing later in childhood.[135] This contradictory data may be due in part to the nonspecific identification of beta-glucan, which is found in both bacteria and fungi.

Recent studies have used fungal cultures to quantify and describe fungal exposure, and have found that different fungal communities likely have different effects. Two pediatric case-control trials found that high cultured fungus levels in dust samples from play areas and mattresses were significantly associated with current asthma.[136,137] A large cohort study by Gunnbjornsdottir and colleagues,[138] among 3 European cohorts, found that increased levels of culturable fungi were associated with increased bronchial responsiveness. In contrast, a pediatric case-control study from China found that air quality, as defined by CO_2 and particulate matter, had associations with asthma severity, whereas culturable fungi levels did not.[139] A pediatric case-control study found no significant difference in mean fungal concentrations between the homes of asthmatics versus nonasthmatics.[140] Recent literature on cultured fungi and asthma has thus attempted to stratify types of fungus. An adult case-control study found that total levels of culturable fungi were not associated with asthma, but the presence of certain genus groups (including *Aspergillus fumigatus* and *Penicillium*) were associated with severe asthma.[141] Two birth cohort studies found that increased levels of yeast, a type of fungus, on the bedroom floor is protective against wheezing at any age.[142,143] Fungal culture studies of bedroom floor dust have found an increased risk of wheeze with exposure to indoor *Alternaria*,[142] *Penicillium*,[141,142,144] *Cladosporium*,[142,145,146] and *Aspergillus*,[141,147] as well as outdoor *Cladosporium*.[142] This overall suggests that rather than fungal levels, there are likely specific fungal communities that may predispose to or protect against asthma development.

In other attempts to identify fungal culprits, studies have used qPCR to quantify and identify fungal exposure. A birth cohort study found that higher fungal diversity for young children reduced risk of ever wheezing through to age 6 years, but these effects were attenuated in later childhood through age 10 years.[148] This was also seen in another birth cohort study where high microbial diversity scores that accounts for both bacterial and fungal qPCRs, have a protective effect against developing asthma.[149] Another interesting cohort study using qPCR found that associations between mold burden and asthma control was different among males and females; specifically, that concentrations of some molds were protective in males but not in females.[150] A large pediatric cohort study out of Europe found that several fungal taxa may be protective against childhood asthma; these authors proposed this may be due to the bioactivity of molds, which may have beneficial immunoregulatory capacities that could be therapeutically targeted.[151] These conflicting data again suggest that there are likely either fungal communities or specific pathogens that may carry the risk or protection for susceptible individuals.[149]

Other literature has focused on the ERMI (see **Table 3**), a score based on qPCR-based assessment focused on fungi found in water-damaged homes, and again found contradictory data. These studies have generally found that older homes have higher scores, and that central air conditioning can help lower this score.[152] In contrast to endotoxin data, where early-life exposure may be protective, there are birth cohorts in fungal studies suggesting that a higher ERMI in an infant's home can increase the risk of developing asthma.[54,133,153] Some pediatric studies have found that the association of an increased ERMI with asthma diminishes as children get older,[153] whereas others have identified an increased ERMI as a consistent risk factor into early adulthood.[55,154–156] When we look at the adult population, there are multiple studies demonstrating that higher ERMI scores (ie, a higher ratio of group 1 molds found in water-damaged homes) are associated with asthma symptoms and/or severity,[157,158] whereas others show no statistically significant associations.[159] Other cross-sectional studies have found median ERMI values are higher in the homes of asthmatics compared with the homes of nonasthmatics.[160]

Another method to measure and identify fungal exposures is through sequencing to identify the indoor fungal mycobiome. A pediatric cohort study by Dannemiller and colleagues[94] using amplicon sequencing found an increased asthma severity with exposure to high summed allergenic fungal species levels. They also found that, in atopic children, specific fungal community composition was associated with asthma severity, with the fungal genus *Volutella* emerging as a culprit.[94] Interestingly, there was a protective effect with exposure to yeast genus *Kondoa*,[94] similar to the culture data above, suggesting that yeast may have a protective effect. In contrast, another birth cohort study found that lower fungal diversity in the home was associated with increased risk of asthma development.[57] Specifically, decreased diversity within the genus *Cryptococcus* was associated with asthma risk.[57]

There have been reports investigating whether sensitization to molds (ie, having positive skin testing or allergen-specific IgE) relates to asthma rates. Two cohort studies of adults with allergic asthma found that skin sensitization toward *Cladosporium* was associated with severe asthma.[161,162] Other studies have found higher incidence of IgE seropositivity to *Penicillium* and *Fusarium* species among asthma patients,[163,164] and some have found that sensitization to *Aspergillus alternata* was associated with frequent wheeze.[165]

With regard to modifiable factors, there have been data about the effect of cleaning of work environments and reduced symptoms.[132] Other pediatric studies have shown that education about cleaning visible mold can help reduce hospital visits for asthma.[166] Some studies have found that the number of household residents correlates with the amount of mold in the home.[167] One unique study evaluated the effect of moving children from a high ERMI home environment to a low ERMI forest environment for a few days, and noted improved lung function in the children.[168] Much like gene-by-environmental interactions with bacterial exposure, there have been data demonstrating asthma rates linked to a specific polymorphism of the interleukin-4 promoter and visible mold exposure.[169]

THE MICROBIOME AND CHRONIC OBSTRUCTIVE LUNG DISEASE

Chronic obstructive lung disease, known as COPD, is an adult pulmonary disease characterized by progressive airway inflammation, usually associated with tobacco inhalation.[170] Tobacco smoke is the most well-established risk factor; however, there is emerging evidence from developing countries that other substantial risk factors exist, including biomass from fuel exposure, and potentially colonization of the lower airway with pathogenic bacteria.[170] Studies examining the association of microbial exposures with COPD have again used different methods for exposure assessment.

A large cohort study in patients with COPD found that endotoxin levels were not significantly associated with COPD symptoms or severity,[171] and that in vitro whole-blood assays demonstrated that endotoxin exposure was not a primary trigger for interleukin-1β release, thought to be the primary driver of the inflammatory response.[171] A well-designed case-control study by Ghosh and colleagues[170] compared the microbiome profile of tobacco exposure-related patients with COPD, to the microbiome of biomass-related patients with COPD. Specific examination was performed of bacterial load by potentially pathogenic bacteria (defined by *Streptococcus pneumoniae*, *Haemophilus influenza*, *Moraxella*, and *Pseudomonas aeruginosa*); the biomass-related patients with COPD had higher loads of potentially pathogenic bacteria. Very interestingly, the patients with higher pathogenic bacterial loads were noted to have defective phagocytosis by macrophages, which may explain the chronic inflammatory state.[170] Higher rates of COPD have been observed in professional farmers[172]; 1 case-control study noted that this seemed to be largely related to livestock, including swine, goat or sheep.[173] A recent large case-control study found that livestock farmers were more likely to have COPD, and that this effect seems to be potentiated by concurrent exposure to ammonia, hydrogen sulfide, inorganic dust, and organic dust.[174] Another cross-sectional study confirmed that farmers are exposed to higher levels and different populations of bacteria; however, the IgG and IgE sensitivities did not match the different populations of bacteria to explain COPD rates.[172] Thus, it seems that increased environmental microbial exposure is associated with some phenotypes of COPD, although the best method of quantification (ie, endotoxin versus culture versus sequencing) has not yet been identified.

The data on fungal disease with association to COPD are again sparse; 2 large case-control studies by Pahwa and colleagues[175] noted a greater prevalence of chronic bronchitis associated with self-reported mold in the home. This effect was potentiated by concurrent tobacco use,[175] similar to the effects seen in asthma with bacterial exposures.

SUMMARY

As we reviewed above, there is substantial conflict in the literature regarding the effects of environmental microbial exposures on chronic lung diseases, with the bulk of the literature focused on obstructive lung diseases, such as asthma or COPD. This may be due to factors, such as coexposures or gene-by-environment interactions, or due to inconsistent exposure measurement approaches and a gap in our knowledge about which method of exposure assessment is most pertinent to human health. Advances in sequencing technology have allowed us to better characterize the composition and potential function of environmental microbial communities. This has shed light on the limitations of exposure assessment in previous studies. Future studies incorporating multiple methods of assessing environmental microbial exposures, with standardized reporting of methods and results, are likely to be critical in understanding how to promote healthy microbial environments to reduce the burden of lung disease.

DISCLOSURE

■

REFERENCES

1. Braun-Fahrlander C, Riedler J, Herz U, et al. Environmental exposure to endotoxin and its relation to asthma in school-age children. N Engl J Med 2002;347(12):869–77.
2. Campo P, Kalra HK, Levin L, et al. Influence of dog ownership and high endotoxin on wheezing and atopy during infancy. J Allergy Clin Immunol 2006;118(6):1271–8.
3. Carlsten C, Ferguson A, Dimich-Ward H, et al. Association between endotoxin and mite allergen exposure with asthma and specific sensitization at age 7 in high-risk children. Pediatr Allergy Immunol 2011;22(3):320–6.
4. Douwes J, van Strien R, Doekes G, et al. Does early indoor microbial exposure reduce the risk of asthma? The Prevention and Incidence of Asthma and Mite Allergy birth cohort study. J Allergy Clin Immunol 2006;117(5):1067–73.
5. El-Sharif N, Douwes J, Hoet P, et al. Childhood asthma and indoor aeroallergens and endotoxin in Palestine: a case-control study. J Asthma 2006;43(3):241–7.
6. Gehring U, Strikwold M, Schram-Bijkerk D, et al. Asthma and allergic symptoms in relation to house dust endotoxin: phase two of the international study on asthma and allergies in childhood (ISAAC II). Clin Exp Allergy 2008;38(12):1911–20.
7. Karvonen AM, Hyvärinen A, Gehring U, et al. Exposure to microbial agents in house dust and wheezing, atopic dermatitis and atopic sensitization in early childhood: a birth cohort study in rural areas. Clin Exp Allergy 2012;42(8):1246–56.
8. Stein MM, Hrusch CL, Gozdz J, et al. Innate immunity and asthma risk in Amish and Hutterite farm children. N Engl J Med 2016;375(5):411–21.
9. Bolte G, Bischof W, Borte M, et al. Early endotoxin exposure and atopy development in infants: results of a birth cohort study. Clin Exp Allergy 2003;33(6):770–6.
10. Celedon JC, Milton DK, Ramsey CD, et al. Exposure to dust mite allergen and endotoxin in early life and asthma and atopy in childhood. J Allergy Clin Immunol 2007;120(1):144–9.
11. Gillespie J, Wickens K, Siebers R, et al. Endotoxin exposure, wheezing, and rash in infancy in a New Zealand birth cohort. J Allergy Clin Immunol 2006;118(6):1265–70.
12. Lai PS, Sheehan WJ, Gaffin JM, et al. School endotoxin exposure and asthma morbidity in inner-city children. Chest 2015;148(5):1251–8.
13. Perzanowski MS, Miller RL, Thorne PS, et al. Endotoxin in inner-city homes: associations with wheeze and eczema in early childhood. J Allergy Clin Immunol 2006;117(5):1082–9.
14. Smit LA, Heederik D, Doekes G, et al. Occupational endotoxin exposure reduces the risk of atopic sensitization but increases the risk of bronchial hyperresponsiveness. Int Arch Allergy Immunol 2010;152(2):151–8.
15. Tavernier GO, Fletcher GD, Francis HC, et al. Endotoxin exposure in asthmatic children and matched healthy controls: results of IPEADAM study. Indoor Air 2005;15(Suppl 10):25–32.
16. Thorne PS, Kulhánková K, Yin M, et al. Endotoxin exposure is a risk factor for asthma: the national survey of endotoxin in United States housing. Am J Respir Crit Care Med 2005;172(11):1371–7.
17. Ege MJ, Frei R, Bieli C, et al. Not all farming environments protect against the development of asthma and wheeze in children. J Allergy Clin Immunol 2007;119(5):1140–7.
18. Gehring U, Heinrich J, Jacob B, et al. Respiratory symptoms in relation to indoor exposure to mite and cat allergens and endotoxins. Indoor Factors and Genetics in Asthma (INGA) Study Group. Eur Respir J 2001;18(3):555–63.
19. Rullo VE, Arruda LK, Cardoso MR, et al. Respiratory infection, exposure to mouse allergen and breastfeeding: role in recurrent wheezing in early life. Int Arch Allergy Immunol 2009;150(2):172–8.
20. Wickens K, Lane JM, Fitzharris P, et al. Farm residence and exposures and the risk of allergic diseases in New Zealand children. Allergy 2002;57(12):1171–9.
21. Tischer C, Casas L, Wouters IM, et al. Early exposure to bio-contaminants and asthma up to 10 years of age: results of the HITEA study. Eur Respir J 2015;45(2):328–37.
22. Eder W, Klimecki W, Yu L, et al. Opposite effects of CD 14/-260 on serum IgE levels in children raised in different environments. J Allergy Clin Immunol 2005;116(3):601–7.
23. Lai PS, Massoud AH, Xia M, et al. Gene-environment interaction between an IL4R variant and school endotoxin exposure contributes to asthma symptoms in inner-city children. J Allergy Clin Immunol 2018;141(2):794–6.e3.
24. Martinez FD. CD14, endotoxin, and asthma risk: actions and interactions. Proc Am Thorac Soc 2007;4(3):221–5.

25. Levin J, Bang FB. A description of cellular coagulation in the limulus. Bull Johns Hopkins Hosp 1964; 115:337–45.
26. Levin J, Bang FB. The role of endotoxin in the extracellular coagulation of limulus blood. Bull Johns Hopkins Hosp 1964;115:265–74.
27. Nakamura S, Morita T, Iwanaga S, et al. A sensitive substrate for the clotting enzyme in horseshoe crab hemocytes. J Biochem 1977;81(5):1567–9.
28. Dehus O, Hartung T, Hermann C. Endotoxin evaluation of eleven lipopolysaccharides by whole blood assay does not always correlate with Limulus amebocyte lysate assay. J Endotoxin Res 2006; 12(3):171–80.
29. Gutsmann T, Howe J, Zähringer U, et al. Structural prerequisites for endotoxic activity in the Limulus test as compared to cytokine production in mononuclear cells. Innate Immun 2010;16(1):39–47.
30. Gangloff SC, Hijiya N, Haziot A, et al. Lipopolysaccharide structure influences the macrophage response via CD14-independent and CD14-dependent pathways. Clin Infect Dis 1999;28(3): 491–6.
31. Vatanen T, Kostic AD, d'Hennezel E, et al. Variation in microbiome LPS immunogenicity contributes to autoimmunity in humans. Cell 2016; 165(6):1551.
32. Lee YK, Mazmanian SK. Has the microbiota played a critical role in the evolution of the adaptive immune system? Science 2010;330(6012):1768–73.
33. Macher J, Chen B, Rao C. Field evaluation of a personal, bioaerosol cyclone sampler. J Occup Environ Hyg 2008;5(11):724–34.
34. Solomon WR. A simplified application of the Andersen sampler to the study of airborne fungus particles. J Allergy 1970;45(1):1–13.
35. Roszak DB, Colwell RR. Survival strategies of bacteria in the natural environment. Microbiol Rev 1987;51(3):365–79.
36. Stewart EJ. Growing unculturable bacteria. J Bacteriol 2012;194(16):4151–60.
37. Hochstein HD, Mills DF, Outschoorn AS, et al. The processing and collaborative assay of a reference endotoxin. J Biol Stand 1983;11(4):251–60.
38. DECOS. Endotoxins: health based recommended exposure limit. A report of the Health Council of the Netherlands, in publication no 2010/040SH. The Hague (The Netherlands): Health Council of the Netherlands; 2010.
39. Silhavy TJ, Kahne D, Walker S. The bacterial cell envelope. Cold Spring Harb Perspect Biol 2010; 2(5):a000414.
40. Brown S, Santa Maria JP Jr, Walker S. Wall teichoic acids of Gram-positive bacteria. Annu Rev Microbiol 2013;67:313–36.
41. Sebastian A, Larsson L. Characterization of the microbial community in indoor environments: a chemical-analytical approach. Appl Environ Microbiol 2003;69(6):3103–9.
42. Manter DK, Vivanco JM. Use of the ITS primers, ITS1F and ITS4, to characterize fungal abundance and diversity in mixed-template samples by qPCR and length heterogeneity analysis. J Microbiol Methods 2007;71(1):7–14.
43. Woese CR, Fox GE, Zablen L, et al. Conservation of primary structure in 16S ribosomal RNA. Nature 1975;254(5495):83–6.
44. Fox GE, Magrum LJ, Balch WE, et al. Classification of methanogenic bacteria by 16S ribosomal RNA characterization. Proc Natl Acad Sci U S A 1977; 74(10):4537–41.
45. Marchesi JR, Ravel J. The vocabulary of microbiome research: a proposal. Microbiome 2015;3: 31.
46. Knight R, Vrbanac A, Taylor BC, et al. Best practices for analysing microbiomes. Nat Rev Microbiol 2018;16(7):410–22.
47. Gilbert JA, Blaser MJ, Caporaso JG, et al. Current understanding of the human microbiome. Nat Med 2018;24(4):392–400.
48. Human Microbiome Project. Structure, function and diversity of the healthy human microbiome. Nature 2012;486(7402):207–14.
49. Miller JD, McMullin DR. Fungal secondary metabolites as harmful indoor air contaminants: 10 years on. Appl Microbiol Biotechnol 2014;98(24): 9953–66.
50. Bush RK, Portnoy JM, Saxon A, et al. The medical effects of mold exposure. J Allergy Clin Immunol 2006;117(2):326–33.
51. Baxi SN, Portnoy JM, Larenas-Linnemann D, et al. Exposure and health effects of fungi on humans. J Allergy Clin Immunol Pract 2016;4(3): 396–404.
52. Baxi SN, Sheehan WJ, Sordillo JE, et al. Association between fungal spore exposure in inner-city schools and asthma morbidity. Ann Allergy Asthma Immunol 2019;122(6):610–5.e1.
53. Vesper S, McKinstry C, Ashley P, et al. Quantitative PCR analysis of molds in the dust from homes of asthmatic children in North Carolina. J Environ Monit 2007;9(8):826–30.
54. McSharry C, Vesper S, Wymer L, et al. Decreased FEV1% in asthmatic adults in Scottish homes with high environmental relative moldiness index values. Clin Exp Allergy 2015;45(5):902–7.
55. Reponen T, Lockey J, Bernstein DI, et al. Infant origins of childhood asthma associated with specific molds. J Allergy Clin Immunol 2012;130(3):639–44. e5.
56. Pitkaranta M, Meklin T, Hyvärinen A, et al. Molecular profiling of fungal communities in moisture damaged buildings before and after remediation—a comparison of culture-dependent and

culture-independent methods. BMC Microbiol 2011;11:235.

57. Dannemiller KC, Mendell MJ, Macher JM, et al. Next-generation DNA sequencing reveals that low fungal diversity in house dust is associated with childhood asthma development. Indoor Air 2014; 24(3):236–47.
58. Kusel MM, de Klerk NH, Kebadze T, et al. Early-life respiratory viral infections, atopic sensitization, and risk of subsequent development of persistent asthma. J Allergy Clin Immunol 2007;119(5): 1105–10.
59. Wu P, Hartert TV. Evidence for a causal relationship between respiratory syncytial virus infection and asthma. Expert Rev Anti Infect Ther 2011;9(9): 731–45.
60. Barnett DJM, Mommers M, Penders J, et al. Intestinal archaea inversely associated with childhood asthma. J Allergy Clin Immunol 2019;143(6): 2305–7.
61. Mendy A, Cohn RD, Thorne PS. Endotoxin exposure, serum vitamin D, asthma and wheeze outcomes. Respir Med 2016;114:61–6.
62. Bacharier LB, Beigelman A, Calatroni A, et al. Longitudinal phenotypes of respiratory health in a high-risk urban birth cohort. Am J Respir Crit Care Med 2019;199(1):71–82.
63. Tischer C, Dadvand P, Basagana X, et al. Urban upbringing and childhood respiratory and allergic conditions: a multi-country holistic study. Environ Res 2018;161:276–83.
64. Leung TF, Wong YS, Chan IH, et al. Indoor determinants of endotoxin and dust mite exposures in Hong Kong homes with asthmatic children. Int Arch Allergy Immunol 2010;152(3):279–87.
65. Mendy A, Wilkerson J, Salo PM, et al. Exposure and sensitization to pets modify endotoxin association with asthma and wheeze. J Allergy Clin Immunol Pract 2018;6(6):2006–13.e4.
66. Sordillo JE, Hoffman EB, Celedón JC, et al. Multiple microbial exposures in the home may protect against asthma or allergy in childhood. Clin Exp Allergy 2010;40(6):902–10.
67. Ege MJ, Mayer M, Normand AC, et al. Exposure to environmental microorganisms and childhood asthma. N Engl J Med 2011;364(8):701–9.
68. Timm S, Frydenberg M, Janson C, et al. The urban-rural gradient in asthma: a population-based study in Northern Europe. Int J Environ Res Public Health 2015;13(1):13.
69. Campbell B, Raherison C, Lodge CJ, et al. The effects of growing up on a farm on adult lung function and allergic phenotypes: an international population-based study. Thorax 2017;72(3): 236–44.
70. Feng M, Yang Z, Pan L, et al. Associations of early life exposures and environmental factors with asthma among children in rural and urban areas of Guangdong, China. Chest 2016;149(4): 1030–41.
71. Lawson JA, Dosman JA, Rennie DC, et al. Endotoxin as a determinant of asthma and wheeze among rural dwelling children and adolescents: a case-control study. BMC Pulm Med 2012;12:56.
72. Morcos MM, Morcos WM, Ibrahim MA, et al. Environmental exposure to endotoxin in rural and urban Egyptian school children and its relation to asthma and atopy. Minerva Pediatr 2011;63(1):19–26.
73. Lawson JA, Dosman JA, Rennie DC, et al. Relationship of endotoxin and tobacco smoke exposure to wheeze and diurnal peak expiratory flow variability in children and adolescents. Respirology 2011; 16(2):332–9.
74. Oluwole O, Rennie DC, Senthilselvan A, et al. The association between endotoxin in house dust with atopy and exercise-induced bronchospasm in children with asthma. Environ Res 2018;164:302–9.
75. Oluwole O, Rennie DC, Senthilselvan A, et al. The association between endotoxin and beta-(1→3)-D-glucan in house dust with asthma severity among schoolchildren. Respir Med 2018;138: 38–46.
76. Moniruzzaman S, Hägerhed Engman L, James P, et al. Levels of endotoxin in 390 Swedish homes: determinants and the risk for respiratory symptoms in children. Int J Environ Health Res 2012;22(1): 22–36.
77. Delfino RJ, Staimer N, Tjoa T, et al. Relations of exhaled nitric oxide and FEV1 to personal endotoxin exposure in schoolchildren with asthma. Occup Environ Med 2015;72(12):830–6.
78. Jacobs J, Borràs-Santos A, Krop E, et al. Dampness, bacterial and fungal components in dust in primary schools and respiratory health in schoolchildren across Europe. Occup Environ Med 2014;71(10):704–12.
79. Bertelsen RJ, Carlsen KC, Carlsen KH, et al. Childhood asthma and early life exposure to indoor allergens, endotoxin and beta(1,3)-glucans. Clin Exp Allergy 2010;40(2):307–16.
80. Norback D, Hashim JH, Markowicz P, et al. Endotoxin, ergosterol, muramic acid and fungal DNA in dust from schools in Johor Bahru, Malaysia—associations with rhinitis and sick building syndrome (SBS) in junior high school students. Sci Total Environ 2016;545-546:95–103.
81. Tischer C, Gehring U, Chen CM, et al. Respiratory health in children, and indoor exposure to (1,3)-β-D-glucan, EPS mould components and endotoxin. Eur Respir J 2011;37(5):1050–9.
82. Mendy A, Gasana J, Vieira ER, et al. Endotoxin exposure and childhood wheeze and asthma: a meta-analysis of observational studies. J Asthma 2011;48(7):685–93.

83. Thorne PS, Mendy A, Metwali N, et al. Endotoxin exposure: predictors and prevalence of associated asthma outcomes in the United States. Am J Respir Crit Care Med 2015;192(11):1287–97.
84. Carnes MU, Hoppin JA, Metwali N, et al. House dust endotoxin levels are associated with adult asthma in a U.S. farming population. Ann Am Thorac Soc 2017;14(3):324–31.
85. Bakolis I, Doekes G, Heinrich J, et al. Respiratory health and endotoxin: associations and modification by CD14/-260 genotype. Eur Respir J 2012; 39(3):573–81.
86. Jacobs JH, Krop EJ, de Wind S, et al. Endotoxin levels in homes and classrooms of Dutch school children and respiratory health. Eur Respir J 2013;42(2):314–22.
87. Lai PS, Allen JG, Hutchinson DS, et al. Impact of environmental microbiota on human microbiota of workers in academic mouse research facilities: an observational study. PLoS One 2017;12(7): e0180969.
88. Birzele LT, Depner M, Ege MJ, et al. Environmental and mucosal microbiota and their role in childhood asthma. Allergy 2017;72(1):109–19.
89. Lynch SV, Wood RA, Boushey H, et al. Effects of early-life exposure to allergens and bacteria on recurrent wheeze and atopy in urban children. J Allergy Clin Immunol 2014;134(3):593–601.e12.
90. Karvonen AM, Kirjavainen PV, Täubel M, et al. Indoor bacterial microbiota and development of asthma by 10.5 years of age. J Allergy Clin Immunol 2019;144(5):1402–10.
91. Ciaccio CE, Barnes C, Kennedy K, et al. Home dust microbiota is disordered in homes of low-income asthmatic children. J Asthma 2015;52(9): 873–80.
92. Ege MJ, Mayer M, Schwaiger K, et al. Environmental bacteria and childhood asthma. Allergy 2012;67(12):1565–71.
93. Pekkanen J, Valkonen M, Täubel M, et al. Indoor bacteria and asthma in adults: a multicentre case-control study within ECRHS II. Eur Respir J 2018;51(2):51.
94. Dannemiller KC, Gent JF, Leaderer BP, et al. Indoor microbial communities: influence on asthma severity in atopic and nonatopic children. J Allergy Clin Immunol 2016;138(1):76–83.e1.
95. Lai PS, Kolde R, Franzosa EA, et al. The classroom microbiome and asthma morbidity in children attending 3 inner-city schools. J Allergy Clin Immunol 2018;141(6):2311–3.
96. Choi H, Schmidbauer N, Bornehag CG. Volatile organic compounds of possible microbial origin and their risks on childhood asthma and allergies within damp homes. Environ Int 2017;98:143–51.
97. Sorensen M, Wickman M, Sollid JU, et al. Allergic disease and *Staphylococcus aureus* carriage in adolescents in the Arctic region of Norway. Pediatr Allergy Immunol 2016;27(7):728–35.
98. Davis MF, Ludwig S, Brigham EP, et al. Effect of home exposure to *Staphylococcus aureus* on asthma in adolescents. J Allergy Clin Immunol 2018;141(1):402–5.e10.
99. Sintobin I, Siroux V, Holtappels G, et al. Sensitisation to staphylococcal enterotoxins and asthma severity: a longitudinal study in the EGEA cohort. Eur Respir J 2019;54(3):1900198.
100. Loss G, Apprich S, Waser M, et al. The protective effect of farm milk consumption on childhood asthma and atopy: the GABRIELA study. J Allergy Clin Immunol 2011;128(4):766–73.e4.
101. Kljaic-Bukvic B, Blekic M, Aberle N, et al. Genetic variants in endotoxin signalling pathway, domestic endotoxin exposure and asthma exacerbations. Pediatr Allergy Immunol 2014;25(6): 552–7.
102. Lawson JA, Dosman JA, Rennie DC, et al. The association between endotoxin and lung function among children and adolescents living in a rural area. Can Respir J 2011;18(6):e89–94.
103. Mumm J, Mahr TA. Indoor pollutant exposures modify the effect of airborne endotoxin on asthma in urban children. Pediatrics 2014;134(Suppl 3): S144–5.
104. Matsui EC, Hansel NN, Aloe C, et al. Indoor pollutant exposures modify the effect of airborne endotoxin on asthma in urban children. Am J Respir Crit Care Med 2013;188(10):1210–5.
105. Athavale A, Iyer H, Punwani AD, et al. Association of environmental factors, prevalence of asthma and respiratory morbidity in Mumbai: need of a public health policy. J Assoc Physicians India 2017;65(6):48–54.
106. Khan MS, Coulibaly S, Matsumoto T, et al. Association of airborne particles, protein, and endotoxin with emergency department visits for asthma in Kyoto, Japan. Environ Health Prev Med 2018; 23(1):41.
107. Mendy A, Wilkerson J, Salo PM, et al. Synergistic association of house endotoxin exposure and ambient air pollution with asthma outcomes. Am J Respir Crit Care Med 2019;200(6):712–20.
108. Mendy A, Wilkerson J, Salo PM, et al. Endotoxin predictors and associated respiratory outcomes differ with climate regions in the U.S. Environ Int 2018;112:218–26.
109. Strassle PD, Smit LAM, Hoppin JA. Endotoxin enhances respiratory effects of phthalates in adults: results from NHANES 2005–6. Environ Res 2018; 162:280–6.
110. Mendy A, Metwali N, Perry SS, et al. Household endotoxin reduction in the Louisa Environmental Intervention Project for rural childhood asthma. Indoor Air 2020;30(1):88–97.

111. Norback D, Lu C, Zhang Y, et al. Onset and remission of childhood wheeze and rhinitis across China—associations with early life indoor and outdoor air pollution. Environ Int 2019;123:61–9.
112. Moses L, Morrissey K, Sharpe RA, et al. Exposure to indoor mouldy odour increases the risk of asthma in older adults living in social housing. Int J Environ Res Public Health 2019;16(14):2600.
113. Norback D, Lampa E, Engvall K. Asthma, allergy and eczema among adults in multifamily houses in Stockholm (3-HE study)—associations with building characteristics, home environment and energy use for heating. PLoS One 2014;9(12):e112960.
114. Sharpe RA, Thornton CR, Nikolaou V, et al. Higher energy efficient homes are associated with increased risk of doctor diagnosed asthma in a UK subpopulation. Environ Int 2015;75:234–44.
115. Wen XJ, Balluz L, Mokdad A. Do obese adults have a higher risk of asthma attack when exposed to indoor mold? A study based on the 2005 Behavioral Risk Factor Surveillance System. Public Health Rep 2009;124(3):436–41.
116. Hsu J, Chen J, Mirabelli MC. Asthma morbidity, comorbidities, and modifiable factors among older adults. J Allergy Clin Immunol Pract 2018;6(1):236–43.e7.
117. Shorter C, Crane J, Pierse N, et al. Indoor visible mold and mold odor are associated with new-onset childhood wheeze in a dose-dependent manner. Indoor Air 2018;28(1):6–15.
118. Hu Y, Liu W, Huang C, et al. Home dampness, childhood asthma, hay fever, and airway symptoms in Shanghai, China: associations, dose-response relationships, and lifestyle's influences. Indoor Air 2014;24(5):450–63.
119. Cai J, Li B, Yu W, et al. Household dampness-related exposures in relation to childhood asthma and rhinitis in China: a multicentre observational study. Environ Int 2019;126:735–46.
120. Azalim S, Camargos P, Alves AL, et al. Exposure to environmental factors and relationship to allergic rhinitis and/or asthma. Ann Agric Environ Med 2014;21(1):59–63.
121. Lin Z, Norback D, Wang T, et al. The first 2-year home environment in relation to the new onset and remission of asthmatic and allergic symptoms in 4246 preschool children. Sci Total Environ 2016;553:204–10.
122. Norback D, Zock J-P, Plana E, et al. Mould and dampness in dwelling places, and onset of asthma: the population-based cohort ECRHS. Occup Environ Med 2013;70(5):325–31.
123. Tischer C, Zock JP, Valkonen M, et al. Predictors of microbial agents in dust and respiratory health in the Ecrhs. BMC Pulm Med 2015;15:48.
124. Weinmayr G, Gehring U, Genuneit J, et al. Dampness and moulds in relation to respiratory and allergic symptoms in children: results from phase two of the international study of asthma and allergies in childhood (ISAAC phase two). Clin Exp Allergy 2013;43(7):762–74.
125. Han YY, Lee YL, Guo YL. Indoor environmental risk factors and seasonal variation of childhood asthma. Pediatr Allergy Immunol 2009;20(8):748–56.
126. Wen HJ, Chiang TL, Lin SJ, et al. Predicting risk for childhood asthma by pre-pregnancy, perinatal, and postnatal factors. Pediatr Allergy Immunol 2015;26(3):272–9.
127. Tischer CG, Hohmann C, Thiering E, et al. Meta-analysis of mould and dampness exposure on asthma and allergy in eight European birth cohorts: an ENRIECO initiative. Allergy 2011;66(12):1570–9.
128. Karvonen AM, Hyvärinen A, Korppi M, et al. Moisture damage and asthma: a birth cohort study. Pediatrics 2015;135(3):e598–606.
129. Chen YC, Tsai CH, Lee YL. Early-life indoor environmental exposures increase the risk of childhood asthma. Int J Hyg Environ Health 2011;215(1):19–25.
130. Thacher JD, Gruzieva O, Pershagen G, et al. Mold and dampness exposure and allergic outcomes from birth to adolescence: data from the BAMSE cohort. Allergy 2017;72(6):967–74.
131. Norback D, Zock JP, Plana E, et al. Lung function decline in relation to mould and dampness in the home: the longitudinal European Community Respiratory Health Survey ECRHS II. Thorax 2011;66(5):396–401.
132. Karvala K, Toskala E, Luukkonen R, et al. Prolonged exposure to damp and moldy workplaces and new-onset asthma. Int Arch Occup Environ Health 2011;84(7):713–21.
133. Bernstein DI. Diesel exhaust exposure, wheezing and sneezing. Allergy Asthma Immunol Res 2012;4(4):178–83.
134. Iossifova YY, Reponen T, Ryan PH, et al. Mold exposure during infancy as a predictor of potential asthma development. Ann Allergy Asthma Immunol 2009;102(2):131–7.
135. Seo S, Choung JT, Chen BT, et al. The level of submicron fungal fragments in homes with asthmatic children. Environ Res 2014;131:71–6.
136. Oluwole O, Kirychuk SP, Lawson JA, et al. Indoor mold levels and current asthma among school-aged children in Saskatchewan, Canada. Indoor Air 2017;27(2):311–9.
137. Carreiro-Martins P, Papoila AL, Caires I, et al. Effect of indoor air quality of day care centers in children with different predisposition for asthma. Pediatr Allergy Immunol 2016;27(3):299–306.

138. Gunnbjornsdottir MI, Norbäck D, Björnsson E, et al. Indoor environment in three North European cities in relationship to atopy and respiratory symptoms. Clin Respir J 2009;3(2):85–94.
139. Huang C, Wang X, Liu W, et al. Household indoor air quality and its associations with childhood asthma in Shanghai, China: on-site inspected methods and preliminary results. Environ Res 2016;151:154–67.
140. Jones R, Recer GM, Hwang SA, et al. Association between indoor mold and asthma among children in Buffalo, New York. Indoor Air 2011;21(2): 156–64.
141. Vincent M, Corazza F, Chasseur C, et al. Relationship between mold exposure, specific IgE sensitization, and clinical asthma: a case-control study. Ann Allergy Asthma Immunol 2018;121(3):333–9.
142. Behbod B, Sordillo JE, Hoffman EB, et al. Wheeze in infancy: protection associated with yeasts in house dust contrasts with increased risk associated with yeasts in indoor air and other fungal taxa. Allergy 2013;68(11):1410–8.
143. Behbod B, Sordillo JE, Hoffman EB, et al. Asthma and allergy development: contrasting influences of yeasts and other fungal exposures. Clin Exp Allergy 2015;45(1):154–63.
144. Rosenbaum PF, Crawford JA, Anagnost SE, et al. Indoor airborne fungi and wheeze in the first year of life among a cohort of infants at risk for asthma. J Expo Sci Environ Epidemiol 2010;20(6):503–15.
145. Bundy KW, Gent JF, Beckett W, et al. Household airborne penicillium associated with peak expiratory flow variability in asthmatic children. Ann Allergy Asthma Immunol 2009;103(1):26–30.
146. Vicendese D, Dharmage SC, Tang ML, et al. Bedroom air quality and vacuuming frequency are associated with repeat child asthma hospital admissions. J Asthma 2015;52(7):727–31.
147. Zubairi AB, Azam I, Awan S, et al. Association of airborne *Aspergillus* with asthma exacerbation in Southern Pakistan. Asia Pac Allergy 2014;4(2): 91–8.
148. Tischer C, Weikl F, Probst AJ, et al. Urban dust microbiome: impact on later atopy and wheezing. Environ Health Perspect 2016;124(12):1919–23.
149. Karvonen AM, Hyvärinen A, Rintala H, et al. Quantity and diversity of environmental microbial exposure and development of asthma: a birth cohort study. Allergy 2014;69(8):1092–101.
150. Segura-Medina P, Vargas MH, Aguilar-Romero JM, et al. Mold burden in house dust and its relationship with asthma control. Respir Med 2019;150: 74–80.
151. Mueller-Rompa S, Janke T, Schwaiger K, et al. Identification of fungal candidates for asthma protection in a large population-based study. Pediatr Allergy Immunol 2017;28(1):72–8.
152. Reponen T, Levin L, Zheng S, et al. Family and home characteristics correlate with mold in homes. Environ Res 2013;124:67–70.
153. Reponen T, Vesper S, Levin L, et al. High environmental relative moldiness index during infancy as a predictor of asthma at 7 years of age. Ann Allergy Asthma Immunol 2011;107(2):120–6.
154. Vesper S, Barnes C, Ciaccio CE, et al. Higher environmental relative moldiness index (ERMI) values measured in homes of asthmatic children in Boston, Kansas city, and San Diego. J Asthma 2013; 50(2):155–61.
155. Vesper S, Choi H, Perzanowski MS, et al. Mold populations and dust mite allergen concentrations in house dust samples from across Puerto Rico. Int J Environ Health Res 2016;26(2):198–207.
156. Vesper S, Robins T, Lewis T, et al. Use of Medicaid and housing data may help target areas of high asthma prevalence. J Asthma 2017;54(3):230–8.
157. Eiffert S, Noibi Y, Vesper S, et al. A citizen-science study documents environmental exposures and asthma prevalence in two communities. J Environ Public Health 2016;2016:1962901.
158. Sinclair R, Russell C, Kray G, et al. Asthma risk associated with indoor mold contamination in hispanic communities in Eastern Coachella Valley, California. J Environ Public Health 2018;2018: 9350370.
159. Rosenbaum PF, Crawford JA, Hunt A, et al. Environmental relative moldiness index and associations with home characteristics and infant wheeze. J Occup Environ Hyg 2015;12(1):29–36.
160. Blanc PD, Quinlan PJ, Katz PP, et al. Higher environmental relative moldiness index values measured in homes of adults with asthma, rhinitis, or both conditions. Environ Res 2013; 122:98–101.
161. Hayes D Jr, Jhaveri MA, Mannino DM, et al. The effect of mold sensitization and humidity upon allergic asthma. Clin Respir J 2013;7(2):135–44.
162. Cazzoletti L, Marcon A, Corsico A, et al. Asthma severity according to Global Initiative for Asthma and its determinants: an international study. Int Arch Allergy Immunol 2010;151(1):70–9.
163. Bezerra GF, de Almeida FC, Neto da Silva MA, et al. Respiratory allergy to airborne fungi in São Luís-MA: clinical aspects and levels of IgE in a structured asthma program. J Asthma 2014; 51(10):1028–34.
164. Gent JF, Kezik JM, Hill ME, et al. Household mold and dust allergens: exposure, sensitization and childhood asthma morbidity. Environ Res 2012; 118:86–93.
165. Soffer N, Green BJ, Acosta L, et al. Alternaria is associated with asthma symptoms and exhaled NO among NYC children. J Allergy Clin Immunol 2018;142(4):1366–8.e10.

166. Barnes CS, Amado M, Portnoy JM. Reduced clinic, emergency room, and hospital utilization after home environmental assessment and case management. Allergy Asthma Proc 2010;31(4):317–23.
167. Ceylan E, Doruk S, Genc S, et al. The role of molds in the relation between indoor environment and atopy in asthma patients. J Res Med Sci 2013; 18(12):1067–73.
168. Seo SC, Park SJ, Park CW, et al. Clinical and immunological effects of a forest trip in children with asthma and atopic dermatitis. Iran J Allergy Asthma Immunol 2015;14(1):28–36.
169. Hwang BF, Liu IP, Huang TP. Gene-environment interaction between interleukin-4 promoter and molds in childhood asthma. Ann Epidemiol 2012; 22(4):250–6.
170. Ghosh B, Gaike AH, Pyasi K, et al. Bacterial load and defective monocyte-derived macrophage bacterial phagocytosis in biomass smoke-related COPD. Eur Respir J 2019;53(2):1702273.
171. Bose S, Rivera-Mariani F, Chen R, et al. Domestic exposure to endotoxin and respiratory morbidity in former smokers with COPD. Indoor Air 2016; 26(5):734–42.
172. Barrera C, Rocchi S, Degano B, et al. Microbial exposure to dairy farmers' dwellings and COPD occurrence. Int J Environ Health Res 2019;29(4): 387–99.
173. Smit LA, Hooiveld M, van der Sman-de Beer F, et al. Air pollution from livestock farms, and asthma, allergic rhinitis and COPD among neighbouring residents. Occup Environ Med 2014; 71(2):134–40.
174. Eduard W, Pearce N, Douwes J. Chronic bronchitis, COPD, and lung function in farmers: the role of biological agents. Chest 2009;136(3): 716–25.
175. Pahwa P, Karunanayake C, Willson PJ, et al. Prevalence of chronic bronchitis in farm and nonfarm rural residents in Saskatchewan. J Occup Environ Med 2012;54(12):1481–90.

Electronic Cigarettes

Past, Present, and Future: What Clinicians Need to Know

Stephen R. Baldassarri, MD, MHS

KEYWORDS

• Electronic cigarette • Tobacco • Smoking • Nicotine • Addiction

KEY POINTS

- Electronic cigarettes (ECs) are battery-operated devices that heat and aerosolize a liquid solution that may contain nicotine.
- Some ECs deliver nicotine rapidly and have addictive potential.
- ECs have inherent toxicity and unknown long-term health effects.
- ECs are substantially less toxic than combustible cigarettes.
- ECs likely have a role in smoking cessation and harm reduction in a subset of people who smoke combustible cigarettes.
- Some people use EC devices to consume tetrahydrocannabinol and other psychoactive substances.

INTRODUCTION: WHAT ARE ELECTRONIC CIGARETTES AND VAPING?

Electronic cigarettes (ECs) are battery-operated devices that heat and aerosolize a liquid solution that typically contains nicotine. ECs do not refer to a single device or product but to a heterogeneous class of products. Despite their heterogeneity, ECs all contain the same basic features: (1) a battery to provide heat; (2) a metal heating element; and (3) a liquid solution (**Fig. 1**).[1]

Vaping is the act of inhaling a heated, aerosolized substance. It is critical to distinguish vaping from smoking. Smoking is the inhalation of a burned substance. The main difference between the 2 processes is that smoking occurs at much higher temperatures (ie, >540°C [1000°F]) compared with vaping (120°C–240°C [250°F–500°F]). This difference in temperature has significant implications for the relative toxicities of the 2 activities and for the chemical mixtures that are produced in the process.[2] Smoking leads to a much more complex mixture of chemicals compared with vaping.[3]

E-liquids are the liquid solutions contained in ECs that users vape. E-liquids usually contain the same basic elements: alcohol-based solvents (propylene glycol and vegetable glycerin), flavorings, and (typically, although not exclusively) nicotine.[4] Although e-liquids are simple mixtures, the aerosol that forms following heating becomes much more complex.[5] Many chemicals of concern in combustible cigarettes have been found in ECs, although at much lower levels.[3]

WHY ARE ELECTRONIC CIGARETTES CONTROVERSIAL? THE DILEMMA OF YOUTH USE AND ADULT HARM REDUCTION

The emergence of ECs has polarized physicians, public health experts, and governments.[6] In the United States, ECs evoke memories of so-called Big Tobacco (tobacco industry firms): its betrayal of public trust, and its contribution to an epidemic of smoking-related diseases despite knowledge of the consequences.[7] The tobacco industry's explicit targeting of young people strikes a particularly noxious chord in the United States.[8] ECs

Funded by: NIH / NIDA. Grant number(s): K23DA045957. NIHMS-ID: 1626416.
Department of Internal Medicine, Section of Pulmonary, Critical Care, and Sleep Medicine, Yale School of Medicine, 300 Cedar Street, TAC-455 South, New Haven, CT 06520, USA
E-mail address: stephen.baldassarri@yale.edu

Clin Chest Med 41 (2020) 797–807
https://doi.org/10.1016/j.ccm.2020.08.018

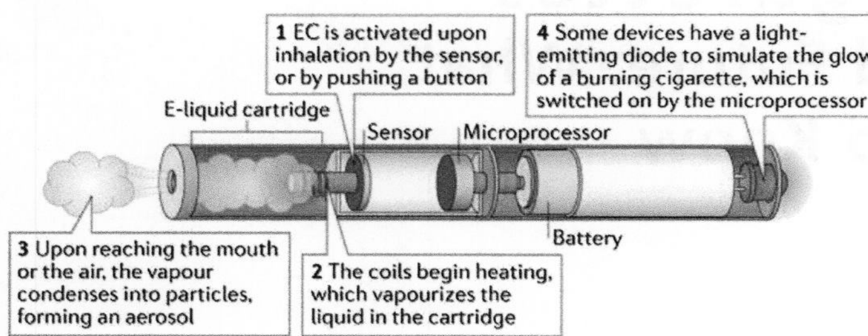
1 EC is activated upon inhalation by the sensor, or by pushing a button
4 Some devices have a light-emitting diode to simulate the glow of a burning cigarette, which is switched on by the microprocessor
E-liquid cartridge
Sensor
Microprocessor
Battery
3 Upon reaching the mouth or the air, the vapour condenses into particles, forming an aerosol
2 The coils begin heating, which vapourizes the liquid in the cartridge

Fig. 1. Components of an electronic cigarette (EC). (*From* Benowitz, NL, Fraiman JB. Cardiovascular effects of electronic cigarettes. Nature Reviews Cardiology 2017; 14(8):447; with permission.)

represent both an opportunity and a threat. The opportunity is harm reduction, which is the less harmful form of drug use or less harmful route of drug administration. If ECs are substantially less harmful than combustible cigarettes and an acceptable alternative to current smokers, the public health benefits to the adult population could be large. In the best-case scenario, ECs might lead to a reduction in combustible cigarette use and lower levels of heart, lung, and oncologic diseases.[9,10] However, whether harm reduction will occur on a broad scale remains unknown. In contrast, ECs pose a threat of reversing progress in tobacco control efforts that have occurred over the past 70 years.[11] The products may pose a risk of engendering a new epidemic of nicotine addiction, with unknown long-term health harms among young people.[12,13] In the worst-case scenario, ECs could lead to millions of new people using a harmful, addictive product that not only causes disease but does not reduce (and perhaps even increases) combustible cigarette smoking.

Economically, the EC industry has grown rapidly and poses an existential threat to combustible tobacco products. Although the EC market still pales compared with the combustible cigarette market ($11.5 billion vs $125 billion in 2018), Big Tobacco has taken notice and is adapting accordingly (https://www.wsj.com/articles/altria-takes-4-1-billion-writedown-on-juul-investment-11580386578). With so much at stake, it is not surprising that the EC debate has been spotlighted in the media and has received significant attention in the political sphere. The EC question has proved to be as much a political issue as a scientific one. To more clearly understand the present issues surrounding ECs, it is necessary first to take a look at the past.

BIG VAPES? A BRIEF HISTORY OF ELECTRONIC CIGARETTES

Contrary to popular belief, ECs were initially launched into commercial markets independently of the tobacco companies. It was not until much later in the evolution of ECs that Big Tobacco decided to take a stake in an industry that threatened to make the combustible cigarette obsolete. The first EC available for commercial use is usually attributed to Hon Lik, a Chinese pharmacist.[14] Hon sought to design a smoking-cessation product that could mimic the look, feel, and experience of smoking without the associated toxicities. Thus, the first EC later became known as a cig-alike. Cig-alikes could mimic the behavioral elements of smoking. They were roughly the same size as a cigarette and usually had a red light-emitting diode (LED) attached to the end of it. However, these products had problems for users. The battery life was short and unreliable. The e-liquid chamber was small (ie, 1 mL or less), meaning that heavy users needed to change products frequently. Perhaps most importantly, for many users, cig-alikes simply did not deliver nicotine fast enough or in high enough quantity to provide an effective smoking substitute.[15,16]

Thus, second-generation ECs were designed to address many of these issues. Second-generation ECs are now commonly associated with the term vape pens, given their penlike shape. Two innovations were important. First, the battery was significantly larger compared with cig-alikes, which allowed longer, more frequent use, and a larger amount of aerosol and nicotine delivery to users.[15] Second, refillable tank systems were introduced. Tank systems allowed users to fill and refill the EC with e-liquids of varying nicotine strengths and flavorings. This development led to the rapid expansion of the e-liquid industry and its thousands of available (and unregulated) flavors.[17] From the user perspective, it provided an increased amount of flexibility and customizability to the vaping experience. Furthermore, it permitted the use of other substances, such as tetrahydrocannabinol (THC; the psychoactive chemical in cannabis) oils,[18,19] which came to prominence late in 2019 (described in more detail later).[20]

Over time, it became clear that aerosol production was a significant factor in the user experience and increasing the efficiency of nicotine delivery. Thus, the third generation of ECs, commonly referred to as modifiable ECs (mods) or personal vaporizers, pair a tank system with a significantly larger battery compared with the second-generation devices. Larger batteries could provide a greater amount of electrical power to the liquid, leading a bigger aerosol "hit" to users, more rapid nicotine delivery,[21] and less frequent need for battery charging. One additional consequence of the proliferation of higher-powered devices was a shift by consumers to lower-strength nicotine e-liquids,[21] which were less harsh on the throat.

Most recently (as of the year 2020), the EC market was disrupted once more with the development of fourth-generation pod-style ECs[22]. These products captured a large portion of the US market as of 2020.[23] There were some key differences between pod-style ECs and prior EC products. First, the new devices were small, rectangular, and resembled a computer thumb drive. They were portable and very easy toaccess and conceal.[24] Second, the e-liquid mixture contained benzoic acid, an additive used to decrease the chemical pH of nicotine.[25] Because the high pH contained in many commercially available e-liquids could be harsh on the throat, a lower pH could make the product less harsh and more appealing. Over just a few years, pod-style products have become very popular among youth, raising significant public health concerns.[26,27,28]

ARE ELECTRONIC CIGARETTES ADDICTIVE?

As commonly used, ECs (particularly later-generation products) have addictive potential through rapid delivery of nicotine to the brain.[29] Though other psychoactive drugs such as THC may be used via vaping devices,[30] the discussion that follows focuses on the role of nicotine-containing ECs. Nicotine is a central nervous system stimulant that is highly reinforcing when delivered rapidly and at high dose.[31] Its role in perpetuating combustible cigarette addiction has been well established.[32] When considering the addictive properties of psychoactive drugs, several factors are critical, including (1) pharmacologic effect, (2) route of administration, (3) speed of delivery, (4) development of tolerance (requiring more of the drug for pharmacologic effect), and (5) severity of withdrawal. Differences in these factors show why 2 nicotine-containing products may vary substantially with respect to addictive risk. On one hand, conventional cigarettes deliver nicotine via inhalation through the pulmonary circulation,[33] which leads to rapid drug delivery to the brain within several seconds, resulting in a highly reinforcing effect. Furthermore, the ability of users to titrate the drug dose by varying puff volume and speed contributes significantly to abuse liability and reinforcement.[34] In contrast, the nicotine patch delivers nicotine slowly via the transdermal route over a period of 24 hours.[35] The onset is gradual and there is no ability to rapidly titrate the dose. As a result, the patch does not have significant reinforcing effects or abuse liability.

ECs are capable of providing nicotine delivery rapidly and in a manner similar to combustible cigarettes, at least under some circumstances.[36,37] The new generation of ECs are more efficient nicotine delivery systems compared with older ECs.[15] Nicotine exposure among adolescents who use pod-style ECs seems to be substantial, and similar in magnitude to prior studies of teen smokers.[25,38] Furthermore, ease of use relating to the newer products may be another factor increasing addiction risk.

In addition to the drug effects of nicotine, a multitude of other environmental and social factors mediate addiction, including product characteristics (ie, design, flavor, image), social influences (ie, behaviors of friends and family, advertising, health warnings/messaging), beliefs regarding harms and benefits, underlying host comorbidities and vulnerabilities (ie, mental illness), and sensation seeking.[39] All of these factors, in combination with nicotine delivery, may affect the risk of addiction at the individual level.

In summary, ECs have addictive potential through their rapid delivery of nicotine to the brain, ease of use, and associated environmental influences.

ARE ELECTRONIC CIGARETTES TOXIC AND DO THEY HAVE HEALTH EFFECTS?

EC aerosol is inherently toxic, although exceedingly less so than combustible cigarettes comparing the products puff for puff[3] (**Fig. 2**). Unlike cigarettes, EC aerosol does not contain combustion products such as carbon monoxide and tar. Nonetheless, both clinical and preclinical data suggest that EC aerosol inhalation has adverse effects on the airways and lungs (**Fig. 3**). In human epidemiologic studies, adolescents using ECs more frequently reported symptoms of chronic cough or sputum production compared with non-EC users.[40,41] Studies of changes in spirometry following acute EC use have been mixed, with some studies showing obstructive effects and others not.[42,43] These varying effects could depend on preexisting host comorbidities

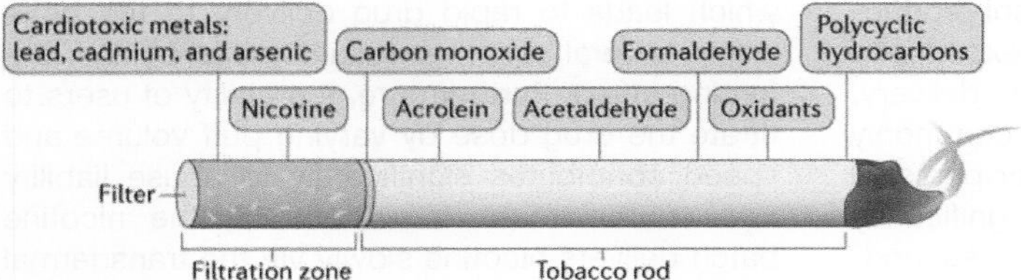

Fig. 2. Tobacco combustion products. (*From* Benowitz NL, Fraiman JB. Cardiovascular effects of electronic cigarettes. *Nature Reviews Cardiology.* 2017;14(8):447; with permission.)

and other environmental factors. Bronchoscopies of healthy EC users have shown erythema of airway mucosa and altered airway epithelial cell gene expression patterns.[44] In a 3-way comparison of bronchoalveolar lavage (BAL) inflammatory cell count and gene expression among EC users, smokers, and nonusers, the EC users showed gene expression patterns that were closer to never-smokers than to smokers.[45] They also had inflammatory cell counts that were intermediate between smokers and never-smokers. Preclinical animal and cell culture studies have shown a variety of potentially adverse effects of ECs, including increased airway reactivity, alterations in mucus production and clearance, and alteration of normal immune function.[46–48] The adverse effects of ECs on the cardiovascular system are less well characterized but remain a significant concern. Particular EC emissions of concern include aldehydes, particulates, oxidizing chemicals, and nicotine.[49]

In summary, ECs are toxic and carry health risks for the development of pulmonary disease, and possibly also cardiovascular and oncologic diseases. Compared with combustible cigarettes, ECs seem to be substantially less toxic considered puff for puff (ie, equal volumes of smoke vs aerosol consumed). The long-term health effects of EC use are currently unknown.

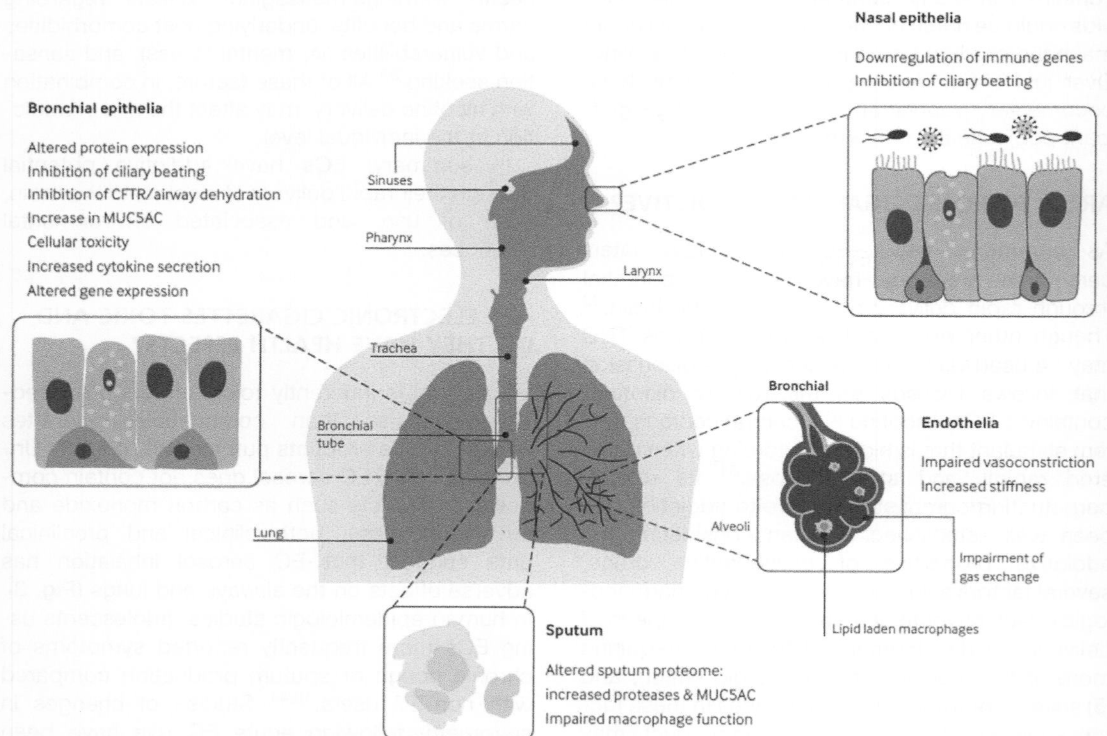

Fig. 3. Pulmonary effects of vaping. MUC5AC, mucin 5AC; CFTR, cystic fibrosis transmembrane conductance regulator. (*From* Gotts JE, Jordt S-E, McConnell R, et al. What are the respiratory effects of e-cigarettes? *BMJ (Clinical research ed.).* 2019;366:l5275; with permission.)

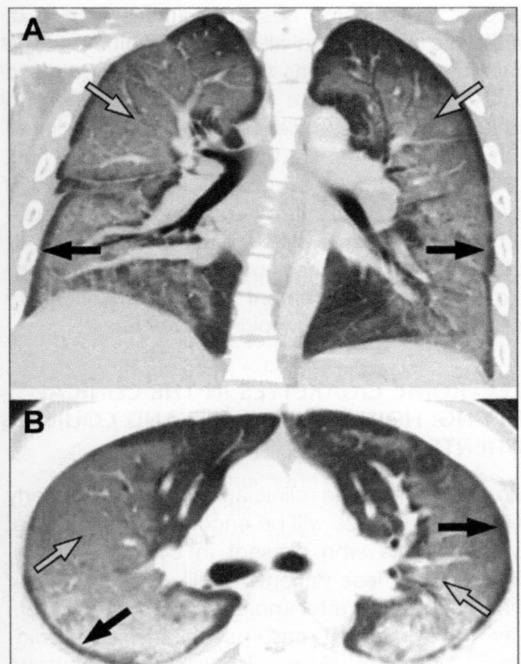

Fig. 4. High-resolution CT imaging. This patient has e-cigarette, or vaping, product use associated lung injury, with diffuse bilateral ground glass opacities (*green arrows*) in a peribronchial distribution, with subpleural sparing (*black arrows*). (*From* Kalininskiy A, Bach CT, Nacca NE, et al. E-cigarette, or vaping, product use associated lung injury (EVALI): case series and diagnostic approach. Lancet Respiratory Medicine. 2019; 7(12):p.1017-1026; Reprinted with permission from Elsevier.)

ELECTRONIC CIGARETTE, OR VAPING, PRODUCT USE–ASSOCIATED LUNG INJURY

Beginning approximately June 2019, the US Centers for Disease Control and Prevention (CDC) began receiving reports of severe acute lung injury occurring in the setting of EC use. As of April 2020, more than 2800 cases of EC, or vaping, product use–associated lung injury (EVALI) had been reported[50] (**Fig. 4**). Several EVALI case series were first described beginning around September 2019.[51–53] The largest series, involving patients in Illinois and Wisconsin,[51] reported that 84% of the cases involved the vaping of THC, the psychoactive chemical in marijuana. A wide variety of products and devices were reported, and a single causal agent could not be clearly identified. For the purpose of surveillance, case definitions were created. A confirmed case was defined as meeting 4 criteria: (1) use of an EC (vaping) within 90 days of symptom onset, (2) pulmonary infiltrate on chest imaging, (3) absence of pulmonary infection on initial work-up, and (4) no evidence in the medical record of alternative plausible diagnoses (ie, heart failure, rheumatic, or malignant processes). Probable cases were defined similarly except that there was evidence of pulmonary infection present and, despite this, the treating physicians thought infection was not the sole cause of the patient's respiratory failure.

Cases typically involved young people, with a median age of 19 years, although a wide age range was reported (16–53 years). There was a male predominance (83%) of unknown significance. In addition to the near-universal presence of respiratory and constitutional symptoms, more than 80% of people reported prominent gastrointestinal symptoms such as nausea or vomiting. The typical course in some cases led to the development of the acute respiratory distress syndrome, and approximately one-third of patients required mechanical ventilation. A range of pathologic findings were reported, complicating efforts to identify a clear precipitant and disease mechanism. Half of BAL specimens noted lipid-laden macrophages with oil red O stain, raising the possibility of lipoid pneumonia. This pattern was subsequently seen commonly in patients from North Carolina and Utah.[52,53] Other early reports noted a wide range of pathologic patterns that were more consistent with chemical pneumonitis.[54] Improvement following the administration of steroids was noted in many patients.

The key takeaway from the EVALI outbreak was that it revealed people were using EC devices to vape substances other than nicotine, such as THC oils. The use of street-bought (ie, illegal) or modified EC products was commonly reported, suggesting that low-quality, unregulated products were the primary source of the problem. Vitamin E acetate, an oil-based cutting agent added to THC oils, was discovered by CDC in many of the BAL samples analyzed.[55] Although this was one of likely several chemicals causing the illness, it showed the problems with an unregulated marketplace. To date, a comprehensive understanding of EVALI is still lacking, although vitamin E acetate is heavily suspected as a culprit.[55]

The increase of EVALI reports turned out to be politically consequential. Under intense political pressure and with persistent media coverage, the US Food and Drug Administration (FDA) chose to ban flavorings in pod-style ECs (https://www.fda.gov/news-events/press-announcements/trump-administration-combating-epidemic-youth-e-cigarette-use-plan-clear-market-unauthorized-non). Whether such action will reduce youth EC use, push adult EC users back toward combustible cigarette use, contribute to illegal EC markets, or have no effect on current trends remains to be seen. Nonetheless, bold policy, taken in part because of EVALI reporting, will likely be viewed as a significant event in the history of ECs when viewed retrospectively.

DO ELECTRONIC CIGARETTES PROMOTE SMOKING CESSATION?

The role of ECs for the purpose of smoking cessation has been controversial. After a few years following the introduction of ECs into commercial markets, physicians were solidly divided regarding whether ECs are helpful for smoking cessation and whether the products should be used for harm reduction in instances when patients fail to respond to conventional smoking-cessation medications and behavioral support.[56] The lack of understanding of the true risks of EC has made it difficult to provide adequate counsel for patients. Furthermore, balancing the values of promoting health, reducing harm, and echoing public health messages creates communication challenges for clinicians.

Nonetheless, as noted earlier, ECs originated in large part as a means to treat smoking addiction and are commonly used for this purpose outside of medical settings.[57] Several lines of epidemiologic evidence suggest that intensive EC use is associated with greater odds of smoking cessation,[58,59] and, importantly, smoking rates have continued to decline in the United States since the introduction of ECs into commercial markets.[60] It is now clear that ECs help some people with cessation of combustible tobacco.[61] Earlier EC trials studied cig-alike ECs in both motivated and unmotivated smokers, finding quit rates equivalent or nonstatistically higher than the nicotine patch, and reductions in cigarettes smoked per day.[62,63] However, the overall smoking quit rates were low, and the studies may have been underpowered to detect differences between groups. The most consequential study to date was a multicenter randomized controlled trial conducted in the United Kingdom from 2015 to 2018 comparing second-generation ECs with traditional combination nicotine replacement (eg, nicotine patch, gum, lozenge).[64] Eight-hundred and eighty-six study participants were smokers who were open to quitting smoking and had no strong preference regarding the use of nicotine replacement therapy (NRT) or ECs. The subjects were randomized to receive a 3-month supply of either an EC starter kit that included choice of different e-liquid strengths and flavors or their preferred nicotine-replacement products. Behavioral support for smoking cessation (the standard of care) was provided to all study participants. The major study finding was that subjects randomized to the EC group were nearly twice as likely to achieve smoking abstinence at week 52 compared with the NRT group (18.0% vs 9.9%; relative risk, 1.75 [1.24–2.46]). Adverse events were similar among groups. Importantly, around 80% of subjects in the EC group were still using their EC products at the end of the study, showing that long-term nicotine replacement is likely a necessary condition to maintain smoking abstinence.

ELECTRONIC CIGARETTES IN THE CLINICAL SETTING: HOW TO EVALUATE AND COUNSEL PATIENTS

For adult medicine clinicians, it is now nearly certain that EC use will be encountered in at least some patients who present in clinical settings. Almost all of these patients are likely to be former combustible cigarette smokers, and many of them may have medical and psychiatric comorbidities.[65] Some of them will also be concurrent smokers of tobacco and other substances (eg, marijuana/THC). However, in the near future, providers are likely to see EC users who have never smoked combustible cigarettes. How should they evaluate and counsel these patients?

A strong history is the initial key step and helps identify the patient's level of risk and other related comorbidities that require attention. A simple screening question can follow the smoking history typically taken as part of the patient's social history: "Do you vape or use e-cigarettes?" Follow-up questions to a positive response help to clarify health risks and the level of nicotine dependence. It is important to understand which devices are being used, which e-liquids are vaped (ie, nicotine content, flavorings, or other drugs, especially THC), where the products were obtained (ie, authorized retailers or from informal sources such as friends), and the duration and frequency of use. Clinicians must seek to understand the patients' reasons for use, including the patients' perceived benefits and risks of use, as well as desire and willingness to stop. Concurrent use of combustible tobacco products is important, because studies have shown that any combustible product use significantly increases toxic exposure compared with EC-only use.[66] Similarly, understanding the role that ECs have played for the patient in maintaining abstinence from combustible cigarette smoking is crucial.

How should the advice be framed? In an ideal world, the only thing people should inhale is clean air. This advice is reasonable to give to patients, but it does not fully account for the complexities of the real world, in which addiction and other comorbidities and environmental factors interact to create behaviors that are very difficult to modify. Long-term abstinence rates from cigarette smoking are low, particularly among patients who have difficulty achieving abstinence for at least 3 months.[67] A nuanced message is important for patients who switched from combustible cigarettes to ECs for the purpose of harm reduction. Although the long-term effects of ECs are unknown, the devastating effects of continued combustible cigarette use are known.[11] ECs do have health risks, but these risks are likely substantially less compared with combustible cigarettes.[68–70] Permanent and complete cessation from combustible products should be highly prioritized. If the patient is using ECs successfully for this purpose, clinicians should acknowledge and applaud their efforts to stop smoking.

If the patient is solely using ECs (and not using combustible products), clinicians should inquire whether the patient wishes to discontinuing vaping as well. The optimal approach to nicotine vaping cessation is unknown. In the absence of clear evidence, the combination of behavioral and pharmacologic treatments, which is the standard of care for the treatment of cigarette smoking addiction, is a reasonable starting point despite a lack of evidence of effectiveness in people who vape. It is not clear whether gradually reducing the nicotine level in e-liquids is a beneficial strategy to promote cessation from vaping. There is some evidence that, as with people who smoke, those who vape might engage in compensatory puffing behavior (ie, bigger or longer puffs) to maintain similar nicotine intake from ECs that contain less nicotine.[37] Studies examining effective interventions to promote cessation from nicotine vaping are needed to provide definitive guidance for clinicians.

WHAT ELSE NEEDS TO BE LEARNED ABOUT ELECTRONIC CIGARETTES?

If the story of ECs is a book, clinicians are currently at the beginning of the first chapter of a very long narrative. For context, tobacco smoking has been present in the Americas for centuries, if not millennia.[71] The consumption of liquid nicotine via ECs is a distinctly twenty-first century phenomenon that will likely continue to grow. Although the emotions surrounding the increase of EC use run high, facts and knowledge remain scarce.[72] What are the key areas where more clarity is needed?

First, and perhaps most importantly, clinicians need to understand the long-term health effects of chronic EC use. Will it lead to chronic lung, heart, and oncologic diseases in the way cigarette smoking does? Does it cause a different disease phenotype, such as chronic bronchitis, or increased susceptibility to pulmonary infection?[44,73–75] Clinicians especially need to understand how these risks compare with chronic cigarette smoking, the current leading cause of preventable death in the United States. Longitudinal cohort studies exploring key health outcomes including heart, lung, and oncologic diseases will help clinicians to understand both the absolute and relative risks of chronic EC use. Related to this point is figuring out which features of ECs themselves contribute to the risks of both addiction and toxicity. As mentioned earlier, ECs are a heterogeneous group of products that likely carry differential risks depending on the device type, electrical power, and type of e-liquid used. Understanding the factors that influence these health risks will help authorities to properly regulate the products and inform the public.

Second, clinicians need to understand how to optimize use of ECs for smoking cessation[64] and harm reduction[9] in individuals who fail to stop smoking cigarettes through conventional methods. Which individuals or populations are most likely to respond to harm-reduction strategies? What is the optimal timing for offering harm-reduction strategies? How can complete product switching be optimized to eliminate all combustible cigarette consumption?

Third, developing an understanding of the environmental effects of EC emissions will be important for protecting the public. Again, comparing their polluting effects with combustible cigarettes is critical for proper regulation and protection of the public.

Fourth, do ECs create a gateway into cigarette smoking or provide an adequate substitute to reduce smoking at the population level? Some association studies have suggested an increased risk of combustible cigarette use following initiation of ECs.[76] Although not causal, the data raise concerns about what the increasing prevalence of ECs in youth means for long-term tobacco control efforts to prevent combustible tobacco use. In contrast, ECs might prevent combustible cigarette smoking simply by being a more satisfying alternative to would-be smokers and inhibiting smoking initiation. It will be critical to continue monitoring trends in cigarette smoking, which have continued to decline among adults and youth since the introduction of ECs.[26]

WHAT IS THE FUTURE OF ELECTRONIC CIGARETTES?

There is no doubt that the emergence of ECs marks a profound event in the history of human consumption of nicotine and tobacco products. On the one hand, ECs offer hope for harm reduction among people with smoking addiction who cannot or will not stop smoking using conventional methods. In the best-case scenario, ECs might help people reduce their chronic exposure to toxins, reduce disease burden, and save lives. The products might eventually make combustible cigarettes obsolete. In contrast, ECs threaten to reverse the significant advances made in tobacco control over the past half century. In the worst-case scenario, harm reduction gains fail to materialize and a new generation of young people develop chronic addiction to a potent nicotine delivery system with significant health consequences. What does the future hold?

ECs will likely continue to evolve in terms of design, drug delivery efficiency, and user experience. They will eventually be regulated by the FDA, which has begun to take steps to protect youth (https://www.fda.gov/news-events/press-announcements/fda-finalizes-enforcement-policy-unauthorized-flavored-cartridge-based-e-cigarettes-appeal-children) but has not yet finalized a regulatory paradigm. Research to inform optimal FDA strategies is ongoing.

From the perspective of industry, the end point is clear: to create products that are highly profitable. The industry playbook has been well characterized[77] and involves extensive promotion efforts: aggressive advertising and marketing (particularly to youth, who are more likely to develop addiction than adults), public relations promotions, sponsored "friendly" research via universities and nonprofit organizations, government lobbying, and legal action against regulation.

Public health advocates will push back with equally clear end points: to prevent a health epidemic caused by vaping and to prevent a resurgence of cigarette smoking. Antivaping legislation has already been introduced in many countries and localities. Education efforts have been aimed at youth and other at-risk groups.[78] Clean indoor air laws have been passed.[79] Warning signals have been sounded.[80,81] This push and pull of markets and social forces inherent to society will ultimately determine the influence of ECs and their role in human history. This struggle has been playing out in the political arena in all branches of government, and will continue to do so for the years ahead.

REFERENCES

1. National Academies of Sciences E, Medicine. Public health consequences of E-cigarettes. Washington, DC: The National Academies Press; 2018.
2. Kosmider L, Sobczak A, Fik M, et al. Carbonyl compounds in electronic cigarette vapors: effects of nicotine solvent and battery output voltage. Nicotine Tob Res 2014;16(10):1319–26.
3. Goniewicz ML, Knysak J, Gawron M, et al. Levels of selected carcinogens and toxicants in vapour from electronic cigarettes. Tob Control 2014;23(2):133–9.
4. Callahan-Lyon P. Electronic cigarettes: human health effects. Tob Control 2014;23(suppl 2):ii36–40.
5. Cheng T. Chemical evaluation of electronic cigarettes. Tob Control 2014;23(suppl 2):ii11–7.
6. Green SH, Bayer R, Fairchild AL. Evidence, policy, and e-cigarettes—will England reframe the debate? N Engl J Med 2016;374(14):1301–3.
7. Glantz SA, Barnes DE, Bero L, et al. Looking through a keyhole at the tobacco industry: the Brown and Williamson documents. JAMA 1995;274(3):219–24.
8. Ling PM, Glantz SA. Why and how the tobacco industry sells cigarettes to young adults: evidence from industry documents. Am J Public Health 2002;92(6):908–16.
9. Cahn Z, Siegel M. Electronic cigarettes as a harm reduction strategy for tobacco control: a step forward or a repeat of past mistakes? J Public Health Policy 2011;32(1):16–31.
10. Polosa R, Rodu B, Caponnetto P, et al. A fresh look at tobacco harm reduction: the case for the electronic cigarette. Harm Reduct J 2013;10(1):19.
11. National Center for Chronic Disease P, Health Promotion Office on S, Health. Reports of the Surgeon general. The health consequences of smoking-50 years of progress: a report of the surgeon general. Atlanta (GA): Centers for Disease Control and Prevention (US); 2014.
12. Kong G, Morean ME, Cavallo DA, et al. Reasons for electronic cigarette experimentation and discontinuation among adolescents and young adults. Nicotine Tob Res 2015;17(7):847–54.
13. Camenga DR, Delmerico J, Kong G, et al. Trends in use of electronic nicotine delivery systems by adolescents. Addict Behav 2014;39(1):338–40.
14. Hon L. Electronic cigarette. Google Patents; 2013.
15. Farsalinos KE, Spyrou A, Tsimopoulou K, et al. Nicotine absorption from electronic cigarette use: comparison between first and new-generation devices. Sci Rep 2014;4:4133.
16. Eissenberg T. Electronic nicotine delivery devices: ineffective nicotine delivery and craving suppression after acute administration. Tob Control 2010;19(1):87–8.

17. Allen JG, Flanigan SS, LeBlanc M, et al. Flavoring chemicals in e-cigarettes: diacetyl, 2, 3-pentanedione, and acetoin in a sample of 51 products, including fruit-, candy-, and cocktail-flavored e-cigarettes. Environ Health Perspect 2016;124(6):733–9.
18. Borodovsky JT, Crosier BS, Lee DC, et al. Smoking, vaping, eating: is legalization impacting the way people use cannabis? Int J Drug Policy 2016;36: 141–7.
19. Spindle TR, Bonn-Miller MO, Vandrey R. Changing landscape of cannabis: novel products, formulations, and methods of administration. Curr Opin Psychol 2019;30:98–102.
20. Kalininskiy A, Bach CT, Nacca NE, et al. E-cigarette, or vaping, product use associated lung injury (EVALI): case series and diagnostic approach. Lancet Respir Med 2019;7(12):1017–26.
21. Wagener TL, Floyd EL, Stepanov I, et al. Have combustible cigarettes met their match? The nicotine delivery profiles and harmful constituent exposures of second-generation and third-generation electronic cigarette users. Tob Control 2016;26(e1): e23–8.
22. Fadus MC, Smith TT, Squeglia LM. The rise of e-cigarettes, pod mod devices, and JUUL among youth: factors influencing use, health implications, and downstream effects. Drug Alcohol Depend 2019; 201:85–93.
23. Huang J, Duan Z, Kwok J, et al. Vaping versus JUULing: how the extraordinary growth and marketing of JUUL transformed the US retail e-cigarette market. Tob Control 2019;28(2):146–51.
24. Ramamurthi D, Chau C, Jackler RK. JUUL and other stealth vaporisers: hiding the habit from parents and teachers. Tob Control 2019;28(6):610–6.
25. Goniewicz ML, Boykan R, Messina CR, et al. High exposure to nicotine among adolescents who use Juul and other vape pod systems ('pods'). Tob Control 2019;28(6):676–7.
26. Arrazola RA, Singh T, Corey CG, et al. Tobacco use among middle and high school students - United States, 2011-2014. MMWR Morb Mortal Wkly Rep 2015;64(14):381–5.
27. Gentzke AS, Creamer M, Cullen KA, et al. Vital signs: tobacco product use among middle and high school students—United States, 2011–2018. MMWR Morb Mortal Wkly Rep 2019;68(6):157.
28. Dyer O. FDA considers regulatory action as vaping among US teens jumps 78% in a year. British Medical Journal Publishing Group; 2019.
29. Baldassarri SR, Bernstein SL, Chupp GL, et al. Electronic cigarettes for adults with tobacco dependence enrolled in a tobacco treatment program: a pilot study. Addict Behav 2018;80:1–5.
30. Morean ME, Kong G, Camenga DR, et al. High school students' use of electronic cigarettes to vaporize cannabis. Pediatrics 2015;136(4):611–6.
31. Benowitz NL. Pharmacology of nicotine: addiction and therapeutics. Annu Rev Pharmacol Toxicol 1996;36(1):597–613.
32. Benowitz NL. Nicotine addiction. N Engl J Med 2010;362(24):2295–303.
33. Henningfield JE, Stapleton JM, Benowitz NL, et al. Higher levels of nicotine in arterial than in venous blood after cigarette smoking. Drug Alcohol Depend 1993;33(1):23–9.
34. Gritz ER, Baer-Weiss V, Jarvik ME. Titration of nicotine intake with full-length and half-length cigarettes. Clin Pharmacol Ther 1976;20(5):552–6.
35. Perkins KA, Lerman C, Keenan J, et al. Rate of nicotine onset from nicotine replacement therapy and acute responses in smokers. Nicotine Tob Res 2004;6(3):501–7.
36. Ramôa CP, Hiler MM, Spindle TR, et al. Electronic cigarette nicotine delivery can exceed that of combustible cigarettes: a preliminary report. Tob Control 2016;25(e1):e6.
37. Baldassarri SR, Hillmer AT, Anderson JM, et al. Use of electronic cigarettes leads to significant beta2-nicotinic acetylcholine receptor occupancy: evidence from a PET imaging study. Nicotine Tob Res 2017;20(4):425–33.
38. Benowitz NL, Nardone N, Jain S, et al. Comparison of urine 4-(methylnitrosamino)-1-(3) pyridyl-1-butanol and cotinine for assessment of active and passive smoke exposure in urban adolescents. Cancer Epidemiol Biomarkers Prev 2018;27(3):254–61.
39. Carey FR, Rogers SM, Cohn EA, et al. Understanding susceptibility to e-cigarettes: a comprehensive model of risk factors that influence the transition from non-susceptible to susceptible among e-cigarette naïve adolescents. Addict Behav 2019;91: 68–74.
40. Wang MP, Ho SY, Leung LT, et al. Electronic cigarette use and respiratory symptoms in Chinese adolescents in Hong Kong. JAMA Pediatr 2016;170(1): 89–91.
41. McConnell R, Barrington-Trimis JL, Wang K, et al. Electronic cigarette use and respiratory symptoms in adolescents. Am J Respir Crit Care Med 2017; 195(8):1043–9.
42. Vardavas CI, Anagnostopoulos N, Kougias M, et al. Short-term pulmonary effects of using an electronic cigarette: impact on respiratory flow resistance, impedance, and exhaled nitric oxide. Chest 2012; 141(6):1400–6.
43. Ferrari M, Zanasi A, Nardi E, et al. Short-term effects of a nicotine-free e-cigarette compared to a traditional cigarette in smokers and non-smokers. BMC Pulm Med 2015;15(1):120.
44. Ghosh A, Coakley RC, Mascenik T, et al. Chronic e-cigarette exposure alters the human bronchial epithelial proteome. Am J Respir Crit Care Med 2018;198(1):67–76.

45. Song M-A, Freudenheim JL, Brasky TM, et al. Biomarkers of exposure and effect in the lungs of smokers, nonsmokers, and electronic cigarette users. Cancer Epidemiol Biomarkers Prev 2020;29(2):443–51.
46. Lee H-W, Park S-H, Weng M-w, et al. E-cigarette smoke damages DNA and reduces repair activity in mouse lung, heart, and bladder as well as in human lung and bladder cells. Proc Natl Acad Sci U S A 2018;115(7):E1560–9.
47. Khosravi M, Lin R-L, Lee LY. Inhalation of electronic cigarette aerosol induces reflex bronchoconstriction by activation of vagal bronchopulmonary C-fibers. Am J Physiol Lung Cell Mol Physiol 2018;315(4):L467–75.
48. Sussan TE, Gajghate S, Thimmulappa RK, et al. Exposure to electronic cigarettes impairs pulmonary anti-bacterial and anti-viral defenses in a mouse model. PLoS One 2015;10(2):e0116861.
49. Benowitz NL, Fraiman JB. Cardiovascular effects of electronic cigarettes. Nat Rev Cardiol 2017;14(8):447.
50. Outbreak of lung disease associated with E-cigarette use, or vaping. Centers for disease control and prevention. 2019. Available at: https://www.cdc.gov/tobacco/basic_information/e-cigarettes/severe-lung-disease.html.
51. Layden JE, Ghinai I, Pray I, et al. Pulmonary illness related to E-cigarette use in Illinois and Wisconsin - preliminary report. N Engl J Med 2020;382(10):903–16.
52. Davidson K. Outbreak of electronic-cigarette–associated acute lipoid pneumonia—North Carolina, July–August 2019. MMWR Morb Mortal Wkly Rep 2019;68:784–6.
53. Lewis N. E-cigarette use, or vaping, practices and characteristics among persons with associated lung injury—Utah, April–October 2019. MMWR Morb Mortal Wkly Rep 2019;68:953–6.
54. Butt YM, Smith ML, Tazelaar HD, et al. Pathology of vaping-associated lung injury. N Engl J Med 2019;381(18):1780–1.
55. Blount BC, Karwowski MP, Morel-Espinosa M, et al. Evaluation of bronchoalveolar lavage fluid from patients in an outbreak of E-cigarette, or vaping, product use-associated lung injury - 10 States, August-October 2019. MMWR Morb Mortal Wkly Rep 2019;68(45):1040–1.
56. Baldassarri SR, Chupp GL, Leone FT, et al. Practice patterns and perceptions of chest health care providers on electronic cigarette use: an in-depth discussion and report of survey results. J Smok Cessat 2017;13(2):72–7.
57. Hartmann-Boyce J, Begh R, Aveyard P. Electronic cigarettes for smoking cessation. BMJ 2018;360:j5543.
58. Zhu S-H, Zhuang Y-L, Wong S, et al. E-cigarette use and associated changes in population smoking cessation: evidence from US current population surveys. BMJ 2017;358:j3262.
59. Biener L, Hargraves JL. A longitudinal study of electronic cigarette use among a population-based sample of adult smokers: association with smoking cessation and motivation to quit. Nicotine Tob Res 2015;17(2):127–33.
60. Jamal A, Homa DM, O'Connor E, et al. Current cigarette smoking among adults - United States, 2005-2014. MMWR Morb Mortal Wkly Rep 2015;64(44):1233–40.
61. Rahman MA, Hann N, Wilson A, et al. E-cigarettes and smoking cessation: evidence from a systematic review and meta-analysis. PLoS One 2015;10(3):e0122544.
62. Caponnetto P, Campagna D, Cibella F, et al. EffiCiency and Safety of an eLectronic cigAreTte (ECLAT) as tobacco cigarettes substitute: a prospective 12-month randomized control design study. PLoS One 2013;8(6):e66317.
63. Bullen C, Howe C, Laugesen M, et al. Electronic cigarettes for smoking cessation: a randomised controlled trial. Lancet 2013;382(9905):1629–37.
64. Hajek P, Phillips-Waller A, Przulj D, et al. A randomized trial of E-cigarettes versus nicotine-replacement therapy. N Engl J Med 2019;380(7):629–37.
65. Rojewski AM, Baldassarri S, Cooperman NA, et al. Exploring issues of comorbid conditions in people who smoke. Nicotine Tob Res 2016;18(8):1684–96.
66. Shahab L, Goniewicz ML, Blount BC, et al. Nicotine, carcinogen, and toxin exposure in long-term e-cigarette and nicotine replacement therapy users: a cross-sectional study. Ann Intern Med 2017;166(6):390–400.
67. Gilpin EA, Pierce JP, Farkas AJ, et al. Duration of smoking abstinence and success in quitting. J Natl Cancer Inst 1997;89(8):572.
68. D'Ruiz CD, Graff DW, Yan XS. Nicotine delivery, tolerability and reduction of smoking urge in smokers following short-term use of one brand of electronic cigarettes. BMC Public Health 2015;15:991.
69. Goniewicz ML, Gawron M, Smith DM, et al. Exposure to nicotine and selected toxicants in cigarette smokers who switched to electronic cigarettes: a longitudinal within-subjects observational study. Nicotine Tob Res 2016;19(2):160–7.
70. McRobbie H, Phillips A, Goniewicz ML, et al. Effects of switching to electronic cigarettes with and without concurrent smoking on exposure to nicotine, carbon monoxide, and Acrolein. Cancer Prev Res 2015;8(9):873–8.
71. Mackay J, Eriksen M, Eriksen MP. The tobacco atlas. World Health Organization; 2002.
72. Bernstein SL. Electronic cigarettes: more light, less heat needed. Lancet Respir Med 2016;4(2):85–7.

73. Ghosh A, Coakley RD, Ghio AJ, et al. Chronic E-cigarette use increases neutrophil elastase and matrix metalloprotease levels in the lung. Am J Respir Crit Care Med 2019;200(11):1392–401.
74. Chun LF, Moazed F, Calfee CS, et al. Pulmonary toxicity of e-cigarettes. Am J Physiol Lung Cell Mol Physiol 2017;313(2):L193–206.
75. Gotts JE, Jordt S-E, McConnell R, et al. What are the respiratory effects of e-cigarettes? BMJ 2019;366:l5275.
76. Leventhal AM, Strong DR, Kirkpatrick MG, et al. Association of electronic cigarette use with initiation of combustible tobacco product smoking in early adolescence. JAMA 2015;314(7):700–7.
77. Proctor RN, Proctor R. Golden holocaust: origins of the cigarette catastrophe and the case for abolition. Univ of California Press; 2011.
78. Dobbs PD, Hammig B, Sudduth A. 2015 legislative update of e-cigarette youth access and exposure laws. Prev Med 2016;88:90–4.
79. Gourdet CK, Chriqui JF, Chaloupka FJ. A baseline understanding of state laws governing e-cigarettes. Tob Control 2014;23(suppl 3):iii37–40.
80. Murthy VH. E-cigarette use among youth and young adults: a major public health concern. JAMA Pediatr 2017;171(3):209–10.
81. Roditis M, Lee J, Halpern-Felsher BL. Adolescent (mis) perceptions about nicotine addiction: results from a mixed-methods study. Health Educ Behav 2016;43(2):156–64.

The Respiratory Risks of Ambient/Outdoor Air Pollution

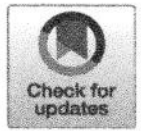

Gary Adamkiewicz, PhD[a], Jahred Liddie, BA[a],
Jonathan M. Gaffin, MD, MMSc[b,*]

KEYWORDS

- Ambient air pollution • Air pollutants • COPD • Asthma • Childhood asthma • Air quality
- Pollutant sources • Epidemiology

KEY POINTS

- Ambient air pollution is emitted primarily as a result of fossil fuel combustion and atmospheric chemical reactions.
- Ambient air pollution exposure is responsible for premature mortality due to its effect on multiple organ systems, particularly the respiratory and cardiovascular system.
- Outdoor pollutant exposure is highly associated with impaired lung development and accelerated lung function decline.
- Outdoor air pollution is a potent modifiable risk factor for exacerbations of asthma, COPD, and acute bronchopulmonary infections.

INTRODUCTION

Humans are exposed to a wide range of air pollutants known to be associated with adverse health effects. These pollutants can be associated with a wide range of activities and sources, including the burning of fossil fuels, traffic-related emissions, industrial activities, agricultural activities, and wildfires, as well as a diverse group of pollutants that originate indoors (**Fig. 1**). For an individual, their totality of exposure is determined by concentrations of pollutants in the various microenvironments where they spend time (eg, home, school, work), and their time activity patterns (how much time is spent in each of these spaces). Indoor exposures are strongly influenced by the characteristics of the building, its location, and ambient sources, due to the exchange of air between indoor and outdoor spaces. Because of these relationships, and because most individuals spend most of their time indoors, most of human exposure to pollutants of outdoor origin actually occurs indoors. This review focuses on ambient pollutants, those that are emitted or formed in the atmosphere and primarily measured by outdoor monitoring stations or models that depend on outdoor metrics.

Any process that includes fossil fuel combustion is likely releasing pollutants that have been shown to cause health effects. Traffic-related emissions (including diesel), combustion related to electricity production (eg, coal, natural gas), and other fuel burning can release particulate matter, oxides of nitrogen and other pollutants into the atmosphere. Once released, these pollutants can be transported, removed, and/or chemically transformed.

Air pollution exposure has been implicated in myriad disease processes in almost every organ system[1] and is currently the fifth highest risk factor for mortality worldwide.[2] A recent estimate shows that outdoor air pollution, mostly by driven by

Funding sources: This article is supported by NIH grants R01 ES 030100, K23AI106945 (PI, Dr J.M. Gaffin).
[a] Department of Environmental Health, Harvard T.H. Chan School of Public Health, Boston, MA 02115, USA;
[b] Division of Pulmonary Medicine, Boston Children's Hospital, Harvard Medical School, Boston, MA 02115, USA
* Corresponding author.
E-mail address: jonathan.gaffin@childrens.harvard.edu

Clin Chest Med 41 (2020) 809–824
https://doi.org/10.1016/j.ccm.2020.08.013
0272-5231/20/

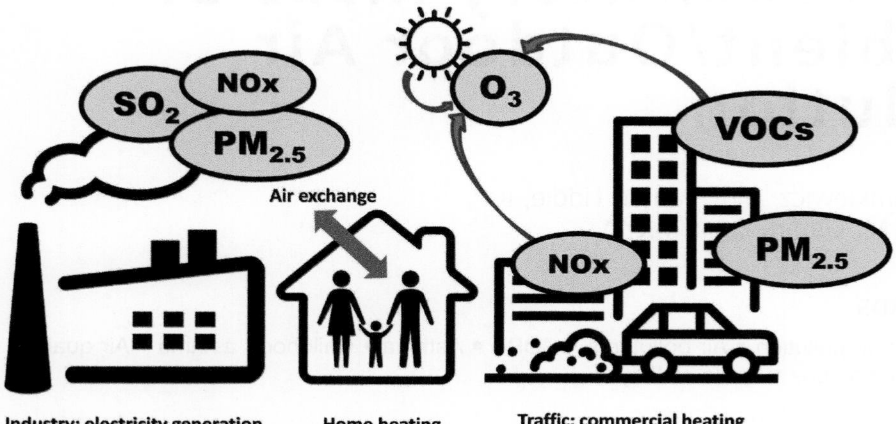

Fig. 1. Key sources of ambient air pollutants. Schematic of source apportionment for major ambient/outdoor air pollutants.

exposure to fine particulate matter ($PM_{2.5}$, described later in this article), leads to 3.3 (95% confidence interval 1.61–4.81) million premature deaths per year worldwide, with most of these deaths occurring in Asia.[3] These risks are in addition to the significant global burden of disease from household air pollution from the burning of solid fuels for cooking and heating.[4] In general, ambient air pollution levels have increased in low-income and middle-income countries,[2] whereas notable progress has been made in the United States.[5] In addition to these global differences in exposure and health effects, many studies have highlighted the disproportionate burden of air pollution within low-income populations and communities of color in the United States.[6]

We focus this article on key air pollutants (**Table 1**) that have an extensive evidence base linking exposure to respiratory health effects, with the exception of wildfire smoke, which is addressed elsewhere in this issue. We aim to describe the most important ambient pollutants implicated in human health and disease and discuss the sources of ambient pollution. Recognizing that many of these individual pollutants are encountered as pollutant mixtures, we outline the major respiratory risks of ambient pollution, as a whole and fractioned by pollutant or source where data are available. Focus is on the inception, exacerbation and mortality related to chronic respiratory diseases and vulnerable populations. As the burden of air pollution on respiratory morbidity and mortality is high, clinicians must be aware of the potentially harmful exposures to properly advise vulnerable patients on avoidance strategies and/or affect change through public policy efforts.

AIR POLLUTANTS

Particulate Matter

The term particulate matter (PM) describes the mixture of solid and/or liquid particles suspended in air, which may or may not be visible. These particles are generated through mechanical or chemical processes and can be either directly emitted or can form through chemical reactions in the air. For example, PM can be generated from wildfires, combustion of fossil fuels (eg, oil, gasoline, diesel), industrial sources, as well as from the suspension of road dust and soils. PM is often classified by the size fractions that determine the pattern of capture, deposition and transport in the lung, and thus directly affects the extent of human exposure and related health effects. For example, PM_{10} refers to particles that are smaller than 10 μm in diameter and $PM_{2.5}$ refers to particles smaller than 2.5 μm in diameter. Both of these fractions are considered inhalable, with the smallest particles, such as $PM_{2.5}$ or smaller fractions having a higher likelihood to be deposited deep in the lung.

A recent systematic review[7] summarized the literature that has estimated source apportionment of particulate matter, and found that globally 25% of urban ambient $PM_{2.5}$ is generated by traffic, 15% by industrial activities, 20% by domestic fuel burning, 22% from unspecified sources of human origin, and 18% from natural dust and salt. Similarly, using data from a national network of $PM_{2.5}$ monitors with chemical speciation, Thurston and colleagues[8] identified the major

Table 1
Overview of ambient air pollutant sources and health effects

Key Pollutants	Emission Sources	Key Health Effects
Particulate matter (PM)	• PM is a mixture of solid and/ or liquid particles suspended in air • They have both anthropogenic and natural sources and can be both directly emitted and formed in the atmosphere • Human sources, include traffic, road dust, industrial sources (combustion of fossil fuels, metallurgy, ceramics, and others), domestic fuel combustion, and other human activities[7] • PM can form in the atmosphere as a result of chemical reactions of certain compounds like sulfur dioxide and nitrogen oxides • Natural sources, including wildfires, soil dust, and sea salt	• Associated with all-cause daily mortality and more highly associated with mortality from respiratory conditions[19] • Lowered life expectancy[20] • Asthma symptoms and exacerbation[89] • Coughing, wheezing, and breathlessness[27,39] • Impaired lung development in children[45] and impaired lung function in adults[55–57] • Exacerbation of chronic obstructive pulmonary disease (COPD)[96]
Ozone (O_3)	• Not emitted directly, but formed as a product of chemical reactions between sunlight, nitrogen oxides (NO_x), and volatile organic compounds (VOCs) • These primary or "precursor" pollutants can be emitted from various sources, including traffic, power plants, refineries, chemical plants, and other sources[130]	• Emphysema and decreased forced expiratory volume over one second (FEV1)[105] • Asthma symptoms and exacerbation[89] • Allergic responses with co-exposure to allergens[37]
Nitrogen dioxide (NO_2)	• Formed in high-temperature combustion processes, including power plants, traffic, and off-road vehicles[131]	• Decreased lung function[63,64] • Allergic responses with co-exposure to allergens[37]
Sulfur dioxide (SO_2)	• Human sources include combustion of sulfur-containing fuels (such as coal) in power plants and other industrial process, metal extraction, and heavy vehicles[132] • Natural sources, including volcanic eruptions	• Eye and upper airway irritation[1] • Alterations to lung function, loss of smell, headaches, dizziness, and decreased fertility[133]
Traffic-related air pollution (TRAP)	• Combustion of diesel and gasoline in motor vehicles • Significant sources include roadways, especially those with high traffic density	• Decreased lung function[63,64] • Asthma symptoms and exacerbations[89]

Data from Refs.[7,19,20,27,37,39,45,55–57,63,64,89,96,105,130–133]

$PM_{2.5}$ sources in the United States as (in no particular order) motor vehicle traffic, metals industry, crustal/soil particles, steel industry, coal combustion, oil combustion, salt particles, and biomass burning. Although motor vehicle emissions were ubiquitous, the relative contribution of these sources varied significantly by region.

Although significant progress has been made in reducing $PM_{2.5}$ in the United States, exposure disparities across economic and racial lines are notable. A 2018 analysis of PM-emitting facilities in the United States showed that those living in poverty had 1.35 times higher burden than did the overall population, and that Black populations had a 1.54 times higher burden than did the overall population.[9,10] A recent study focused on ambient monitoring data in Massachusetts showed that racial disparities in population-weighted concentrations increased over time, although overall exposures have decreased during the same period. Due to the effects of urbanization, differences in motor vehicle fleets, fuel usage patterns and other factors, the global exposure picture is troubling. A 2018 assessment showed that 95% of the world's population lived in areas where ambient $PM_{2.5}$ levels exceeded the World Health Organization 10 μg/m^3 (annual average) guideline.[11]

It has long been known that the size and composition of airborne particles can strongly influence exposure and the observed patterns of health effects.[12] Another fraction, ultrafine particles (UFP), defined as particles smaller than 0.1 μm in diameter, have been suggested as an important component of airborne particles that may be mechanistically responsible for some health effects.[13] Although ultrafine particles are not regulated (like $PM_{2.5}$ and other particulate matter fractions), the health effects of these exposures remain an active and important area of investigation.

Ozone

Ozone, a key component of smog, is not emitted directly, but rather is formed in the atmosphere through complex series of photochemical reactions involving two other classes of pollutants: oxides of nitrogen (NOx) and volatile organic compounds (VOCs). In addition to its health effects, ozone is known to affect agricultural output and damage materials. Because of the photochemical origins of ozone, large urban areas located in warmer climates are more likely to experience high ozone levels. Ozone hotspots are frequently located downwind of emission sources, due to the timescales of the underlying chemical reactions.

Nitrogen Dioxide

Nitrogen dioxide (NO_2) is formed during high-temperature combustion and is both relevant for its direct effects on health as well as its role as a precursor of ozone. In urban areas, the most significant contributor to the levels and patterns of nitrogen dioxide exposure is traffic. Power plants and other industrial sources that burn fossil fuels are also major emitters of NO_2 (and other oxides of nitrogen). Personal exposures to nitrogen dioxide are influenced by these ambient sources, as well as indoor combustion sources, such as emissions from gas stoves.

Sulfur Dioxide

When burned, sulfur-containing fuels, such as coal, can release significant quantities of sulfur dioxide. Although sulfur dioxide (SO_2) can be released naturally (eg, volcanoes), most emissions are anthropogenic, from power plants, pulp and paper production, smelter and steel mill operations, and other industrial operations.[14] Historically, the focus on controlling SO_2 emissions was based on its presumed contributions to acid rain, and not health effects.

Traffic-related Air Pollution/Diesel

Given the range of pollutants released from gasoline-powered and diesel-powered vehicles and the potential range of health effects, it has been convenient to refer to this pollutant mix as traffic-related air pollution, or TRAP. This designation is aligned with the large body of evidence that shows a consistent pattern of health effects associated with being exposed to high traffic density or living close to major roadways. Numerous exposure-focused studies have documented the influence of roadways on the concentration gradients for several air pollutants near these sources.[15]

The ability to estimate human exposure to ambient pollutants has evolved substantially over the past several decades. The primary measurement direct measurement devices for population-based pollution research have been central monitoring sites that are able to measure real-time and filter-based particle and gas composition in the local environment. However, sophisticated modeling that incorporates land use, green space, and other factors that affect the local exposure profiles have greatly enhanced the precision of these measures and ability to extrapolate from central monitors to discrete nearby locations. The use of satellite imagery to further enhance predictive models has led to accurate ground estimates as small as 1 km across large portions of the United States More recently, the availability of low-cost sensors allows for more fine-scale or personal assessment of exposure to pollutants released by traffic and other urban sources. For example, recent studies reveal the small-scale variation of air pollution at the neighborhood level, and the potential associations with health.[16,17]

HEALTH EFFECTS

Population Health

Air pollution health effects are seen on a population scale in both healthy and vulnerable subjects. The World Health Organization estimates that ambient pollution is responsible for 4.2 million premature deaths annually.[18] Several studies in the developed and developing world have consistently demonstrated a higher risk of all-cause mortality in people exposed to high levels of pollutants. Liu and colleagues[19] from the Multi-City Multi-Country (MCC) Collaborative Research Network recently reported on the effects of daily particulate exposure with daily mortality among 652 cities from 24 countries or regions. Daily mortality increased 0.68% for each 10 $\mu g/m^3$ increase in $PM_{2.5}$. A recent study incorporating data from counties across the United States from 1999 to 2015 observed excess $PM_{2.5}$ was responsible for approximately 30,000 premature deaths, lowering the estimated national life expectancy by 0.15 years.[20] In counties where $PM_{2.5}$ was reduced over the 15-year period, so did mortality. Highlighting these health effects, changes in emissions as a result of the US Clean Air Act and its amendments over a 20-year period from 1980 to 2000 revealed that a 10 $\mu g/m^3$ improvement in $PM_{2.5}$ resulted in mean increased life expectancy of greater than 7 months across 51 US cities, which accounted for 15% of improved longevity overall.[5,21] These findings are consistent with other cohort studies over the same time period.[22,23] In 2011, the US Environmental Protection Agency (EPA) estimated that improved PM exposure would result in 230,000 adult lives saved by 2020.[24] Most notably, the dose-response of the relationship between particulate exposure and mortality is fairly consistent across concentration ranges, even at ambient levels below national and international thresholds.[19,20]

Respiratory-specific mortality is an even higher individual risk. In the MCC data investigated by Liu and colleagues,[19] the corresponding increase in daily mortality from respiratory events was 0.74% for each 10 $\mu g/m^3$ increase in $PM_{2.5}$, higher than both all-cause and cardiovascular mortality attribution. Respiratory mortality is driven by chronic obstructive pulmonary disease (COPD) and lung cancer, for which the estimates of respiratory mortality from the Global Burden of Disease study are greater than 800,0000 persons and 280,000 in 2015, respectively.[2] However, in contrast to these provocative mortality data, a recent prospective study with individual level data within the multicenter European Study of Cohorts for Air Pollution Effects (ESCAPE) found no significant association of air pollution exposure with non-malignant respiratory mortality among 1559 deaths from 307,553 subjects across 16 cohorts.[25]

Pollutant Transport to the Respiratory Tree

The size of the particulate and the solubility of the pollutant dictate the type of symptoms that are induced by pollutant exposure. Generally speaking, large particles are filtered by impaction in the upper airway and natural cleaning mechanisms in the nose (nasal hair and turbulent flow) and upper airway. Particle sizes 10 μm and larger tend to be deposited in the upper airway and may cause nasal congestion and/or mucous membrane irritation of the eye. $PM_{2.5}$ is small enough to reach the small airways and deposit as deep as the alveolar space. For this reason, $PM_{2.5}$ is most highly associated with lower respiratory tract diseases, including asthma and airway infections. Ultrafine particles freely cross the alveolar capillary membranes and can be transported to all organ systems. For gaseous pollutants, tissue specificity depends more on solubility profile. For example, water-soluble pollutants, such as sulfur dioxide, cause eye and mucous membrane irritation in the upper airway. NO_2 and O_3 are less soluble and therefore penetrate deeper into the lower respiratory tract and lung.[1] However, it is important to recognize that real-world encounters with ambient pollutants are largely with pollutant mixtures that may contain a variety of particle sizes and gaseous components. Many studies have attempted to disentangle the effects of different pollutants in multipollutant models, but this is complicated by the number of contaminants and the variety of elemental components[26,27] that contribute to particle mass at different levels.

Mechanism of Biological Effects

Mechanistic studies to determine how air pollution affects human health have uncovered several plausible pathways,[28] including oxidative stress and damage, innate[29] and adaptive immunologic/inflammatory responses, allergic sensitization and Th2 airways inflammation, alteration of epigenetic loci that influences airways development, and direct effects on neuromuscular function of the airways.

Air pollution exposure may cause a variety of inflammatory changes in the airways, which depend on the type of pollutant exposure, elemental composition of the particles, and concurrent exposures. In addition, host factors may play a significant role in the type of the inflammatory response. The inflammatory response to naturally occurring pollutant mixtures and coexposure to other environmental factors are inherently difficult to systematically study due to the countless variables that would need to be accounted, so inferences are drawn from carefully designed single and coexposure cell, animal, and human studies. Perhaps the most ubiquitous response to air pollution exposure found in human studies has been the association with airways and lung injury via oxidative stress,[30,31] mechanisms that increase neutrophilic airway inflammation. Controlled human exposure studies have demonstrated increased levels of inflammatory cells, primarily neutrophils, but also mast cells and lymphocytes, along with increased inflammatory mediators, such as interleukin (IL)-8 and IL-13 in healthy volunteers.[32,33] Gene variants in the glutathione pathway have been shown to influence the effect of ambient pollutant exposure on lung function in children,[34,35] further supporting the role of oxidative stress as a mechanism in the adverse health effects of pollution exposure.

At-risk populations of patients with underlying asthma and atopy have found increased allergic responses, such as nasal and airway eosinophilia in response to exposure.[36] Moreover, studies of coexposure of NO_2 or PM with allergens has found these pollutants to have an adjuvant effect on allergic inflammatory response. Fine particles may be important conduits in which adherent allergens may reach the lower respiratory tract or cause epithelial disruption due to oxidative stress.[37]

In addition, diesel exhaust particles, a major component of urban pollution, have been shown to affect the vagal afferent nerves in in vitro and in vivo models by depolarization of the vagus nerve via airway c-fiber afferents, which could lead to respiratory symptoms by a direct neurostimulatory effect on airway smooth muscle.[38]

Respiratory Symptoms

These biologic mechanisms affect respiratory symptoms in both general and vulnerable populations. In studies involving general populations of children and adults, exposure to particulate pollution has been associated with regular cough, wheezing, and breathlessness,[27,39] which improve with reduction of pollutant levels.[40] A few case-control studies in children and adults have demonstrated higher rates of noninfectious conjunctivitis and conjunctival irritation associated with urban pollutant exposure.[41,42] Moreover, chronic exposure to air pollutants have been associated with dry eye disease across populations.[43,44]

Alteration of lung function

Chronic exposure to ambient pollution has been linked to impaired lung growth in children and progressive lung function decline in adult populations. Rice and colleagues[45] evaluated chronic pollutant effects on early lung function development in a large birth cohort study and found that both proximity to roadway and home address estimates of black carbon (BC) and $PM_{2.5}$ in the first 7 years of life was associated with low forced vital capacity (FVC) and forced expiratory volume in 1 second (FEV_1) without significantly impacting the ratio of FEV_1/FVC. These data suggest that early-life exposure to pollutants affects lung growth in a restrictive pattern rather than airway obstruction. In adolescence, the effects are similar. Perhaps the most demonstrative examples are from the California Health Study, which demonstrated across 3 distinct time periods the association of ambient NO_2, $PM_{2.5}$, and BC with poor lung function in children.[46,47] Although the most significant effects were reported for FEV_1, the effect on FVC and maximal mid-expiratory flows were similarly reduced. Importantly, for children who moved from high exposure locations to lower exposures, there was a significant improvement in lung function,[48] highlighting that intervention on an individual level can alter long-term lung growth. These findings extend to the prenatal period in which maternal exposure is associated with lower lung function in the child, as well as preterm birth,[49] which itself is associated with poor lung function outcomes.[50] These data suggest that perhaps alteration in DNA methylation is responsible for altered lung formation rather than direct effects of airway inflammation.[51] However, these associations have not been found in all cohorts.[52] The summation of the prenatal and pediatric findings are particularly salient as more and more data support that long-term lung function trajectories are determined in childhood.[53,54]

In adults, several longitudinal studies have demonstrated exposure to particulate pollutants are associated with lower lung function in cross-sectional and longitudinal analyses.[55–57] Moreover, across repeated measures, the Normative Aging Study found higher annual BC concentration was associated with accelerated rate of decline in

FEV_1 and FVC for elderly men living in Boston, MA.[55] Results from studies documenting the improvement in lung function in concert with decreased ambient PM add more convincing evidence of the causal effect of long-term pollution on lung function outcomes.[58,59] The SAPALDIA study, a Swiss population-based study sampling more than 9000 adults, demonstrated a 10 $\mu g/m^3$ decrease in PM_{10} concentration was associated with a 9% decrease in annual FEV_1.[58]

AMBIENT POLLUTION AND RESPIRATORY DISEASE

The effects of ambient pollutant exposure on respiratory symptoms and lung function in the general population are amplified in vulnerable populations of adults and children with existing lung disease. Moreover, for many chronic lung diseases, ambient exposure to particulates and gaseous pollutants have been implicated in the inception of the disease process. In the following sections, we detail the relationship of ambient pollution exposure to the inception and exacerbation of chronic lung diseases, focusing primarily on asthma and COPD, which represent the most common noncancer lung diseases of childhood and adulthood. **Fig. 2** illustrates respiratory diseases affected by ambient air pollutants.

Asthma

Asthma inception

The relationship between air pollution and the development of asthma has been found in population studies across all age groups. Prenatal exposure to ambient pollution may lead to epigenetic modifications that can be transmitted from mother to child in a nongenomic hereditary manner.[60] The Asthma Coalition on Community, Environment and Social Stress (ACCESS) project, an urban pregnancy cohort, found that exposure to BC and $PM_{2.5}$, particularly in the second trimester were associated with infantile wheeze and childhood asthma, especially for boys.[61]

The Southern California Children's Health Study identified home and school air pollution as a significant contributor to incident asthma in kindergarten and first-grade students who were asthma and wheeze-free at the start of the study.[62] Similarly, a Swedish birth cohort found that TRAP and NO_2 encountered in the first year of life had significant effects on lung function later in childhood and adolescence.[63,64] Although a longitudinal European study incorporating multiple birth cohorts found no association between childhood air pollutant exposure and asthma prevalence,[65] the vast majority of studies from the developed world support the relationship.[66–71] Moreover, a population-based study including more than 14,000 children from prospective birth cohorts in Germany, Sweden, and the Netherlands extended the findings from childhood asthma measured primarily during early childhood to adolescents. They found a significant association of NO_2 and BC (measured as $PM_{2.5}$ absorbance) at the birth address with higher odds of incident asthma up to age 14 to 16 years.[72] Overall, these findings (1) demonstrate that long-term associations persist between early-life pollutant exposure and asthma, and (2) add confidence to the association at an age when asthma is more reliably diagnosed. The breadth of pediatric data strongly supports the relationship between ambient pollution and the inception of asthma in childhood across regions of the world and racial/ethnic differences, with a suggestion that early-life exposures are the most important with different studies identifying differential effects of gender, allergic sensitization and

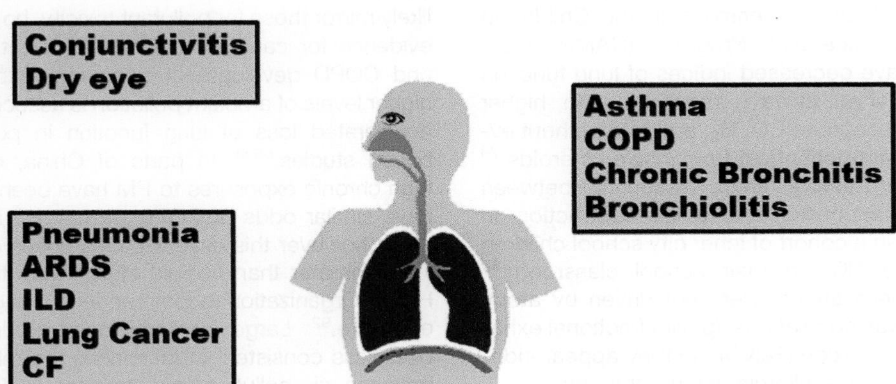

Fig. 2. Respiratory diseases affected by ambient air pollutants. Schematic of respiratory diseases affected by ambient pollutant exposure. CF, cystic fibrosis.

family history of atopy that may modify the relationship.

Fewer data are available for adult-onset asthma.[73,74] A study by Bowatte and colleagues[74] identified that in the Tasmanian Longitudinal Health Study there was a significant association between home NO_2 exposure or living within 200 m from a major road and current wheeze and asthma. The highest risk group had the null genotype of GSTT1, suggesting that lack of antioxidant activity may be a susceptibility factor for developing airways disease and thereby highlighting the role of an oxidative stress mechanism in explaining harm from pollutants. Aside from the association with the inception of adult asthma, exposure to ambient pollution may influence the development of asthma-COPD overlap syndrome (ACOS), which is noted to have higher morbidity and lung function decline than either condition alone. The prospective Canadian Community Healthy Survey study identified an almost threefold higher incidence of developing ACOS in those residing in locations with higher cumulative $PM_{2.5}$ and 31% higher in areas of higher O_3.[75]

Asthma morbidity

Human controlled exposure studies in subjects with allergic asthma have shown both increased airway hyperresponsiveness to subsequent allergen challenge[76] and reduced lung function after exposure to ambient pollutants at levels encountered in routine urban life.[77] The lung function deficits were accompanied by elevated markers of neutrophilic airways inflammation and acidification.

Epidemiologic studies extend these findings to demonstrate consistent alterations in lung function, increased symptoms and emergency health care services use in relation to short-term increases in ambient pollutant exposures, primarily those included in TRAP, ozone, NO_2, and PM.[78] Children with asthma enrolled in the Childhood Asthma Management Program (CAMP) were found to have decreased indices of lung function and heightened airways reactivity with higher ambient exposure to CO, O_3, and NO_2 without evidence of treatment effect from inhaled steroids.[79] We similarly found a direct relationship between elevated levels of NO_2 and airflow obstruction on spirometry in a cohort of inner city school children exposed to NO_2 in their school classroom.[80] Notably, these affects were not driven by atopy and there was no relationship with fractional exhalation of nitric oxide (FeNO), so they appear independent of typical allergic asthma triggers.

Emergency department (ED) visits for pediatric asthma have been highly associated with spikes in ambient pollution in urban environments[81,82]; this relationship is potentially stronger in asthmatic patients with premature birth or from low-income and Latino populations.[83,84] Time series analyses confirm increased emergency room visits for children and young adults with asthma exacerbations in concert with elevations in ambient pollutants.[84] Although it is difficult to differentiate individual pollutants from pollutant mixtures, ozone appears to have the most potent effect on asthma exacerbations[85] and is consistently found to be associated with ED visits.[86,87] In a study assessing asthma exacerbations presenting to emergency departments across Seoul, Korea, multiple triggers were assessed in time series analysis, stratified by age (infant, preschool children, school-aged children, adults and elderly [60 years or older]).[88] The most provocative association for asthma morbidity was air pollutant exposure, measured as individual gaseous or particle pollutants, which exceeded the effect of viral infection or environmental allergens. Moreover, in each age stratification, 7-day O_3 exposure had the highest relative risk of asthma exacerbation, greater than any allergen, weather or viral factor. In summary, pollutant exposures, including particles, gases (ozone and NO_2, primarily) and TRAP are strongly and consistently associated with increased asthma symptoms, lung function decline, and exacerbations of asthma across all ages.[89]

Chronic Obstructive Pulmonary Disease

Chronic obstructive pulmonary disease inception

COPD is the second most common chronic respiratory disease in adults worldwide, affecting more than 170 million people, but has a disproportionately high rate of associated morbidity and mortality.[90] Cigarette smoking is the predominant etiology for the development of COPD; the mechanisms responsible likely mirror those for pollutant toxicity, however the evidence for causality between ambient pollution and COPD development is limited. Exposure to higher levels of ambient pollution is associated with accelerated loss of lung function in population-based studies.[55,56] In parts of China, extremely high chronic exposures to PM have been found to have similar odds of COPD prevalence as smoking[91]; however this association is observed at PM levels greater than fivefold higher than the World Health Organization recommended average annual exposure.[92] Large epidemiologic studies have been less consistent in identifying the relationship between air pollution and incident COPD. Initial COPD hospital admission over a 10-year period in a prospective Danish cohort of 53,000 subjects was associated with 35-year mean NO_2 level at home residence.[93] However, a subsequent large English[94] study with more than 800,000 subjects did not find an association and an analysis of European cohorts included in the ESCAPE project found positive but nonsignificant associations between COPD incidence and prevalence with air pollution measure.[95] When using the GOLD (Global Initiative for Chronic Obstructive Lung Disease) criteria to define COPD, there was a significant association with traffic intensity near the home and suggested that female and never-smoker subgroups may be more strongly affected.[95]

Chronic Obstructive Pulmonary Disease Morbidity

The association of ambient pollution with exacerbation of COPD is much more consistent. A recent meta-analysis by Li and colleagues[96] report a 3.1% increase in COPD related hospitalization and 2.5% increase in COPD mortality for each 10 $\mu g/m^3$ increase in daily $PM_{2.5}$ exposure. In Chile, COPD ED admissions increase by up to 19% in association with increased pollutants by an interquartile range.[97]

Several panel studies of patients with COPD reporting person-level outcomes have demonstrated variable associations with air pollution and COPD morbidity. Several studies have demonstrated increased symptoms and exacerbations,[98–100] whereas the effects on lung function parameters[101,102] are less consistent.[98] A large East London cohort with COPD identified a significant increase in symptoms with pollutant exposure and nonsignificant trends for exacerbations associated with local ambient pollutant exposure in East London.[103] Even moderate exercise in high traffic areas may reduce the benefits of exercise in patients with COPD.[104]

Perhaps the most convincing evidence of the relationship of exposure with disease progression comes from a recent longitudinal cohort from the Multi-Ethnic Study of Atherosclerosis (MESA) and Lung Studies. In this study, investigators found significant associations between ambient pollutant exposure and increases in percent emphysema measured on chest computed tomography (CT) scans over a 10-year period.[105] Concentrations of O_3, $PM_{2.5}$, NOx, and BC, while only O_3 and NOx at follow-up, were significantly associated with the 10-year change in percent emphysema. O_3 was also significantly associated with decrease in FEV_1 over the 10-year time period.

Other Respiratory Disorders

Although most air pollution respiratory literature focuses on asthma and COPD, it is important to highlight a few respiratory conditions in which there is evidence suggesting the influence of ambient air pollution: lung cancer, acute respiratory infection, acute respiratory distress syndrome (ARDS), and interstitial lung disease (ILD). Cancer incidence and cancer mortality are also both associated with exposure to high levels of ambient air pollution. The International Agency for Research on Cancer estimates that between 3% and 5% of lung cancer cases are attributable to ambient air pollution. The independent effect of pollution on lung cancer mortality is estimated at more than 62,000 per year.[2]

A recently emerging body of evidence links ambient pollution exposure to risk of ARDS after trauma, an association that suggests pollutant exposure confers respiratory vulnerability in otherwise healthy adults such that a nonrespiratory event that stresses the respiratory system can be overwhelming. Reilly and colleagues[106] found that among 996 critically ill patients with acute trauma, both short and long-term exposures with ambient pollutants were highly associated with development of ARDS. These exposure levels were largely within acceptable ranges per US and European Union air quality standards. The findings were mirrored in a separate cohort of critically ill patients with a specific risk associated with ozone exposure at their home location.[107]

Several studies have documented the increased risk of respiratory infection associated with air pollution exposure. The odds of acute lower respiratory tract infections, particularly bronchiolitis, following short-term elevations in PM increase by 7% to 15%[108,109] and even higher for infants born preterm. Short-term increases in air pollution have been associated with acute respiratory infection emergency visits and hospitalization in children and adults.[110–112]

Globally, increased levels of indoor and ambient pollutants are risk factors for pneumonia across the ages.[113,114] For patients with cystic fibrosis, a genetic disease of dysfunction chloride transport, which leads to airways inflammation and chronic and acute infection, exposure to ambient pollution is significantly associated with respiratory exacerbations[115–117] and decline in FEV_1.[115]

Although the full narrative on environmental and social determinants is unfolding, some early analyses suggest that Coronavirus Disease 2019 (COVID)-related outcomes are related to ambient air pollution. Recently published studies from both China[118] and Italy[119] have demonstrated significant relationships between regions of high ambient particle and gaseous pollution and rates of COVID-19 infection. In a cross-sectional study using county-level US data,[120] COVID-related mortality was highest in locations where long-term air pollution concentrations have been highest, adjusting for some key area-level risk factors, such as population size, age distribution, and population density. A similar study in the United Kingdom[121] showed association between COVID mortality and ambient levels of nitrogen oxides and ozone.

The development of ILDs from exposure to occupational or intense environmental exposures have been well documented for conditions such as hypersensitivity pneumonitis, silicosis, asbestosis, and other pneumoconioses. More recently, outdoor air pollution has emerged as a plausible contributor to ILDs.[122] Gaseous pollutants, O_3, and NO_2 have been associated with idiopathic pulmonary fibrosis (IPF) exacerbations,[123,124] whereas PM has been associated with decline in lung function[125] and mortality.[126] In a longitudinal study by Johannson and colleagues, [127] with weekly symptom and spirometry measures over 40 consecutive weeks, air pollution was associated with lower lung function across the study period, but not short-term variations in lung function.

HOW CLINICIANS CAN APPROACH POLLUTION AND RESPIRATORY HEALTH

The summation of basic science, human exposure panel studies, cohort, and large epidemiologic research overwhelmingly supports both the health risks to humans from exposure to ambient air pollution at levels encountered in industrialized and developing countries, alike. The risks are even higher for vulnerable populations with underlying chronic lung diseases, such as asthma and COPD. So how does the clinician coerce the breadth of research findings into daily practice? This, too, can be addressed on many levels. As the source apportionment of harmful environmental contaminants are derived largely from the burning of fossil fuels for industry, home, and transportation uses, efforts to promote curtailing these practices should be encouraged.

Air Quality Index Levels of Health Concern	Numerical Value	Meaning
Good	0 to 50	Air quality is considered satisfactory, and air pollution poses little or no risk.
Moderate	51 to 100	Air quality is acceptable; however, for some pollutants there may be a moderate health concern for a very small number of people who are unusually sensitive to air pollution.
Unhealthy for Sensitive Groups	101 to 150	Members of sensitive groups may experience health effects. The general public is not likely to be affected.
Unhealthy	151 to 200	Everyone may begin to experience health effects; members of sensitive groups may experience more serious health effects.
Very Unhealthy	201 to 300	Health alert: everyone may experience more serious health effects.
Hazardous	301 to 500	Health warnings of emergency conditions. The entire population is more likely to be affected.

Fig. 3. Schematic of AQI. (*From* U.S. EPA's AirNow Program. *From* U.S. EPA's AirNow ProgramAir Quality Index (AQI) Basics. Available at: https://airnow.gov/index.cfm?action=aqibasics.aqi. Accessed February 11, 2020; with permission.)

Supporting local, regional and national policies to encourage clean energy production and utilization and regulations to minimize emissions of pollutants may lead to improved air quality. Alterations in personal use, such as minimizing gas and oil dependency in favor of renewable sources of energy for home (solar) and personal transportation (electric vehicles, public transportation, cycling, and walking) can minimize the personal contribution to environmental pollution.

Health care providers have a unique relationship with patients with chronic disease. The office visit serves to assess and manage the individual's physical disability but also offers a discrete opportunity to offer guidance on minimizing harmful exposures. One such publicly available tool providers can use for anticipatory guidance for patients is the air quality index (AQI). AirNow is a program by the US EPA that is the national repository for real-time air quality data derived from federal ambient sampling sites for ozone and particle pollution with coverage of all 50 states, 6 Canadian provinces, and 24 US national parks.[128] The AQI is presented in a color-coded graphic to represent the air quality rating and levels of health concerns, specifically identifying conditions that may affect sensitive populations[129] (**Fig. 3**), and can be accessed by Web site, social media feed, and iPhone and Android apps. For individual patients, this daily information and forecasting of air quality can help provide advanced warning for adverse conditions for which the patient will want to avoid being outside and consider using an air cleaning device indoors.

SUMMARY

Air quality is an important influence on human health and disease. Our understanding of these relationships are limited by the complex interactions between exposure dynamics (eg, pollutant mixtures, concentrations, the duration and intensity of exposure) and personal characteristics (eg, age at exposure, underlying disease, genetic predisposition). Although the adverse respiratory effects of air pollutants encountered in the *outdoor* environment presented in this article highlight the negative impact of pollutants on chronic disease and lung function growth and decline, it is important to note that human exposure to air pollution is not so neatly compartmentalized; sources of pollutants are ubiquitous in the indoor and outdoor environment and mixing of ambient and indoor air occurs constantly. Nevertheless, there are clear risks that poor ambient air quality presents to the development and exacerbation of chronic lung disease, especially COPD and asthma. Clinicians should be aware of the health effects of these environmental factors, as well as the publicly available resources to monitor them, to provide optimal guidance for their patients.

CLINICS CARE POINTS

- Clinicians should consider poor air quality when evaluating triggers for exacerbations of chronic lung disease, especially asthma and COPD.
- Healthcare providers should consider advising patients with chronic lung disease on how to minimize exposure to high levels of air pollution.
- The Air Quality Index (US EPA) may be useful in daily assessment of local outdoor air quality to inform patients of the potential exposure to air pollutants.

DISCLOSURE

None of the authors have any commercial/financial conflicts of interest.

REFERENCES

1. Schraufnagel DE, Balmes JR, Cowl CT, et al. Air pollution and noncommunicable diseases: a review by the forum of international respiratory societies' environmental committee, Part 1: the damaging effects of air pollution. Chest 2019;155(2):417–26.
2. Cohen AJ, Brauer M, Burnett R, et al. Estimates and 25-year trends of the global burden of disease attributable to ambient air pollution: an analysis of data from the Global Burden of Diseases Study 2015. Lancet 2017;389(10082):1907–18.
3. Lelieveld J, Evans JS, Fnais M, et al. The contribution of outdoor air pollution sources to premature mortality on a global scale. Nature 2015; 525(7569):367–71.
4. Landrigan PJ, Fuller R, Acosta NJR, et al. The Lancet Commission on pollution and health. Lancet 2018. https://doi.org/10.1016/S0140-6736(17)32345-0.
5. Pope CA 3rd, Ezzati M, Dockery DW. Fine-particulate air pollution and life expectancy in the United States. N Engl J Med 2009;360(4):376–86.
6. Hajat A, Hsia C, O'Neill MS. Socioeconomic disparities and air pollution exposure: a global review. Curr Environ Health Rep 2015. https://doi.org/10.1007/s40572-015-0069-5.
7. Karagulian F, Belis CA, Dora CFC, et al. Contributions to cities' ambient particulate matter (PM): a systematic review of local source contributions at global level. Atmos Environ 2015;120:475–83. https://doi.org/10.1016/j.atmosenv.2015.08.087.

8. Thurston GD, Ito K, Lall R. A source apportionment of U.S. fine particulate matter air pollution. Atmos Environ 2011;45(24):3924–36.
9. Mikati I, Benson AF, Luben TJ, et al. Disparities in distribution of particulate matter emission sources by race and poverty status. Am J Public Health 2018;108(4):480–5.
10. Rosofsky A, Levy JI, Zanobetti A, et al. Temporal trends in air pollution exposure inequality in Massachusetts. Environ Res 2018. https://doi.org/10.1016/j.envres.2017.10.028.
11. Shaddick G, Thomas ML, Amini H, et al. Data Integration for the assessment of population exposure to ambient air pollution for global burden of disease assessment. Environ Sci Technol 2018;52(16):9069–78.
12. Kelly FJ, Fussell JC. Size, source and chemical composition as determinants of toxicity attributable to ambient particulate matter. Atmos Environ 2012. https://doi.org/10.1016/j.atmosenv.2012.06.039.
13. Delfino RJ, Sioutas C, Malik S. Potential role of ultrafine particles in associations between airborne particle mass and cardiovascular health. Environ Health Perspect 2005. https://doi.org/10.1289/ehp.7938.
14. US EPA O. Integrated Science Assessment (ISA) for Sulfur Oxides - Health Criteria.
15. Karner AA, Eisinger DS, Niemeier DA. Near-roadway air quality: synthesizing the findings from real-world data. Environ Sci Technol 2010. https://doi.org/10.1021/es100008x.
16. Alexeeff SE, Roy A, Shan J, et al. High-resolution mapping of traffic related air pollution with Google street view cars and incidence of cardiovascular events within neighborhoods in Oakland, CA. Environ Health 2018. https://doi.org/10.1186/s12940-018-0382-1.
17. Apte JS, Messier KP, Gani S, et al. High-resolution air pollution mapping with google street view cars: exploiting big data. Environ Sci Technol 2017. https://doi.org/10.1021/acs.est.7b00891.
18. Ambient (outdoor) air pollution. Available at: https://www.who.int/en/news-room/fact-sheets/detail/ambient-(outdoor)-air-quality-and-health. Accessed February 4, 2020.
19. Liu C, Chen R, Sera F, et al. Ambient particulate air pollution and daily mortality in 652 cities. N Engl J Med 2019;381(8):705–15.
20. Bennett JE, Tamura-Wicks H, Parks RM, et al. Particulate matter air pollution and national and county life expectancy loss in the USA: a spatiotemporal analysis. PLoS Med 2019;16(7):e1002856.
21. Jerrett M, Burnett RT, Pope CA 3rd, et al. Long-term ozone exposure and mortality. N Engl J Med 2009;360(11):1085–95.
22. Hart JE, Garshick E, Dockery DW, et al. Long-term ambient multipollutant exposures and mortality. Am J Respir Crit Care Med 2011;183(1):73–8.
23. Laden F, Schwartz J, Speizer FE, et al. Reduction in fine particulate air pollution and mortality: extended follow-up of the Harvard Six Cities Study. Am J Respir Crit Care Med 2006. https://doi.org/10.1164/rccm.200503-443OC.
24. Epa U, of Policy Analysis O. The benefits and costs of the clean air Act from 1990 to 2020, final report, Revision A, April 2011 2011. Available at: https://www.epa.gov/sites/production/files/2015-07/documents/fullreport_rev_a.pdf.
25. Dimakopoulou K, Samoli E, Beelen R, et al. Air pollution and nonmalignant respiratory mortality in 16 cohorts within the ESCAPE project. Am J Respir Crit Care Med 2014;189(6):684–96.
26. Bell ML, Ebisu K, Peng RD, et al. Hospital admissions and chemical composition of fine particle air pollution. Am J Respir Crit Care Med 2009;179(12):1115–20.
27. Patel MM, Hoepner L, Garfinkel R, et al. Ambient metals, elemental carbon, and wheeze and cough in New York City children through 24 months of age. Am J Respir Crit Care Med 2009;180(11):1107–13.
28. Gowers AM, Cullinan P, Ayres JG, et al. Does outdoor air pollution induce new cases of asthma? Biological plausibility and evidence; a review. Respirology 2012;17(6):887–98.
29. Bauer RN, Diaz-Sanchez D, Jaspers I. Effects of air pollutants on innate immunity: the role of Toll-like receptors and nucleotide-binding oligomerization domain-like receptors. J Allergy Clin Immunol 2012;129(1):14–6.
30. Ciencewicki J, Trivedi S, Kleeberger SR. Oxidants and the pathogenesis of lung diseases. J Allergy Clin Immunol 2008;122(3):456–70.
31. Huang W, Wang G, Lu S-E, et al. Inflammatory and oxidative stress responses of healthy young adults to changes in air quality during the Beijing Olympics. Am J Respir Crit Care Med 2012;186(11):1150–9.
32. Kim CS, Alexis NE, Rappold AG, et al. Lung function and inflammatory responses in healthy young adults exposed to 0.06 ppm ozone for 6.6 hours. Am J Respir Crit Care Med 2011;183(9):1215–21.
33. Wu W, Jin Y, Carlsten C. Inflammatory health effects of indoor and outdoor particulate matter. J Allergy Clin Immunol 2018;141(3):833–44.
34. Breton CV, Salam MT, Vora H, et al. Genetic variation in the glutathione synthesis pathway, air pollution, and children's lung function growth. Am J Respir Crit Care Med 2011;183(2):243–8.
35. Dai X, Bowatte G, Lowe AJ, et al. Do glutathione S-Transferase Genes modify the link between indoor air pollution and asthma, allergies, and lung

function? A systematic review. Curr Allergy Asthma Rep 2018;18(3):20.

36. Noah TL, Zhou H, Zhang H, et al. Diesel exhaust exposure and nasal response to attenuated influenza in normal and allergic volunteers. Am J Respir Crit Care Med 2012;185(2):179–85.
37. Diaz-Sanchez D, Garcia MP, Wang M, et al. Nasal challenge with diesel exhaust particles can induce sensitization to a neoallergen in the human mucosa. J Allergy Clin Immunol 1999. https://doi.org/10.1016/S0091-6749(99)70011-4.
38. Robinson RK, Birrell MA, Adcock JJ, et al. Mechanistic link between diesel exhaust particles and respiratory reflexes. J Allergy Clin Immunol 2018; 141(3):1074–84.e9.
39. Ryan PH, Bernstein DI, Lockey J, et al. Exposure to traffic-related particles and endotoxin during infancy is associated with wheezing at age 3 years. Am J Respir Crit Care Med 2009;180(11):1068–75.
40. Schindler C, Keidel D, Gerbase MW, et al. Improvements in PM10 exposure and reduced rates of respiratory symptoms in a cohort of Swiss adults (SAPALDIA). Am J Respir Crit Care Med 2009; 179(7):579–87.
41. Gutiérrez MA, Giuliani D, Porta AA, et al. Relationship between ocular surface alterations and concentrations of aerial particulate matter. J Ophthalmic Vis Res 2019;14(4):419–27.
42. Nucci P, Sacchi M, Pichi F, et al. Pediatric conjunctivitis and air pollution exposure: a prospective observational study. Semin Ophthalmol 2017; 32(4):407–11.
43. Alves M, Novaes P, Morraye M de A, et al. Is dry eye an environmental disease? Arq Bras Oftalmol 2014;77(3):193–200.
44. Mo Z, Fu Q, Lyu D, et al. Impacts of air pollution on dry eye disease among residents in Hangzhou, China: a case-crossover study. Environ Pollut 2019;246:183–9.
45. Rice MB, Rifas-Shiman SL, Litonjua AA, et al. Lifetime exposure to ambient pollution and lung function in children. Am J Respir Crit Care Med 2016; 193(8):881–8.
46. Gauderman WJ, McConnell R, Gilliland F, et al. Association between air pollution and lung function growth in southern California children. Am J Respir Crit Care Med 2000;162(4 Pt 1): 1383–90.
47. Gauderman WJ, Urman R, Avol E, et al. Association of improved air quality with lung development in children. N Engl J Med 2015;372(10):905–13.
48. Avol EL, Gauderman WJ, Tan SM, et al. Respiratory effects of relocating to areas of differing air pollution levels. Am J Respir Crit Care Med 2001; 164(11):2067–72.
49. Wu J, Ren C, Delfino RJ, et al. Association between local traffic-generated air pollution and preeclampsia and preterm delivery in the South Coast air basin of California. Environ Health Perspect 2009;117(11):1773–9.
50. Korten I, Ramsey K, Latzin P. Air pollution during pregnancy and lung development in the child. Paediatr Respir Rev 2017;21:38–46.
51. Janssen BG, Byun H-M, Gyselaers W, et al. Placental mitochondrial methylation and exposure to airborne particulate matter in the early life environment: an ENVIRONAGE birth cohort study. Epigenetics 2015;10(6):536–44.
52. Fuertes E, Bracher J, Flexeder C, et al. Long-term air pollution exposure and lung function in 15 year-old adolescents living in an urban and rural area in Germany: the GINIplus and LISAplus cohorts. Int J Hyg Environ Health 2015;218(7):656–65.
53. McGeachie MJ, Yates KP, Zhou X, et al. Patterns of growth and decline in lung function in persistent childhood asthma. N Engl J Med 2016;374(19): 1842–52.
54. Martinez FD. Early-life origins of chronic obstructive pulmonary disease. N Engl J Med 2016; 375(9):871–8.
55. Lepeule J, Litonjua AA, Coull B, et al. Long-term effects of traffic particles on lung function decline in the elderly. Am J Respir Crit Care Med 2014; 190(5):542–8.
56. Rice MB, Ljungman PL, Wilker EH, et al. Long-term exposure to traffic emissions and fine particulate matter and lung function decline in the Framingham heart study. Am J Respir Crit Care Med 2015;191(6):656–64.
57. Ackermann-Liebrich U, Leuenberger P, Schwartz J, et al. Lung function and long term exposure to air pollutants in Switzerland. Study on air pollution and lung diseases in adults (SAPALDIA) Team. Am J Respir Crit Care Med 1997;155(1):122–9.
58. Downs SH, Schindler C, Liu L-JS, et al. Reduced exposure to PM10 and attenuated age-related decline in lung function. N Engl J Med 2007; 357(23):2338–47.
59. Boogaard H, Fischer PH, Janssen NAH, et al. Respiratory effects of a reduction in outdoor air pollution concentrations. Epidemiology 2013;24(5): 753–61.
60. Burbank AJ, Sood AK, Kesic MJ, et al. Environmental determinants of allergy and asthma in early life. J Allergy Clin Immunol 2017;140(1):1–12.
61. Hsu H-HL, Chiu Y-HM, Coull BA, et al. Prenatal particulate air pollution and asthma onset in urban children. Identifying sensitive windows and sex differences. Am J Respir Crit Care Med 2015; 192(9):1052–9.
62. McConnell R, Islam T, Shankardass K, et al. Childhood incident asthma and traffic-related air pollution at home and school. Environ Health Perspect 2010;118(7):1021–6.

63. Schultz ES, Hallberg J, Bellander T, et al. Early-life exposure to traffic-related air pollution and lung function in adolescence. Am J Respir Crit Care Med 2016;193(2):171–7.
64. Schultz ES, Gruzieva O, Bellander T, et al. Traffic-related air pollution and lung function in children at 8 years of age: a birth cohort study. Am J Respir Crit Care Med 2012;186(12):1286–91.
65. Molter A, Simpson A, Berdel D, et al. A multicentre study of air pollution exposure and childhood asthma prevalence: the ESCAPE project. Eur Respir J 2015;45(3):610–24.
66. Nishimura KK, Iwanaga K, Oh SS, et al. Early-life ozone exposure associated with asthma without sensitization in Latino children. J Allergy Clin Immunol 2016;138(6):1703–6.e1.
67. Gehring U, Wijga AH, Brauer M, et al. Traffic-related air pollution and the development of asthma and allergies during the first 8 years of life. Am J Respir Crit Care Med 2010;181(6):596–603.
68. Jerrett M, Shankardass K, Berhane K, et al. Traffic-related air pollution and asthma onset in children: a prospective cohort study with individual exposure measurement. Environ Health Perspect 2008; 116(10):1433–8.
69. Nishimura KK, Galanter JM, Roth LA, et al. Early-life air pollution and asthma risk in minority children. The GALA II and SAGE II studies. Am J Respir Crit Care Med 2013;188(3):309–18.
70. Brunst KJ, Ryan PH, Brokamp C, et al. Timing and duration of traffic-related air pollution exposure and the risk for childhood wheeze and asthma. Am J Respir Crit Care Med 2015; 192(4):421–7.
71. Bowatte G, Lodge C, Lowe AJ, et al. The influence of childhood traffic-related air pollution exposure on asthma, allergy and sensitization: a systematic review and a meta-analysis of birth cohort studies. Allergy 2015;70(3):245–56.
72. Gehring U, Wijga AH, Hoek G, et al. Exposure to air pollution and development of asthma and rhinoconjunctivitis throughout childhood and adolescence: a population-based birth cohort study. Lancet Respir Med 2015;3(12):933–42.
73. Young MT, Sandler DP, DeRoo LA, et al. Ambient air pollution exposure and incident adult asthma in a nationwide cohort of U.S. women. Am J Respir Crit Care Med 2014;190(8):914–21.
74. Bowatte G, Lodge CJ, Knibbs LD, et al. Traffic-related air pollution exposure is associated with allergic sensitization, asthma, and poor lung function in middle age. J Allergy Clin Immunol 2017; 139(1):122–9.e1.
75. To T, Zhu J, Larsen K, et al. Progression from asthma to chronic obstructive pulmonary disease. Is air pollution a risk factor? Am J Respir Crit Care Med 2016;194(4):429–38.
76. Svartengren M, Strand V, Bylin G, et al. Short-term exposure to air pollution in a road tunnel enhances the asthmatic response to allergen. Eur Respir J 2000;15(4):716–24.
77. McCreanor J, Cullinan P, Nieuwenhuijsen MJ, et al. Respiratory effects of exposure to diesel traffic in persons with asthma. N Engl J Med 2007; 357(23):2348–58.
78. Burbank AJ, Peden DB. Assessing the impact of air pollution on childhood asthma morbidity: how, when, and what to do. Curr Opin Allergy Clin Immunol 2018;18(2):124–31.
79. Ierodiakonou D, Zanobetti A, Coull BA, et al. Ambient air pollution, lung function, and airway responsiveness in asthmatic children. J Allergy Clin Immunol 2016;137(2):390–9.
80. Gaffin JM, Hauptman M, Petty CR, et al. Nitrogen dioxide exposure in school classrooms of inner-city children with asthma. J Allergy Clin Immunol 2017. https://doi.org/10.1016/j.jaci.2017.08.028.
81. Strickland MJ, Darrow LA, Klein M, et al. Short-term associations between ambient air pollutants and pediatric asthma emergency department visits. Am J Respir Crit Care Med 2010;182(3):307–16.
82. Zheng XY, Ding H, Jiang LN, et al. Association between air pollutants and asthma emergency room visits and hospital admissions in time series studies: a systematic review and meta-analysis. PLoS One 2015;10(9):e0138146.
83. Strickland MJ, Klein M, Flanders WD, et al. Modification of the effect of ambient air pollution on pediatric asthma emergency visits: susceptible subpopulations. Epidemiology 2014;25(6): 843–50.
84. Byers N, Ritchey M, Vaidyanathan A, et al. Short-term effects of ambient air pollutants on asthma-related emergency department visits in Indianapolis, Indiana, 2007-2011. J Asthma 2016;53(3): 245–52.
85. Gass K, Klein M, Sarnat SE, et al. Associations between ambient air pollutant mixtures and pediatric asthma emergency department visits in three cities: a classification and regression tree approach. Environ Health 2015;14:58.
86. Noh J, Sohn J, Cho J, et al. Short-term effects of ambient air pollution on emergency department visits for asthma: an assessment of effect modification by prior allergic disease history. J Prev Med Public Heal 2016;49(5):329–41.
87. Tétreault L-F, Doucet M, Gamache P, et al. Severe and moderate asthma exacerbations in asthmatic children and exposure to ambient air pollutants. Int J Environ Res Public Health 2016;13(8):771.
88. Lee SW, Yon DK, James CC, et al. Short-term effects of multiple outdoor environmental factors on risk of asthma exacerbations: age-stratified time-

series analysis. J Allergy Clin Immunol 2019. https://doi.org/10.1016/j.jaci.2019.08.037.
89. Guarnieri M, Balmes JR. Outdoor air pollution and asthma. Lancet 2014;383(9928):1581–92.
90. GBD 2015 Chronic Respiratory Disease Collaborators. Global, regional, and national deaths, prevalence, disability-adjusted life years, and years lived with disability for chronic obstructive pulmonary disease and asthma, 1990-2015: a systematic analysis for the Global Burden of Disease Study 2015. Lancet Respir Med 2017;5(9): 691–706.
91. Wang C, Xu J, Yang L, et al. Prevalence and risk factors of chronic obstructive pulmonary disease in China (the China Pulmonary Health [CPH] study): a national cross-sectional study. Lancet 2018;391(10131):1706–17.
92. World Health Organization Regional Office for Europe. 2006. Available at: www.euro.who.int. Accessed February 10, 2020.
93. Andersen ZJ, Hvidberg M, Jensen SS, et al. Chronic obstructive pulmonary disease and long-term exposure to traffic-related air pollution: a cohort study. Am J Respir Crit Care Med 2011; 183(4):455–61.
94. Atkinson RW, Carey IM, Kent AJ, et al. Long-term exposure to outdoor air pollution and the incidence of chronic obstructive pulmonary disease in a national English cohort. Occup Environ Med 2015; 72(1):42–8.
95. Schikowski T, Adam M, Marcon A, et al. Association of ambient air pollution with the prevalence and incidence of COPD. Eur Respir J 2014;44(3): 614–26.
96. Li M-H, Fan L-C, Mao B, et al. Short-term exposure to ambient fine particulate matter increases hospitalizations and mortality in COPD: a systematic review and meta-analysis. Chest 2016;149(2): 447–58.
97. Arbex MA, de Souza Conceição GM, Cendon SP, et al. Urban air pollution and chronic obstructive pulmonary disease-related emergency department visits. J Epidemiol Community Health 2009;63(10): 777–83.
98. Harré ESM, Price PD, Ayrey RB, et al. Respiratory effects of air pollution in chronic obstructive pulmonary disease: a three month prospective study. Thorax 1997. https://doi.org/10.1136/thx.52.12.1040.
99. Desqueyroux H, Pujet JC, Prosper M, et al. Effects of air pollution on adults with chronic obstructive pulmonary disease. Arch Environ Health 2002. https://doi.org/10.1080/00039890209602088.
100. Van Der Zee SC, Hoek G, Boezen MH, et al. Acute effects of air pollution on respiratory health of 50-70 yr old adults. Eur Respir J 2000. https://doi.org/10.1034/j.1399-3003.2000.15d13.x.
101. Lagorio S, Forastiere F, Pistelli R, et al. Air pollution and lung function among susceptible adult subjects: a panel study. Environ Health 2006. https://doi.org/10.1186/1476-069X-5-11.
102. Trenga CA, Sullivan JH, Schildcrout JS, et al. Effect of particulate air pollution on lung function in adult and pediatric subjects in a Seattle panel study. Chest 2006. https://doi.org/10.1378/chest.129.6.1614.
103. Peacock JL, Anderson HR, Bremner SA, et al. Outdoor air pollution and respiratory health in patients with COPD. Thorax 2011;66(7):591–6.
104. Sinharay R, Gong J, Barratt B, et al. Respiratory and cardiovascular responses to walking down a traffic-polluted road compared with walking in a traffic-free area in participants aged 60 years and older with chronic lung or heart disease and age-matched healthy controls: a randomised, cross. Lancet 2018; 391(10118):339–49.
105. Wang M, Aaron CP, Madrigano J, et al. Association between long-term exposure to ambient air pollution and change in Quantitatively assessed emphysema and lung function. JAMA 2019;322(6): 546–56.
106. Reilly JP, Zhao Z, Shashaty MGS, et al. Low to moderate air pollutant exposure and acute respiratory distress syndrome after Severe trauma. Am J Respir Crit Care Med 2019;199(1):62–70.
107. Ware LB, Zhao Z, Koyama T, et al. Long-term ozone exposure increases the risk of developing the acute respiratory distress syndrome. Am J Respir Crit Care Med 2016;193(10):1143–50.
108. Horne BD, Joy EA, Hofmann MG, et al. Short-term elevation of fine particulate matter air pollution and acute lower respiratory infection. Am J Respir Crit Care Med 2018;198(6):759–66.
109. Girguis MS, Strickland MJ, Hu X, et al. Exposure to acute air pollution and risk of bronchiolitis and otitis media for preterm and term infants. J Expo Sci Environ Epidemiol 2018;28(4):348–57.
110. Darrow LA, Klein M, Flanders WD, et al. Air pollution and acute respiratory infections among children 0-4 years of age: an 18-year time-series study. Am J Epidemiol 2014;180(10):968–77.
111. Barnett AG, Williams GM, Schwartz J, et al. Air pollution and child respiratory health: a case-crossover study in Australia and New Zealand. Am J Respir Crit Care Med 2005;171(11):1272–8.
112. Cakmak S, Dales RE, Gultekin T, et al. Components of particulate air pollution and emergency department visits in Chile. Arch Environ Occup Health 2009;64(3):148–55.
113. Pirozzi CS, Jones BE, VanDerslice JA, et al. Short-term air pollution and incident pneumonia. A case-crossover study. Ann Am Thorac Soc 2018;15(4): 449–59.

114. Nhung NTT, Amini H, Schindler C, et al. Short-term association between ambient air pollution and pneumonia in children: a systematic review and meta-analysis of time-series and case-crossover studies. Environ Pollut 2017;230:1000–8.
115. Goss CH, Newsom SA, Schildcrout JS, et al. Effect of ambient air pollution on pulmonary exacerbations and lung function in cystic fibrosis. Am J Respir Crit Care Med 2004;169(7):816–21.
116. Farhat SCL, Almeida MB, Silva-Filho LVRF, et al. Ozone is associated with an increased risk of respiratory exacerbations in patients with cystic fibrosis. Chest 2013;144(4):1186–92.
117. Goeminne PC, Kiciński M, Vermeulen F, et al. Impact of air pollution on cystic fibrosis pulmonary exacerbations: a case-crossover analysis. Chest 2013;143(4):946–54.
118. Zhu Y, Xie J, Huang F, et al. Association between short-term exposure to air pollution and COVID-19 infection: evidence from China. Sci Total Environ 2020;727:138704.
119. Fattorini D, Regoli F. Role of the chronic air pollution levels in the Covid-19 outbreak risk in Italy. Environ Pollut 2020;264:114732.
120. Wu X, Nethery RC, Sabath BM, et al. Exposure to air pollution and COVID-19 mortality in the United States: a nationwide cross-sectional study. medRxiv 2020. https://doi.org/10.1101/2020.04.05.20054502.
121. Travaglio M, Popovic R, Yu Y, et al. Links between air pollution and COVID-19 in England. medRxiv 2020. https://doi.org/10.1101/2020.04.16.20067405.
122. Johannson KA, Balmes JR, Collard HR. Air pollution exposure: a novel environmental risk factor for interstitial lung disease? Chest 2015;147(4):1161–7.
123. Sese L, Annesi-Maesano I, Nunes H. Impact of particulate matter on the natural history of IPF: a matter of concentrations? Chest 2018;154(3):726–7.
124. Johannson KA, Vittinghoff E, Lee K, et al. Acute exacerbation of idiopathic pulmonary fibrosis associated with air pollution exposure. Eur Respir J 2014;43(4):1124–31.
125. Winterbottom CJ, Shah RJ, Patterson KC, et al. Exposure to ambient particulate matter is associated with accelerated functional decline in idiopathic pulmonary fibrosis. Chest 2018;153(5):1221–8.
126. Sesé L, Nunes H, Cottin V, et al. Role of atmospheric pollution on the natural history of idiopathic pulmonary fibrosis. Thorax 2018;73(2):145–50.
127. Johannson KA, Vittinghoff E, Morisset J, et al. Air pollution exposure is associated with lower lung function, but not changes in lung function, in patients with idiopathic pulmonary fibrosis. Chest 2018;154(1):119–25.
128. About AirNow. Available at: https://airnow.gov/index.cfm?action=topics.about_airnow. Accessed February 11, 2020.
129. Air quality index (AQI) basics. Available at: https://airnow.gov/index.cfm?action=aqibasics.aqi. Accessed February 11, 2020.
130. Ground-level ozone basics | ground-level ozone pollution | US EPA. Available at: https://www.epa.gov/ground-level-ozone-pollution/ground-level-ozone-basics. Accessed May 24, 2020.
131. Basic information about NO2 | nitrogen dioxide (NO2) pollution | US EPA. Available at: https://www.epa.gov/no2-pollution/basic-information-about-no2#What is NO2. Accessed May 24, 2020.
132. Sulfur dioxide basics | sulfur dioxide (SO2) pollution | US EPA. Available at: https://www.epa.gov/so2-pollution/sulfur-dioxide-basics. Accessed May 24, 2020.
133. Sulfur dioxide: your environment, your health | National Library of Medicine. Available at: https://toxtown.nlm.nih.gov/chemicals-and-contaminants/sulfur-dioxide. Accessed May 24, 2020.

Indoor Air Pollution and Respiratory Health

Sarath Raju, MD, MPH*,[1], Trishul Siddharthan, MD[1], Meredith C. McCormack, MD, MHS

KEYWORDS

• Asthma • Chronic obstructive pulmonary disease • Indoor air pollution • Household air pollution • Respiratory health effects • Respiratory tract infections • Lung function • Lung development

KEY POINTS

- More than 4 million people die prematurely annually due to household air pollution.
- A large number of factors contribute to household air pollution including household characteristics (ventilation, dampness, humidity), behaviors (cooking practices and use of solid fuels), as well as allergens related to pests.
- Indoor air pollution is associated with impaired lung development, increased risk for respiratory tract infection, and increased prevalence of and morbidity attributable to asthma and chronic obstructive pulmonary disease.
- Research is ongoing into effective strategies to reduce pollutant exposure and improve lung health.

INTRODUCTION: WHY INDOOR AIR POLLUTION IS IMPORTANT

The World Health Organization (WHO) estimates that household air pollution (HAP) accounts for an estimated 4.3 million premature deaths annually and 110 million disability-adjusted life years lost.[1] This largely preventable exposure has been listed by the Comparative Risk Assessment for the 2010 Global Burden of Diseases the third leading risk factor for morbidity and mortality worldwide, representing about 4.5% of global burden of disease.[2] Even in industrialized settings, the home represents a critical source of pollutant exposure, with individuals spending approximately 90% of their time indoors, the majority of that being in the home.[3–5] Although a significant source of morbidity related to HAP is from cardiovascular disease, HAP has a wide range of respiratory sequela across the lifespan, adversely affecting lung development early in life to potentially increasing the risk of chronic obstructive pulmonary disease (COPD) in adulthood. The impact on respiratory health has been observed across a variety of settings and disease processes, in both low-middle income and high-income countries. Today, organizations including the WHO, United Nations, American Thoracic Society, and European Respiratory Society have begun to invest in developing strategies to reduce the global respiratory health effects of HAP.[6,7] This article outlines sources of indoor air pollution, the respiratory effects of indoor air pollution in low-middle income and high-income countries, as well as strategies to reduce pollutant exposure in both settings (**Fig. 1**).

INDOOR AIR POLLUTION IN LOW-MIDDLE INCOME COUNTRIES

In low-middle income countries (LMICs), nearly 3 billion people rely on biomass fuels for cooking and heating daily.[8] Biomass fuels, often referred to as solid fuels, include wood, dung, agricultural crop waste, and coal. Biomass is the main domestic energy source for ∼40% of all households and

Division of Pulmonary and Critical Care Medicine, Johns Hopkins University, Johns Hopkins School of Medicine, 1830 East Monument Street Fifth Floor, Baltimore, MD, 21287, USA
[1] These authors contributed equally to the publication.
* Corresponding author.
E-mail address: sraju3@jhmi.edu

Clin Chest Med 41 (2020) 825–843
https://doi.org/10.1016/j.ccm.2020.08.014

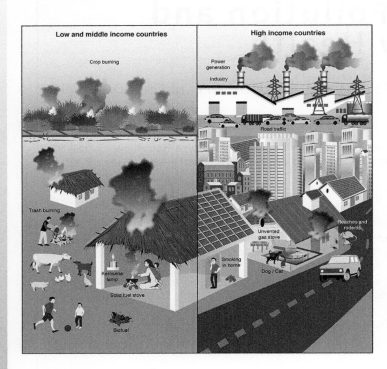

Fig. 1. Sources of indoor air pollution in low-middle income and home income countries.

~90% of rural households in LMICs. Solid fuels are often burned in inefficient and poorly vented combustion devices (ie, open fires, traditional stoves). Multiple respiratory health outcomes have been associated with HAP in LMICs, including preterm birth; low birth weight and attenuated lung function; childhood respiratory infection; as well as increased risk for development of asthma, COPD, lung cancer, and exacerbations of existing diseases.[9,10]

INDOOR AIR POLLUTION IN HIGH-INCOME COUNTRIES

Although respiratory health effects of pollution are most prominent in LMICs, significant mortality has been observed at lower pollutant concentrations typical of high-income countries, including the United States and Canada. In 2016, the WHO estimated that nearly 400,000 deaths in high-income countries were attributable to HAP, due to ongoing use of solid fuels, as well as other sources of pollution relevant to high-income countries. Currently 6.5 million people in the United States still rely on solid fuels for heating, particularly those living in rural areas. Moreover, urbanization and the expanding built environment predispose individuals in high-income settings to other pollutants indoors, including indoor particulate matter (PM), environmental tobacco smoke, gases such as nitrogen dioxide (NO_2) from cooking and heating, allergens from indoor pests, toxic cleaning chemicals, and molds related to increased indoor humidity and dampness. These important sources of indoor air pollution are outlined in the following section.

SOURCES OF INDOOR AIR POLLUTION

Indoor air includes pollutants that penetrate from the outdoors, as well as sources that are unique to the indoor environment. Thus, indoor pollution differs from outdoor pollution in source, composition, and concentration, and as a result the effects of indoor air pollution cannot be easily extrapolated from studies of outdoor air pollution.[11] The burning of solid fuels represents a significant source of household pollution across the globe, whereas numerous household activities more common in urban environments have also been associated with the generation of pollutants.[12,13] Environmental tobacco smoke (ETS) from primary and secondhand smoke remains an important source of household air pollution. In this review, we primarily discuss nontobacco sources of pollution that are often overlooked. However, initiatives to reduce smoking and environment tobacco smoke remain imperative and a continued high priority. We focus on household behaviors and practices associated with increased production of pollutants (solid fuel combustion, cooking and heating practice, cleaning, and indoor smoking) in both LMICs and high-income countries. Other sources of interest include general housing characteristics that directly influence (dampness, humidity, pests, and allergens) and modify exposures (ventilation).

Household Behaviors and Practices: Smoking, Solid Fuel Combustion, Cooking and Heating, Cleaning

Smoking

Tobacco smoke is a major source of indoor particulate matter, accounting for 50% to 90% of indoor PM concentrations in high-income countries.[14,15] Indoor tobacco smoke is a critical driver of environmental health disparities with as many as half of all children and up to 70% of African American children exposed to secondhand smoke in the United States.[16]

Solid fuel combustion

A significant body of evidence related to HAP and respiratory health has been generated from studies concerning the combustion of solid fuels, used for cooking and heating. The combustion products include gases (ie, NO_2 and carbon monoxide [CO]) and particulate matter, including particles with median diameter less than $10_{\mu m}$ (PM_{10}) and those with median diameter less than $2.5_{\mu m}$ ($PM_{2.5}$). In addition, formaldehyde, airborne endotoxins, and a number of toxic organic compounds (eg, benzene; 1,3 butadiene; benzo[a] pyrene, and other polycyclic aromatic hydrocarbons) are present in biomass smoke. Although household pollution from the burning of biomass and solid fuels has been thought to mostly affect individuals from LMICs, data from the US Census Bureau's American Community Survey has indicated that 6.5 million people in the United States live in homes heated primarily by wood or coal.[17] The burden of household pollution from solid fuels in the United States has been shown to disproportionately affect those living in poor communities, with 53% to 65% of homes that primarily heat with wood or coal also facing household $PM_{2.5}$ concentrations that exceed the WHO 24-hour particulate matter guidelines.[17–20]

Cooking and heating

Even in homes that do not use solid fuels, other common heating and cooking practices can increase household pollutant concentrations. Combustion of fuels used for cooking and heating can produce NO_2, volatile organic compounds, sulfur dioxide (SO_2), CO_2, CO, and PM. Exposure concentrations are driven by factors that include ventilation, duration of use of the cooking or heating equipment, and individual proximity to the source of pollutants. NO_2 is of particular interest for homes that use gas stoves for cooking.[13] One study indicated that each hour of gas stove or furnace use was associated with an 18 ppb increase in 24-h NO_2 concentrations.[21] NO_2 levels are even greater in poorly ventilated homes using unvented gas stoves. In addition to NO_2, other studies have demonstrated that the frequency of stove use is also associated with significant increases in household $PM_{2.5}$ concentrations.[12]

Cleaning

Cleaning represents a common household activity that can lead to the mobilization of particles and allergens. One study demonstrated indoor sweeping, which resuspends settled dust, was associated with increased household $PM_{2.5}$ and PM_{10}.[12] In addition, cleaning products and pesticides have direct toxic health effects that are discussed in more detail in the in a separate chapter of this issue.

Housing Characteristics: Ventilation, Humidity, Dampness, and Allergens from Pests

Ventilation

One global factor that impacts household pollution concentrations is ventilation, as diminished indoor-outdoor air exchange rates can result in the accumulation of indoor pollutants. As insulation has improved, household air exchange rates have diminished.[22] The relationship between sources of pollution, air exchange rates, and health outcomes is an important consideration in understanding the respiratory health effects of indoor air pollution. In LMICs, poor ventilation, particularly around biomass stoves, results in increased levels of indoor air pollution.[23,24] Ventilation in LMIC settings, primarily in tropical and subtropical regions of the world, often includes direct openings to the outdoors, and is typically greater compared with high-income areas.[25] Households that use enclosed metal heating or cooking stoves with chimneys have significantly lower indoor pollutant concentrations than those that use open fires.[26,27] A number of studies have additionally demonstrated associations between ventilation and respiratory outcomes. Qian and colleagues[24] demonstrated higher household ventilation was associated with lower reporting of persistent cough, phlegm, bronchitis, and wheeze among school children in 4 Chinese cities. Household ventilation, as well as more efficient ventilated stoves has been outlined by the WHO as an important health intervention in LMICs.

Humidity and dampness

Humidity and dampness are also important factors that influence indoor air quality. A number of daily activities including showering, cooking, and humidifier use, can affect indoor moisture and humidity. Many homes additionally experience leaks and some degree of water damage over their lifetime. Molds, bacteria, insects, and mites thrive in humid and damp environments.[28] These pathogens in particular have been linked to a number of respiratory disorders including asthma, chronic rhino sinusitis, and hypersensitivity pneumonitis, along with increased respiratory symptoms (cough, wheeze, and exacerbations of underlying respiratory disease).[29]

Allergens from household pests

Exposure to household allergens from animals and pests represent significant but modifiable contributors to respiratory disease, particularly asthma and allergic rhinitis. In urban environments allergens from house dust mites, cockroaches, and mouse infestations are important to consider. House dust mites represent a significant source of allergens, with 13 different species found in household dust.[4] Allergens arise from mite bodies and feces. Dust mites are most commonly found on furniture, carpet, and bedding. House dust mite growth further increases in high humidity and temperature environments.[30] Similar to dust mites, allergens from cockroaches are increased in high temperature environments.[4] Mouse allergen can be found in small particle sizes between 0.5 and 10 μm and can remain airborne once resuspended from settled dust.[31] Mouse allergen has been detected in high concentration in settled dust from homes of children with asthma living in urban areas, as well as in air samples, where as many as a quarter of children had airborne mouse concentrations similar to those in mouse facilities.[32] Pest allergen, including cockroach and mouse represent important drivers of childhood asthma in urban environments.[33,34] Other sources to consider, not included in this review, include allergens from pets and domestic animals that can also contribute to morbidity.

Other important housing factors to consider include residential crowding, along with proximity to roadways and high traffic corridors, which can lead to increases in indoor PM and NO_2 due to penetration from the outdoor environment.

CONSEQUENCE OF INDOOR AIR POLLUTION

The respiratory consequences of HAP are wide ranging, affecting lung development in childhood, incidence of lower respiratory tract infection, and both disease development and morbidity for COPD and asthma. The known impacts of HAP are described for each of these processes in both LMICs and high-income countries.

Mechanisms

There have been a number of mechanisms proposed by which indoor air pollution results in pulmonary disease and alters host immune responses, leading to chronic respiratory conditions. Exposure to HAP results in proinflammatory states with associated increases in neutrophilic inflammation, proteolytic activity of matrix metalloproteinases, oxidative stress and apoptosis[35–37] (**Box 1**). Loss of lung function from prolonged exposure to air pollution has been proposed as a leading cause of COPD globally.[38] In addition, recurrent respiratory infections have been associated with increased levels of HAP, likely due to underlying immune dysregulation. HAP has been demonstrated to impair macrophage phagocytosis and surface adherence, reduce bacterial and mucociliary clearance, and disrupt the alveolar-capillary barrier in the lungs.[39–41] A number of effects also relate to alterations in the airway microbiome as well as immune dysregulation and host response to commensals.[6] In particular, *Streptococcus pneumoniae* carriage, the most common cause of bacterial pneumonia, is thought to be increased in individuals with high HAP exposure. One study demonstrated that PM exposure from wood smoke decreased macrophage phagocytosis of *S pneumoniae* and increased the duration and density of pneumococcal carriage.[42] In addition, immune responses to respiratory viruses may be impaired, with prior literature

Box 1
Mechanism by which household pollution can impact respiratory health

- Neutrophilic inflammation
- Reduced bacterial clearance and alterations in microbiome
- Increased matrix metalloproteinase activity and gene expression
- Greater oxidative stress
- Increased apoptosis
- Pulmonary surfactant deactivation
- Reduced mucociliary clearance
- Epigenetic changes: DNA damage and methylation
- Disruption of lung endothelial cell barrier

demonstrating that increased PM_{10} exposure can blunt alveolar macrophage responses to respiratory syncytial virus.[43] As a result, recent literature has focused on the impacts of HAP on both viral and bacterial acute lower respiratory tract infection (ALRI). Air pollution additionally may result in genetic and epigenetic changes that alter inflammatory and oxidative stress responses even after the exposure is removed.[44]

Lung Development in Children

Lung development begins in utero and by the fourth week of development nascent bronchi form. By gestation, only a small fraction of primary alveoli has developed, a process, which increases linearly up to the age of 18, with 85% to 90% of alveoli formed within the first 6 months of life. Fetal and adolescent lung development is a critical period, which predicts future lung function. Low lung function in infancy and childhood is associated with respiratory health sequela including, wheeze, airway hyperreactivity, asthma, and COPD in adulthood.[45,46] Although a comprehensive review of secondhand smoke (SHS) exposure is beyond the scope of this article, there is a large body of evidence concerning SHS as a contributor to indoor air pollution and lung development. SHS has been identified as a risk factor for low lung function in several studies.[47,48] A study of 2500 children followed over 6 decades demonstrated that parental smoking during childhood is a determinant of low lung function trajectories, low lung function in adulthood and eventual development of COPD[47,49]

Studies related to ambient air pollution have demonstrated associations between prenatal exposures, lower lung function at birth and the likelihood of respiratory disease in adolescence and adulthood. However, few studies related to in utero exposures have evaluated HAP or assessed personal exposure monitoring.[50,51] In an LMIC setting, Lee and colleagues[52] examined the association between maternal carbon monoxide exposure (CO) from cookstove sources (traditional 3 stone fires with wood as the dominant fuel) and infant lung function at 30 days, and found a dose response relationship between elevated maternal CO exposure and reduced peak tidal expiratory flow to expiratory time and higher minute ventilation. Furthermore, the authors found this increase in minute ventilation was associated with increased risk for physician-assessed pneumonia and severe pneumonia in the first year of life.[52] Further works needs to be done to confirm the contribution of early exposure to household pollutants, outside of secondhand smoke, to early lung development.

Respiratory Tract Infections

A number of studies have demonstrated a strong association between HAP and the risk of childhood ALRI globally. It has been hypothesized that the contribution of HAP to lung development, along with the development of COPD and chronic bronchitis, is related to repeated infections over time.

Low-middle income countries

In LMIC settings, HAP results in an estimated half a million deaths among children younger than 5 annually, specifically from pneumonia. Dherani and colleagues[53] demonstrated exposure to HAP from solid fuel use during childhood increased the risk of ALRIs by 78% (pooled odds ratio [OR] 1.78; 95% confidence interval [CI] 1.45–2.18) in a meta-analysis of 24 studies. As a result of the high prevalence and associated mortality, pediatric pneumonia has been a primary clinical outcome for interventions aiming to mitigate pollution exposure with mixed results (see Cookstove Interventions). While a number of studies have examined the association between HAP and pediatric pneumonia, the relationship with ALRI in adults is less clear. A recent systematic review limited to adults found mixed results, though some evidence of an increased risk of adult ALRI from exposure to HAP.[54]

High-income countries

Within high-income countries more research exists on the association between outdoor pollution and health care encounters for ALRI among children and infants. A study by Horne and colleagues[55] explored the relationship between rises in outdoor air pollution in Utah between 1999 and 2016 and odds of health care utilization related to lower respiratory tract infections. The study demonstrated that a 10 $\mu g/m^3$ increase in ambient $PM_{2.5}$ was associated with increased health care utilization for ALRIs (OR 1.15; 95% CI 1.12–1.19). Most individuals included in this study were again young children (0–2 years), though effects were still observed to the age of 18. These results have been replicated in other areas of the United States, including among adults in New York State, where increases in outdoor $PM_{2.5}$ were associated with higher rates of influenza and culture-negative pneumonia.[56] In contrast to the literature on ambient pollution, studies surrounding the association between household pollution and ALRI in high-income countries are much less robust, limited primarily to survey data with inconsistent findings.[54] The association between HAP and ALRI in high-income countries still requires further investigation.

Asthma

Prior meta-analyses conducted across continents have demonstrated that early secondhand smoke exposure is associated with the childhood asthma development and subsequent increased risk for adult asthma.[57] As a result, many have hypothesized that particulate from other sources of HAP and airway irritants may lead to asthma development and increased morbidity for children living with asthma.

Low-middle income countries

Studies in LMICs to date have been inconsistent regarding HAP from solid fuel smoke and asthma among children and adults. Po and colleagues[58,59] did not find a statistically significant association (children: OR 0.50, 95% CI 0.12–1.98; adults: OR 1.34, 95% CI 0.93–1.93) among 25 studies. Chronic exposure to HAP is associated with increased levels of airway hyperresponsivness.[60] In addition, HAP exposure can result in airway remodeling and inflammation with similar patterns of small airway disease seen in asthma. HAP from biomass contains known endotoxins and organic compounds, which increase the risk for asthma.[61] Air pollution from solid fuel combustion and existing allergens can become amalgamated resulting in increased serum immunoglobulin (Ig)E, eosinophils and neutrophils.[62] Nonetheless, the lack of consistent findings related to the association between HAP and asthma in LMICs require additional investigation.

High-income settings

Within high-income countries, studies of solid fuels and asthma development are limited to rural settings, where heating with wood and coal is relatively more common. One survey of adults in Southeastern Kentucky, conducted as part of the Burden of Lung Disease (BOLD) study, described an association between cooking with wood or coal and pediatric asthma (OR 2.3; 95% CI 1.1–5.0). The study demonstrated no effect of heating with solid fuels on asthma development (OR 0.8; 95% CI 0.4–1.8).[63] Research from Noonan and Ward[64] investigated the association between woodstove use for heating and asthma symptoms among children in Libby, Montana, where woodstoves were the primary source of home heating in 33% of households. Their findings suggested that woodstove use was associated with greater odds of wheezing (OR 1.74; 95% CI 0.55–5.56) although findings were not statistically significant.[64]

There is more consistent evidence to suggest household pollution may increase respiratory morbidity among children with asthma in both urban and rural environments. Among populations with asthma, elevated levels of $PM_{2.5}$ and PM_{10} are associated with higher rates of asthma attacks, medication use, and emergency department visits.[18,65,66] One study of household pollution in an urban inner-city environment, where the use of solid fuels is less common, demonstrated that increases in indoor $PM_{2.5}$ were associated with greater asthma morbidity for children with both atopic and nonatopic forms of asthma.[67] In this study of 133 children ages 2 to 6, with repeated measured of household pollutants ($PM_{2.5}$, PM_{coarse}), higher PM_{coarse} and $PM_{2.5}$ concentrations were associated with greater risk for wheezing, rescue inhaler use, and nocturnal symptoms.[66]

In addition to PM, higher levels of elevated household NO_2 may lead to greater asthma morbidity. Higher NO_2 exposure has been tied to lower peak flow measurements in a nationwide analysis of urban asthmatic children in the National Cooperative Inner-City Asthma Study (NCICAS).[68] A longitudinal study of asthmatic children in Baltimore demonstrated that each 20-ppb increase in NO_2 exposure over a 72-hour period was associated with an increase in the number of days with limited speech (incidence rate ratio [IRR] 1.15; 95% CI 1.05–1.25), cough (IRR 1.10; 95% CI 1.02–1.18), and nocturnal symptoms (IRR 1.09; 95% CI 1.02–1.16), after adjustment for potential confounders.[13] Paulin and colleagues[21] demonstrated that daily changes in household NO_2 exposure were associated with gas stove/oven use and led to worsened asthma symptoms and nighttime inhaler use among children with asthma. Studies of school classrooms have also demonstrated that indoor NO_2 is associated with increased airflow obstruction among children with asthma.[69]

There are still certain populations that are known to be more susceptible to the health effects of household pollution. Being overweight or obese may be risk factors that increases susceptibility to indoor $PM_{2.5}$ and NO_2 among children with asthma.[70] Studies have indicated that being overweight has been associated with a oxidative stress and inflammation, which may affect the ability to defend against oxidative and proinflammatory exposures, such as that from particulate and gaseous pollutants.[71,72] To investigate the hypothesis that obesity increases susceptibility to air pollution health effects, Lu and colleagues[70] examined the effects of household $PM_{2.5}$ and NO_2 exposure. They observed that compared with normal-weight children with asthma, overweight children experienced greater symptoms (cough, wheeze, and chest tightness) and rescue medication use, when faced with similar increases in household $PM_{2.5}$ and NO_2. Wu and colleagues[73] similarly observed that overweight and obesity increased susceptibility to household secondhand smoke exposure among children with asthma. These findings suggest that diet and weight loss, in addition to pollution reduction, may be important targets in efforts to reduce the respiratory health effects of indoor air pollution among children with asthma. Investigations of differential responses to air pollution by weight may provide insights as to pathways by which air pollutants elicit respiratory health effects. Most of the studies of household pollution and asthma morbidity are conducted among children, and further research is needed to demonstrate whether these results can be extrapolated to adults.

Multiple studies have proposed a synergistic relationship between allergen and pollutant exposure but have focused on outdoor air pollution exposures. A prospective cohort study of children followed from infancy to 4 years demonstrated that exposure to traffic-related diesel exhaust was associated with increased risk of aeroallergen sensitization.[74] Controlled exposure studies in atopic volunteers have demonstrated that diesel exhaust increases markers of allergic and non-allergic inflammation and that allergen and diesel exhaust have exposure specific responses.[75,76] Previous studies have demonstrated that increased ambient $PM_{2.5}$, NO_2, and ozone exposure are associated with a significant increases in risk for asthma and allergic rhinitis among children with allergic sensitization.[77,78] Several studies of children living in urban settings have demonstrated that pest allergen, including mouse and cockroach, are associated with increased asthma morbidity.[34,79,80] Children are often coexposed to high levels of indoor $PM_{2.5}$, NO_2, and dust allergens.[81] The combined effects of indoor air pollution and allergen exposure are not well understood and can provide insight as to priority targets for multi-faceted intervention studies.

Chronic Obstructive Pulmonary Disease

Low-middle income countries

There have been a number of studies that have examined the association between biomass and COPD in LMICs, with heterogeneity in exposure history and outcomes.[60,82] A meta-analysis of 23 papers by Kurmi and colleagues[38] found an increased odds of COPD (OR 2.80; 95% CI 1.85–4.0) and chronic bronchitis (OR 2.32; 95% CI 1.92–2.80). Similarly, Hu and colleagues[83] demonstrated a similar association (OR 2.44; 95% CI 1.9–3.33) between HAP and COPD, relative to those not exposed to biomass smoke. While the vast majority of studies related to COPD pertain to tobacco exposure in high-income settings, less is known about how HAP can lead to COPD development in LMICs. Although evidence of direct causal relationship between HAP and COPD is not definitive, it is likely that HAP exposure over the course of the lifespan has direct and indirect effects (recurrent ALRI, low socioeconomic status) on lung function that predispose to COPD.[84]

Individuals with biomass-related COPD demonstrate a distinct pattern of lung injury with increased anthracosis, small airway thickening and peripheral fibrosis on lung biopsy compared with individuals with tobacco smoke–mediated COPD.[6] Women with biomass-related COPD have lower rates of emphysema and higher rates of air trapping and bronchiectasis compared with those with tobacco-related disease.[85] In addition, individuals with biomass-related COPD have distinct patterns of airway disease, which may be related to the size of particles deposited in the airways during biomass exposure.[86] This phenotype is marked by increased cough, phlegm on respiratory symptom questionnaire, as well as higher rates of bronchodilator reversibility and hyperresponsiveness, signifying an elevated degree of airway inflammation.[60] Biomass-related COPD results in a different inflammatory profile, with higher circulating levels of CD4 inflammatory mediators (TH2, interleukin [IL]-4, and IL-10) than tobacco-related disease.[87] Furthermore, those with biomass-related COPD have higher levels of malonylaldehyde and superoxide dismutase, measures of oxidative stress that correlate inversely to FEV_1.[88]

High-income countries

Given lower utilization of solid fuels in high-income countries the relationship between household use of solid fuels and COPD development in high-income studies has not been as intensively investigated. However, a few studies have demonstrated a potential link between the utilization of solid fuels for heating and COPD development in the United States. A 2010 study by Sood and colleagues[89] demonstrated that self-reported wood smoke exposure was associated with greater odds of airflow obstruction and chronic bronchitis (OR 1.96; 95% CI 1.52–2.54) and 1.64 (95% 1.36–2.06), respectively. This study was limited to a cohort of primarily smokers in New Mexico. A subsequent, nationally representative study, which used the National Health Interview Survey for data on COPD prevalence and the US Census for information on community use of solid fuels (coal and wood) for heating, demonstrated that higher use of coal for heating, at the community level, was associated with greater odds of self-reported COPD (OR 1.09; $P<.001$), among never-smokers.[90] A similar study that used data from the National Health and Nutrition Examination Survey demonstrated that increased use of wood for heating, at the community level, was associated with greater odd of COPD, defined by spirometry (OR 1.12; $P<.001$), among never-smokers. Both of these studies demonstrated that living in a rural region of the United States was associated with greater odds of COPD, even after taking account traditional risk factors such as smoking, community-level poverty and individual socioeconomic status. Rural regions notably reported a higher percentage of homes using solid fuels (wood and coal) for heating, which may be an explanation for this disparity. All 3 of these studies were limited by a lack of information on individual level exposures, as they relied on the census level data, and did not contain direct measurement of pollutants. As a result, there remains a significant gap in our knowledge of the contribution of these household pollutants to COPD development in high-income settings.

Among individuals living with COPD indoor air pollution has been associated with increased respiratory morbidity, even in communities that do not use solid fuels for heating or cooking. Hansel and colleagues[91] demonstrated in an urban cohort of 84 former smokers with COPD that increases in $PM_{2.5}$ and NO_2 are associated with worsened COPD morbidity. An increase of 10 $\mu g/m^3$ $PM_{2.5}$ in the main living area was independently associated with increases in nocturnal symptoms, wheeze, worse respiratory status based on St. George Respiratory Questionnaire scores, and greater odds of severe exacerbation (OR 1.50; 95% CI 1.04–2.18). A 20 ppb increase in NO_2 in the main living area was associated with increased modified medical research council (mMRC) dyspnea scores while a similar increase in bedroom NO_2 was associated with increased odds of severe exacerbations (OR 2.71; 95% CI 1.05–6.93). One notable thing about this study is that these effects were seen despite relatively low household pollutant concentrations (median [interquartile range] $PM_{2.5}$ 8.3 [4.9–14.4] $\mu g/m^3$ and NO_2 6.8 [4.2–14.5] ppb), which are typical of high-income countries. These studies did not show an effect of $PM_{2.5}$ or NO_2 on FEV_1, though the follow-up period was limited to 6 months. In addition to $PM_{2.5}$ and NO_2, studies have highlighted the impact of household allergen sensitization on COPD morbidity. Data from an urban COPD cohort demonstrated that sensitization to allergens from mouse, cockroach, cat, dog, and dust mites increased respiratory morbidity.[92] In this study, the authors measured detectable IgE levels for the aforementioned allergens, as well as markers of allergen exposure and sensitization, among 77 participants with COPD. After adjusting for confounders, an increasing number of sensitizations was associated higher risk for cough, wheeze, and nocturnal dyspnea, though the effects were primarily observed among those with 3 or more sensitizations. Those with only 1 to 2 sensitization still had greater odds of reporting an ED visit (OR 10.0; 95% CI 1.6–60.7). This study was limited by a small sample size, with broad effect estimates, but still provides evidence to suggest that household allergen exposure and sensitization can lead to increased morbidity for those with COPD.

Certain factors can also increase susceptibility to the impact of household pollutants for those living with COPD. Similar to what has been observed among children with asthma, obesity may increase susceptibility to the effects of HAP among adults with COPD. One study of 84 participants with moderate to severe COPD demonstrated that obese individuals had exaggerated increases in nocturnal symptoms, dyspnea and rescue medication use compared with nonobese in response to $PM_{2.5}$ and PM_{coarse}.[93] Other studies have demonstrated that extremes of temperature, both hot and cold, may also influence the effects of indoor pollution on COPD morbidity.[94,95] One study in particular demonstrated that high heat increased the effect of $PM_{2.5}$ and NO_2 exposures on rescue inhaler use, cough, and sputum production.[96] We do note that most of the data presented here regarding the effects of household pollution on COPD morbidity in high-income countries are from urban environments. To date there are few studies, with direct measurements of household pollutants, in rural regions of the United States that have studied the effects of household pollution on COPD morbidity. Although the literature is suggestive of this, we do not know if there is a difference in the impact of HAP between urban and rural environments in the United States remains an important area for future study. The present studies have also not shown that increases in household $PM_{2.5}$ or NO_2 exposure are associated with more accelerated lung function decline for those with COPD. This may ultimately be related to relatively short-term follow-up (<1-year follow-up) in the studies performed to date.

STRATEGIES FOR REDUCING HOUSEHOLD AIR POLLUTION

A number of strategies have been attempted to reduce pollutant exposure in diverse settings. Interventions have been attempted to reduce a wide range of indoor pollutants including, PM, gases, allergens, and mold (**Table 1**). Certain strategies outlined focus on source reduction (ie, liquified petroleum gas [LPG] stove interventions and smoking bans) whereas others focus on secondary reduction (air cleaner interventions).

Cookstove Interventions

Over the past decade, a number of studies have attempted to lower the levels of HAP through cleaner-burning biomass stoves. RESPIRE was one of the first randomized controlled trials to demonstrate a reduction in deleterious health outcomes, in their case severe pediatric pneumonia.[97] Romieu and colleagues[98] demonstrated reduced respiratory symptoms (OR 0.29; 95% CI 0.11–0.77; for wheeze) and declines in lung function (31 mL vs. 62 mL over 1 year, $P = .01$) over a 12-month period among those randomized to cook stove intervention, though few other studies have replicated these results despite evidence of increased cookstove uptake (**Table 2**).

Design of stove interventions to reduce the burden of disease has additionally been challenged by a limited understanding of exposure-response relationships.[102] Many studies were limited by small samples size, limited length of follow-up, variability in intervention and level of adoption, as well as protocol deviations.[103] Importantly, most studies have failed to capture meaningful exposure reduction to gain a complete understanding of exposure-response across a range of relevant and targeted exposures. Few HAP studies have included low exposure groups (ie, clean fuel users) to demonstrate the maximum benefit that can be expected. Because of financial and technical constraints associated with performing large-scale HAP measurements in LMIC settings, many studies have relied on imprecise, proxy exposure measures. Measurement of fine particulate matter ($PM_{2.5}$), the best exposure indicator of health risk, has been particularly challenging due to the limitations of affordable, feasible, and reliable instrumentation.[104,105]

The evidence from clinical trials to date do not support the efficacy of cleaner-burning cook stoves to improve pulmonary health or reduce mortality in LMICs.[103] LPG stoves may sufficiently reduce HAP levels to deliver meaningful health gains. Ongoing trials using LPG stoves with inclusion of participants across the lifespan (fetal, childhood, and elderly participants), sufficient follow-up and exposure monitoring may add additional value in understanding the pulmonary benefits of reduction in HAP. A multicenter randomized controlled trial, funded by the National Institutes of Health, with sites in Rwanda, Peru, Guatemala, and India, aims to address additional gaps in evidence.[106]

Air Cleaner Interventions

Portable air cleaner devices may be effective for reducing HAP in high-income countries. Air cleaner interventions have been studied in both urban and rural regions of the United States including both high-efficiency particle air (HEPA) cleaners and HEPA and activated carbon filters to address household gases (ie, NO_2) (**Table 3**).

Although air purifiers have been shown to improve indoor air quality and reduce household $PM_{2.5}$ concentrations, the long-term health benefits of these devices are still being uncovered. A study of healthy adults in woodsmoke-impacted community, demonstrated improved endothelial function (based on the reactive hyperemia index) and decreased concentrations of inflammatory biomarkers (serum C-reactive protein) after a weeklong HEPA filter intervention.[107] As noted previously, studies of air purifier interventions have shown promise for improving childhood asthma outcomes. Two trials in urban settings have shown improvements in symptom-free days and health care utilization with air cleaner interventions.[108,109] In contrast, for adults with COPD, the effects of an air cleaner intervention remain unknown, given a lack of high-quality intervention trials. The effects of an area cleaner intervention for adults with COPD remains an area in need of ongoing research and studies are under way.[110]

Integrated Approaches for Pollutant and Allergen Reduction

Integrated approaches have additionally been attempted that combine education on allergen reduction and remediation, pest management, and air cleaners to reduce household particulates. These studies have primarily focused on children with asthma, and their effects on other populations are not yet known. One multicenter randomized trial of 937 inner-city children with asthma demonstrated improvements with a 12-month environment intervention centered around the bedroom that included HEPA air cleaners, allergen remediation, and allergen prevention education for caretakers.[111] Children who underwent this intervention saw an improvement in the symptom-free days during the intervention year

Table 1
Common strategies for reducing household pollutants

Pollutant	Interventions
Particulate matter ($PM_{2.5}$, PM_{10})	Cookstove exchanges (in homes burning biomass fuels), air cleaner interventions, woodstove replacement
Gases (NO_2)	Air cleaners (HEPA with carbon filter), gas stove replacement, vented hoods for stoves
Allergens	Air cleaners, integrated pest management, pest education
Molds	Remediation of household dampness and humidity
Environmental tobacco smoke	Smoking cessation, indoor smoking bans

(3.39 vs 4.20 days, $P<.001$) and the year after (2.62 vs 3.21 days, $P<.001$). This was accompanied by a significant reduction in dust mite and cockroach allergens. A smaller study that used air cleaners and cockroach extermination among 100 asthmatic children, demonstrated a 51% reduction in cockroach allergen along with a 36% reduction in $PM_{2.5}$ at 1-year follow-up.[112] In this study, participants who received the intervention reported fewer daytime symptoms (OR 0.55; 95% CI 0.31–0.97). Studies that have focused solely on pest allergen reduction have had mixed results.[29,79,113,114] A more recent randomized trial did not demonstrate a benefit of an integrated pest management intervention over providing pest management education alone to families of children with asthma.[29] However, a post hoc analysis demonstrated that mouse allergen reduction was associated with greater increases in lung function over a year, suggesting that allergen exposure reduction may improve lung growth.[115] In this study, pest management education alone (providing written material and demonstration about and pest management and housekeeping practices) resulted in a 65% reduction in household mouse antigen, suggesting that detailed education may provide benefit in reducing environmental exposures.

Community-Level Interventions

Community-level strategies, bolstered by policy, have been used to reduce sources of pollution in high-income countries. Successful campaigns have been implemented to reduce pollution from solid fuels and address the use of wood stoves, in rural communities. One community-wide wood stove exchange program in Libby, Montana, led to a 27.6% (95% CI 3.0%–44.5%) decrease in ambient $PM_{2.5}$ levels, with an associated decrease in odds of both wheeze and respiratory infections among school children in this community.[116] A similar study in Tasmania, Australia, observed a significant reduction in outdoor PM_{10} (from 43.6 $\mu g/m^3$ to 27.0 $\mu g/m^3$), after community-wide efforts to replace wood-burning stoves with cleaner electric appliances. Community-level woodstove exchange programs have also been effective in reducing ambient concentration of phenolics and PAHs.[117] Despite observed improvements in ambient pollutant levels and potential health benefits, there has not been a consistent long-term decrease in household $PM_{2.5}$ from these efforts alone.[118] Given that significant legislative and regulatory action is often required to implement similar community-level interventions, further research is needed to confirm their long-term benefits.

Smoke-free legislation provides examples of successful interventions with the potential to impact health at a population level. For example, meta-analyses of studies investigating the effect of smoke-free legislation in North America and Europe have demonstrated reductions in emergency department visits for asthma and hospitalizations for asthma and respiratory tract infections.[119,120] Recent legislation on smoking bans in public housing more specifically addresses residential smoke exposure. Effective February 2017, the US Department of Housing and Urban Development published a rule requiring each public housing agency to implement a smoke-free policy within 18 months.[121] Implementation of this rule poses challenges and studies investigating health effects are not yet available.

Schools represent another venue for community-level interventions. Despite the strong evidence base for health effects of air pollution, including indoor air pollution, on children's respiratory health, there has been relatively little investigation of interventions in schools. Children spend a substantial proportion of their time in schools and, thus, school environments represent an opportunity to improve

Table 2
Cookstove interventions to improve respiratory health

Author, Year	Intervention	Location/Participants	Findings
Romieu et al,[98] 2009	RCT of chimney stove vs traditional open fire *Primary Outcomes:* Respiratory symptoms and lung function	Rural Mexico, n = 552 women	No statistically significant effect seen in intention-to-treat (ITT) analyses, although a significant effect on both cough and annual rate of decline in forced expiratory volume in 1 s (FEV_1; 31 vs 62 mL) was observed for women who reported using the chimney stove.
Smith et al,[97] 2011	RCT of chimney stove vs traditional open fire *Primary Outcomes:* Physician-diagnosed pneumonia	Rural Guatemala, n = 518 children younger than 19 mo	No statistically significant effect on physician-diagnosed pneumonia was found, although physician-diagnosed severe pneumonia (defined by the presence of hypoxemia) was significantly reduced among children in the intervention group. The chimney stove intervention was reported to improve respiratory symptoms in the mothers of the study children, but not rate of decline in lung function in ITT analyses. A subsequent analysis demonstrated reduced carbon monoxide exposure was associated with a lower rate of decline in FEV_1
Tielsch et al,[99] 2016	Cluster-randomized, step-wedge, community-based trial of a cleaner-burning biomass stove vs traditional open stove *Primary outcome:* Acute lower respiratory tract infection	Rural Nepal, n = 5254 children younger than 3 y	No statistically significant effect on the incidence of acute lower respiratory tract infection in the intervention compared with the control group (relative risk = 0.87 [95% confidence interval = 0.67–1.13]). Potentially beneficial effects were seen in selected secondary analyses on cough, wheeze, and burn injury.

(*continued on next page*)

Table 2
(continued)

Author, Year	Intervention	Location/Participants	Findings
Asante et al,[100] 2019	Three-arm household-level RCT of liquefied petroleum gas vs a cleaner-burning biomass-fueled cookstove *Primary Outcome:* Birthweight and physician-diagnosed severe pneumonia in the first year of life	Rural Ghana, n = 1415 pregnant women	Although children born to mothers with higher HAP CO exposures during pregnancy were at increased risk for impaired lung function measured 1 mo after birth, no significant difference in birth weight or physician-assessed IMCI pneumonia in either of the intervention arms in ITT analysis
Mortimer et al,[101] 2017	Community-level C-RCT of 2 cleaner-burning, biomass-fueled cookstoves with a solar charger vs traditional open fire *Primary Outcome*: Pneumonia	Rural Malawi, n = 10,750 children younger than 5 y	No effect of the intervention on the primary outcome of WHO Integrated Management of Childhood Illness–defined pneumonia in an ITT analysis.

Abbreviations: HAP, household air pollution; IMCI, integrated management of childhood illness; RCT, randomized controlled trial; WHO, World Health Organization.
Data from Refs.[97–101]

Table 3
Air cleaner interventions to improve respiratory health

Author, Year	Intervention	Location/Participants	Findings
Ward et al,[125] 2017	Randomized placebo-controlled trial of woodstove change out and air filtration *Primary Outcomes:* PM2.5 and CO concentration	Missoula, Montana, n = 98 households	Homes randomized to the air purifier intervention had a 63% (95% CI 47%–75%) reduction in household $PM_{2.5}$. The air purifier intervention arm was more efficacious and less expensive than a using a woodstove changeout, which resulted in no significant change in household $PM_{2.5}$.
Butz et al,[108] 2011	RCT of health coaching and high-efficiency particle air (HEPA) filter vs HEPA filter vs control *Primary Outcomes:* Change in PM, air nicotine, urine cotinine concentration and symptom-free days	Baltimore, MD, n = 125 children with asthma who resided with smokers	Homes randomized to receive an air cleaner observed a 50% reduction in $PM_{2.5}$, representing a change of ~$20_{ug/m^3}$ for children living in smoking homes. These improvements were observed with only modest adherence (59%) to the intervention itself. No reduction was observed in markers of tobacco exposure; air nicotine levels or cotinine measurements. The intervention still led to an improvement in symptom-free days (1.36; $P = .03$), though did not result in a significant improvement in nocturnal symptoms or a reduction in acute asthma events
Paulin et al,[126] 2014	RCT of gas stove replacement with electric stoves vs instillation of hood over existing stoves vs placement of HEPA and carbon purifiers in the house *Primary Outcomes:* Indoor NO_2 concentrations	Baltimore, MD, n = 100 households	Homes where the air cleaners were placed in the kitchen and bedroom of homes using gas stoves had an immediate decrease in median NO_2 concentrations in both the kitchen (27%; $P<.01$) and bedroom (22%, $P = .02$). However, at 3-mo follow-up improvements were only observed in the kitchen (20%; $P = .05$). Notably in this study, adherence data were missing from the bedroom air purifier, which potentially could account for the lack of long-term benefit

Abbreviations: CI, confidence interval; PM, particulate matter; RCT, randomized controlled trial.

health at a population level by reducing harmful exposures. The School Inner-City Asthma Study demonstrated that mouse allergen exposure in schools was associated with increased asthma symptoms and decreased lung function.[80] Studies of school-based environmental interventions are logistically challenging but studies, some of which are currently under way, are needed in order to provide evidence of the magnitude of potential health benefits for children.[122,123]

FUTURE AREAS FOR STUDY

Today there are robust data to suggest that indoor air pollution is associated with a multitude of respiratory effects across the lifespan, including impaired lung development in childhood, greater risk for acute lower respiratory tract infections, risk for developing chronic lung disease and increased morbidity related to asthma and COPD. Although longitudinal cohort studies of participants followed for decades has informed our understanding of the effects of outdoor air pollution and the benefits of pollution reduction, analogous studies of the long-term health effects of indoor air pollution are lacking.[124] Although there are a relatively limited number of studies investigating interventions to reduce household pollutants, existing evidence has been inconsistent in demonstrating benefit. Challenges of studying the health effects of indoor air pollution include the need for individual exposure assessment, and interventions that require long-term implementation at the household level. Opportunities to longitudinally study the health effects of legislation aimed at improving indoor air quality and interventions at community levels with the potential to improve health of local populations provide a means of efficiently understanding the health benefits of improved indoor air quality. As individuals spend most of their time indoors and most of their time in the home environment, this continues to be an important target for improving respiratory health. Ongoing investigations are needed to more clearly identify targetable mechanisms by which indoor pollutants may influence respiratory morbidity, interventions with long-term benefit, and susceptible populations who are most likely to benefit from these interventions.

SUMMARY

Indoor air pollution, from sources that include indoor tobacco smoke, the burning of solid fuels, and noxious gases from cooking and heating, is associated with greater risk for chronic lung disease development and respiratory morbidity worldwide. Although the impact is most pronounced in LMICs, significant health effects are still observed at lower pollutant concentrations typical of high-income settings. It is important to raise awareness of common sources of pollution among clinicians, policy makers, and patients with chronic respiratory disease alike, to improve health education and promote efforts that can reduce pollutant exposure across households and address environmental health disparities. Although the long-term benefits of efforts to reduce indoor air pollution are yet to be defined, multiple intervention strategies at the household and community levels (including indoor smoking bans and air cleaner interventions) have been effective in reducing pollutant exposure. Future research may help to define optimal strategies for reducing indoor air pollution at the individual, household, community, and population levels to improve long-term lung health and reduce health disparities.

CLINICS CARE POINTS

- Indoor air pollution can contribute to increases in respiratory symptoms for patients in both low-middle and high-income countries.
- Evaluation of household pollutants should be considered in the care of patients with chronic respiratory disease.
- Potential strategies to reduce household pollutants include indoor smoking bans and air cleaner interventions, with research ongoing to determine the most effective interventions.

DISCLOSURE

T. Siddharthan is supported through the NHLBI (1K23HL146946). M.C. McCormack is supported by NIMHD P50MD010431/EPA 83615001, NIEHS P50ES018176/EPA 83615201, and EPA 83563901. S. Raju is supported by NHLBI K12HL143957 and NIAID P30AI094189.

REFERENCES

1. World Health Organization. World Health Organization: air pollution. Available at: https://www.who.int/health-topics/air-pollution#tab=tab_1. Accessed December 15, 2019.
2. Lim SS, Vos T, Flaxman AD, et al. A comparative risk assessment of burden of disease and injury attributable to 67 risk factors and risk factor clusters in 21 regions, 1990-2010: a systematic analysis for the Global Burden of Disease Study 2010. Lancet 2012;380(9859):2224–60.

3. Richardson G, Eick S, Jones R. How is the indoor environment related to asthma? Literature review. J Adv Nurs 2005;52(3):328–39.
4. Ho LA, Kuschner WG. Respiratory health in home and leisure pursuits. Clin Chest Med 2012;33(4): 715–29.
5. Smith KR, Peel JL. Mind the gap. Environ Health Perspect 2010;118(12):1643–5.
6. Sood A, Assad NA, Barnes PJ, et al. ERS/ATS workshop report on respiratory health effects of household air pollution. Eur Respir J 2018;51(1): 1700698.
7. Balmes JR. Household air pollution from domestic combustion of solid fuels and health. J Allergy Clin Immunol 2019;143(6):1979–87.
8. Bonjour S, Adair-Rohani H, Wolf J, et al. Solid fuel use for household cooking: country and regional estimates for 1980-2010. Environ Health Perspect 2013;121(7):784–90.
9. Smith KR, Bruce N, Balakrishnan K, et al. Millions dead: how do we know and what does it mean? Methods used in the comparative risk assessment of household air pollution. Annu Rev Public Health 2014;35(1):185–206.
10. Gordon SB, Bruce NG, Grigg J, et al. Respiratory risks from household air pollution in low and middle income countries. Lancet Respir Med 2014;2(10): 823–60.
11. Wallace LA, Mitchell H, O'Connor GT, et al. Particle concentrations in inner-city homes of children with asthma: the effect of smoking, cooking, and outdoor pollution. Environ Health Perspect 2003; 111(9):1265–72.
12. McCormack MC, Breysse PN, Hansel NN, et al. Common household activities are associated with elevated particulate matter concentrations in bedrooms of inner-city Baltimore pre-school children. Environ Res 2008;106(2): 148–55.
13. Hansel NN, Breysse PN, McCormack MC, et al. A longitudinal study of indoor nitrogen dioxide levels and respiratory symptoms in inner-city children with asthma. Environ Health Perspect 2008; 116(10):1428–32.
14. Baldacci S, Maio S, Cerrai S, et al. Allergy and asthma: effects of the exposure to particulate matter and biological allergens. Respir Med 2015; 109(9):1089–104.
15. Centers for Disease Control and Prevention. The health consequences of involuntary exposure to tobacco smoke: a report of the Surgeon General. Atlanta (GA): US Department of Health and Human Services; 2006.
16. Quinto KB, Akinbami LJ. Environmental tobacco smoke exposure in children aged 3–19 years with and without asthma in the United States, 1999-2010. NCHS Data Brief 2013;(126):1–8.
17. Rogalsky DK, Mendola P, Metts TA, et al. Estimating the number of low-income americans exposed to household air pollution from burning solid fuels. Environ Health Perspect 2014;122(8):806–10.
18. Noonan CW, Ward TJ. Asthma randomized trial of indoor wood smoke (ARTIS): rationale and methods. Contemp Clin Trials 2012;33(5):1080–7.
19. Ward T, Boulafentis J, Simpson J, et al. Lessons learned from a woodstove changeout on the Nez Perce Reservation. Sci Total Environ 2011;409(4): 664–70.
20. Bunnell JE, Garcia LV, Furst JM, et al. Navajo coal combustion and respiratory health near Shiprock, New Mexico. J Environ Public Health 2010;2010: 260525.
21. Paulin LM, Williams D'AL, Peng R, et al. 24-h Nitrogen dioxide concentration is associated with cooking behaviors and an increase in rescue medication use in children with asthma. Environ Res 2017;159:118–23.
22. Heinrich J. Influence of indoor factors in dwellings on the development of childhood asthma. Int J Hyg Environ Health 2011;214(1):1–25.
23. Barnes B, Mathee A, Moiloa K. Assessing child time – activity patterns in relation to indoor cooking fires in developing countries: a methodological comparison. Int J Hyg Environ Health 2005; 208(3):219–25.
24. Qian Z, Zhang J, Korn LR, et al. Factor analysis of household factors: are they associated with respiratory conditions in Chinese children? Int J Epidemiol 2004;33(3):582–8.
25. Smith KR, Samet JM, Romieu I, et al. Indoor air pollution in developing countries and acute lower respiratory infections in children. Thorax 2000; 55(6):518–32.
26. Regalado J, Pérez-Padilla R, Sansores R, et al. The effect of biomass burning on respiratory symptoms and lung function in rural mexican women. Am J Respir Crit Care Med 2006;174(8):901–5.
27. Samet JM, Spengler JD. Indoor environments and health: moving into the 21st century. Am J Public Health 2003;93(9):1489–93.
28. Mendell MJ, Mirer AG, Cheung K, et al. Respiratory and allergic health effects of dampness, mold, and dampness-related agents: a review of the epidemiologic evidence. Environ Health Perspect 2011; 119(6):748–56.
29. Matsui EC, Perzanowski M, Peng RD, et al. Effect of an integrated pest management intervention on asthma symptoms among mouse-sensitized children and adolescents with asthma: a randomized clinical trial. JAMA 2017;317(10):1027–36.
30. Roche N, Chinet T, Huchon G. Allergic and nonallergic interactions between house dust mite allergens and airway mucosa. Eur Respir J 1997; 10(3):719.

31. Ohman JL, Hagberg K, MacDonald MR, et al. Distribution of airborne mouse allergen in a major mouse breeding facility. J Allergy Clin Immunol 1994;94(5):810–7.
32. Matsui EC, Simons E, Rand C, et al. Airborne mouse allergen in the homes of inner-city children with asthma. J Allergy Clin Immunol 2005;115(2):358–63.
33. Ahluwalia SK, Peng RD, Breysse PN, et al. Mouse allergen is the major allergen of public health relevance in Baltimore City. J Allergy Clin Immunol 2013;132(4):830–5.e52.
34. Matsui EC, Eggleston PA, Buckley TJ, et al. Household mouse allergen exposure and asthma morbidity in inner-city preschool children. Ann Allergy Asthma Immunol 2006;97(4):514–20.
35. Rinne S, Rodas E, Rinne M, et al. Use of biomass fuel is associated with infant mortality and child health in trend analysis. Am J Trop Med Hyg 2007;76:585–91.
36. Loke J, Paul E, Virgulto JA, et al. Rabbit lung after acute smoke inhalation: cellular responses and scanning electron microscopy. Arch Surg 1984;119(8):956–9.
37. Feldbaum DM, Wormuth D, Nieman GF, et al. Exosurf treatment following wood smoke inhalation. Burns 1993;19(5):396–400.
38. Kurmi OP, Semple S, Simkhada P, et al. COPD and chronic bronchitis risk of indoor air pollution from solid fuel: a systematic review and meta-analysis. Thorax 2010;65(3):221.
39. Stockfelt L, Sallsten G, Olin A-C, et al. Effects on airways of short-term exposure to two kinds of wood smoke in a chamber study of healthy humans. Inhal Toxicol 2012;24(1):47–59.
40. Barregard L, Sällsten G, Andersson L, et al. Experimental exposure to wood smoke: effects on airway inflammation and oxidative stress. Occup Environ Med 2008;65(5):319.
41. Fick RB, Paul ES, Merrill WW, et al. Alterations in the antibacterial properties of rabbit pulmonary macrophages exposed to wood smoke. Am Rev Respir Dis 1984;129(1):76–81.
42. Rylance J, Fullerton DG, Scriven J, et al. Household air pollution causes dose-dependent inflammation and altered phagocytosis in human macrophages. Am J Respir Cell Mol Biol 2014;52(5):584–93.
43. Susanne Becker JMS. Exposure to urban air particulates alters the macrophage-mediated inflammatory response to respiratory viral infection. J Toxicol Environ Health A 1999;57(7):445–57.
44. Danielsen PH, Møller P, Jensen KA, et al. Oxidative stress, DNA damage, and inflammation induced by ambient air and wood smoke particulate matter in human A549 and THP-1 cell lines. Chem Res Toxicol 2011;24(2):168–84.
45. Berry CE, Billheimer D, Jenkins IC, et al. A distinct low lung function trajectory from childhood to the fourth decade of life. Am J Respir Crit Care Med 2016;194(5):607–12.
46. Martinez FD. Early-life origins of chronic obstructive pulmonary disease. N Engl J Med 2016;375(9):871–8.
47. Bui DS, Lodge CJ, Burgess JA, et al. Childhood predictors of lung function trajectories and future COPD risk: a prospective cohort study from the first to the sixth decade of life. Lancet Respir Med 2018;6(7):535–44.
48. Belgrave DCM, Granell R, Turner SW, et al. Lung function trajectories from pre-school age to adulthood and their associations with early life factors: a retrospective analysis of three population-based birth cohort studies. Lancet Respir Med 2018;6(7):526–34.
49. Bui DS, Walters HE, Burgess JA, et al. Childhood respiratory risk factor profiles and middle-age lung function: a prospective cohort study from the first to sixth decade. Ann Am Thorac Soc 2018;15(9):1057–66.
50. Latzin P, Röösli M, Huss A, et al. Air pollution during pregnancy and lung function in newborns: a birth cohort study. Eur Respir J 2009;33(3):594.
51. Gauderman WJ, Urman R, Avol E, et al. Association of improved air quality with lung development in children. N Engl J Med 2015;372(10):905–13.
52. Lee AG, Kaali S, Quinn A, et al. Prenatal household air pollution is associated with impaired infant lung function with sex-specific effects. Evidence from GRAPHS, a cluster randomized cookstove intervention trial. Am J Respir Crit Care Med 2018;199(6):738–46.
53. Dherani M, Pope D, Mascarenhas M, et al. Indoor air pollution from unprocessed solid fuel use and pneumonia risk in children aged under five years: a systematic review and meta-analysis. Bull World Health Organ 2008;86(5):390–398C.
54. Jary H, Simpson H, Havens D, et al. Household air pollution and acute lower respiratory infections in adults: a systematic review. PLoS One 2016;11(12):e0167656.
55. Horne BD, Joy EA, Hofmann MG, et al. Short-term elevation of fine particulate matter air pollution and acute lower respiratory infection. Am J Respir Crit Care Med 2018;198(6):759–66.
56. Croft DP, Zhang W, Lin S, et al. The association between respiratory infection and air pollution in the setting of air quality policy and economic change. Ann Am Thorac Soc 2019;16(3):321–30.
57. Vork Kathleen L, Broadwin Rachel L, Blaisdell Robert J. Developing asthma in childhood from exposure to secondhand tobacco smoke: insights from a meta-regression. Environ Health Perspect 2007;115(10):1394–400.

58. Po JYT, FitzGerald JM, Carlsten C. Respiratory disease associated with solid biomass fuel exposure in rural women and children: systematic review and meta-analysis. Thorax 2011;66(3):232.
59. Kumar R, Nagar JK, Raj N, et al. Impact of domestic air pollution from cooking fuel on respiratory allergies in children in India. Asian Pac J Allergy Immunol 2008;26(4):213–22.
60. Siddharthan T, Grigsby MR, Goodman D, et al. Association between household air pollution exposure and chronic obstructive pulmonary disease outcomes in 13 low- and middle-income country settings. Am J Respir Crit Care Med 2018;197(5):611–20.
61. Semple S, Devakumar D, Fullerton DG, et al. Airborne endotoxin concentrations in homes burning biomass fuel. Environ Health Perspect 2010;118(7):988–91.
62. Behrendt H, Kasche A, Ebner von Eschenbach C, et al. Secretion of proinflammatory eicosanoid-like substances precedes allergen release from pollen grains in the initiation of allergic sensitization. Int Arch Allergy Immunol 2001;124(1–3):121–5.
63. Barry AC, Mannino DM, Hopenhayn C, et al. Exposure to indoor biomass fuel pollutants and asthma prevalence in Southeastern Kentucky: results from the Burden of Lung Disease (BOLD) study. J Asthma 2010;47(7):735–41.
64. Noonan CW, Ward TJ. Environmental tobacco smoke, woodstove heating and risk of asthma symptoms. J Asthma 2007;44(9):735–8.
65. Breysse PN, Diette GB, Matsui EC, et al. Indoor air pollution and asthma in children. Proc Am Thorac Soc 2010;7(2):102–6.
66. McCormack MC, Breysse PN, Matsui EC, et al. In-home particle concentrations and childhood asthma morbidity. Environ Health Perspect 2009;117(2):294–8.
67. McCormack MC, Breysse PN, Matsui EC, et al. Indoor particulate matter increases asthma morbidity in children with non-atopic and atopic asthma. Ann Allergy Asthma Immunol 2011;106(4):308–15.
68. Kattan M, Gergen PJ, Eggleston P, et al. Health effects of indoor nitrogen dioxide and passive smoking on urban asthmatic children. J Allergy Clin Immunol 2007;120(3):618–24.
69. Gaffin JM, Hauptman M, Petty CR, et al. Nitrogen dioxide exposure in school classrooms of inner-city children with asthma. J Allergy Clin Immunol 2018;141(6):2249–55.e2.
70. Lu KD, Breysse PN, Diette GB, et al. Being overweight increases susceptibility to indoor pollutants among urban children with asthma. J Allergy Clin Immunol 2013;131(4):1017–23.e3.
71. Holguin F, Fitzpatrick A. Obesity, asthma, and oxidative stress. J Appl Physiol (1985) 2009;108(3):754–9.
72. Keaney John F, Larson Martin G, Vasan Ramachandran S, et al. Obesity and systemic oxidative stress. Arterioscler Thromb Vasc Biol 2003;23(3):434–9.
73. Wu TD, Brigham EP, Peng R, et al. Overweight/obesity enhances associations between secondhand smoke exposure and asthma morbidity in children. J Allergy Clin Immunol Pract 2018;6(6):2157–9.e5.
74. Codispoti CD, LeMasters GK, Levin L, et al. Traffic pollution is associated with early childhood aeroallergen sensitization. Ann Allergy Asthma Immunol 2015;114(2):126–33.e3.
75. Carlsten C, Blomberg A, Pui M, et al. Diesel exhaust augments allergen-induced lower airway inflammation in allergic individuals: a controlled human exposure study. Thorax 2016;71(1):35–44.
76. Biagioni BJ, Tam S, Chen Y-WR, et al. Effect of controlled human exposure to diesel exhaust and allergen on airway surfactant protein D, myeloperoxidase and club (Clara) cell secretory protein 16. Clin Exp Allergy 2016;46(9):1206–13.
77. Morgenstern V, Zutavern A, Cyrys J, et al. Atopic diseases, allergic sensitization, and exposure to traffic-related air pollution in children. Am J Respir Crit Care Med 2008;177(12):1331–7.
78. Wang I-J, Tung T-H, Tang C-S, et al. Allergens, air pollutants, and childhood allergic diseases. Int J Hyg Environ Health 2016;219(1):66–71.
79. Eggleston PA. Cockroach allergy and urban asthma. J Allergy Clin Immunol 2017;140(2):389–90.
80. Sheehan WJ, Permaul P, Petty CR, et al. Association between allergen exposure in inner-city schools and asthma morbidity among students. JAMA Pediatr 2017;171(1):31–8.
81. Breysse PN, Buckley TJ, Williams D, et al. Indoor exposures to air pollutants and allergens in the homes of asthmatic children in inner-city Baltimore. Environ Res 2005;98(2):167–76.
82. Amaral AFS, Patel J, Kato BS, et al. Airflow obstruction and use of solid fuels for cooking or heating. BOLD (Burden of Obstructive Lung Disease) results. Am J Respir Crit Care Med 2017;197(5):595–610.
83. Hu G, Zhou Y, Tian J, et al. Risk of COPD from exposure to biomass smoke: a metaanalysis. Chest 2010;138(1):20–31.
84. Rinne ST, Rodas EJ, Bender BS, et al. Relationship of pulmonary function among women and children to indoor air pollution from biomass use in rural Ecuador. Respir Med 2006;100(7):1208–15.
85. Camp PG, Ramirez-Venegas A, Sansores RH, et al. COPD phenotypes in biomass smoke versus tobacco smoke-exposed Mexican women. Eur Respir J 2014;43(3):725.
86. Diette GB, Accinelli RA, Balmes JR, et al. Obstructive lung disease and exposure to burning biomass

fuel in the indoor environment. Glob Heart 2012; 7(3):265–70.
87. Pérez-Padilla R, Ramirez-Venegas A, Sansores-Martinez R. Clinical characteristics of patients with biomass smoke-associated COPD and chronic bronchitis, 2004-2014. Chronic Obstr Pulm Dis 2014;1(1):23–32.
88. Montaño M, Cisneros J, Ramírez-Venegas A, et al. Malondialdehyde and superoxide dismutase correlate with FEV1 in patients with COPD associated with wood smoke exposure and tobacco smoking. Inhal Toxicol 2010;22(10):868–74.
89. Sood A, Petersen H, Blanchette CM, et al. Wood smoke exposure and gene promoter methylation are associated with increased risk for COPD in smokers. Am J Respir Crit Care Med 2010;182(9): 1098–104.
90. Raju S, Keet CA, Paulin LM, et al. Rural residence and poverty are independent risk factors for COPD in the United States. Am J Respir Crit Care Med 2019;199(8):961–9.
91. Hansel NN, McCormack MC, Belli AJ, et al. In-home air pollution is linked to respiratory morbidity in former smokers with chronic obstructive pulmonary disease. Am J Respir Crit Care Med 2013; 187(10):1085–90.
92. Jamieson DB, Matsui EC, Belli A, et al. Effects of allergic phenotype on respiratory symptoms and exacerbations in patients with chronic obstructive pulmonary disease. Am J Respir Crit Care Med 2013;188(2):187–92.
93. McCormack MC, Belli AJ, Kaji DA, et al. Obesity as a susceptibility factor to indoor particulate matter health effects in COPD. Eur Respir J 2015;45(5): 1248–57.
94. Hansel NN, McCormack MC, Kim V. The effects of air pollution and temperature on COPD. COPD 2016;13(3):372–9.
95. McCormack MC, Paulin LM, Gummerson CE, et al. Colder temperature is associated with increased COPD morbidity. Eur Respir J 2017;49(6):1601501.
96. McCormack MC, Belli AJ, Waugh D, et al. Respiratory effects of indoor heat and the interaction with air pollution in chronic obstructive pulmonary disease. Ann Am Thorac Soc 2016;13(12):2125–31.
97. Smith KR, McCracken JP, Weber MW, et al. Effect of reduction in household air pollution on childhood pneumonia in Guatemala (RESPIRE): a randomised controlled trial. Lancet 2011;378(9804): 1717–26.
98. Romieu I, Riojas-Rodríguez H, Marrón-Mares AT, et al. Improved biomass stove intervention in rural Mexico. Am J Respir Crit Care Med 2009;180(7): 649–56.
99. Tielsch JM, Katz J, Khatry SK, et al. Effect of an improved biomass stove on acute lower respiratory infections in young children in rural Nepal: a cluster-randomised, step-wedge trial. Lancet Glob Health 2016;4:S19.
100. Asante KP, Wylie B, Chilrude S, et al. The Ghana Randomized Air Pollution and Health Study (GRAPHS): a cluster randomized trial of Liquified petroleum gas (LPG) and efficient biomass cookstoves delivered during pregnancy. Environ Epidemiol 2019;3:296. Available at: https://journals.lww.com/environepidem/Fulltext/2019/10001/The_Ghana_Randomized_Air_Pollution_and_Health.903.aspx.
101. Mortimer K, Ndamala CB, Naunje AW, et al. A cleaner burning biomass-fuelled cookstove intervention to prevent pneumonia in children under 5 years old in rural Malawi (the Cooking and Pneumonia Study): a cluster randomised controlled trial. Lancet 2017;389(10065):167–75.
102. Clark ML, Peel JL, Balakrishnan K, et al. Health and household air pollution from solid fuel use: the need for improved exposure assessment. Environ Health Perspect 2013;121(10):1120–8.
103. Mortimer K, Balmes JR. Cookstove trials and tribulations: what is needed to decrease the burden of household air pollution? Ann Am Thorac Soc 2018;15(5):539–41.
104. Naeher LP, Brauer M, Lipsett M, et al. Woodsmoke health effects: a review. Inhal Toxicol 2007;19(1): 67–106.
105. Northcross AL, Hwang N, Balakrishnan K, et al. Assessing exposures to household air pollution in public health research and program evaluation. Ecohealth 2015;12(1):57–67.
106. Steenland K, Pillarisetti A, Kirby M, et al. Modeling the potential health benefits of lower household air pollution after a hypothetical liquified petroleum gas (LPG) cookstove intervention. Environ Int 2018;111:71–9.
107. Allen RW, Carlsten C, Karlen B, et al. An air filter intervention study of endothelial function among healthy adults in a woodsmoke-impacted community. Am J Respir Crit Care Med 2011;183(9): 1222–30.
108. Butz AM, Matsui EC, Breysse P, et al. A randomized trial of air cleaners and a health coach to improve indoor air quality for inner-city children with asthma and secondhand smoke exposure. Arch Pediatr Adolesc Med 2011; 165(8):741–8.
109. Lanphear BP, Hornung RW, Khoury J, et al. Effects of HEPA air cleaners on unscheduled asthma visits and asthma symptoms for children exposed to secondhand tobacco smoke. Pediatrics 2011; 127(1):93–101.
110. Hansel NN. Clinical trial of air cleaners to improve indoor air quality and COPD health. Available at: https://clinicaltrials.gov/ct2/show/NCT02236858. Accessed March 5, 2020.

111. Morgan WJ, Crain EF, Gruchalla RS, et al. Results of a home-based environmental intervention among urban children with asthma. N Engl J Med 2004;351(11):1068–80.
112. Eggleston PA, Butz A, Rand C, et al. Home environmental intervention in inner-city asthma: a randomized controlled clinical trial. Ann Allergy 2005;95:7.
113. Gergen PJ, Mortimer KM, Eggleston PA, et al. Results of the National Cooperative Inner-City Asthma Study (NCICAS) environmental intervention to reduce cockroach allergen exposure in inner-city homes. J Allergy Clin Immunol 1999;103(3):501–6.
114. Gøtzsche PC, Hammarquist C, Burr M. House dust mite control measures in the management of asthma: meta-analysis. BMJ 1998;317(7166): 1105–10 [discussion: 1110].
115. Grant T, Phipatanakul W, Perzanowski M, et al. Reduction in mouse allergen exposure is associated with greater lung function growth. J Allergy Clin Immunol 2020;145(2):646–53.e1.
116. Noonan CW, Ward TJ, Navidi W, et al. A rural community intervention targeting biomass combustion sources: effects on air quality and reporting of children's respiratory outcomes. Occup Environ Med 2012;69(5):354.
117. Ward TJ, Palmer CP, Houck JE, et al. Community woodstove changeout and impact on ambient concentrations of polycyclic aromatic hydrocarbons and phenolics. Environ Sci Technol 2009;43(14): 5345–50.
118. Noonan CW, Navidi W, Sheppard L, et al. Residential indoor PM2.5 in wood stove homes: follow-up of the Libby changeout program. Indoor Air 2012; 22(6):492–500.
119. Faber T, Kumar A, Mackenbach JP, et al. Effect of tobacco control policies on perinatal and child health: a systematic review and meta-analysis. Lancet Public Health 2017;2(9):e420–37.
120. Been JV, Nurmatov UB, Cox B, et al. Effect of smoke-free legislation on perinatal and child health: a systematic review and meta-analysis. Lancet 2014;383(9928):1549–60.
121. HUD. Federal Register,U.S. Department of Housing and Urban Development (HUD). Instituting Smoke-Free Public Housing.81FR87430. 2016. Available at: www.federalregister.gov/documents/2016/12/05/2016-28986/instituting-smoke-free-public-housing. Accessed February 6, 2017.
122. Phipatanakul W. School inner-city asthma intervention study (SICAS-2) (SICAS-2). Available at: https://clinicaltrials.gov/ct2/show/NCT02291302?term=Phipatanakul&draw=2&rank=2. Accessed January 5, 2020.
123. Phipatanakul W, Koutrakis P, Coull BA, et al. The school inner-city asthma intervention study: design, rationale, methods, and lessons learned. Contemp Clin Trials 2017;60:14–23.
124. Cromar KR, Gladson LA, Ewart G. Trends in excess morbidity and mortality associated with air pollution above American Thoracic Society–Recommended Standards, 2008–2017. Ann Am Thorac Soc 2019;16(7):836–45.
125. Ward TJ, Semmens EO, Weiler E, et al. Efficacy of interventions targeting household air pollution from residential wood stoves. J Expo Sci Environ Epidemiol 2017;27(1):64–71.
126. Paulin LM, Diette GB, Scott M, et al. Home interventions are effective at decreasing indoor nitrogen dioxide concentrations. Indoor Air 2014;24(4): 416–24.

UNITED STATES POSTAL SERVICE®

Statement of Ownership, Management, and Circulation (All Periodicals Publications Except Requester Publications)

1. Publication Title	2. Publication Number	3. Filing Date
CLINICS IN CHEST MEDICINE	000 – 706	9/18/2020
4. Issue Frequency	**5. Number of Issues Published Annually**	**6. Annual Subscription Price**
MAR, JUN, SEP, DEC	4	$388.00

7. Complete Mailing Address of Known Office of Publication *(Not printer) (Street, city, county, state, and ZIP+4®)*
ELSEVIER INC.
230 Park Avenue, Suite 800
New York, NY 10169

Contact Person
Malathi Samayan
Telephone *(Include area code)*
91-44-4299-4507

8. Complete Mailing Address of Headquarters or General Business Office of Publisher *(Not printer)*
ELSEVIER INC.
230 Park Avenue, Suite 800
New York, NY 10169

9. Full Names and Complete Mailing Addresses of Publisher, Editor, and Managing Editor *(Do not leave blank)*

Publisher *(Name and complete mailing address)*

Editor *(Name and complete mailing address)*
JOANNA COLLETT, ELSEVIER INC.
1600 JOHN F KENNEDY BLVD. SUITE 1800
PHILADELPHIA, PA 19103-2899

Managing Editor *(Name and complete mailing address)*
PATRICK MANLEY, ELSEVIER INC.
1600 JOHN F KENNEDY BLVD. SUITE 1800
PHILADELPHIA, PA 19103-2899

10. Owner *(Do not leave blank. If the publication is owned by a corporation, give the name and address of the corporation immediately followed by the names and addresses of all stockholders owning or holding 1 percent or more of the total amount of stock. If not owned by a corporation, give the names and addresses of the individual owners. If owned by a partnership or other unincorporated firm, give its name and address as well as those of each individual owner. If the publication is published by a nonprofit organization, give its name and address.)*

Full Name	Complete Mailing Address
WHOLLY OWNED SUBSIDIARY OF REED/ELSEVIER, US HOLDINGS	1600 JOHN F KENNEDY BLVD. SUITE 1800 PHILADELPHIA, PA 19103-2899

11. Known Bondholders, Mortgagees, and Other Security Holders Owning or Holding 1 Percent or More of Total Amount of Bonds, Mortgages, or Other Securities. If none, check box ☐ None

Full Name	Complete Mailing Address
N/A	

12. Tax Status *(For completion by nonprofit organizations authorized to mail at nonprofit rates) (Check one)*
The purpose, function, and nonprofit status of this organization and the exempt status for federal income tax purposes:
☒ Has Not Changed During Preceding 12 Months
☐ Has Changed During Preceding 12 Months *(Publisher must submit explanation of change with this statement)*

13. Publication Title: CLINICS IN CHEST MEDICINE

14. Issue Date for Circulation Data Below: JUNE 2020

15. Extent and Nature of Circulation		Average No. Copies Each Issue During Preceding 12 Months	No. Copies of Single Issue Published Nearest to Filing Date
a. Total Number of Copies *(Net press run)*		391	338
b. Paid Circulation *(By Mail and Outside the Mail)*	(1) Mailed Outside-County Paid Subscriptions Stated on PS Form 3541 (Include paid distribution above nominal rate, advertiser's proof copies, and exchange copies)	228	208
	(2) Mailed In-County Paid Subscriptions Stated on PS Form 3541 *(Include paid distribution above nominal rate, advertiser's proof copies, and exchange copies)*	0	0
	(3) Paid Distribution Outside the Mails Including Sales Through Dealers and Carriers, Street Vendors, Counter Sales, and Other Paid Distribution Outside USPS®	117	92
	(4) Paid Distribution by Other Classes of Mail Through the USPS (e.g., First-Class Mail®)	0	0
c. Total Paid Distribution *[Sum of 15b (1), (2), (3), and (4)]* ▶		345	300
d. Free or Nominal Rate Distribution *(By Mail and Outside the Mail)*	(1) Free or Nominal Rate Outside-County Copies included on PS Form 3541	26	20
	(2) Free or Nominal Rate In-County Copies Included on PS Form 3541	0	0
	(3) Free or Nominal Rate Copies Mailed at Other Classes Through the USPS (e.g., First-Class Mail)	0	0
	(4) Free or Nominal Rate Distribution Outside the Mail *(Carriers or other means)*	0	0
e. Total Free or Nominal Rate Distribution *(Sum of 15d (1), (2), (3) and (4))*		26	20
f. Total Distribution *(Sum of 15c and 15e)* ▶		371	320
g. Copies not Distributed *(See Instructions to Publishers #4 (page #3))* ▶		20	18
h. Total *(Sum of 15f and g)*		391	338
i. Percent Paid *(15c divided by 15f times 100)* ▶		92.99%	93.75%

* If you are claiming electronic copies, go to line 16 on page 3. If you are not claiming electronic copies, skip to line 17 on page 3

16. Electronic Copy Circulation	Average No. Copies Each Issue During Preceding 12 Months	No. Copies of Single Issue Published Nearest to Filing Date
a. Paid Electronic Copies ▶		
b. Total Paid Print Copies (Line 15c) + Paid Electronic Copies (Line 16a) ▶		
c. Total Print Distribution (Line 15f) + Paid Electronic Copies (Line 16a) ▶		
d. Percent Paid (Both Print & Electronic Copies) (16b divided by 16c × 100) ▶		

☒ **I certify that 50% of all my distributed copies (electronic and print) are paid above a nominal price.**

17. Publication of Statement of Ownership
☒ If the publication is a general publication, publication of this statement is required. Will be printed in the DECEMBER 2020 issue of this publication. ☐ Publication not required.

18. Signature and Title of Editor, Publisher, Business Manager, or Owner
Malathi Samayan - Distribution Controller — *Malathi Samayan* — Date 9/18/2020

I certify that all information furnished on this form is true and complete. I understand that anyone who furnishes false or misleading information on this form or who omits material or information requested on the form may be subject to criminal sanctions (including fines and imprisonment) and/or civil sanctions (including civil penalties).

Printed and bound by CPI Group (UK) Ltd, Croydon, CR0 4YY
08/05/2025
01864691-0011